144.00

3690276945

KU-407-165

Lymphedema

Byung-Boong Lee
John Bergan
Stanley G. Rockson

Editors

Lymphedema

A Concise Compendium
of Theory and Practice

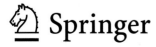 Springer

Editors
Byung-Boong Lee, MD
Department of Surgery
Division of Vascular Surgery
George Washington University School
of Medicine
Washington, DC
USA

John Bergan, MD
Vein Institute of La Jolla
University of California
La Jolla, CA
USA

Stanley G. Rockson, MD
Division of Cardiovascular Medicine
Stanford University School of Medicine
Falk Cardiovascular Research Center
Stanford, CA
USA

ISBN 978-0-85729-566-8   e-ISBN 978-0-85729-567-5
DOI 10.1007/978-0-85729-567-5
Springer London Dordrecht Heidelberg New York

British Library Cataloguing in Publication Data
A catalogue record for this book is available from the British Library

Library of Congress Control Number: 2011928401

Cover design: SPI Publisher Services

Printed on acid-free paper

Springer is part of Springer Science+Business Media (www.springer.com)

Foreword

Alistair Mackenzie
Wishaw General Hospital
50 Netherton Street
Wishaw
ML2 0DP

The entire field of vascular diseases has experienced phenomenal progress during the past few decades. Multiple books and journal publications are silent witnesses to the dramatic advances in the diagnosis and management of arterial and venous diseases. Endovascular prosthesis, bare and covered stents, and complex endoluminal techniques dealing with the devastating sequelae of atherosclerosis have dramatically changed our approach to abdominal and thoracic aneurysms, obstructive coronary and carotid lesions, as well as arterial occlusion of the extremities. The same technological revolution has reached the field of venous diseases. The traditional "long and short" saphenous stripping for varicose veins that many of us performed during decades of vascular surgery practice, have been replaced by foam sclerotherapy, radiofrequency, and laser catheters. Dermatologists, interventional radiologists, cardiologists, and other non-surgical specialists have entered the endovenous therapy field en masse. Prestigious societies devoted to the study and care of patients with venous diseases have sprouted worldwide for the benefit of the millions of patients suffering from diseases of the veins. The majority of papers published in vascular journals deal with arterial topics, a few on venous diseases, and even fewer on lymphatic disorders.

The recently published third edition of *The Handbook of Venous Disorders* of the American Venous Forum dedicates only 42 of its 744 pages to lymphatic diseases. The prestigious *Journal of Vascular Surgery* publishes annually a relatively small number of papers on the lymphatic system.

If venous diseases are the Cinderella of the vascular field, as the late Michael Hume, former President of the American Venous Forum called them, then lymphatic malformations are Cinderella's poor cousin.

There has been, however, a revival of Cinderella's cousin and this book is a welcome update of the significant progress observed in the lymphatic field during the past 20 years. The monumental work of early pioneers in the field of lymphatic circulation, such as Servelle, Kinmonth, Casley-Smith, Olszewski and Nielubowicz, Földi, and many others, has established the basis and served as a stepping-stone for many of the subjects covered by recognized specialists in this book. One of the most important obstacles in the study of the lymphatics has been its visualization. On the trail of visual lymphography using intradermal injections of Patent Blue (alphazurine) to visualize cutaneous and deeper lymphatics, followed the technique of oil lymphography and lymphadenography, as described by Kinmonth. These techniques were a useful tool in the study of the lymphatic vasculature and served as a basis for a working classification of lymphedemas. The tedious and time-consuming lymphography has been replaced by new nuclear medicine imaging techniques, radionuclide lymphoscintigraphy, multislice CT, magnetic resonance imaging, and computerized axial tomography. These techniques have contributed to guiding the clinician in the process of establishing a rational diagnosis and dictating appropriate treatment. Advances in diagnosis have been followed by an array of therapeutic techniques. Many of them are described in this book by their original authors. Because of my long-time interest in the subject, I have had personal experience in some of the diagnostic and surgical techniques described in this book, such as oil lymphography, lymphoscintigraphy, lymphovenous anastomosis, and debulking procedures for massive lymphedema. I consider, however, that at present, a program of complex manual decongestive technique associated with properly applied intermittent pneumatic compression and followed by well-supervised compression therapy in a compliant patient may achieve long-lasting edema control without the need for surgery. The role of surgery, as described in surgical books and texts on vascular surgery, has been relegated to a few cases of severe fibro-lymphedema and to reconstructive plastic surgery to excise and remodel the redundant skin folds resulting from a good lymphatic manual decompression program of the extremities.

The field of genetics has found fertile ground in the lymphatic vasculature. I am certain that as genetic research on the phenotypes of different lymphedema conditions advances, our thoughts and concepts on the nature and classification of some primary lymphedemas will change. The same will occur in those cases of lymphedemas associated with other vascular and nonvascular anomalies. We are on the threshold of a true revolution in our understanding of the Kinmonth lymphedemas for the benefit of our own understanding of the disease, and hopefully for the benefit of many unfortunate patients suffering from the disabling pathophysiology of the lymphatic circulation.

Bethesda, USA   J. Lionel Villavicencio

Preface I

Management of chronic swelling of the limbs is a continuing challenge to patients and clinicians. In recent years, there has been progress in diagnoses and treatment of this disabling condition. The goal of this present volume is to collect between two covers the best guidelines for treatment, followed by detailed descriptions of the most effective tests and modern treatments for the disabling condition best called chronic lymphedema.

Chronic lymphedema is a common condition that can be easily recognized and effectively treated according to the guidelines collected in this volume. Several national and international societies are primarily concerned with this condition, and they have periodic meetings that make exchange of useful information possible. Clinical experience has promoted the development of guidelines and statements of principle, which guide diagnosis and treatment of this chronic condition.

Because of the nature of the abnormalities that cause lymphedema, there is no established cure. There are, however, many methods that, when used in their aggregate, can correct and ameliorate limb swelling. These methods provide guidelines and prescription for effective treatment. The stated objectives of this volume are to describe the guidelines for thorough diagnosis and effective treatment of patients with disabling lymphedema.

Each of the presenters who write in this volume comes from a different background and draws on different wells of knowledge about lymphedema. Their aggregate experience is enormous; it has accumulated over many years through the mechanisms of international, local, and regional scientific meetings. This book states clearly the thoughts and varied experiences of friends and colleagues, all of whom have established canonical treatment principles for a variety of manifestations of this deadly condition.

The authors have hoped to assemble discussions of the many types of lymphedema. In each discussion displayed in the chapter below, it is hoped that new ideas will develop, which, in the aggregate, will improve accuracy of diagnosis and effectiveness of medical and surgical care.

John Bergan, MD

Preface II

It is truly fortunate that, as we enter the twenty-first century, the fields of lymphatic biology and medicine are experiencing a highly anticipated renaissance. This much-needed emphasis upon the study of the lymphatic system is predicted to have a transformative impact upon our understanding of physiology, health, and disease.

Inexplicably, the lymphatic system has been the subject of passive neglect for centuries of medical development. This is, indeed, paradoxical, considering that such a very important component of the human circulation plays an equally important role in the normal functioning of the immune apparatus.

Awareness of the importance of lymphatic mechanisms to the continuum of human biology and disease is growing. This "lymphatic continuum" now easily encompasses cardiovascular disease, obesity, autoimmune disease, respiratory and other forms of chronic inflammation, and chronic transplant rejection, among many other expressions of human pathology.

Lymphedema is a central manifestation of both peripheral and visceral diseases of the lymphatic circulation. Any pathological condition of the lymphatic vasculature, whether superficial or internal, regional, or systemic, is predominated by the appearance of the characteristic type of tissue edema that occurs when lymphatic dysfunction supervenes. While there is a broad spectrum of lymphatic vascular diseases, the most common diagnosis in lymphatic medicine is, of course, lymphedema. This patient population is large and, historically, under-served by the medical community.

At last, after decades and centuries of relative neglect, these patients are increasingly receiving attention. It is very timely, and gratifying, that there is now a clinical need for a comprehensive textbook that addresses the problem of lymphedema, and it is equally gratifying to acknowledge that this compendium has called upon the expertise of so many authorities to contribute their collective wisdom.

I am especially honored to collaborate with such an inspiring group of colleagues and, in particular, to have had the privilege to work so closely with my esteemed co-editors, Drs. John Bergan and Byung-Boong Lee.

It is an honor to dedicate this volume to the current and future well-being of our patients with lymphedema.

Stanley G. Rockson, MD

Contents

Part XI   Lymphedema and Congenital Vascular Malformation

Part XII   Management of Chylous Reflux

Part XIII   Filariasis Lymphedema

Part XIV   Genetic Prospects for Lymphedema Management

Part XV   Oncology and Lymphedema

Part XVI   Phlebolymphedema

Part XVII   Lymphedema Health Care Delivery

Part XVIII   Epilogue

Contributors

Claudio Allegra, M.D. Angiology Department, San Giovanni Hospital, Rome, Italy

Mauro Andrade, M.D., Ph.D. Department of Surgery, University of São Paulo Medical School, São Paulo, Brazil

Richard G. Azizkhan, M.D., Ph.D. Department of Surgery and Pediatrics, Cincinnati Children's Hospital Medical Center, Cincinnati, OH, USA

Michelangelo Bartolo, M.D. Angiology O.U., Department of Medical Sciences, San Giovanni Hospital, Rome, Italy

Ruediger G.H. Baumeister, M.D., Ph.D. Professor of Surgery, the Ludwig Maximilians University, Munich, Germany Consultant of Lymphology, Chirurgische Klinik Muenchen Bogenhausen, Muenchen, Bavaria, Germany

Corinne Becker, M.D. Department of Academy of Surgery, Hopital Universitaire Europeen Georges Pompidou, Paris, France and Department of Plastic Surgery, Jouvenet Hospital, Paris, France

John Bergan, M.D. Vein Institute of La Jolla, University of California, La Jolla, CA, USA

Michael J. Bernas, M.S. Department of Surgery, University of Arizona College of Medicine, Tucson, AZ, USA

Franciene Blei, M.D., M.B.A. Vascular Birthmark Institute, Roosevelt Hospital, New York, NY, USA

Francesco Boccardo, M.D., Ph.D. Department of Surgery – Unit of Lymphatic Surgery, University of Genoa, Genoa, Italy

Pierre Bourgeois, M.D., Ph.D. Service of Nuclear Medicine, Institute Jules Bordet, Université Libre de Bruxelles, Brussels, Belgium

Håkan Brorson, M.D., Ph.D. Department of Clinical Sciences in Malmö, Lund University, Plastic and Reconstructive Surgery, Skåne University Hospital, Malmö, Sweden

Department of Plastic and Reconstructive Surgery, Skåne University Hospital, Malmö, Sweden

Nisha Bunke, M.D. Clinical Instructor of Surgery, Director, La Jolla Vein Care, La Jolla, CA, USA

Corradino Campisi, M.D., Ph.D. Department of Surgery, Section of Lymphology and Microsurgery, University Hospital "San Martino", Genoa, Italy

Marco Cardone San Giovanni Battista Hospital, Rome, Italy

Anita Carlizza, M.D. Angiology O.U., Department of Medical Sciences, San Giovanni Hospital, Rome, Italy

Attilio Cavezzi, M.D. Vascular Unit, Poliambulatorio Hippocrates and Clinica Stella Maris, San Benedetto del Tronto (AP), Italy

Wendy Chaite, J.D. Lymphatic Research Foundation, Glen Cove, NY, USA

Robert J. Damstra, M.D., Ph.D. Department of Dermatology, Phlebology and Lympho-Vascular Medicine, Nij Smellinghe Hospital, Drachten, The Netherlands

Alessandro Failla San Giovanni Battista Hospital, Rome, Italy

Etelka Földi, M.D. Clinic for Lymphology, Földiklinik, Hinterzarten, Baden-Württemberg, Germany

Martha Földi, M.D. Clinic for Lymphology, Földiklinik, Hinterzarten, Baden-Württemberg, Germany

LeAnne M. Fox, M.D., M.P.H., DTM&H. Division of Parasitic Dieases and Malaria, Center for Global Health, Center for Dieases Control and Prevention, Atlanta, GA, USA

Claude Franceschi, M.D. Dispensaire Marie Therese, Hopital Saint Joseph, Paris, France

Peter Gloviczki, M.D. Division of Vascular and Endovascular Surgery, Gonda Vascular Center, Mayo Clinic, Rochester, MN, USA

Kathleen C. Horst, M.D. Department of Radiation Oncology, Stanford University, Stanford, CA, USA

Emily Iker, M.D. Lymphedema Center of Santa Monica, California, CA, USA

Kimberly A. Jones, M.D. Department of Medicine, Huntsman Cancer Institute, University of Utah, Salt Lake City, UT, USA

Sharon L. Kilbreath, Ph.D., M.C.I.Sc., B.Sc. Breast Cancer Research Group of the Faculty of Health Sciences, University of Sydney, Lidcombe, NSW, Australia

Victor S. Krylov, M.D., Ph.D., Dr.h.c. Vascular Research Laboratory, Department of Surgery, University of Tennessee, Graduate School of Medicine, Knoxville, TN, USA

James Laredo, M.D., Ph.D. Department of Surgery, Division of Vascular Surgery, George Washington University Medical Center, Washington, DC, USA

Albert Leduc, Ph.D. Institut des Sciences de la Motricité, Université Libre de Bruxelles and Vrije Universiteit Brussel, Brussels, Belgium

Olivier Leduc, Ph.D. Department of Physical Therapy, Unité de lympho-phlébologie, Haute Ecole P.H. Spaak, Brussels, Belgium

Byung-Boong Lee, M.D. Department of Surgery, Division of Vascular Surgery, George Washington University School of Medicine, Washington, DC, USA

Mi-Joung Lee, Ph.D. Division of Cardiovascular Medicine, Stanford University School of Medicine, Falk Cardiovascular Researgh Center, Stanford, CA, USA

Dirk A. Loose, M.D. Department of Vascular Surgery, European Center for the Diagnosis and Treatment of Vascular Malformations, Die Facharztklinik Hamburg, Hamburg, Germany

Gurusamy Manokaran, M.B.B.S., M.S., M.Ch (Plastic Surg.) FICS Department of Plastic and Reconstructive Surgery and Lymphologist, Apollo Hospitals, Chennai, India

Raul Mattassi, M.D. Director, Center for Vascular Malformations "Stefan Belov", Clinical Institute Humanitas "Mater Domini", Castellanza (Varese), Italy

Erica Menegatti, Ph.D. Vascular Disease Center, University of Ferrara, Ferrara, Italy

Sandro Michelini, M.D. San Giovanni Battista Hospital, Rome, Italy

Takki A. Momin, M.D. Vascular Surgery Fellow, Georgetown University/ Washington Hospital Center, Washington, DC, USA

Giovann Moneta, M.D. San Giovanni Battista Hospital, Rome, Italy

Cheryl L. Morgan, Ph.D. Department of Rehabilitation Medicine, Therapy Concepts Inc., Leawood, KS, USA

Richard F. Neville, M.D. Department of Surgery, Division of Vascular Surgery, George Washington University Medical Center, Washington, DC, USA

Magdalene Ochart, B.S. Department of Nuclear Medicine, University Medical Center, Tucson, AZ, USA

Waldemar L. Olszewski, M.D., Ph.D., Department of Surgical Research and Transplantology, Medical Research Centre, Warsaw, Poland

Cristobal Miguel Papendieck, M.D. Angiopediatria, Buenos Aires, Argentina

Neil B. Piller, Ph.D., B.Sc(hons), FACP Lymphoedema Assessment Clinic, Department of Surgery, School of Medicine, Flinders University and Medical Centre, Bedford Park, SA, Australia

Gael Piquilloud, M.D. Department of Academy of Surgery,
Hopital Universitaire Europeen Georges Pompidou, Paris, France
Department of Plastic Surgery, Jouvenet Hospital, Paris, France

Stanley G. Rockson, M.D. Division of Cardiovascular Medicine,
Stanford University School of Medicine, Falk Cardiovascular Research Center,
Stanford, CA, USA

Győző Szolnoky, Ph.D. Department of Dermatology and Allergology,
University of Szeged, Szeged, Hungary

Jesse A. Taylor, M.D. Department of Plastic and Reconstructive Surgery,
University of Pennsylvania, Philadelphia, PA, USA

Saskia R.J. Thiadens, R.N. National Lymphedema Network, Inc.,
San Francisco, CA, USA

Anne-Marie Vaillant-Newman, P.T., M.A. Division of Cardiovascular
Medicine, Stanford University School of Medicine, Falk Cardiovascular Research
Center, Stanford, CA, USA

J. Leonel Villavicencio, B.S., M.D. Distinguished Professor of Surgery,
Department of Surgery, Uniformed Services, University School of Medicine,
Director Emeritus Venous and Lymphatic Teaching Clinics,
Walter Reed Army and National Naval Medical Centers,
Washington DC and Bethesda, MD, USA

Leigh C. Ward, B.Sc., Ph.D., R.Nutr. School of Chemistry and Molecular
Biosciences, The University of Queensland, Queensland, Australia

Walter H. Williams, Ph.D., M.D. Department of Radiology,
University of Arizona College of Medicine, Tucson, AZ, USA

Marlys H. Witte, M.D. Department of Surgery, University of Arizona
College of Medicine, Tucson, AZ, USA

Charles L. Witte, M.D. Department of Surgery, University of Arizona
College of Medicine, Tucson, AZ, USA

Paolo Zamboni, M.D. Vascular Disease Center, University of Ferrara,
Ferrara, Italy

Introductory Note

The Editors are very proud to have assembled a book that we believe to be the first comprehensive, practical compendium of lymphatic medicine, both diagnostic and therapeutic. It is our hope that this volume will further the application of sound medical principles in the general approach to the lymphatic patient. However, we also recognize that this is a medical field that, relatively speaking, is in its infancy. Many of the theories and observations are in very dynamic flux. It will be apparent to the reader that, within individual chapters, there are seeming "truths" that conflict with similar statements in parallel chapters. The editors have not constrained the individual authors to adhere to a universal set of facts or opinions and, accordingly, their chapters reflect their individual interpretations of their own work and the work of others.

It is our fervent hope that, as the field of lymphatic medicine matures, these seeming inconsistencies will be resolved and that the discipline will achieve the goal of providing the best possible diagnostic and therapeutic approaches to a very large and complex patient population.

Byung-Boong Lee
John Bergan
Stanley G. Rockson

Part I
Introduction

Chapter 1
General Considerations

John Bergan and Nisha Bunke

Lymphedema is a progressive, usually unrelenting, and variably painful swelling of the limbs and/or genitalia resulting from lymphatic system insufficiency and deranged lymphatic transport. At the physical level, lymphedema is characterized by swelling of the tissues and eventual thickening and hardening of the skin and soft tissue. At the microvascular level, inadequate clearance of lymph causes the abnormal accumulation of interstitial fluid, which incites cellular proliferation and inflammation.[1] Chronic inflammation of lymphatic structures and surrounding tissue results in subcutaneous and lymph vessel fibrosis with irreversible structural damage.[2,3] As a result of underlying lymphatic damage, normal immune defenses are diminished. Therefore, lymphedema can best be described as a condition of impaired immunity, and a process of degeneration and chronic inflammation of the lymphatic structures and surrounding tissue.

Understanding of lymphatic system insufficiency depends on an understanding of normal lymphatic anatomy and physiology. The lymphatic system is a specialized network of vessels that regulates fluid homeostasis and immune defense. The prime function of the lymphatic system is to maintain fluid balance by clearing the interstitial spaces of excess water, large molecules, lipids, antigens, immune cells, and particulate matter. A large proportion of plasma proteins pass through the capillary wall daily, and not all of these return directly to the circulation. These are returned to the intravascular circulation by way of the lymphatic system.[4]

The lymphatic system is not a true circulatory system, but instead is a transport system for interstitial fluid. In contrast to the cardiovascular system, the lymphatic system is a low-pressure system that lacks a central pump and is not closed. Uptake of interstitial fluid begins in initial lymphatic vessels. The lymphatic capillaries are similar to blood capillaries, but there are gaps between the endothelial cells that allow the molecules that are too large for venous uptake to be reabsorbed.

J. Bergan (✉)
Vein Institute of La Jolla, University of California, La Jolla, CA, USA

B.-B. Lee et al. (eds.), *Lymphedema*,
DOI 10.1007/978-0-85729-567-5_1, © Springer-Verlag London Limited 2011

In collecting lymphatic vessels, valves facilitate the unidirectional movement of lymph by propulsion from external forces. A series of lymph nodes periodically interrupts the transporting vessels, which filter lymph as well as provide an immunological function.

Failure of any part of the lymphatic system causes the lymphatic load to exceed its transport capacity and causes fluid to accumulate in the interstitium. Inadequate clearance of lymph can occur in three distinct states; *dynamic insufficiency* (lymphatic system overload), *mechanical insufficiency* (intrinsic abnormality), or a combination of both mechanical and dynamic insufficiency, termed *safety valve insufficiency*.

Dynamic insufficiency of the lymphatic system, or high lymph flow failure, occurs when the normal functioning lymphatic structures are burdened with an increased load of microvascular filtrate, which reduces lymphatic transport capacity. Mechanical insufficiency, or low-output failure, refers to decreased lymphatic transport due to an intrinsic defect. Safety valve insufficiency occurs from the combined effect of increased lymph flow and a defective lymphatic system. The lymphatic defect may be due to an inherited abnormality, termed primary lymphedema, or an acquired cause, referred to as secondary lymphedema.

Classification of Lymphedema

Primary Lymphedema

Primary lymphedema encompasses a group of lymphatic disorders caused by inborn abnormalities of the lymphatic system, combined with abnormal structural development caused by mutant genes. Developmental lymphedema disorders may be caused by a single gene defect, chromosomal abnormality, or multifactorial inheritance.[5] Several genes have been identified as playing a role in embryonic and postnatal lymphatic development, including FOXC2, EphrinB2, VEGFR-3, VEGF-C, angiopoietin-2, Prox-1, and podoplanin.[6]

Most primary lymphedemas are actually truncular lymphatic malformations, arising during the later stages of lymphangiogenesis.[7,8] Many primary lymphedemas are congenital in nature. Lymphatic developmental disorders can be associated with combined malformations, arteriovenous malformations, and/or capillary malformations.[9]

Classification of primary lymphedema is based on several parameters, such as age at onset, anatomical variations, or pathophysiological phenomena. The most familiar system of classification used to describe primary lymphedema, however, is based on age at presentation; *congenital lymphedema*, also known as Milroy's disease if it is familial in an apparently autosomal dominant pattern of transmission, presents at birth or prior to age 2; *lymphedema praecox*, termed Meige disease, presents between ages 2 and 35; and *lymphedema tarda* presents after age 35.

Patients with known genetic mutations may develop lymphedema at puberty or at later stages of life. Therefore, classifying lymphedema into praecox or tarda is potentially misleading in understanding the etiology of these particular lymphedemas; the terms themselves may soon prove redundant. The future of the diagnosis and classification of primary lymphedema is likely to be determined by further insight into the genetic basis of this condition.

Secondary Lymphedema

Secondary lymphedema refers to an acquired cause of lymphedema, which may arise from the surgical removal of the lymph nodes or damage to lymphatic vessels by surgery, radiation, parasitic infiltration, malignancy, infection, inflammation, or filiariasis, the most common cause of secondary lymphedema worldwide. Filiariasis refers to infection by the parasitic nematode *Wuchereria Bancrofti*. Following transmission by a mosquito vector, the adult filarial worms lodge in the lymphatic vessels and initiate an immune response and subsequent activation of vascular endothelial growth factors (VEGF), thus promoting lymph vessel hyperplasia and inflammation as a result of the immune response.[10,11] Filariasis can be associated with lymphedema in the upper or lower extremities, breasts or male genitalia.

In developed countries, malignant neoplasms and their therapies are the most common cause of lymphedema. In the United States, breast cancer-related lymphedema of the arm is the most prevalent form. Nodal dissections and/or radiation therapy for gynecological, genitourinary, and head/neck malignancies have been implicated in the development of lymphedema. Nodal infiltration or metastasis to lymph nodes can occur from primary malignancies, such as lymphoma, melanoma, and a variety of gynecological and urological malignancies.

Interruption of the lymphatic vasculature during vein stripping surgery, vein harvesting procedures, recurrent cellulitis infections, and trauma are other mechanisms by which damage to lymphatic structures may occur.[12] Lastly, just as obstruction may occur in limb lymphatics, defects in central, abdominal or thoracic collecting trunks may cause either lymphedema in the limbs or chylous reflux in the body cavities. The latter phenomenon is described as chylous ascites when it affects the peritoneum, chylothorax when it affects pleura, chyluria when it affects renal lymphatics, and chylous metrorrhagia when it affects the uterus.

Clinical Presentation

The presentation of lymphedema may be at birth or in middle age; it may be sudden, or slow to develop. Edema is often painless at first, beginning on the dorsum of the foot or in the hand or forearm, and progressing proximally. Early in the presentation, it subsides during recumbency and worsens towards the end of the waking day. The swelling becomes permanent with the passage of time, accompanied by architectural changes in the tissues. Early in the presentation, as the edema attacks the dorsum of the feet, the toes may become swollen also. The forefoot comes to resemble a buffalo hump and the skin on the dorsum of the toes thickens. The resulting inability to pinch the skin fold of the second toe is referred to as Stemmer's sign.[13]

As fibrosis ensues and the skin and subcutaneous tissues become thick and firm, edema no longer pits and the skin develops a *peau d'orange* (orange peel) appearance. The skin may become darkened and develop multiple warty projections. This is referred to as lymphostatic verrucosis. Elephantiasis nostras verrucosa (ENV) can be a late sequela of non-filarial lymphedema, although it is uncommon. A "pebbly" or cobblestone appearance, papules, verrucous lesions, enlargement, and woody fibrosis of the affected area characterize this condition.[14] Papillomas may result from local dermal lymphostasis and can be seen in other conditions associated with chronic limb edema.[15,16]

Lymphedema Staging

Lymphedema staging is based on the physical condition of the affected limb. Although there is some debate about staging, The International Society of Lymphology categorizes three stages of lymphedema.[17] The first stage is characterized by non-fibrotic edema that puts pressure on the affected limb and can be reduced by leg elevation. The second stage is characterized by lymphedema in which some degree of fibrosis is present. As a result, the edema does not put on pressure or reduce with leg elevation. Lymphedema in the third stage is associated skin and subcutaneous fibrosis and is irreversible (lymphostatic elephantiasis).

An additional stage of lymphedema (stage 0) has been introduced to represent the sub-clinical condition where swelling is not evident, although impaired lymph transport is present. Therefore, stage 0 may exist for months to years before overt lymphedema is present. For example, symptoms of lymphedema, such as limb heaviness, in breast cancer patients have been observed to occur long before gross edema.[18] None of the available systems includes tissue tenderness, limb shape, disability, or complications arising from lymphedema, such as skin breakdown and malignancy in lymphedema staging.

Diagnosis

Diagnosis of lymphedema can be determined by the clinical history and physical examination. History should include age at onset, travel to tropical countries, and a complete history inquiring into all possible causes of secondary lymphedema.

History of temporary edema of the affected area must be noted, and a detailed family history of limb swelling should be recorded. The examination should assess the distribution of edema, the condition of the skin, varicose veins, signs of lymphangitis or other skin lesions, past or present. The characteristic signs of lymphedema as described earlier in this chapter should be documented. Lymph vesicles, drainage of fluid, clear or milky, and yellow discoloration or other abnormalities of the nails must be noted. Finally, any complications, such as cellulitis, lymphangitis, malnutrition, immunodeficiency, or, rarely, suspected malignancy, must be documented.

Lymphedema in its early stages may be difficult to distinguish from other causes of non-pitting limb edema. Peripheral edema is most commonly caused by cardiac, hepatic or renal disease, or it can be induced by medication. Venous edema is more common than lymphedema. Lipedema can be confused with lymphedema, but can be clinically distinguished by its symmetrical distribution and characteristic sparing of the feet.

Confirmatory Testing

When the diagnosis is uncertain, the appropriate combination of non-to-minimally invasive tests should be able to provide all of the information necessary to ensure adequate diagnosis and lead to correct multi-disciplinary targeted treatment strategies.

X-rays of bones will identify limb length discrepancies, bony abnormalities, or phleboliths in patients with combined lymphatic and vascular malformations. Venous duplex studies will confirm any associated venous anomalies such as valvular incompetence, obstruction, ectasia, or localized dilations, and aneurysms. These studies should exclude venous obstruction as a cause or a contributing factor to the lymphedema.

Radionuclide lymphoscintigraphy (LSG) has largely replaced conventional oil contrast lymphography for visualizing the lymphatic network. LSG, performed with injection of 99mTc-labeled human serum albumin or 99MTc-labeled sulfur colloid subcutaneously into the first and second web-space of the toes and fingers is the test of choice to confirm or exclude lymphedema as the cause of the chronic limb swelling. Appearance time of the activity at the knee, groin, or axilla, as well as the absence or presence of major lymphatic collectors, numbers and size of vessels and nodes, and the presence or absence of dermal back flow should be looked for and carefully noted.[19] The presence of collaterals and reflux, as well as symmetrical activity in the opposite limb, must be recorded and used for interpretation. It can be easily repeated with minimal risk.[20,21]

Magnetic resonance imaging (MRI)/computed tomography (CT), typically of the pelvis and abdomen, can be useful to exclude underlying malignancy and for the differential diagnosis, and can differentiate amongst lymphedema and lipedema, chronic venous changes, vascular anomalies, and soft tissue hypertrophy. MR/CT angiography is useful to exclude vascular anomalies, proximal obstruction, extrinsic iliac or vena caval compression.

Some invasive tests may be required to provide more information for an accurate differential diagnosis. Biopsy of an enlarged regional lymph node in the setting of chronic lymphedema is seldom needed to confirm the diagnosis, but is occasionally required for a differential diagnosis. Fine needle aspiration with cytological recommendations is strongly recommended as a substitute for excisional biopsy to minimize aggravation of the edema.

Finally, genetic testing may play a greater role in the future diagnosis of lymphedema to identify specific hereditary syndromes with genetic mutations.

Therapy

Physical and Non-Operative Therapy

The ultimate goal of treatment is to achieve better social, functional, and psychological adaptation in lymphedema patients. Therefore, therapy should improve the physical characteristics of the limb, alleviate symptoms, and reduce disease progression and secondary complications. The initial treatment for lymphedema is combined physical therapy (CPT) or complete/complex decongestive therapy (CDT), a two-stage treatment program. The first stage consists of manual lymphatic drainage (MLD), decongestive exercises and multilayer bandaging for compression. MLD is a specialized massage technique using specific pressures to stimulate lymphatic flow, redistribute fluid, which ultimately reduces limb volume.[22] As an adjunct to MLD, special short-stretch bandages, pneumatic sequential pumps, and other devices may be used for compression to promote venous and lymphatic flow.

The second phase is self-treatment with the above techniques for maintenance and prevention of re-accumulation of lymph. Prevention of infection can be accomplished with self-surveillance of the skin for early signs of infection, good hygiene, and skin care. Immediate antiseptic care of minor wounds and antibiotic treatment for early signs of infection is warranted. Antibiotic prophylaxis should be considered in patients who have had two or more attacks of cellulitis per year. The role of pharmacotherapy in treating symptoms of lymphedema has not been established.

Operative Therapy

Surgical treatment may benefit patients who remain refractory to all other treatment. There are three general surgical approaches to primary lymphedema: (1) Reconstructive surgery with microsurgical interventions (2) Debulking, ablative, or excisional surgery, and (3) Liposuction. Indications for reconstructive surgery include failure to respond to therapy in the early stages of lymphedema, progression of the disease to the advanced stages, presence of chylous reflux or recurrent infections. The objective of debulking, ablative, or excisional surgery is to reduce the subcutaneous fat and fibrous overgrowth. Liposuction is designed to obliterate the epifacscial compartment by removal of excessive adipose tissue. Candidates for palliative excisional surgery should be in the late stages of lymphedema with grotesquely disfigured limbs and/or have failed conservative therapy.

Complications of Lymphedema

Patients with lymphedema are prone to repeated episodes of infection and inflammation of the skin, soft tissue, and lymphatic vessels. Gram-positive bacteria are the usual pathogen in attacks of cellulitis, lymphangitis, and erysipelas. Recurrent skin infections may be an early presentation of lymphedema before overt signs are present.[23] Dermatolymphangioadenitis (DLA) can occur as a complication of obstructive peripheral lymphedema. The clinical characteristics of acute DLA are local tenderness and erythema of the skin, red streaks that follow the distribution of the superficial lymphatics, enlarged inguinal lymph nodes, and systemic symptoms such as fever and chills.

A rare, but potentially lethal complication of chronic lymphedema is the development of a cutaneous malignancy, referred to as Stewart–Treves syndrome. Stewart–Treves syndrome is an aggressive lymphangiosarcoma that was originally described in women who had chronic lymphedema of the upper limb following mastectomy and axillary lymph node dissection for breast cancer.[24,25] Other neoplasms associated with chronic lymphedema are Kaposi sarcoma, B-cell lymphoma, squamous cell carcinoma, and malignant fibrous histiocytoma.

Conclusions

Lymphedema is fundamentally a failure of fluid transport and is usually diagnosed by its physical features. The hallmark of lymphedema is fibrosis of the skin and subcutaneous tissues, and progression to non-pitting edema. History and physical findings dictate its classification and grading. Specific testing is used only in difficult cases in which imaging studies clarify the diagnosis, although genetic testing will likely play a role in the future diagnosis of primary lymhedema. Treatment is primarily non-surgical. Surgical intervention may be of benefit to a few, well-selected individuals. Future therapy for primary lymphedema will likely involve molecular interventions and increased efforts to prevent secondary lymphedema.

References

1. Rockson SG. The unique biology of lymphatic edema. *Lymphat Res Biol*. 2009;7(2):97-100.
2. Kobayashi MR, Miller TA. Lymphedema. *Clin Plast Surg*. 1987;14:303-313.
3. Warren AG, Brorson H, Borud LJ, Slavin SA. Lymphedema: a comprehensive review. *Ann Plast Surg*. 2007;59:464-472.
4. Bergan JJ. Lymphatic disease. In: Gloviczki P, Yao J, eds. *Handbook of Venous Disorders: Guidelines of the American Venous Forum*. 2nd ed. London, UK: Hodder Arnold; 2001.
5. Rockson SG. Lymphedema. *Curr Treat Options Cardiovasc Med*. 2000 June; 2(3):237-242.
6. Lee BB, Kim YW, Seo JM, et al. Current concepts in lymphatic malformation. *Vasc Endovasc Surg*. 2005;39(1):67-81. Review.
7. Lee BB. Lymphatic malformation. In: Tretbar LL, Morgan CL, Lee BB, Simonian SJ, Blondeau B, eds. *Lymphedema: Diagnosis and Treatment*. London: Springer; 2008.
8. Lee BB, Villavicencio JL. Primary lymphoedema and lymphatic malformation: are they the two sides of the same coin? *Eur J Vasc Endovasc Surg*. 2010;39(5):646-653. Review.
9. Damstra RJ, Mortimer PS. Diagnosis and therapy in children with lymphoedema. *Phlebology*. 2008;23(6):276-286.
10. Bennuru S, Nutman TB. Lymphangiogenesis and lymphatic remodeling induced by filarial parasites: implications for pathogenesis. *PLoS Pathog*. 2009;5(12):e1000688.
11. Pfarr KM et al. Filariasis and lymphoedema. *Parasite Immunol*. 2009;31(11):664-672.
12. Van Bellen B et al. Lymphatic disruption in varicose vein surgery. *Surgery*. 1977;82(2): 257-259.
13. Stemmer R. A clinical symptom for the early and differential diagnosis of lymphedema. *Vasa*. 1976;5:261-262.
14. Sisto K, Khachemoune A. Elehantiasis nostras verrucosa: a review. *Am J Clin Dermatol*. 2008;9(3):141-146.
15. Stoberl C, Partsch H. Congestive lymphostatic papillomatosis. *Hautarzt*. 1988;39(7): 441-446.
16. Schultz-Ehrenburg U, Niederauer HH, Tiedjen KU. Stasis papillomatosis. Clinical features, etiopahtogenesis and radiological findings. *J Dermatol Surg Oncol*. 1993;19(5):440-446.
17. International Society of Lymphology. The diagnosis and treatment of peripheral lymphedema: 2009 Consensus document of the International Society of Lymphology. *Lymphology*. 2009; 53-54.
18. Stanton AW, Levick JR, Mortimer PS. Chronic arm edema following breast cancer treatment. *Kidney Int Suppl*. 1997;59:S76.
19. Szuba A, Shin WS, Strauss HW, Rockson S. The third circulation: radionuclide lymphoscintigraphy in the evaluation of lymphedema. *J Nucl Med*. 2003;44:43-57.
20. Scarsbrook AF, Ganeshan A, Bradley KM. Pearls and pitfalls of radionuclide imaging of the lymphatic system. II. Evaluation of extremity lymphedema. *Br J Radiol*. 2007;80:219-226.
21. Witte CL, Witte MH, Unger EC, et al. Advances in imaging of lymph flow disorders. *Radiographics*. 2000;20:1697.
22. Kasseroller RG. The Vodder School: the Vodder method. *Cancer*. 1998;83(12 Suppl American):2840-2842. Review.
23. Damstra RJ, van Steensel MA, Boomsma JH, Nelemans P, Veraart JC. Erysipelas as a sign of subclinical primary lymphoedema: a prospective quantitative scintigraphic study of 40 patients with unilateral erysipelas of the leg. *Br J Dermatol*. 2008;158(6):1210-1215.
24. Chung KC, Kim HJ, Jeffers LL. Lymphangiosarcoma (Stewart-Treves syndrome) in post-mastectomy patients. A review. *J Hand Surg*. 2000;25:1163-1168.
25. Stewart FW, Treves N. Lymphangiosarcoma in postmastectomy lymphedema: a report of six cases in elephantiasis chirurgica. *Cancer*. 1948;1:64-81.

Chapter 2
Etiology and Classification of Lymphatic Disorders

Stanley G. Rockson

Beyond lymphedema, in its diverse manifestations, there is a spectrum of human disease that directly or indirectly alters lymphatic structure and function. Not surprisingly, the symptomatic and objective presentation of these patients is quite heterogeneous. Diagnosis and differential diagnosis pose distinct challenges. In this overview, the various categories of lymphatic disease are enumerated and viewed through the prism of lymphatic embryological development (Chap. 4).

Embryological Development of the Lymphatic System

The lymphatic progenitors are believed to arise from among the endothelial cells within the embryonic venous structures. Lymphatic endothelial cell specification involves the expression of the distinguishing molecular markers that impose the unique phenotype of this cell. As the lymphatic endothelial cells attain a higher level of differentiation, additional lymphatic-specific markers are expressed, with concomitant suppression of blood vascular expression profiles.[1] The committed lymphatic cell population achieves complete autonomy from the local venous microenvironment and migrates peripherally. Budding and migration precede the formation of primary lymph sacs throughout the embryo. Secondary budding and migration mark the final stages of lymphatic development.

S.G. Rockson
Division of Cardiovascular Medicine, Stanford University School of Medicine,
Falk Cardiovascular Research Center, Stanford, CA, USA

B.-B. Lee et al. (eds.), *Lymphedema*,
DOI 10.1007/978-0-85729-567-5_2, © Springer-Verlag London Limited 2011

Lymphatic Vascular Disease Classification

The newly derived insights into molecular embryology have significantly advanced our comprehension of lymphatic vascular development. The spectrum of lymphatic vascular disease is broad, and, ideally, insights into classification and treatment will ultimately be increasingly tied to growing insights drawn from developmental biology. In fact, until quite recently, disease classification and risk stratification have been very imprecise, and comprehension of disease natural history and epidemiology has been disappointingly primitive.[2,3] The recognized categories and representative subsidiary diseases are summarized in Table 2.1.

Lymphedema

Lymphedema is unquestionably the most common diagnostic entity among the lymphatic vascular diseases. It is encountered in both acquired and heritable forms.[2] Traditionally, a distinction is drawn among primary and secondary causes of lymphedema.[4] In this schema, primary lymphedemas encompass both the sporadic and hereditary forms, as well as those that are syndrome associated; secondary lymphedema is either malignant (i.e., associated with direct neoplastic invasion or obstruction of the vascular channels and nodes) or benign (acquired as a consequence of infection, trauma, or iatrogenic causes). More recent attitudes surrounding lymphedema suggest that the boundaries may be blurred: primary cases often declare themselves after a "secondary" provocation, and evolving clinical data suggest that there might be a genetic predisposition for the development of lymphedema, even when the inciting secondary events are easy to identify.[5]

Heritable congenital lymphedema of the lower extremities was first described in 1891[6]; in 1892, Milroy[7] described the familial distribution of congenital lymphedema, noting the involvement of 26 persons in a single family, spanning six generations. Nonne–Milroy's lymphedema is characterized by unilateral or bilateral swelling of the legs, arms, and/or face with gradual and irreversible fibrotic changes. Additional, distinct variants of heritable lymphedema have subsequently been described. In 1898, Meige reported cases of lymphedema in which the age of onset was after puberty and that often appeared alongside acute cellulitis.[8] In 1964, another variety of pubertal-onset lymphedema was reported, in which the affected individuals had distichiasis (i.e., an auxiliary set of eyelashes).[9]

In addition to the isolated gene mutations responsible for Milroy's disease and lymphedema distichiasis, there is an array of syndromic heritable disorders that are associated with dysfunction of the lymphatic vasculature. Often, these syndromes are associated with abnormal facial and mental development.

A useful organizational schema is to classify the disorders by their autosomal dominant (Noonan syndrome, Adams–Oliver syndrome, and neurofibromatosis) or autosomal recessive (Hennekam's syndrome, the Prader–Willi syndrome, and Aagenaes' syndrome) modes of genetic transmission.

Table 2.1 Lymphatic disease classification (Modified from Radhakrishnan and Rockson)[11]

Disease	Symptoms	Signs	Genetic features	Pathology
I. Primary lymphedema				
Nonne–Milroy lymphedema	Pitting/brawny swellings of ankles and shins apparent at birth or infancy	Firm edema of lower limbs	Autosomal dominant	Inadequate lymphatic drainage (insufficient development of lymphatic vessels)
Milroy disease	Congenital swelling of the lower limbs	Lymphedema confined to lower limbs	Autosomal dominant	Hypoplasia of lymphatic capillary network; fibrosis of limb tissues
Lymphedema tarda (Meige's disease)		Lymphedema of lower extremity; becomes clinically evident near age 35	No family history	Hyperplastic pattern, with tortuous lymphatics increased in caliber and number; absent or incompetent valves
Klippel–Trenaunay syndrome: combination of cutaneous capillary malformation, varicose veins, and hypertrophy of bone and soft tissue		Capillary hemangioma/ port-wine stain: distinct, linear border; nevus flammeus (salmon pink patch); large, lateral, superficial vein beginning at foot/lower leg and travels proximally until entering the thigh/gluteal area; bony/soft tissue hypertrophies: limb hypertrophies/ discrepancies		

(continued)

Table 2.1 (continued)

Disease	Symptoms	Signs	Genetic features	Pathology
Noonan syndrome; (congenital)	Decreased appetite Frequent or forceful vomiting Difficulty swallowing Severe joint or muscle pain	Facial abnormalities, webbing of the neck, and deformities of the chest Heart murmur Mental retardation	Autosomal dominant or sporadic	
Neurofibromatosis	Coffee-colored skin spots, freckling in non-sun exposed areas, back pain	Neurofibromas Optic glioma hamartomas on the iris Distinctive bony lesions	Autosomal dominant (half of cases have no family history, high mutation rate)	Vasculopathy (arterial stenoses due to proliferation of cells in intima) Fibro-muscular hyperplasia of arteries leads to renal artery stenosis, cerebral infarction, aneurysm (rare)
Lymphedema distichiasis	Onset of edema commonly at or near the time of puberty	Distichiasis Pitting edema	Autosomal dominant inheritance	Abnormal development of intra-lymphatic valves; enhanced recruitment of vascular mural cells to lymphatic capillaries
Protein-losing enteropathy	Swelling of the legs or other areas Diarrhea Weight loss Abdominal pain	Edema Ascites Pleural effusion Pericardial effusion		
Lymphedema/hypo-parathyroidism		Symmetrical congenital lymphedema with pulmonary lymphangiectasia	Pleiotropic effect of an autosomal or X-linked recessive gene	

Turner's syndrome	Short stature Congenital edema of hands/feet at birth; Webbed neck; ptosis; a "shield-shaped", broad, flat chest; absent or incomplete development at puberty, including sparse pubic hair and small breasts. Infertility Dry eyes Absent menstruation, absent normal moisture in vagina; painful intercourse	Ovarian failure Hypoplastic or hyperconvex nails Underdeveloped breasts and genitalia, webbed neck, short stature, low hairline in back, simian crease, and abnormal bone development of the chest	X-linked dominant inheritance	Absence of one set of genes from the short arm of one X chromosome
Klinefelter syndrome (supplementary X chromosome)	Infertility, gynecomastia	Lack secondary sexual characteristics lack facial/body/sexual hair, high-pitched voice, female type of fat distribution; testicular dysgenesis		Small, firm testes with seminiferous tubular hyalinization, sclerosis, degenerated Leydig cells; histology of gynecomastic breasts shows hyperplasia of interductal tissue

(continued)

Table 2.1 (continued)

Disease	Symptoms	Signs	Genetic features	Pathology
Patau syndrome	Scalp defects	Holoprosencephaly (brain does not divide completely into halves)		
Trisomy chromosome 13	Cleft lip/palate Facial defects (absent or malformed nose) Hernias	Hypotelorism Microphthalmia Anophthalmia Rocker-bottom feet Microphthalmia Cutis aplasia Omphalocele		
Edwards syndrome (trisomy 18)	Stop breathing, poor feeding	Apneic episodes, marked failure to thrive; severe growth retardation, mental retardation Malformations (e.g., microcephaly, cerebellar hypoplasia, hypoplasia/aplasia of corpus callosum, holoprosencephaly)		
Triploidy syndrome		General dysmaturity, muscular hypotonia, large posterior fontanel, hypertelorism, microphthalmia, colobomata, cutaneous syndactyly Abnormalities of the skull, face, limbs, genitalia (male karyotype), various internal organs Fetal hypoplasia, microstomia, low-set ears		Triploid cell lines may have disappeared from peripheral blood so evidence of triploidy can only be found in the cultured skin fibroblasts

Yellow nail syndrome	Yellow nails Edema	Triad of lymphedema (symmetrical, non-pitting), slow-growing yellow nails, pleural effusion	Heterogeneous inheritance, both autosomal dominant and recessive	Hypoplastic lymphatics
Adams liver syndrome	Rare syndrome of defects of the scalp and cranium associated with distal limb anomalies and occasional mental retardation		Most autosomal dominant; some autosomal recessive/sporadic	
Proteus syndrome	Partial gigantism, long face, wide nasal bridge, mouth open at rest, upper body wasting, learning disabilities, occasional seizures	Cutaneous and subcutaneous lesions including vascular malformations, lipomas, hyperpigmentation, and several types of nevi	Somatic mosaicism for a dominant lethal gene yet to be identified; mosaicism: a fraction of cells have mutation, a fraction do not	Connective tissue nevi resemble tightly compacted, collagen-rich connective tissue. Epidermal nevi generally exhibit a combination of hyperkeratosis, parakeratosis, acanthosis, and papillomatosis
Hennekam syndrome	Edema Facial anomalies Moderate developmental problems	Lymphedema, lymphangiectasia, facial anomalies, delayed onset of puberty Moderate mental retardation	In one report of ten familial cases, equal sex ratio, increased parental consanguinity, no vertical transmission; consistent with autosomal recessive	
Aagenaes' syndrome (cholestasis with malabsorption)	Predominantly in patients in Norway, jaundice, severe itching	Enlarged liver	Possibly autosomal recessive	Generalized lymphatic anomaly (lymphedema due to lymph vessel hypoplasia) giant-cell hepatitis with fibrosis of the portal tract

(continued)

Table 2.1 (continued)

Disease	Symptoms	Signs	Genetic features	Pathology
Prader-Willi syndrome: genomic imprinting; genes expressed differentially based upon parent of origin (loss of paternal gene or maternal disomy)	Floppy newborn infant (hypotonic), small for gestational age, undescended testicles in the male infant, delayed motor development, slow mental development, very small hands and feet in comparison to body, rapid weight gain, insatiable appetite, food craving, almond-shaped eyes, narrow bifrontal skull, morbid obesity, skeletal (limb) abnormalities, striae	Hypotonia, hypomentia, hypogonadism, obesity	Genomic imprinting; genes expressed differentially based upon parent of origin (loss of paternal gene or maternal disomy)	

II. Acquired lymphedema

Stewart–Treves syndrome (Cutaneous angiosarcoma induced by radical mastectomy to treat breast cancer; tumor develops 5–15 years after mastectomy)	Recurrent erysipelas	Severe chronic edema of an upper extremity; first appears on the arm on the side operated on; gradually extends from arm to forearm and the dorsal aspect of the hand/fingers		Proliferating vascular channels; tumor endothelial cells lining these channels show marked hyperchromatism and pleomorphism Mitoses commonly seen in these tumor cells; lymphangiosarcoma cells surrounded by complete basal lamina

Hodgkin's disease (potentially curable malignant lymphoma)	Unexplained weight loss, fever, night sweats; Chest pain, cough, and/or shortness of breath; hemoptysis; Pruritus; Intermittent fever; Alcohol-induced pain at sites of nodal disease	Asymptomatic lymph-adenopathy; splenomegaly; Hepatomegaly; Superior vena cava syndrome (rare); CNS symptoms (cerebellar degeneration, neuropathy)	
Filariasis	Fever, inguinal or axillary lymphadenopathy, testicular and/or inguinal pain, skin exfoliation, and limb or genital swelling; cloudy, milk-like urine	Episodic attacks of fever associated with inflammation of the inguinal lymph nodes, testis, spermatic cord, lymphedema, or a combination of these; abscess formation at nodes; cellular invasion with plasma cells/eosinophils/macrophages with hyperplasia of lymphatic endothelium; lymphatic damage and chronic leakage of protein-rich lymph in the tissues, thickening of skin, chronic infections contribute to the appearance of elephantiasis	Fibrosis of affected lymph nodes; stenosis and obstruction of lymphatics with creation of collateral channels; cutaneous hyperkeratosis, acanthosis, loss of elastin fibers, and fibrosis

(continued)

Table 2.1 (continued)

Disease	Symptoms	Signs	Genetic features	Pathology
III. Lymphangiectasia				
Pulmonary lymphangiectasia	May present at birth, tachypnea, cough, wheeze	Increased respiratory effort with inspiratory crackle, respiratory distress, cyanosis; pleural effusion (chylous), lymphedema	Sporadic, a few autosomal recessive	Lung histology reveals large, cystic endothelial-lined lymphatic channels
Intestinal lymphangiectasia	Intermittent diarrhea, nausea, vomiting, steatorrhea, Peripheral edema	Growth retardation	Most sporadic	Diffuse or localized ectasia of enteric lymphatics
Lymphangiomatosis	Presents in late childhood, can occur in any tissue in which lymphatics are normally found, predilection for thoracic and neck involvement; wheezes (misdiagnosed as asthma)			Multiple lymphangiomas (well-differentiated lymphatic tissue that present as multicystic or sponge-like accumulations; benign proliferations of the lymphatic channels with abnormal connections to the lymphatic system); anastomosing endothelial lined spaces along pulmonary lymphatic routes accompanied by asymmetrically spaced bundles of spindle cells

Gorham's disease – proliferation of vascular channels that results in destruction/resorption of osseous matrix	Dull aching pain or insidious onset (limitation of motion, progressive weakness); swelling	Massive bone loss	No familial predisposition	Non-malignant proliferation of thin-walled vessels; proliferative vessels may be capillary/sinusoidal or cavernous Wide capillary-like vessels
Lymphangioleiomyomatosis (LAM)	Shortness of breath, expectoration of chyle or blood Nausea Bloating Abdominal distension Cough Phlegm Crackles Wheezing Chest pain Gurgling in chest	Pneumothorax Chylothorax Chylous, pleural effusions Enlarged lymph nodes	Sporadic	
Diffuse hemangiomatosis	Many newborns have premonitory lesions, such as small red macule, telangiectasias, or blue macule at the hemangioma site	Visceral hemangiomas (in the neonatal period), three or more organ systems were affected, hemangiomas are not malignant Vascular hamartomas	Congenital defect	Lesions have dilated thin-walled channels lined by a single layer of flattened endothelial cells Only a few focal areas of endothelial proliferation, no other cellular hyperplasia or pleomorphism, well formed vascular channels; abnormal capillaries coursing through muscle suggest that hemangiomas are hamartomas

(continued)

Table 2.1 (continued)

Disease	Symptoms	Signs	Genetic features	Pathology
Lymphangitis (Inflammation of the lymphatic channels that occurs as a result of infection at a site distal to the channel)	Red streaks on the skin Fever, chills, malaise Headache, loss of appetite, muscle aches Recent cut/abrasion that appears infected and spreading	Erythematosus and irregular linear streaks extend from primary infection site toward draining regional nodes Tender/warm Blistering of skin Lymph nodes swollen and tender Children may be febrile/tachycardic		
Maffucci syndrome	Soft, blue-colored growths of distal aspects of extremities Short in stature, unequal arm/leg	Enchondroma (benign enlargements of cartilage) with multiple angiomas Bone deformities Dark, irregularly shaped hemangiomas	Sporadic, manifests early in life (~4–5 years); 25% of cases are congenital	Thrombi often form within vessels and develop into phleboliths – appear as calcified vessels under the microscope; chondrosarcomas diagnosed by poorly differentiated pleiomorphic chondrocytes
Blue rubber bleb nevus syndrome (Multiple cutaneous venous malformations in association with visceral lesions, most commonly affecting GI)	Skin lesions multiple, protuberant, dark blue, compressible blebs, look and feel of a rubber nipple	Lesions asymptomatic but may be painful or tender Increased sweating on skin overlying lesion Fatigue from blood loss Hematemesis, melena, or frank rectal bleeding Joint pain Blindness due to cerebral or cerebellar cavernomas that hemorrhage into occipital lobes	Sporadic, autosomal dominant inheritance also reported	Vascular tissue with tortuous, blood-filled ecstatic vessels, lined by single layer of endothelium, with surrounding thin connective tissue; dystrophic calcification may be present

Cystic angiomatosis	Soft tissue masses, localized pain and swelling related to pathological fracture	Vascular malformation of congenital origin	Dilated, cavernous thin-walled vascular channels lined by flat endothelial cells (similar to LAM)
Lymphangioma: (uncommon, hamartomatous, congenital malformations of the lymphatic system that involve skin and subcutaneous tissues) Superficial vesicles: lymphangioma circumscriptum More deep-seated includes cavernous lymphangioma and cystic hygroma	Verrucous changes, warty appearance; clear or solitary rubbery nodule with no skin changes Persistent, multiple clusters of translucent vesicles that contain clear lymph fluid; superficial saccular dilations from underlying lymphatic vessels that occupy papilla and push upward against overlying epidermis		Vesicles are greatly dilated lymph channels that cause dermis to expand Lumen filled with lymphatic fluid often contains red blood cells, lymphocytes, macrophages, neutrophils; lined by flat endothelial cells Large, irregular channels in the reticular dermis, lined by single layer of endothelial cells
Cystic hygroma (develops in first trimester)	Single or multiple fluid-filled lesions that occur at sites of lymphatic-venous connection; primarily in the neck and axilla	Lymphedema Hydrops fetalis	Congenital; autosomal recessive	Dilated, disorganized lymph channels due to failure of lymph sacs to establish venous drainage

(continued)

Table 2.1 (continued)

Disease	Symptoms	Signs	Genetic features	Pathology
IV. Lipedema				
Lipedema	Insidious onset in adolescence; progressive, swollen legs with foot sparing; range of skin, bruises, pain, varicose veins, weight gain	Edema without pitting, Stemmer's sign negative	Sporadic	Fibro-sclerosis, damage to deep venous system

Chromosomal disorders can also result in multiple organ defects, including lymphedema. These disorders are uncommon; hence, the chromosomal basis can be readily overlooked or misdiagnosed. Confirmatory identification can be achieved only through detailed cytogenetic studies. Many of these disorders severely distort lymphatic function. Turner's syndrome and Klinefelter's syndrome are linked to the sex chromosomes, whereas Edwards' syndrome and Patau syndrome are linked to autosomal chromosomes. Triploidy syndrome denotes the presence of an extra copy of all of the chromosomes.

Beyond peripheral lymphedema, the lymphatic spectrum is remarkably diverse. Histologically, the vasculature can display various changes, with pathological dilation of normal structures or abnormal patterns of vascular growth. The pathological alterations can be isolated, regionalized, or diffuse, and can occur in isolation or in concert with other complex vascular lesions.

Lymphangioma

Lymphangioma is a congenital lymphatic malformation that arises during embryological development. These lesions may arise from segments of lymphatic vascular tissue that fail to appropriately anastomose, or they may represent portions of lymph sacs that become grouped together during development.[10] The presence of multiple or widespread lymphatic vascular malformations of this type can be termed *lymphangiomatosis*.[11] The lesions are classified by size and depth of formation, with the smaller, superficial form designated as *lymphangioma circumscriptum*, whereas the deeper lesions have traditionally been called *cavernous lymphangiomas* and *cystic hygromas*.

Protein-Losing Enteropathy and Intestinal Lymphangiectasia

Loss of lymphatic fluid and plasma protein within the lumen of the gastrointestinal tract can lead to edema and hypoproteinemia.[11] Patients with protein-losing enteropathy typically have local lymphatic obstruction and stasis,[12] whereas those with lymphangiectasia have dilated lymphatic vessels in the intestinal villi.[13]

In general, obstruction of the lymphatic vasculature yields increased hydrostatic pressure throughout the lymphatic system of the gastrointestinal tract, resulting in lymph stasis. Protein-rich lymphatic fluid is consequently lost within the lumen of the gastrointestinal tract through the lacteals in the intestinal microvilli.

In specific, intestinal lymphangiectasia is a rare condition characterized by severe edema, thickening of the small bowel wall, protein-losing enteropathy, ascites, and pleural effusion. The condition may be primary, resulting from a congenital lymphatic vascular disorder, or secondary, as a consequence of inflammatory or neoplastic involvement of the lymphatic system.[14] The pathogenesis remains unclear.

Complex Vascular Malformations

Various disorders result from abnormal development of, or insult to, the blood vascular and lymphatic vascular systems.[11]

Cystic angiomatosis is a congenital condition of unknown etiology, defined by the presence of numerous cystic skeletal lesions. The lesions are generally round or oval, and they vary widely in size. The cystic lesions may be due to dilated blood vessels or lymphatic channels, or both. The cysts are encircled by a single, flat layer of endothelial cells.

Maffucci's syndrome is characterized by the presence of hard subcutaneous enchondromas and hemangiomas due to mesodermal dysplasia.[15] Maffucci's syndrome often impairs lymphatic system function, leading to edema and secondary infection. Lesions appear during childhood and may progressively worsen.

Gorham's disease represents the uncontrolled growth of non-malignant vascular channels that lead to lysis of the affected bone.[16] The condition is associated with angiomatosis of blood and lymphatic vessels. Chylous pericardial and pleural effusions are associated with this condition, and chylothorax can sometimes result from dilation of the lymphatic vessels, with reflux into pleural cavity.

Klippel–Trenaunay syndrome consists of a combination of vascular malformations, including capillary anomalies (port wine stain), varicose veins, and hypertrophy of bone and soft tissue.[17] While Klippel–Trenaunay syndrome generally manifests in a single extremity, it can also affect multiple limbs or the entire body. Histologically, the condition is associated with dilated telangiectatic vessels in the upper dermis that do not spontaneously regress.

Beyond lymphedema and the primary defects of lymphatic vasculature, there are numerous additional categories of disease that can be considered to be part of the spectrum of lymphatic vascular disease.

Infectious Diseases

Lymphatic dysfunction can arise as a consequence of invading pathogens.

Globally, more than 129 million patients are afflicted by lymphatic filariasis. This condition is characterized by markedly impaired lymphatic function and lymphangiectasia. Patients are infected by filariae, or parasitic worms, which take up residence in the lymphatic structures. As a result, the lymphatics become compromised; the formation of new lymph channels is impaired by the adenolymphangitis, fibrosis and stenosis of the lymph nodes.

Lymphangitis is caused by the inflammation of lymphatic channels through tissue infection. Pathogenic organisms can include bacteria, fungi, viruses, and protozoa.

Lipedema

Lipedema was first described in 1940 as a bilateral, gradual accumulation of fatty deposition in the lower extremities and buttocks. The body habitus superficially resembles that of bilateral lower extremity lymphedema, although the involvement of the two limbs is substantially more symmetrical than in lymphedema, and there is almost always sparing of the feet. The condition is found almost exclusively in female subjects. Affected individuals often describe a family history of large legs.[18] Lipedema is further characterized by the presence of normal cutaneous architecture, lacking the fibrotic changes often seen in lymphedema. Histological sampling reveals edematous adipose cells that are sometimes hyperplastic. The microlymphatic function can become distorted in lipedema, and a component of secondary lymphedema often supervenes.

Lymphangioleiomyomatosis

Lymphangioleiomyomatosis (LAM) is a hybrid disorder that has, among its attributes, a distinct relationship with the visceral lymphatic vasculature.[19] The disease is characterized by the spread of abnormal smooth muscle cells (LAM cells) through both the pulmonary interstitium and the axial lymphatics, leading to the cystic destruction of the lung, along with lymphatic wall thickening. LAM is also characterized by the presence of pulmonary cysts and angiomyolipomas, tumors consisting of LAM cells, adipose tissue, and underdeveloped blood vessels. LAM chiefly affects women of childbearing age. It is an extremely rare disease, found in fewer than one in a million individuals. The primary clinical presentation associated with LAM is pulmonary, including pneumothorax, progressive dyspnea, chylous pleural effusions, cough, hemoptysis, and chyloptysis. Non-pulmonary findings include lymphangioleiomyomas, the large cystic masses commonly found in the abdominal and retroperitoneal regions, and chylous ascites.[11]

References

1. Wigle JT, Harvey N, Detmar M, et al. An essential role for Prox1 in the induction of the lymphatic endothelial cell phenotype. *EMBO J*. 2002;21(7):1505-1513.
2. Rockson SG. Lymphedema. *Am J Med*. 2001;110(4):288-295.
3. Rockson SG. Diagnosis and management of lymphatic vascular disease. *J Am Coll Cardiol*. 2008;52(10):799-806.
4. Nakamura K, Rockson SG. Molecular targets for therapeutic lymphangiogenesis in lymphatic dysfunction and disease. *Lymphat Res Biol*. 2008;6(3–4):181-189.
5. Rockson SG. The unique biology of lymphatic edema. *Lymphat Res Biol*. 2009;7(2):97-100.
6. Nonne M. Vier Fälle von Elephantiasis congenita hereditaria. *Virchows Arch*. 1891;125: 189-196.

7. Milroy W. An undescribed variety of hereditary oedema. *NY Med J.* 1892;56:505-508.
8. Brice G, Child AH, Evans A, et al. Milroy disease and the VEGFR-3 mutation phenotype. *J Med Genet.* 2005;42(2):98-102.
9. Falls HF, Kertesz ED. A new syndrome combining pterygium colli with developmental anomalies of the eyelids and lymphatics of the lower extremities. *Trans Am Ophthalmol Soc.* 1964;62:248-475.
10. Faul JL, Berry GJ, Colby TV, et al. Thoracic lymphangiomas, lymphangiectasis, lymphangiomatosis, and lymphatic dysplasia syndrome. *Am J Respir Crit Care Med.* 2000;161(3 Pt 1):1037-1046.
11. Radhakrishnan K, Rockson SG. The clinical spectrum of lymphatic disease. *Ann NY Acad Sci.* 2008;1131:155-184.
12. Chiu NT, Lee BF, Hwang SJ, Chang JM, Liu GC, Yu HS. Protein-losing enteropathy: diagnosis with (99 m)Tc-labeled human serum albumin scintigraphy. *Radiology.* 2001;219(1):86-90.
13. Hilliard RI, McKendry JB, Phillips MJ. Congenital abnormalities of the lymphatic system: a new clinical classification. *Pediatrics.* 1990;86(6):988-994.
14. Fox U, Lucani G. Disorders of the intestinal mesenteric lymphatic system. *Lymphology.* 1993;26(2):61-66.
15. Jermann M, Eid K, Pfammatter T, Stahel R. Maffucci's syndrome. *Circulation.* 2001;104(14):1693.
16. Patel DV. Gorham's disease or massive osteolysis. *Clin Med Res.* 2005;3(2):65-74.
17. Kihiczak GG, Meine JG, Schwartz RA, Janniger CK. Klippel-Trenaunay syndrome: a multisystem disorder possibly resulting from a pathogenic gene for vascular and tissue overgrowth. *Int J Dermatol.* 2006;45(8):883-890.
18. Warren AG, Janz BA, Borud LJ, Slavin SA. Evaluation and management of the fat leg syndrome. *Plast Reconstr Surg.* 2007;119(1):9e-15e.
19. Glasgow CG, Taveira-DaSilva A, Pacheco-Rodriguez G, et al. Involvement of lymphatics in lymphangioleiomyomatosis. *Lymphat Res Biol.* 2009;7(4):221-228.

Chapter 3
Hereditary and Familial Lymphedema

Kimberly A. Jones and Marlys H. Witte

Introduction

Just 10 years ago, a chapter could not have been written about the genetic basis of familial or hereditary lymphedema. Whereas the familial or hereditary occurrence of peripheral lymphedema has been described for at least 150 years in the literature, along with numerous syndromes listed in the database Online Mendelian inheritance in Man (OMIM™),[1] it was not until 2000 that the first of a series of unrelated "lymphedema genes" was discovered. The location had been identified on the long arm of chromosome 5 two years earlier by three independent research groups, but was not pinpointed.[2-4] In a few of the other described syndromes, genes contributing to the disease now have been identified using new molecular tools. Together with advances in understanding the growth and development of the lymphatic vasculature (lymphvasculogenesis and lymphangiogenesis) and diverse lymphatic functions, which have uncovered an array of candidate genes underlying these processes, the field is advancing at a much faster pace. Some of the genes identified to date seem to have a clear function related to the lymphatic system such as the mutation in the *FLT4* gene, which encodes the vascular endothelial growth factor receptor-3 gene (*VEGFR3*), important in lymphatic vessel development and function. Other genes (e.g., *FOXC2*) have identified proteins important in lymphatic structures as well as other organs, thus explaining the unique and at times baffling phenotypes of and within these syndromes. Some gene discoveries have been the stimulus to look at new pathways or to fill in steps or interrelationships in established pathways in lymphatic growth, development, and function. Detailed description and improved classification and reporting of these syndromes and further imaging studies to more precisely define lymphatic phenotypes (including carriers who may not exhibit overt lymphedema, but have structurally/functionally abnormal lymphatic vessels) will

M.H. Witte (✉)
Department of Surgery, University of Arizona College of Medicine,
Tucson, AZ, USA

B.-B. Lee et al. (eds.), *Lymphedema*,
DOI 10.1007/978-0-85729-567-5_3, © Springer-Verlag London Limited 2011

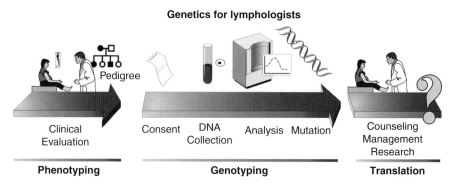

Fig. 3.1 Genetics for lymphologists: the work-up. See text for details (Reproduced with permission, The International Society of Lymphology)

allow use of more precise molecular tools to continue to help identify specific loci responsible for these often multi-system disorders and to carry out pre-natal or post-natal screening for detection. Moreover, once the molecular defects are uncovered and understood, more targeted therapeutic agents are likely to be developed.

Molecular Lymphology

The true incidence of primary lymphangiodysplasias or lymphedema (LE-AD) syndromes is hard to quantify (perhaps as many as one third of all lymphedemas, except in areas endemic for lymphatic filariasis, with hundreds of millions afflicted), and birth registries have not recorded lymphedema incidence. Only a small percentage (an estimated 5–10%) of primary lymphedema patients give a family history of the condition; however, lack of recognition could lead to underreporting. In disorders for which there are multiple congenital abnormalities shared within a family or group of individuals, a common defect(s) early in development is/are most likely compared with disorders for which the abnormalities appear to have a later onset or pubertal onset. Later onset or pubertal onset syndromes are more suggestive of incomplete penetrance, genetic polymorphisms, different molecular deficits within a common pathway, or more complicated variables, such as epigenetics and other environment-related factors.

During the clinical work-up (Fig. 3.1 and see below), once a common lymphedema manifestation and/or lymphovascular phenotype has been described within a family or group of families, a method known as reverse genetics can be applied. DNA from a large family or families can be collected and evaluated for short tandem repeats within each chromosome in an attempt to pinpoint the location of a gene associated with the affected phenotype. Once that location is identified, it can be searched further for possible candidate genes and analyzed for mutations. Forward genetics can be utilized when a candidate gene that is important in lymphatic function has been identified. Animal models can be produced with intentionally absent (knock-out) or overactive (transgenic) gene(s) to see if the expected or observed phenotype can be recapitulated. The function of any potentially involved genes can then be explored in great detail by developing animal models and by studying other genes and proteins related to the known target gene. Environmental influences through the study of proteomics can be performed in these animal models in addition to other in vivo experiments. Well-designed animal models can become the initial testing ground for future therapies.

Work-up

Despite major advances in the understanding of lymphangiogenesis with the discovery of the lymphatic-directed VEGFs (C and D) and related interacting proteins, linkage between the clinical phenotype and genotype is challenging. There are still many unknown genes or epigenetic influences to be discovered. When individuals or families with primary lymphedema in addition to other phenotypic abnormalities are identified, further work-up is a crucial step in understanding these disorders in the future. Referral to a multi-disciplinary group that specializes in the genetics of lymphangiogenesis is an important part of that work-up. Detailed history and phenotypic evaluation of the patient and any or all related family members may be necessary to note other subtle findings. Tools such as high-resolution dynamic lymphangioscintigraphy,[5] fluorescent microlymphangiography,[6] and magnetic resonance imaging,[7] with and without contrast medium administration, can delineate the number, size, and pattern of lymphatic growth or malformation and functional details such as chylous and non-chylous reflux, and these features can be followed over time. Defining the phenotype of the underlying abnormality (primary aplasia, hypoplasia, hyperplasia, or acquired dysplasia) is pertinent for classification of the functional defect and to compare similarities and differences among affected patients and families. High-resolution chromosomal analysis, linkage analysis, fluorescence in situ hybridization, and polymerase chain reaction are all molecular methods that may help identify candidate loci or associated genetic mutations or aberrancies, using both forward and reverse genetics. The type of syndrome (hereditary or sporadic) determines the best method of testing. Mutations can also be somatic (acquired genetic change after conception) and therefore may not be passed on to offspring or affect every organ. For this reason, biopsies of intestinal or pulmonary parenchyma also may be indicated in syndromes primarily affecting visceral organs only. Germline mutations, present at conception, are often passed on to offspring with associated syndromes. Often, mutations, either acquired or inherited, of members in a critical part of a shared pathway, can cause the same clinical consequences. By comparing individuals or families with those with similar syndromes, it is more likely for an error to be identified in a shared pathway of development if they do not share the same mutation. Timely and concise reporting of the findings allow for important collaborations, which are imperative in the study of rare disorders.

All of these efforts, along with the continued study of secondary (acquired) dysfunction and embryological development of the lymphatic system, should ultimately lead to better therapeutic options for those suffering from these disorders.

Syndromes

The definition of a syndrome can be described as any combination of signs and symptoms that are indicative of a particular disease or disorder. Syndromes with an inherited component are often listed in the frequently updated *Online Mendelian Inheritance in Man* (OMIM™) catalog, which focuses mainly on inherited, or heritable, genetic diseases. It lists the associated phenotypes and linked genes when the molecular basis is unknown.[1] When the OMIM™ database I searched, using either "lymphedema" or "lymphangiectasia," over 56 entries are found. Some of these are duplicate entries, variant forms of another syndrome, or do not appear to have primary lymphedema as a major component, leaving a total of 38 syndromes including the two most commonly described syndromes, Milroy and Meige syndrome. In addition, Hennekam presented five more syndromes at the National Lymphedema Network Biennial Conference in Orlando, Florida, September 2000 that were not listed in OMIM™, but which have been previously published and reviewed[8,9] (Fig. 3.2; Table 3.1).

Genes not associated with a particular syndrome have been identified in families with inherited forms of lymphedema and include *HGF*, *MET*,[12] and, most recently, *GJC2*.[13] *HGF* encodes for hepatocyte growth factor and binds with high affinity to its receptor MET. Both genes (*HGF/MET*) were thought to be candidate genes for lymphedema after an observation that they were both expressed in lymphatic endothelial cells, but not blood vascular endothelial cells. Mutational analysis identified six specific mutations in *HGF* and *MET* that were considered to be causal as they were found only in hereditary lymphedema probands and their families, were not present in controls, and caused a mutation in a functional region of the gene thought to disrupt HGF/MET signaling. The phenotypic description of these families or individuals associated with a loss of HGF/MET was not given.[12] Additionally, *GJC2*, the gene for connexin 47 (Cx47), located on chromosome 1q41-q42, was found to be expressed only in lymphatic endothelial cells (LECs) and not blood endothelial cells (BECs), and was also investigated in families with hereditary lymphedema. Six different mutations were identified, but a clearly distinct phenotype was not identified.[13]

Clinical syndromes with altered lymphovascular phenotypes or lymphedema-angiodysplasia (LE-AD) are often described by their inheritance patterns, age at onset, and body sites affected. Within both the families and syndromes, there is clinical variability suggestive of reduced penetrance, genetic heterogeneity, epigenetic and environmental influences, as well as other unrecognized molecular phenomena. Most LE-AD syndromes have congenital onset of lymphedema of the lower limbs. However, others have more extensive edema, chylous ascites, pleural effusions, visceral lymphangiectasias, or other lymphatic growth disturbances such as cystic hygromas, lymphangiomas, fetal hydrops or fetal demise.

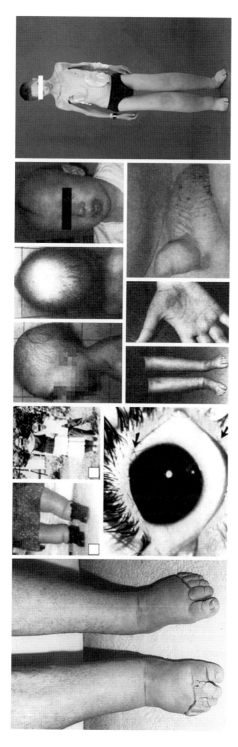

Fig. 3.2 Milroy lymphedema (*left*), lymphedema distichiasis syndrome showing leg lymphedema, tetralogy of Fallot in a young boy, and a double row of eyelashes (*middle left*), hypotrichosis–lymphedema–telangiectasia (*middle right*), and generalized lymphatic dysplasia syndrome (*Hennekam*) (*right*) syndromes demonstrating a wide variation in familial lymphedema phenotypes (Reproduced and composited with permission from Evans et al.[2] [*left*], Irrthum et al.[10] [*middle right*], and Alders et al.[11] [*right*])

Table 3.1 List of lymphedema-associated syndromes and genes identified in hereditary lymphedema

OMIM listed and reference number	
LE–distichiasis	153400
Cholestasis–LE (Aagenaes) (CLS)	214900
LE-Hypoparathryoidism	247410
LE, microcephaly, chorioretinopathy	152950
LE, congenital recessive (Mucke)	247440
LE–ptosis	153000
Hennekam lymphangiectasia	235510
LE, cerebral arteriovenous anomaly	152900
Yellow nail syndrome	153300
LE, ASD, and facial changes	601927
OL-EDA-ID	300301
Noonan syndrome	163950
German syndrome	231080
Campomeilia, cumming type	211890
Fabry disease, variant	301500
Aarskog syndrome, variant	100050
Lissencephaly–cerebellar hypoplasia–LE	257320
Gonadal dysgenesis (GD, XY)	306100
Hydrops fetalis, idiopathic (Njolstadt)	236750
Chylous ascites, autosomal recessive	208300
Prolidase deficiency	170100
Intestinal lymphangiectasia	152800
NAGA deficiency (NAGA)	104170
Aplasia cutis congenita with IL	207731
Mullerian Derivatives – LA–polydactyly (Urioste syndrome)	235255
Pulmonary cystic lymphangiectasia	265300
CDG subtype (Jaeken)	602579
Nevo syndrome	601451
PEHO syndrome	260565
Hypotrichosis–LE–telangiectasia	607823
Tuberous sclerosis, variant	191100
Non-OMIM listed	
Posterior choanal atresia–LE (Sheikh)	
LE–leukaemia–deafness (Emberger) syndrome LE–cleft palate (Figueroa) syndrome	
Microcephaly – cutis verticisggyrata–LE	
Mandibulofacial dysostosis–LE syndrome	
Genes associated with hereditary cases of lymphedema and reference number	
CCBE1- collagen and calcium binding	
EGF-domain containing protein	235510
SOX18- SRY-Box	18 607823
HGF – Hepatocyte growth factor	142409
MET – Met protooncogene	164860
GJC2 – Gap junction protein-gamma2	608803
Chromosomal aberrancies and syndromes associated with lymphedema and reference number	
Turner syndrome (XO)	*many
Noonan syndrome	163950
Down syndrome (trisomy 21)	190685

Mutations in four different genes have been implicated in the origin of four distinct familial lymphedema–angiodysplasia (LE-AD) syndromes (Fig. 3.2). Within these syndromes not all members have the specific mutation, yet appear to share the same phenotype and typical inheritance. Some members of families with autosomal dominant Milroy disease show different mutations within the gene *FLT/VEGFR3* on chromosome 5q35.3.[14,15] VEGFR3 is a tyrosine growth factor receptor for members of the vascular endothelial growth factor family (VEGFC, VEGFD), and these pathways are important in lymphatic vessel growth and remodeling.[16] In autosomal dominant lymphedema–distichiasis (double row of eyelashes) with onset of peripheral lymphedema at puberty, mutations in *FOXC2*, a forkhead transcription factor, on chromosome 16q24.3, have now been consistently documented in more than 30 individuals.[17,18] More recently, one individual with the classic phenotype associated with lymphedema–distichiasis syndrome was found to have a duplicated 5′ region of the *FOXC2* gene, suggesting another mechanism in this pleiotrophic pathway leading to the characteristic phenotype.[19] Hennekam syndrome, an autosomal recessive disorder, characterized by lymphedema, lymphangiectasias, mental retardation, and unusual facies has been well described for years. Linkage analysis on three families with this syndrome has led to the identification of a chromosomal region 18q21.32 that contains the gene for *CCBE1*, the human ortholog of a gene essential for lymphangiogenesis in zebrafish.[11,20] Mutations in *SOX18*, a transcription factor located on chromosome 20q13, have been reported in association with both an autosomal recessive and autosomal dominant (or gonadal mosiacism) form of hypotrichosis–lymphedema–telangiectasia.[10]

The two most common and first described syndromes are Milroy and Meige syndrome. Milroy's (or Type I) is generally inherited in an autosomal dominant fashion and leads to a disabling and disfiguring swelling of the extremities. The usual onset is at birth, and the lymphedema is usually more severe in the lower extremities. There can be variation in this pattern both within and between families that have the same mutation, and some families/individuals have similar phenotypes with lack of mutation. The penetrance is reported to be 80%, and clearly there are many as yet unexplained environmental or biological factors involved.[21] Linkage analysis on large families identified the loci for the gene *FLT4* on chromosome 5q35.3, which encodes the VEGFR3 receptor, and since then several mutations in this gene have been described, all occurring in the tyrosine kinase domain of the VEFR3 receptor.[2,4,21-23] In a search for other possible candidates responsible for this phenotype, ligands for VEFGR3 were evaluated. Mutational screening of the gene that encodes VEGFC, a lymphatic directed endothelial growth factor, failed to identify any mutations in individuals with Milroy disease lacking a mutation in *FLT4*. Unlike other members of the vascular endothelial factor family (VEGFA, VEGFC, VEFGD), Vegfc is crucial for the proper development of the lymphatic system, as demonstrated in mice.[24]

Meige syndrome (or Type II), also inherited in an autosomal dominant-type fashion, presents later in life, usually at the time of puberty, tends to affect patients below the waist, and is not associated with a specific mutation.[25] Other syndromes also have pubertal type onset, but appear to have other specific associated abnormalities. For example, the lymphedema–distichiasis (LD) syndrome mentioned

above presents with later onset lymphedema and has the unique feature of distichiasis, which is a double row of eyelashes. Most patients with this syndrome have a
mutation in the gene for the transcription factor *FOXC2*, which is not seen in patients
with what appears classically to be Meige syndrome. Another syndrome, Yellow
Nail (YNS), can resemble Meige syndrome, with later onset lymphedema affecting
similar areas. However, patients with YNS have affected nails and often have respiratory involvement with chylothorax. YNS is now thought to be a more sporadic
rather than a dominantly inherited condition.[26]

The remaining syndromes with primary lymphedema reported in OMIM™ and
by Hennekam are less common and are frequently associated with other specific
phenotypic abnormalities often in multiple organ systems (Table 3.1). An extensive literature review of the original publications focusing on inheritance, clinical
information, and other reported phenotypic abnormalities in 36 of these syndromes was published by Northup et al. in the journal *Lymphology* in 2003. This
review identified nine syndromes with autosomal dominant inheritance, 21 syndromes with autosomal recessive inheritance, and six syndromes with X-linked
inheritance. The most commonly affected systems outside of the lymphatic system included the ocular system, dysmorphic facies, genitourinary and gastrointestinal systems, skeletal and growth abnormalities, vascular and hematological
disorders, immunological disorders, central nervous system, and dermatological
manifestations.[9] Identifying other abnormalities in other organ systems that appear
to segregate with primary lymphedema can help pinpoint possible defects in similar developmental pathways or pathways affected by similar environmental or epigenetic influences. The careful observation and reporting of associated dysmorphic
features can help better define phenotypes within the LE-AD syndromes.
Abnormalities in several organ systems are commonly reported, and with refined
research into these associated abnormalities, we can identify similar developmental pathways, events during embryogenesis, or perhaps environmental influences
explaining reduced penetrance or later onset. Examples of the types of systems
involved and frequencies are displayed in Fig. 3.3.

Chromosomal Aneuploidies and Sporadic Syndromes

Lymphedema-angiodysplasia syndromes span a wide spectrum of not only familial
disorders, but also those associated with chromosomal abnormalities or mutations
that are of sporadic origin (Table 3.1). Chromosomal aneuploidy (trisomy 13, 18,
21, and 22), Klinefelter XXY, and Turner syndrome (XO), all caused by abnormal
chromosomal division at conception, can be associated with an impaired lymphatic
system and clinical lymphedema. However, not all individuals are affected, and
some of these syndromes, such as Turner's, can improve with time, suggesting that
lymphatic development in utero might be under different influences than other lymphedema syndromes, which either stabilize or worsen over time. Other isolated
reports have implicated other chromosomes.

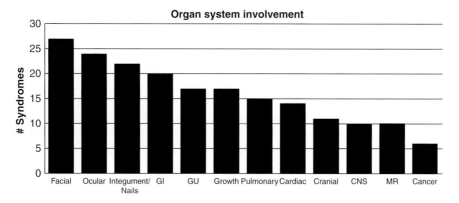

Fig. 3.3 Phenotypic abnormalities (organ system involvement) commonly associated with the 40 OMIM-listed hereditary LE-AD syndromes. *GI* gastrointestinal, *GU* genitalurinary, *MR* mental retardation (Reproduced with permission from Northup et al.[9])

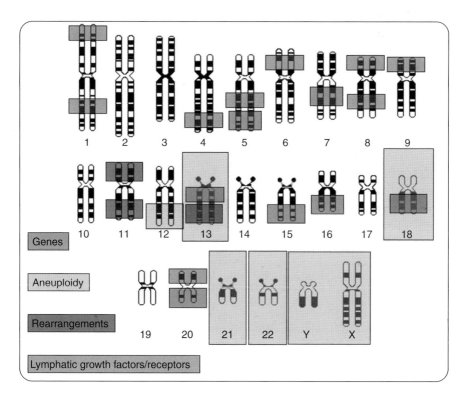

Fig. 3.4 Genomics–proteomics of lymphedema–angiodysplasia syndromes displayed on schematized human chromosomes (Modified with permission, Witte et al.[28])

Figure. 3.4 summarizes the location of documented or suspected candidate genes/ chromosomal abnormalities underlying LE-AD syndromes.

Conclusion

Despite major advances in the understanding of lymphangiogenesis since the first review article in 1997,[27] just prior to the discovery of VEGF-C, there are clearly still many unknown genes or epigenetic influences to be discovered. The high degree of variability and other compounding influences (both genetic with related pathways and environmental) make the ability to define a phenotype from any given genotype nearly impossible at this time. However, advances have been made when individuals or families with primary lymphedema are identified with an appropriate clinical work-up. Referral to a multi-disciplinary group that specializes in the genetics of lymphangiogenesis is an important part of that work-up. Detailed history taking and phenotypic evaluation of the patient and any or all related family members may be necessary to note other subtle findings. Tools such as high-resolution imaging and sophisticated molecular testing, as described above, will continue to provide critical data on the specific structural problem, pattern, and lymphatic dysfunction. Collaborations and timely and concise reporting of the findings from all areas of research are also imperative for advancement. With the rapid development of biological therapeutics, certainly restoration of altered pathways will become a viable possibility, although the obstacles to genetic information and molecular models in clinical applications will remain a formidable challenge.

Acknowledgments Arizona Disease Control Research Commission Contract #9002, I-103, NIH HL 71206, and the International Society of Lymphology.

References

1. Online Mendelian Inheritance in Man, OMIM (™). Johns Hopkins University, Baltimore, MD. MIM Number: World Wide Web URL: http://www.ncbi.nlm.nih.gov/omim
2. Evans AL, Brice G, Sotirova V, et al. Mapping of primary congenital lymphedema to the 5q35.3 region. *Am J Hum Genet.* 1999;64(2):547-555.
3. Witte MH, Erickson R, Bernas M, et al. Phenotypic and genotypic heterogeneity in familial Milroy lymphedema. *Lymphology.* 1998;31(4):145-155.
4. Karkkainen MJ, Ferrell RE, Lawrence EC, et al. Missense mutations interfere with VEGFR-3 signaling in primary lymphedema. *Nat Genet.* 2000;25(2):153-159.
5. McNeil GC, Witte MH, Witte CL, et al. Whole-body lymphangioscintigraphy: the preferred method for the initial assessment of the peripheral lymphatic system. *Radiology.* 1989;172: 495-502.
6. Bolinger A, Jager K, Sgier F, Seglias J. Fluorescence microlymphography. *Circulation.* 1981;64(6):1195-1200.
7. Case TC, Witte CL, Witte MH, Unger EC, Williams WH, et al. Magnetic resonance imaging in human lymphedema: comparison with lymphangioscintigraphy. *Magn Reson Imaging.* 1992;10:549-558.
8. Hennekam R. Syndromic lymphatic maldevelopment. In: Witte M, ed. *Conquering Lymphatic Disease: Setting the Research Agenda.* Tucson: University of Arizona; 2001:70-73.
9. Northup KA, Witte MH, Witte CL. Syndromic classification of hereditary lymphedema. *Lymphology.* 2003;36:162-189.

10. Irrthum A, Devriendt K, Chitayat D, et al. Mutations in the transcription factor gene SOX18 underlie recessive and dominant forms of hypotrichosis-lymphedema-telangiectasia. *Am J Hum Genet.* 2003;72(6):1470-1478.
11. Alders M, Hogan BM, Gjini E, et al. Mutations in CCBE1 cause generalized lymph vessel dysplasia in humans. *Nat Genet.* 2009;41(12):1272-1274.
12. Finegold DN, Schacht V, Kimak MA, et al. HGF and MET mutations in primary and secondary lymphedema. *Lymphat Res Biol.* 2008;6(2):65-68.
13. Ferrell RE, Baty CJ, Kimak MA, et al. GJC2 missense mutations cause human lymphedema. *Am J Hum Genet.* 2010;86:943-948.
14. Irrthum A, Karkkainen MJ, Devriendt K, Alitalo K, Vikkula M. Congenital hereditary lymphedema caused by a mutation that inactivates VEFGFR3 tyrosine kinase. *Am J Hum Genet.* 2000;67:295-301.
15. Connell FC, Ostergaard P, Carver C, et al. Analysis of the coding regions of VEGFR3 and VEGFC in Milroy disease and other primary lymphoedemas. *Hum Genet.* 2009;124(6): 625-631.
16. Lohela M, Saaristo A, Veikkola T, Alitalo K. Lymphangiogenic growth factors, receptors, and therapies. *Thromb Haemost.* 2003;90(2):167-184.
17. Fang J, Dagenais SL, Erickson RP. Mutations in FOXC2 (MFH-1), a forkhead family transcription factor, are responsible for the hereditary lymphedema-distichiasis syndrome. *Am J Hum Genet.* 2000;67:1382-1388.
18. Erickson RP, Dagenais SL, Caulder MS, et al. Clinical heterogeneity in lymphoedema-distichiasis with FOXC2 truncating mutations. *J Med Genet.* 2001;38(11):761-766.
19. Witte MH, Erickson RP, Khalil M, et al. Lymphedema-distichiasis syndrome without FOXC2 mutation: evidence for chromosome 16 duplication upstream of FOXC2. *Lymphology.* 2009;42:152-160.
20. Connell F, Kalidas K, Ostergaard P, et al. Linkage and sequence analysis indicate that *CCBE1* is mutated in recessively inherited generalised lymphatic dysplasia. *Hum Genet.* 2010;127: 231-241.
21. Ferrell RE, Levinson KD, Esman JH, et al. Hereditary lymphedema: evidence for linkage and genetic heterogeneity. *Hum Mol Genet.* 1998;7(13):2073-2078.
22. Evans AL, Bell R, Brice G, et al. Identification of eight novel VEFFR-3 mutations in families with primary lymphoedema. *J Med Genet.* 2003;40(9):697-703.
23. Spiegel R, Ghalamkarpour A, Daniel-Spiegel E, Vikkula M, Shalev SA. Wide clinical spectrum in a family with hereditary lymphedema type I due to a novel missense mutation in VEGFR3. *J Hum Genet.* 2006;51(10):846-850.
24. Karkkainen MJ, Haiko P, Sainio K, et al. Vascular endothelial growth factor C is required for sprouting of the first lymphatic vessels from embryonic veins. *Nat Immunol.* 2004;5(1): 74-80.
25. Meige H. Dystrophie oedemateuse hereditaire. *Presse Méd.* 1898;6:341-343.
26. Hoque SR, Mansour S, Mortimer PS. Yellow nail syndrome: not a genetic disorder? Eleven new cases and review of the literature. *Br J Dermatol.* 2007;156:1230-1234.
27. Witte MH, Way DL, Witte CL, Bernas M. Lymphangiogenesis: mechanisms, significance and clinical implications. In: Goldberg ID, Rosen EM, eds. *Regulation of Angiogenesis.* Basel: Birkhäuser Verlag; 1997:65-112.
28. Witte MH, Bernas M. Lymphatic pathophysiology. In: Cronenwett JL, Johnston KW, eds. *Rutherford's Vascular Surgery.* Philadelphia: W.B. Saunders Company; 2010:177-201.

Part II
Embryology, Anatomy, and Histology

Chapter 4
Embryology of the Lymphatic System and Lymphangiogenesis

Stanley G. Rockson

The lymphatic vasculature was first described by Aselli more than three centuries ago, and the hypothesized embryonic origin of the lymphatic structures was initially investigated in 1902[1]; nevertheless, it only has been recently, during the era of molecular biology, that the mechanisms of mammalian lymphatic development have become well understood.[2,3]

Long a subject of controversy, the developmental origin of the mammalian lymphatic system has been extensively explored over the last decade. Recent molecular and structural insights have helped to shed light on this complex and important topic, which also has distinct implications, not only for molecular therapeutics in lymphatic vascular disease, but also for the broad field of tumor biology.

As a component of the mammalian circulation, the vascular components of the lymphatic system, like all vascular structures, arise from aggregates of endothelial cells through the combined forces of vasculogenesis and angiogenesis (Fig. 4.1). The lymphatic vessels appear substantially later than the blood vascular structures.[4] In human embryos, this occurs at 6–7 weeks, nearly 1 month after the appearance of the first blood vessels.[5] The earliest identifiable lymphatic precursor in the embryo is the jugular lymph sac, a paired structure that can be found adjacent to the jugular section of the cardinal vein.

The origin of these lymph sacs and their relationship to the adjacent cardinal vein have, until recently, remained at the core of the theoretical controversy.[6] The "centrifugal" model, suggested by Florence Sabin, proposed that the primary lymph sacs arise from endothelial cells derived from the embryonic veins, with subsequent endothelial sprouting from the lymph sacs into the surrounding tissues and organs. The contrasting centripetal model of Huntington relies upon the contribution of mesenchymal precursor cells, termed lymphangioblasts, to give rise to the lymph sacs, a process that occurs independently of the veins.

S.G. Rockson
Division of Cardiovascular Medicine, Stanford University School of Medicine,
Falk Cardiovascular Research Center, Stanford, CA, USA

B.-B. Lee et al. (eds.), *Lymphedema*,
DOI 10.1007/978-0-85729-567-5_4, © Springer-Verlag London Limited 2011

Fig. 4.1 The embryonic development of the vasculatures originates from mesodermally-derived endothelial cell precursors, termed vasculogenesis. Subsequently, the developing vessels grow and remodel into a mature vascular network by endothelial sprouting and splitting, the process called angiogenesis. (Adapted from Oliver[15])

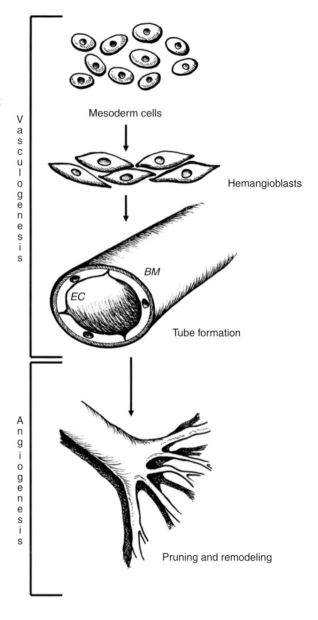

Mesoderm cells

Hemangioblasts

BM

EC

Tube formation

Pruning and remodeling

Although there are lines of evidence to support elements of both of these theories, it seems that the centrifugal model most closely predicts the process in higher mammals. Support for Sabin's centrifugal model was provided by studies in Prox1-deficient mice.[7,8] Prox1 is a homolog of the Drosophila homeobox transcription factor *prospero* 7, serving as a master regulator of lymphatic development. The venous origin of the mammalian lymphatic vasculature recently has been demonstrated by lineage-tracing experiments[9] and supported by studies in zebrafish.[10] However, in Xenopus frogs and avian species,

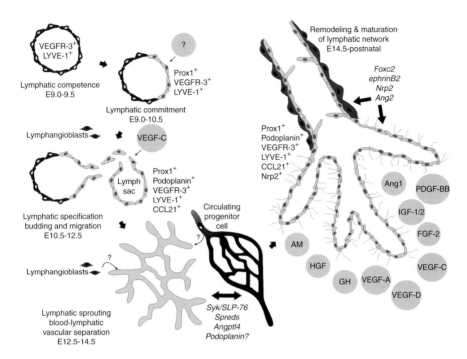

Fig. 4.2 Lymphatic vasculature development and growth. *AM* adrenomedullin; *Ang* angiopoietin; *Angptl* angiopoietin-like protein; *E* mouse embryonic day; *FGF* fibroblast growth factor; *GH* growth hormone; *HGF* hepatocyte growth factor; *IGF* insulin-like growth factor; *Nrp2* neuropilin-2; *PDGF* platelet-derived growth factor; *VEGF* vascular endothelial growth factor. (Reproduced with permission from Cueni and Detmar)[6]

parts of the lymphatic system seem to originate from local lymphangioblasts.[11-13] The potential contribution of lymphangioblasts to mammalian embryonic lymphangiogenesis remains conjectured, but unproven. Nevertheless, mesenchymal cells expressing CD31 and CD45, along with lymphatic endothelial markers (Prox1 and LYVE-1), have been observed in mouse embryos, suggesting that these cells might serve as lymph endothelial precursors.[14]

According to the current prevailing model, lymphatic vasculogenesis would occur in four identifiably distinct stages: lymphatic competence, commitment, specification, and vascular coalescence and maturation (Fig. 4.2).

Lymphatic competence is the capacity of cells to respond to the initial induction signal for lymphatic vascular differentiation.[15] The priming of lymphatic endothelial cells (LECs) to initiate lymphatic development is likely dependent on a form of molecular signaling that is distinct from that found in blood vascular development. LEC competence is recognized through cellular expression of lymphatic vessel endothelial hyaluronan receptor-1 (LYVE1)[7,16] and vascular endothelial growth factor receptor-3 (VEGFR3; also known as Flt-4).[17] Mouse embryos that lack VEGFR-3 die before lymphatics develop. Mouse embryos that lack VEGF-C do not develop lymph sacs.[18]

Lymphatic commitment is characterized developmentally and functionally by the expression of prospero-related homeobox 1 (Prox1). This is a nuclear transcription factor whose expression is exclusive to cells of committed lymphatic lineage.[7] Prox1 expression shifts commitment of venous endothelial cells from the default blood vascular fate to a lymphatic lineage.[8] The mechanism of this differential and ordered expression is still incompletely understood, although, most recently, both SOX18 and COUP-TFII have been identified as potential activators of Prox1 expression.[19-22] As the contributory expression pathways continue to be identified, it is clear that Prox1 is necessary and sufficient for lymphatic commitment. The molecular milieu in which Prox1 operates is still not well understood; neither the downstream initiating and regulatory factors nor the other upstream supplemental events have been entirely identified.

Lymphatic endothelial cell *specification* involves the expression of the distinguishing molecular markers that impose the unique lymphatic endothelial phenotype. As the cells attain a higher level of differentiation, additional lymphatic-specific markers are expressed, with concomitant suppression of blood vascular expression profiles.[8] Through these developmental steps, the committed lymphatic cell population establishes complete autonomy from the local venous microenvironment. Peripheral *migration* occurs. Budding and migration precede the formation of primary lymph sacs throughout the embryo. Secondary budding and migration mark the final stages of lymphatic development. The cells thus form capillaries in a centrifugal fashion, establishing the lymphatic vasculature throughout the bodily tissues and organs.[17]

An important event in lymphatic development is the necessary separation between the flow of blood and lymph. A tyrosine kinase, Syk, and an adapter protein, Slp-76, are critical for lymphatico-venous separation. Deficiency of either *Syk* or *Slp76* has been shown to create abnormal connections between blood vessels and lymphatics, with resultant blood-filled lymphatics and chylous hemorrhage.[23] Most recently, the mechanism of this process has been further elucidated: in the embryo, platelets aggregate at sites of lymphatico-venous connections, triggered by binding of LEC-specific podoplanin to C-type lectin receptor 2 (CLEC-2), which is specifically expressed in platelets; this leads to activation of Syk and Slp-76.[24,25]

After the appearance of the embryonic peripheral lymphatic vasculature, these vessels must experience substantial maturation and remodeling. One of the important maturational events is the development of the valve apparatus. A forkhead transcription factor, FOXC2, is highly expressed in adult lymphatic valves. It seems that FOXC2 specifies a collecting lymphatic vessel phenotype.[26,27]

The ephrins and the angiopoietins may also play a role in lymphatic vascular maturation. In mutant mice, faulty expression of ephrinB2 leads to hyperplasia of the collecting lymphatics, absent valve formation, and failure of lymphatic capillary remodeling[28] Angiopoietin 1 and 2 (Ang1 and Ang2) also participate in the maturation of the lymphatic vasculature.[29-31] In the lymphatics, Ang2 is a Tie2 receptor agonist, in contradistinction to its role in the blood vasculature.[29] Lymphatic valve development apparently also requires normal expression of integrin-alpha9 and deposition of its ligand, fibronectin-EIIIA, in the extracellular matrix.[32]

All of these developmental events are interrelated and complex. New molecular participants in the process continue to be identified. Although lymphangiogenesis is a critical pathway in embryonic development, it has a counterpart in wound healing and inflammation.[33,34] These molecular pathways may also have direct implications for future molecular therapeutics in lymphedema and other lymphatic vascular disorders.[3,35] These concepts are further explored in Chap. 16.

Acknowledgment   The author gratefully acknowledges Shauna Rockson for her artistic contribution to this chapter.

References

1. Kanter MA. The lymphatic system: an historical perspective. *Plast Reconstr Surg*. 1987; 79(1):131-139.
2. Nakamura K, Rockson SG. Biomarkers of lymphatic function and disease: state of the art and future directions. *Mol Diagn Ther*. 2007;11(4):227-238.
3. Nakamura K, Rockson SG. Molecular targets for therapeutic lymphangiogenesis in lymphatic dysfunction and disease. *Lymphat Res Biol*. 2008;6(3–4):181-189.
4. Witte MH, Jones K, Wilting J, et al. Structure function relationships in the lymphatic system and implications for cancer biology. *Cancer Metastasis Rev*. 2006;25(2):159-184.
5. van der Putte S. The development of the lymphatic system in man. *Adv Anat Embryol Cell Biol*. 1975;51:3-60.
6. Cueni LN, Detmar M. The lymphatic system in health and disease. *Lymphat Res Biol*. 2008;6(3–4):109-122.
7. Wigle JT, Oliver G. Prox1 function is required for the development of the murine lymphatic system. *Cell*. 1999;98(6):769-778.
8. Wigle JT, Harvey N, Detmar M, et al. An essential role for Prox1 in the induction of the lymphatic endothelial cell phenotype. *EMBO J*. 2002;21(7):1505-1513.
9. Srinivasan RS, Dillard ME, Lagutin OV, et al. Lineage tracing demonstrates the venous origin of the mammalian lymphatic vasculature. *Genes Dev*. 2007;21(19):2422-2432.
10. Yaniv K, Isogai S, Castranova D, Dye L, Hitomi J, Weinstein BM. Live imaging of lymphatic development in the zebrafish. *Nat Med*. 2006;12(6):711-716.
11. Schneider M, Othman-Hassan K, Christ B, Wilting J. Lymphangioblasts in the avian wing bud. *Dev Dyn*. 1999;216(4–5):311-319.
12. Wilting J, Aref Y, Huang R, et al. Dual origin of avian lymphatics. *Dev Biol*. 2006;292(1):165-173.
13. Ny A, Koch M, Schneider M, et al. A genetic Xenopus laevis tadpole model to study lymphangiogenesis. *Nat Med*. 2005;11(9):998-1004.
14. Buttler K, Kreysing A, von Kaisenberg CS, et al. Mesenchymal cells with leukocyte and lymphendothelial characteristics in murine embryos. *Dev Dyn*. 2006;235(6):1554-1562.
15. Oliver G. Lymphatic vasculature development. *Nat Rev Immunol*. 2004;4(1):35-45.
16. Veikkola T, Karkkainen M, Claesson-Welsh L, Alitalo K. Regulation of angiogenesis via vascular endothelial growth factor receptors. *Cancer Res*. 2000;60(2):203-212.
17. Cueni LN, Detmar M. New insights into the molecular control of the lymphatic vascular system and its role in disease. *J Invest Dermatol*. 2006;126(10):2167-2177.
18. Karkkainen MJ, Haiko P, Sainio K, et al. Vascular endothelial growth factor C is required for sprouting of the first lymphatic vessels from embryonic veins. *Nat Immunol*. 2004;5(1): 74-80.
19. Francois M, Caprini A, Hosking B, et al. Sox18 induces development of the lymphatic vasculature in mice. *Nature*. 2008;456(7222):643-647.

20. Yamazaki T, Yoshimatsu Y, Morishita Y, Miyazono K, Watabe T. COUP-TFII regulates the functions of Prox1 in lymphatic endothelial cells through direct interaction. *Genes Cells.* 2009;14(3):425-434.
21. Lee S, Kang J, Yoo J, et al. Prox1 physically and functionally interacts with COUP-TFII to specify lymphatic endothelial cell fate. *Blood.* 2009;113(8):1856-1859.
22. Srinivasan RS, Geng X, Yang Y, et al. The nuclear hormone receptor Coup-TFII is required for the initiation and early maintenance of Prox1 expression in lymphatic endothelial cells. *Genes Dev.* 2010;24(7):696-707.
23. Abtahian F, Guerriero A, Sebzda E, et al. Regulation of blood and lymphatic vascular separation by signaling proteins SLP-76 and Syk. *Science.* 2003;299(5604):247-251.
24. Bertozzi CC, Hess PR, Kahn ML. Platelets: covert regulators of lymphatic development. *Arterioscler Thromb Vasc Biol.* 2010;30(12):2368-2371.
25. Bertozzi CC, Schmaier AA, Mericko P, et al. Platelets regulate lymphatic vascular development through CLEC-2-SLP-76 signaling. *Blood.* 2010;116(4):661-670.
26. Petrova TV, Karpanen T, Norrmen C, et al. Defective valves and abnormal mural cell recruitment underlie lymphatic vascular failure in lymphedema distichiasis. *Nat Med.* 2004;10(9):974-981.
27. Norrmen C, Ivanov KI, Cheng J, et al. FOXC2 controls formation and maturation of lymphatic collecting vessels through cooperation with NFATc1. *J Cell Biol.* 2009;185(3):439-457.
28. Makinen T, Adams RH, Bailey J, et al. PDZ interaction site in ephrinB2 is required for the remodeling of lymphatic vasculature. *Genes Dev.* 2005;19(3):397-410.
29. Gale N, Thurston G, Hackett S, et al. Angiopoietin-2 is required for postnatal angiogenesis and lymphatic patterning, and only the latter role is rescued by angiopoietin-1. *Dev Cell.* 2002; 3:411-423.
30. Shimoda H, Bernas MJ, Witte MH, Gale NW, Yancopoulos GD, Kato S. Abnormal recruitment of periendothelial cells to lymphatic capillaries in digestive organs of angiopoietin-2-deficient mice. *Cell Tissue Res.* 2007;328(2):329-337.
31. Dellinger M, Hunter R, Bernas M, et al. Defective remodeling and maturation of the lymphatic vasculature in Angiopoietin-2 deficient mice. *Dev Biol.* 2008;319(2):309-320.
32. Bazigou E, Xie S, Chen C, et al. Integrin-alpha9 is required for fibronectin matrix assembly during lymphatic valve morphogenesis. *Dev Cell.* 2009;17(2):175-186.
33. Saaristo A, Tammela T, Farkkila A, et al. Vascular endothelial growth factor-C accelerates diabetic wound healing. *Am J Pathol.* 2006;169(3):1080-1087.
34. Karpanen T, Alitalo K. Molecular biology and pathology of lymphangiogenesis. *Annu Rev Pathol.* 2008;3:367-397.
35. An A, Rockson SG. The potential for molecular treatment strategies in lymphatic disease. *Lymphat Res Biol.* 2004;2(4):173-181.

Chapter 5
Anatomy of the Lymphatic System and Its Disorders

Waldemar L. Olszewski

Definition of the Lymphatic System

Anatomical

The lymphatic system is a bodily complex composed of interstitial space, body cavities, and lymphatics (all of which form the lymphatic space), containing tissue fluid and lymph, migrating immune cells, and organized lymphoid tissue (Fig. 5.1). The total mass comprising extracellular fluid, lymph and lymphoid cells is estimated to be 13 kg. The cell mass alone approximates 1 kg,[1] Lymph nodes and lymphoid cell aggregates, identified as lamina propria and Peyer's patches in the intestine, contain the main aggregates of the recirculating lymphocytes.The lymphoid organs (thymus, spleen and bone marrow) are contained within the blood system and have no lymphatic drainage; however, their cells circulate in the loop of blood–tissue–space–lymphatics–lymphoid tissue–blood. In this sense, they belong to the lymphatic system.[2–4]

Functional

The lymphatic system (a) secures the chemical environment of the tissues, regulating water volume and stabilizing tissue fluid proteins at physiological concentrations; (b) maintains a normal supply of nutrients and removal of waste products from paren-chymatous cells; (c) serves as a reservoir that accumulates surplus tissue fluid under conditions of lymph flow obstruction or excessive lymph production; (d) regulates

W.L. Olszewski
Department of Surgical Research and Transplantology,
Medical Research Centre, Warsaw, Poland

B.-B. Lee et al. (eds.), *Lymphedema*,
DOI 10.1007/978-0-85729-567-5_5, © Springer-Verlag London Limited 2011

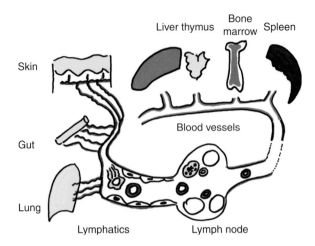

Fig. 5.1 Schematic presentation of the lymphatic system. Skin, gut, and lungs are naturally exposed to the environment and have the highest density of lymphatics draining to the regional lymph nodes. Any environmental antigen that penetrates the epithelial layer of these organs is immediately recognized by local dendritic cells and transported with tissue fluid and the lymph stream to the nodes. Organs such as the thymus, spleen, bone marrow, and even the liver supply the lymph nodes with immune cells. Some of these cells re-circulate among blood–tissues–lymphatics–lymph nodes in the process of immune surveillance. The antigen-laden Langerhans' (veiled) cells and lymphocytes are seen in afferent lymphatics. In the nodes, the antigens stimulate a complex cellular response based on cooperation between various cellular subsets. Moreover, a continuous process of filtration (extravasation) of plasma nutritive and immune proteins takes place in the interstitium. They flow toward the lymphatics. Some proteins are synthesized and secreted by local parenchymatous and migrating cells. In skin, these are keratinocytes and resident immune cells, in the gut, epithelial cells and lymphocytes, and in the lamina propria and in the lung, epithelial cells, and macrophages

the process of recirculation of lymphocytes that survey the integrity of tissue; (e) recognizes microbial antigens through pathogen-associated molecular pattern by immune (dendritic cells, tissue macrophages) and endothelial cells that migrate through the lymph; (f) participates in tumor antigen recognition, active transport of tumor cells to lymph nodes, either eliminating tumor cells or assisting them to proliferate, creating tolerance to tumors; (g) eliminates the host senescent disintegrated cells and cellular debris as well as cellular chemical components from traumatized tissues. Recognition of auto-antigens is achieved through the debris-associated molecular pattern by immune cells contained in lymph.

Lymph Flow Pathways

Lymphatics are found throughout the body, with the exception of the central nervous system (Fig. 5.2). The interstitial space and lymph vessel space form a common "lymph space." The initial lymph spaces are mere intercellular expanses within the

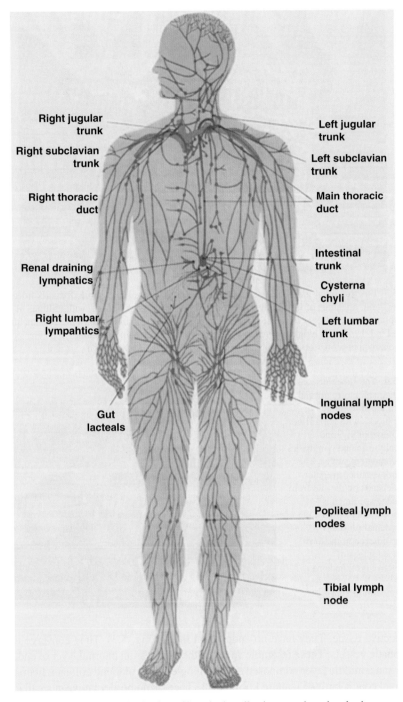

Fig. 5.2 General view of the distribution of lymphatic collecting vessels and nodes in man

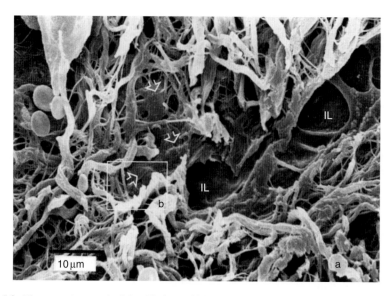

Fig. 5.3 Electron micrograph of the skin interstitial space. There is a network of matrix fibers, and among them, openings of the initial lymphatics (IL). The interstitial space, with millions of small inter-fiber spaces, is freely connected with the initial lymphatics. This allows a free plasma filtrate–tissue fluid flow to the lymphatic vessel system. Endothelial cells in the initial lymphatics possess chemoattractant properties directing immune cell traffic to their lumina

Fig. 5.4 The subepidermal lymphatic plexus in normal lower limb skin stained in tissue blocks with Paris Blue. Note horizontally- and vertically-oriented lymphatics with competent valves. The network is rather irregular. This depends on the site from which the specimen is harvested. Interestingly, the subepidemal plexus is preserved even in the most advanced stages of obstructive lymphedema

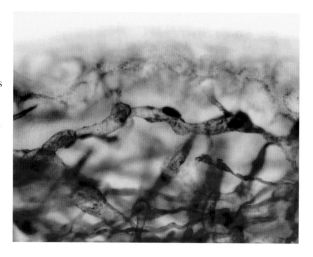

connective tissue. They have no endothelial lining (Fig. 5.3). They converge to the lymphatic vessels. These resemble veins, as they possess an internal layer of endothelium and a middle layer composed of intermingled muscular and collagen fibers. The external coat is built of scattered fibroblasts. There is no border between small (100–500 µ) lymphatics and the surrounding connective tissue. Lymphatics have numerous endothelial unidirectional valves (Fig. 5.4). They divide and anastomose very

Fig. 5.5 Histological
specimen of calf skin with a
lymphatic vessel located in
the dermis, stained for
LYVE1 antigen, specific for
lymphatic endothelial cells.
This vessel is intermediate
between the subepidermal
plexus and collecting trunks.
Close to the lymphatic is a
blood capillary, which is
LYVE1-negative, x 600

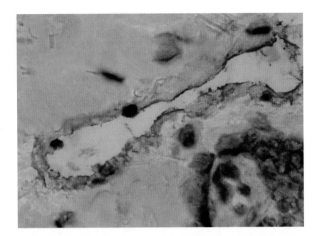

Fig. 5.6 Histological picture
of a normal calf lymphatic
collecting trunk. Note lining
with endothelial cells and
multiple irregularly
distributed muscle cells and
collagen fibers. The irregular
shape of the lumen occurs
because empty lymphatics
collapse under in vivo
conditions. Collecting
lymphatics of the lower leg
usually contain more muscle
fibers than those of the upper
limbs. They contract
rhythmically and propel
lymph centripetally. H&E
stain, x 200

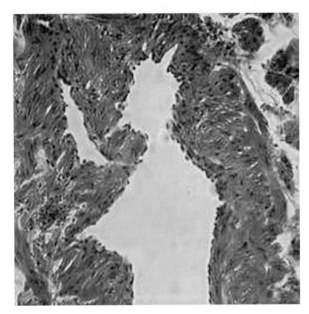

freely, and form a network depending on the local density of connective tissue. The
initial-to-interconnecting dermal lymphatics have LYVE1-positive endothelial cells
(Fig. 5.5). Lymph vessels that are approaching a lymph node are called afferent,
while those leaving are the efferent lymphatics (Fig. 5.6). They are LYVE1-negative.
Each lymph node is supplied with afferent lymph that flows through its vast sinuses
toward the hilum and the efferent vessels (Fig. 5.7). In the intestine, lymphatics are
called lacteals. They begin in the lymphatic spaces in the villi and end up in mesenteric nodes. The efferent vessels merge with the retroperitoneal cysterna chyli. This
is an irregular structure that receives lymph not only from the gut but also from the
liver, the pancreas and the stomach. Its continuation is the main thoracic duct, joining

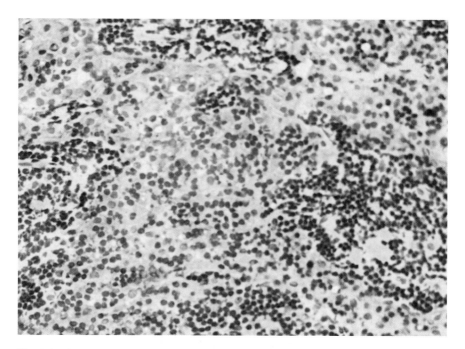

Fig. 5.7 Histological appearance of an inguinal lymph node. Lymphatic endothelial cells in para-cortical sinuses stain red. The sinuses are filled with migrating lymphocyte and large cells, such as Langerhans' and macrophage-like cells. Lymph delivered to the node through afferent lymphatics flows along sinuses to the efferent lymphatics. Note that sinuses cover a large area of the node cross-section. In pathological conditions of long duration, the lymph nodes become fibrotic and sinuses become obstructed. LYVE1 antigen stain, x200

the venous angle where lymph flows to the blood circulation. Lung lymphatics drain into bronchial nodes and further to the right thoracic duct. Lower limb lymphatics are divided into the superficial and deep lymph vasculature. The superficial vessels lead to the inguinal nodes, whereas the deep vessels run along large blood vessels to the deep inguinal nodes. In their transit, they traverse one or two popliteal nodes. Moving cephalad, there are iliac lymphatics that join the distal part of cysterna chyli. Upper limb lymphatics run to the axillary lymph nodes. The exact position of the various groups of nodes is very important from a medical point of view. Damage to the lymphatics and nodes with subsequent obstruction of lymph flow brings about dysfunction of the organ distal to the obstruction. With the passage of time, bacterial colonization, immune cell infiltration and, ultimately, fibrosis develop.

Functional Classification of the Lymphatic Pathways

The lymphatics most commonly affected by noxious factors are those of skin, gut, and lung. These vessels become damaged by infections, trauma, and surgery. The effect is tissue fluid stasis in the interstitial space and stasis of lymph in afferent lymphatics. The levels at which the lymphatic pathways are damaged by noxious factors are: (a) the subepidermal plexus, (b) dermal lymphatics, (c) collecting trunks, and (d) lymph node sinuses. The histological appearance at these sites is depicted in Figs. 5.3, 5.4, 5.5, and 5.6. This classification is important for rational therapy.

Skin and Subcutaneous Tissue

The subepidermal and dermal lymphatics directly participate in soft tissue infections and mechanical injury. (a) The most resistant to the impact of pathological factors are the subepidermal vessels. High plasma filtration rate and lymph formation in the dermal papillae presumably keep these minute vessels open, sometimes forming epidermal vesicles. (b) The collecting trunks become dilated during the acute and chronic phases of skin inflammation and after trauma of soft tissues and bones. With the passage of time, they lose spontaneous contractility and their lumina become obliterated by fibrous elements. (c) Chronic inflammation of soft tissues is reflected by a reaction in lymph nodes. They become depleted of lymphoid cells and replaced by fibrous tissue. Radiotherapy is another factor that damages lymph node structure. The fibrotic lymph nodes are an obstacle to lymph flow (see the chapter on excisional surgery). (d) Following surgical removal of lymph nodes and irradiation (upper and lower limb), the afferent lymphatics gradually become obliterated through their entire length (the die-back phenomenon).

Gut Lymphatics

Inflammatory processes in the gut bring about: (a) Dilatation of vessels and enlargement of mesenteric lymph nodes in the early stages, and (b) Fibrosis of vessels and nodes in the late stages. Intestinal lymph exudes through gut serosa to the peritoneal cavity (chyloperitoneum) (c) Inflammation and mechanical injury may damage the cysterna chili and the thoracic duct. Lack of outflow of the gut lymph to the venous system leads to dilatation of retroperitoneal lymphatics and backflow to the genitals and lower limbs.

Lung Lymphatics

The lung lymphatic system is difficult to evaluate clinically. Histopathologically, fibrosis of lymphatics and bronchial nodes is reported in chronic inflammatory conditions.

References

1. Trepel F. Number and distribution of lymphocytes in man. A critical analysis. *Klin Wschr.* 1974;52:511.
2. Sobotta atlas of human anatomy; head, neck, upper limb, thorax, abdomen, pelvis, lower limb. 14th ed. One volume ed. Ed. by R. Putz and R. Pabst. Elsevier Urban & Fischer. 2009
3. Kubik S. *Atlas of the Lymphatics of the Lower Limbs*. Paris: Servier; 2000.
4. Olszewski WL. *Lymph stasis: pathophysiology, diagnosis and and treatment*. Boca Raton: CRC Press; 1991:3.

Part III
Physiology, Pathophysiology, and Lymphodynamics

Chapter 6
Physiology, Pathophysiology, and Lymphodynamics: General Overview

Stanley G. Rockson

The lymphatic system is a component of both the circulatory and the immune systems. The principal functions of this system include the prevention of edema and maintenance of interstitial fluid homeostasis, immune traffic (transportation of white blood cells and antigen-presenting cells to the lymphoid organs), and lipid absorption from the gastrointestinal tract.[1]

Not surprisingly, this system requires a complex intersection of specific anatomy and physiological function to accomplish these goals. Lymphatics are found throughout the body, with the exception of the central nervous system, in which cerebrospinal fluid fulfills the normal role of lymph. Lymphatic vasculature and lymphoid tissue are prevalent in organs that come into direct contact with the external environment, such as the skin, gastrointestinal tract, and lungs.[2] This distribution likely reflects the protective role of the lymphatics against infectious agents and alien particles. Absorption of fat from the intestine occurs through the lymphatic system, which transports the lipids (chyle) to the liver. The lymphatic system also transports cellular debris, metabolic waste products, and excess fluid (edema safety factor) from local sites back to the systemic circulation.

In the extremities, the lymphatic system consists of a superficial (epifascial) system that collects lymph from the skin and subcutaneous tissue, and a deeper system that drains subfascial structures, such as muscle, bone, and deep blood vessels. The superficial and deep systems of the lower extremities merge within the pelvis, whereas those of the upper extremity merge in the axilla. The two drainage systems function in an interdependent fashion, such that the deep lymphatic system participates in lymph transport from the skin during lymphatic obstruction.[3]

Lymphatic capillaries are lined by a single layer of overlapping endothelial cells with a discontinuous basement membrane.[4] These vascular structures, which lack

S.G. Rockson
Division of Cardiovascular Medicine, Stanford University
School of Medicine, Falk Cardiovascular Research Center,
Stanford, CA, USA

B.-B. Lee et al. (eds.), *Lymphedema*,
DOI 10.1007/978-0-85729-567-5_6, © Springer-Verlag London Limited 2011

either pericytes or smooth muscle cell coverage, begin as blind-ended tubes that interface with the interstitium. Tissue fluid can enter these initial lymphatic vessels between discontinuous button-like cell junctions.[5]

Interendothelial openings may allow cells (macrophages, lymphocytes, erythrocytes) and cellular debris to directly enter lymphatics.[6,7] Fluid transport into the initial lymphatics apparently occurs against a pressure gradient. It is believed that episodic increases in interstitial fluid pressure are created through tissue movement; this combines with suction forces generated through the contraction of the collecting lymphatics.[8]

The lymphatic capillary structures coalesce into progressively larger collecting lymphatic vessels and, ultimately, the cisterna chyli and thoracic duct. Lymph returns to the blood circulation through lymphaticovenous anastomoses. Since the lymphatics lack a central pump, lymph progresses through the concerted effects of respiratory motions, skeletal muscle contraction, and the autocontractility of the mural smooth muscle of the vasculature itself. In skeletal muscle, lymphatics are usually paired with arterioles, so that arterial pulsation can also contribute to the periodic expansion and compression of initial lymphatics to enhance fluid uptake.[9]

Lymph flow in the collectors depends predominantly on lymphatic contraction. The rate of lymph transport can be augmented substantially by humoral and physical factors that influence the rhythm and amplitude of spontaneous contractions. Lymph flow and lymphatic contractility increase in response to tissue edema, hydrostatic pressure (standing position), mechanical stimulation, and exercise.[2]

Failure of adequate lymph transport promotes lymphedema and likely contributes to the pathological presentation of a wide variety of lymphatic vascular diseases. Accordingly, a detailed understanding of lymphatic anatomy, physiology, and dynamics will certainly contribute to an informed response to diagnosis and therapeutic intervention. Similarly, a detailed understanding of normal lymphatic development should allow us to address pathological lymphatic conditions that lead to inflammation, autoimmunity, cancer, and other forms of human disease.[1]

References

1. Oliver G. Lymphatic vasculature development. *Nat Rev Immunol.* 2004;4(1):35-45.
2. Szuba A, Shin WS, Strauss HW, Rockson S. The third circulation: radionuclide lymphoscintigraphy in the evaluation of lymphedema. *J Nucl Med.* 2003;44(1):43-57.
3. Brautigam P, Foldi E, Schaiper I, Krause T, Vanscheidt W, Moser E. Analysis of lymphatic drainage in various forms of leg edema using two compartment lymphoscintigraphy. *Lymphology.* 1998;31(2):43-55.
4. Cueni LN, Detmar M. The lymphatic system in health and disease. *Lymphat Res Biol.* 2008; 6(3-4):109-22.
5. Baluk P, Fuxe J, Hashizume H, et al. Functionally specialized junctions between endothelial cells of lymphatic vessels. *J Exp Med.* 2007;204(10):2349-62.
6. Ikomi F, Hanna GK, Schmid-Schonbein GW. Mechanism of colloidal particle uptake into the lymphatic system: basic study with percutaneous lymphography. *Radiology.* 1995;196(1):107-13.

7. Higuchi M, Fokin A, Masters TN, Robicsek F, Schmid-Schonbein GW. Transport of colloidal particles in lymphatics and vasculature after subcutaneous injection. *J Appl Physiol.* 1999; 86(4):1381-7.
8. Reddy NP, Patel K. A mathematical model of flow through the terminal lymphatics. *Med Eng Phys.* 1995;17(2):134-40.
9. Schmid-Schonbein GW. Microlymphatics and lymph flow. *Physiol Rev.* 1990;70(4):987-1028.

Chapter 7
Lymphodynamics

Stanley G. Rockson

As a tributary of the arteriovenous blood circulation, the lymphatic vasculature plays an exquisite, finely modulated role in the regulation of body fluid homeostasis and interstitial fluid balance. It is estimated that approximately one-sixth of the body's total volume resides in the interstitium (the spaces between cells).[1]

Accordingly, the lymphatic circulation is responsible for unidirectional fluid transport, moving protein-enriched fluid from the interstitium through a complex vascular network that converges upon the thoracic duct(s) and, ultimately, the great veins.[2]

Given the near inaccessibility of the lymphatic vasculature to direct visualization or instrumentation, it is not surprising that insight into the dynamics of this vascular system has been slow to accrue. Nevertheless, substantial strides have been made, particularly in the last 20 years.

Interstitial fluid becomes lymph once it enters the terminal lymphatics. The protein content of lymph is determined by the parenchyma of its origin. In most of the body's tissues, interstitial fluid protein concentration approximates 2 g/dl, but mesenteric lymph protein content approaches 3–4 g/dl and that of the liver is even higher. Accordingly, lymph derived from the thoracic duct reflects the contributions of these various elements, and approximates concentrations of 3–5 g/dl.

At rest, it is estimated that there are 2–3 l/day of lymph formed in the human body. Thus, it is apparent that, in the absence of intact lymphatic transport mechanisms, circulatory collapse would occur in little more than a single day.

Entry of interstitial fluid into the lymphatic capillary is governed chiefly by prevailing interstitial fluid pressure. Under steady-state conditions, the interstitial fluid pressure is typically subatmospheric.[3] If the pressure declines below the normal value of −6 mmHg, lymph flow becomes negligible. At the other end of the

S.G. Rockson
Division of Cardiovascular Medicine, Stanford University School of Medicine,
Falk Cardiovascular Research Center, Stanford, CA, USA

B.-B. Lee et al. (eds.), *Lymphedema*,
DOI 10.1007/978-0-85729-567-5_7, © Springer-Verlag London Limited 2011

spectrum, any physical force that increases interstitial fluid pressure will increase lymph flow. Such factors chiefly reflect the influence of Starling forces, such that increased capillary hydrostatic pressure, decreased plasma oncotic pressure, and increased interstitial oncotic pressure, along with increased capillary permeability can all result in an increase in tissue lymph production. Lymph flow becomes maximal when interstitial pressure is slightly higher than the atmospheric pressure. Nevertheless, paradoxically, the prevailing pressure gradients do not seem to favor fluid entry into the terminal lymphatics.[2] It is conjectured, based upon available evidence, that cyclical changes in prevailing pressure gradients create transient forces that favor fluid entry.[4-6]

Beyond hydrodynamics, in order to drive fluid transport through the vasculature, the lymphatic circulation relies upon the effects of both intrinsic[7] and extrinsic pumps. The latter effect arises through cyclical lymphatic compression and expansion, through the operation of extrinsic tissue forces.[2] Extrinsic forces can include movement of parts of the body, contraction of skeletal musculature, arterial pulsation, and tissue compression by extrinsic forces.

Historically, the effect of physical activity on lymph flow was deduced from direct measurements after direct thoracic duct cannulation but, previously, there have been no studies of thoracic duct flow as a function of exercise intensity. It has now become feasible to surgically instrument the canine thoracic lymph duct with ultrasonic flow transducers and, after surgical recovery, to determine the effect of exercise intensity.[8]

Growing insights such as these are necessary in order to envision our full ability, in future, to harness the forces of lymphatic physiology for enhanced lymphatic imaging, diagnostics, and therapeutics.

References

1. Hall J. *Guyton and Hall Textbook of Medical Physiology.* 12th ed. Philadelphia: Saunders; 2010.
2. Zawieja DC. Contractile physiology of lymphatics. *Lymphat Res Biol.* 2009;7(2):87-96.
3. Aukland K, Reed RK. Interstitial-lymphatic mechanisms in the control of extracellular fluid volume. *Physiol Rev.* 1993;73(1):1-78.
4. Negrini D, Moriondo A, Mukenge S. Transmural pressure during cardiogenic oscillations in rodent diaphragmatic lymphatic vessels. *Lymphat Res Biol.* 2004;2(2):69-81.
5. Moriondo A, Mukenge S, Negrini D. Transmural pressure in rat initial subpleural lymphatics during spontaneous or mechanical ventilation. *Am J Physiol Heart Circ Physiol.* 2005;289(1): H263-9.
6. Grimaldi A, Moriondo A, Sciacca L, Guidali ML, Tettamanti G, Negrini D. Functional arrangement of rat diaphragmatic initial lymphatic network. *Am J Physiol Heart Circ Physiol.* 2006;291(2):H876-85.
7. Olszewski WL, Engeset A. Intrinsic contractility of prenodal lymph vessels and lymph flow in human leg. *Am J Physiol.* 1980;239(6):H775-83.
8. Desai P, Williams AG Jr, Prajapati P, Downey HF. Lymph flow in instrumented dogs varies with exercise intensity. *Lymphat Res Biol.* 2010;8(3):143-8.

Chapter 8
Physiology, Biology, and Lymph Biochemistry

Waldemar L. Olszewski

Tissue Fluid

Tissue fluid is the basic fluid forming lymph. It is the capillary filtrate derived from plasma by diffusion, filtration, and vesicular transport mixed with the preexisting mobile intercellular fluid, containing local cell-produced proteins. It contains all the protein fractions of plasma, but at lower levels. Because of the sieving mechanism that occurs during transport of macromolecules across the capillary wall, the percentage of the total protein that is contributed by the small molecular weight proteins tends to be greater than that in serum. There is still a lack of evidence that, in the steady state, the protein concentration in afferent prenodal lymph differs from that of interstitial fluid. Most authors assume that the lymph protein concentration is identical to that in the interstitium. This applies to both normal and lymphedema conditions.

Tissue fluid proteins under normal conditions and in obstructive lymphedema

Normal mobile tissue fluid is difficult to obtain because of its miniscule volumes. Its mean total protein concentration ranges from 0.5 to 3.5 g%. In lymphedema there is an excess of fluid and large volumes can be collected, allowing changes in protein level to ensue because of the functional changes in the limb. The mean total protein concentration is 2.3 g%, tissue fluid/serum (TF/S) 0.25; of immunoglobulin (Ig) G 0.65 g%, TF/S 0.47, and of C-reactive protein 0.6 mg/L, TF/S 1.2.

W.L. Olszewski
Department of Surgical Research and Transplantology,
Medical Research Centre, Warsaw, Poland

B.-B. Lee et al. (eds.), *Lymphedema*,
DOI 10.1007/978-0-85729-567-5_8, © Springer-Verlag London Limited 2011

Lymph

Physiological Observations

Limb lymph protein concentration undergoes continuous changes depending on the capillary filtration rate. This in turn depends on the capillary hydrostatic pressure, which changes at various body positions, and the metabolic rate of tissues (muscular activity, temperature) increasing the number of dilated capillaries (increase in filtration surface area; Fig. 8.1). The concentration of lymph in individual proteins is inversely proportional to their molecular weight and molecule radius. The larger the molecule the less of it in lymph (molecular sieving mechanism).[1-7]

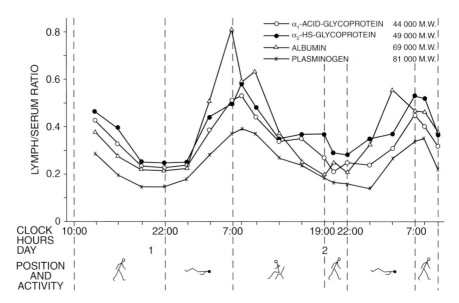

Fig. 8.1 Fluctuation of lymph protein level in the soft tissues of a normal human calf during normal limb activity, expressed as a lymph to serum ratio (L/S). A calf superficial lymphatic was cannulated and lymph was collected over days and nights in various limb physical positions. Lying, standing up, and contracting calf muscles changed the physical conditions for lymph formation, which were expressed at different flow/concentration levels. High venous capillary pressure in an upright position enhanced tissue fluid and lymph formation and subsequently more water with less protein transport, whereas the horizontal position with low capillary pressure acted in an opposite direction. Additionally, the concentrations differed depending on the molecular weight and size of a given protein (see peak levels). The small acid glycoprotein was transported faster than the large IgM. The tissue fluid and afferent lymph protein concentrations change, in contrast to the flowing plasma, from minute to minute in various tissue regions, depending on the actual blood capillary filtration rate (depending on intracapillary hydrostatic and oncotic pressures and filtration surface area), local cell metabolism, the contractility of the lymphangions, and active lymph transport, as well as extrinsic forces propelling lymph (striated muscle contractions)

The mean concentration and lymph to serum ratio (L/S) of some immune proteins in normal lymph, estimated in 24-h collected samples, are listed below. Total protein: 3.5 g% (0.5 during fast walking and 3.8 during night rest), L/S 0.39, and albumin 1.7–3.2 g%, L/S 0.13–0.48. Individual proteins arranged in order of increasing molecular weight reach the following levels: alpha-1-glycoprotein 0.22 g%, L/S 0.45; prealbumin 0.12 g%, L/S 0.35; haptoglobin 0.15 g%, L/S 0.17; beta-lipoprotein 1.11 g%, L/S 0.2; IgM 0.23 g% L/S 0.08. Complement components: C3 0.191 g%, L/S 0.21, and C1q 0.034, L/S 0.15. Cytokines: TNFbeta 12 mg/ml, L/S 1.0; IL1 beta 3.9 pg/ml, L/S 1.4; IL6 8 pg/ml, L/S 1.4; VEGF C 262 pg/ml, L/S 1.1.

Mobile tissue fluid and lymph protein concentration is low and oscillates between 10 and 50% of that of plasma. Admixture of locally synthetized proteins, like cytokines, raises their level to that above plasma with an L/S ratio above 1.0. Protein concentration may be different in different regions of the limb soft tissues because of the local capillary filtration and metabolic rate.

Proteins in Obstructive Lymphedema

Our data are: mean total protein 1.7 g%, L/S 0.25; IgG 350 mg%, L/S 0.28, IgM 23 mg%, L/S 0.1.[8-13]

Generally, tissue fluid and lymph total protein concentration in lymphedema is low. Moreover, there are no statistically significant differences in protein and cytokine concentrations in tissue and fluid lymph between lymphedema and normal samples. This contradicts the anecdotal notion of protein-rich edema. Our studies are the first to be carried out in humans, clearly showing that the homeostatic mechanisms prevent generation of excessive protein concentrations and oncotic pressures. Starling's law clearly shows that an increase in tissue fluid protein leads to a rise in oncotic pressure. The effect of higher tissue oncotic pressure is an immediate attraction of capillary water and dilution of tissue proteins. Increase in water volume expands the tissue space, which is clinically recognized as edema. Expansion of the tissue space is possible because of the high compliance of skin and subcutaneous tissue. Taken together, the total mass of accumulated protein in a lymphedematous tissue is high, but its concentration remains within physiological limits. High tissue fluid and lymph concentrations may be seen only in inflamed tissues with high capillary permeability and an excessive flux of plasma proteins.

Lymph Cytokines in Obstructive Lymphedema

Our data are: TNFalpha 6 pg/ml, L/S 3.5; IL1beta 4.5 pg/ml, L/S 1.4; IL6 60 pg/ml, L/S 20; VEGF C 780 pg/ml, L/S 4.0.

Cytokines are low molecular proteins that easily penetrate the capillary wall. However, they are also produced locally, in the case of skin and subcutaneous tissue, by keratinocytes, fibroblasts, dermal macrophages, dendritic cells, and lymphocytes. The local contribution evidently increases lymph cytokine levels to those above plasma. For example, the lymphatic endothelial-cell-produced VEGF C may be 4–40 times higher in lymph than in plasma.

References

1. Olszewski WL, Engeset A, Sokolowski J. Lymph flow and protein in the normal male leg during lying, getting up, and walking. *Lymphology*. 1977;10(3):178-83.
2. Olszewski W, Engeset A, Jaeger PM, Sokolowski J, Theodorsen L. Flow and composition of leg lymph in normal men during venous stasis, muscular activity and local hyperthermia. *Acta Physiol Scand*. 1977;99(2):149-55.
3. Olszewski WL, Engeset A, Lukasiewicz H. Immunoglobulins, complement and lysozyme in leg lymph of normal men. *Scand J Clin Lab Invest*. 1977;37(8):669-74.
4. Olszewski WL, Engeset A. Haemolytic complement in peripheral lymph of normal men. *Clin Exp Immunol*. 1978;32(3):392-8.
5. Olszewski WL, Engeset A. Immune proteins, enzymes and electrolytes in human peripheral lymph. *Lymphology*. 1978;11(4):156-64.
6. Olszewski WL. *Lymph protein concentration. In Lymph stasis – pathomechanism, diagnosis and therapy*. Boca Raton: CRC Press; 1991:243-56.
7. Interewicz B, Olszewski WL, Leak LV, Petricoin EF, Liotta LA. Profiling of normal human leg lymph proteins using the 2-D electrophoresis and SELDI-TOF mass spectrophotometry approach. *Lymphology*. 2004;37(2):65-72.
8. Plachta J, Olszewski WL, Grzelak I, Engeset A, Cholewka W. Identification of interleukin-1 in normal human lymph derived from skin. *Lymphokine Res*. 1988;7(2):93-7.
9. Olszewski WL, Loe K, Engeset A. Immune proteins and other biochemical constituents of peripheral lymph in patients with malignancy and postirradiation lymphedema. *Lymphology*. 1978;11(4):174-80.
10. Olszewski WL, Jamal S, Lukomska B, Manokaran G, Grzelak I. Immune proteins in peripheral tissue fluid-lymph in patients with filarial lymphedema of the lower limbs. *Lymphology*. 1992;25(4):166-71.
11. Olszewski WL, Pazdur J, Kubasiewicz E, Zaleska M, Cooke CJ, Miller NE. Lymph draining from foot joints in rheumatoid arthritis provides insight into local cytokine and chemokine production and transport to lymph nodes. *Arthritis Rheum*. 2001;44(3):541-9.
12. Olszewski WL. Pathophysiological aspects of lymphedema of human limbs: I Lymph protein composition. *Lymphat Res Biol*. 2003;1(3):235-43.
13. Olszewski WL, Jain P, Ambujam G, Zaleska M, Cakala M. Cytokines in various types of lower limb lymphedema. J Clin Invest 2010 (submitted).

Chapter 9
Physiology – Lymph Flow

Waldemar L. Olszewski

It is in only a few centers that tissue fluid and lymph hydraulics have thus far been studied under normal conditions in the soft tissues of the human limb and in lymphedema.[1-9] Although knowledge of extravascular fluid hydraulics is indispensable for understanding the manual and pneumatic massage events in tissues and after surgical lymphatico-venous anastomoses, few data are available in the pertinent literature.

Tissue Fluid Pressure and Flow

Lymph flow from normal and lymphedematous tissues cannot be analyzed without some knowledge of mobile tissue fluid pressure and movement. Lymph is a product of plasma capillary filtrate. This filtrate forms tissue fluid. A number of tissue humoral and cellular components derived from skin, subcutaneous tissue, fascia, and muscle mix in the interstitial space with the capillary filtrate and flow into the lymphatics. In the lymphatics, the tissue fluid becomes lymph. Forces driving tissue fluid to the lymphatics are responsible for filling vessels and initiating flow.

Pressures in the Normal Limb

Under normal conditions, tissue (interstitial) fluid pressure in the lower limb subcutaneous tissue at rest, when measured, ranges between −3 and +1 mmHg (Fig. 9.1). It is slightly negative, which also has been observed in animals. Active movements of the calf (contractions of muscles) may slightly decrease the pressure due to

W.L. Olszewski
Department of Surgical Research and Transplantology,
Medical Research Centre, Warsaw, Poland

B.-B. Lee et al. (eds.), *Lymphedema*,
DOI 10.1007/978-0-85729-567-5_9, © Springer-Verlag London Limited 2011

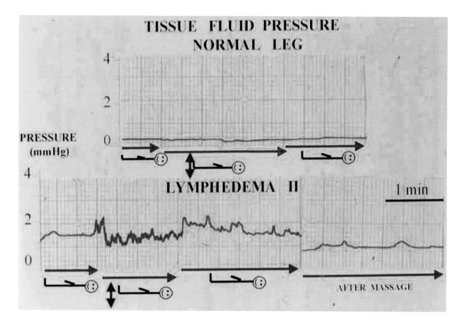

Fig. 9.1 Tissue fluid pressures in the subcutaneous tissues of a normal and a lymphedematous calf in the horizontal position. *Upper panel*: pressure approximating zero, not affected by muscular contractions. *Lower panel*: pressure approximating 2 mmHg, with minor fluctuations, during calf muscle contractions. Tissue fluid pressure is low even in the advanced stages of lymphedema, due to expansion of the interstitial space of the subcutis

emptying of the interstitial space; however, these differences are of no clinical importance (Fig. 9.1).

Pressures in the Lymphedema

In obstructive lymphedema, the resting tissue fluid pressure increases above zero, but remains within a low range, between 1 and 10 mm Hg[9] (Fig. 9.2). Higher pressures are observed in advanced stages (III and IV). There are no significant changes in pressure elicited by the change from a horizontal to an upright position. Moreover, active contractions of calf muscles do not generate higher pressures (Fig. 9.1). Manual massaging of lymphedematous calf soft tissues may even increase the pressure above 100 mm Hg. However, removal of the massaging hand brings about an immediate drop in pressure to zero.

Normal Tissue Fluid Flow

In a normal subcutaneous tissue there is no detectable flow at rest or during walking or massage.[6]

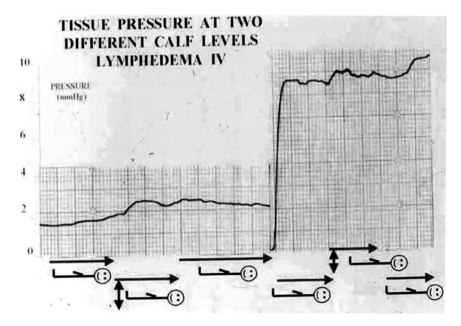

Fig. 9.2 Tissue fluid pressures recorded at the mid-calf (left panel) and ankle level in lymphedema, stage IV. Minor differences depending on the level of measurement. Note lack of effect of muscular contractions and low levels of pressure

Tissue Fluid Flow in Lymphedema

Excess accumulated tissue fluid moves radially from the site of applied force during muscular contractions and massaging, but not unidirectionally toward the root of the extremity. This makes massage of soft tissues without immediate distal compression (bandaging) non-effective. Tissue fluid flow can be seen on lymphoscintigraphy, depicting artificial channels created by deformation of the subcutaneous tissue by the compressed fluid.

Lymph Pressure and Flow

Extrinsic Factors that Propel Lymph

Normal Conditions

Muscular activity, respiratory movements, passive movements and arterial pulsation have no effect on lymph flow.[1-3,5,6] Generally, the lymphatics of the limb are empty, with only a few microliters of lymph in some lymphangions. There is no hydrostatic pressure in normal leg lymphatics in the upright position.[3,6]

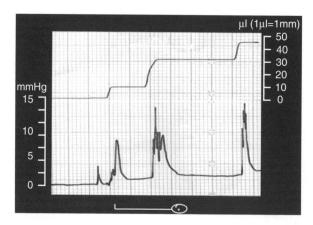

Fig. 9.3 Pressure (lateral) and flow recorded in a normal calf lymphatic vessel. Three pulse waves are seen (*red curve*). They are of different amplitude. Also, the time intervals between contractions are of different duration. The contraction of each lymphangion generated pressures propelling flow (*blue curve*). The ascending component of the curve shows the stroke volume. Flow occurred only during lymphangion contractions

Lymphedema Conditions

Muscular contraction of the foot and calf may increase lymph pressure to values above 100 mmHg. In lymphedema, patent lymphatics are filled with lymph and pressing of the muscles against the skin creates a pressure gradient between the distal and proximal lymphatics.[3,6]

Intrinsic Factors that Propel Lymph

Lymph is propelled by autonomous rhythmic contractions of lymphangions.[1-6] Tissue fluid enters the initial lymphatics to flow into the lymphangions. Stretching of the lymphatic wall by inflowing tissue fluid evokes contractions of the lymphatic wall muscles (according to Starling's law) and generates flow.

Lymph pressures in normal limbs. Lymphatics contract rhythmically with a frequency that depends on the volume of the tissue fluid entering.[3,6] In regions with high capillary filtration rates and tissue fluid formation, the frequency is high. The recorded pressures at rest, without regard to whether they are obtained in the supine or upright position, with free proximal flow (lateral pressure), range between 7 and 30 mmHg and during foot flexion, between 10 and 30 mmHg (Fig. 9.3). The pulse amplitudes are 3–20 mmHg and 5–17 mmHg and the pulse frequencies are 0.6–6/min and 2–8/min respectively.[3,6] The resting end pressures with obstructed flow (e.g. corresponding to lymphatic obstruction in postsurgical lymphedema) range between 15 and 55 mmHg, and during foot flexion 15– 50 mmHg. The pulse amplitudes are 3–35 mmHg and 3–14 mmHg and the pulse frequencies are 2.5–10/min and 3–12/min respectively. Massaging of the foot or tapping of lymph-laden tissues has no effect

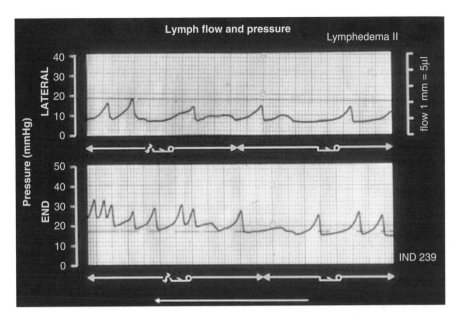

Fig. 9.4 Lymph pressure recorded in a patient with lymphedema, stage III. Spontaneous pressure waves generated by a damaged lymphangion are low and unable to create flow (*flat blue line*)

on lymph pressure. Heating of the foot significantly increases the pressure, amplitude, and frequency of lymphatic contractions.

Pressures in Lymphedematous Limbs

In obstructive lymphedema only a few lymphatic collectors remain patent. The recorded pressures during rest range from 5 to 45 mmHg depending on the surviving contractility force of the damaged lymphatic musculature.[7-9] During calf muscular contractions, pressures are generally low, ranging from 10 to 25 mmHg, although tiptoeing may, in some cases, generate pressures exceeding 200 Hg.

Lymph Flow in Normal Limbs

Flow occurs only during spontaneous contractions of lymphangions.[3]

Lymph Flow in Lymphedematous Limbs

As most collectors are partially or totally obliterated, there might be only some spontaneous flow in patent vessel segments at different levels of the limb.[7,8] Correlation of pressures and flow, in most cases, demonstrates the ineffectiveness of the lymphangions' contractions (Fig. 9.4). This is the consequence of the destruction of vessel musculature and valves.

General Remarks

In post-inflammatory, post-surgical, and post-traumatic lymphedema, as well as in the so-called idiopathic lymphedema (i.e., lymphedema of unknown etiology), the intra-lymphatic pressures and flow are abnormal due to: a) destruction of lymph vessel muscle cells, b) destruction of valves, or c) partial or total lumen obstruction. Tissue fluid finds its way to the non-swollen parts of the limb along hydraulically created tissue channels.

References

1. Olszewski WL, Engeset A. Intrinsic contractility of leg lymphatics in man. Preliminary communication. *Lymphology.* 1979;12:81-4.
2. Olszewski WL. Lymphatic contractions. *N Engl J Med.* 1979;8(300):316.
3. Olszewski WL, Engeset A. Intrinsic contractility of prenodal lymph vessels and lymph flow in human leg. *Am J Physiol.* 1980;239:H775-83.
4. Armenio S, Cetta F, Tanzini G, Guercia C. Spontaneous contractility in the human lymph vessels. *Lymphology.* 1981;14:173-8.
5. Sjöberg T, Norgren L, Steen S. Contractility of human leg lymphatics during exercise before and after indomethacin. *Lymphology.* 1989;22:186-93.
6. Olszewski WL. *Lymph vessel contractility. In Lymph stasis – pathomechanism, diagnosis and therapy.* Boca Raton: CRC Press; 1991:115-154.
7. Olszewski WL. Contractility patterns of normal and pathologically changed human lymphatics. *Ann NY Acad Sci.* 2002;979:52-63.
8. Olszewski WL. Contractility patterns of human leg lymphatics in various stages of obstructive lymphedema. *Ann NY Acad Sci.* 2008;1131:110-8.
9. Olszewski WL, Jain P, Ambujam G, Zaleska M, Cakala M. Tissue fluid pressure and flow during pneumatic massage of lymphedematous lower limbs. Lymphatic Res Biol. 8; 2010 (in press).

Chapter 10
Pathology and Histochemistry

Waldemar L. Olszewski

Immune processes in lymphatics and nodes

The pathological changes observed in the lymphatics in lymphedema can be caused by infection or trauma and include damage of the endothelial and muscular cells, subsequently leading to obliteration of the lumen by fibroblasts, the price the lymphatic system pays for its own function in the body changes. The system is devoted to elimination of microbes and clearance of damaged cells and, in a feedback fashion, to the healing of parenchymatous tissues. The inflammatory process has a destructive effect on the host's cells. The pathological events in the skin and reaction of the regional lymphatic system are shown schematically in Fig. 10.1. The lymph cells participating in the immune response are presented in Fig. 10.2.[1-3]

Classification of Lymphedema of Lower Limbs

The pathological changes observed on lymphoscintigrams, magnetic resonance images and histological specimens depend on the factors responsible for the development of lymphedema. Today, the sole term "lymphedema" does not provide enough information about the etiology of the condition. Lymphedema is not a separate entity, it is a symptom. The term "lymphedema" should be preceded by a qualifying term that refers to the cause (Fig. 10.3). The histological pictures of lymphatics and tissues differ depending on the primary cause.

Human limb lymphedema is characterized by tissue changes[4-6]:

Obstructive lymphedema: (1) obliteration of lymphatic collectors and fibrosis of lymph nodes (Fig. 10.4), (2) hyperkeratosis of epidermis (Fig. 10.5), (3) immune

W.L. Olszewski
Department of Surgical Research and Transplantology,
Medical Research Centre, Warsaw, Poland

B.-B. Lee et al. (eds.), *Lymphedema*,
DOI 10.1007/978-0-85729-567-5_10, © Springer-Verlag London Limited 2011

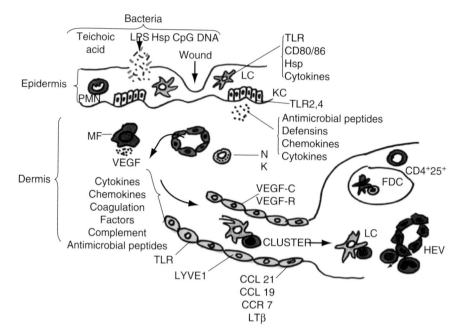

Fig. 10.1 Schematic presentation of immune events in the skin, draining lymphatics and nodes. Bacteria and/or trauma of the epidermis damage the superficial layers of keratinocytes. The bacterial antigens and cellular debris are immediately recognized by Langerhans' cells present among keratinocytes. A cascade of natural immune events is initiated. Multiple non-specific humoral and cellular factors participate in the process. Yellow cells line out afferent lymphatics. *LPS* lipopolysaccharide, *hsp* heat-shock protein, *CpG DNA* bacterial DNA fragment, *LC* Langerhans' cell, *KC* keratinocytes, *TLR* toll-like receptor, *MF* macrophage, *NK* natural killer cell, *VEGF* vascular endothelial growth factor (R-receptor), *LYVE 1* hyaluronate receptor specific for lymphatic endothelial cells, *CCL* lymphocyte chemoattracting cytokine, *LT* lymphocytotoxin attracting lymphocytes, *FDC* follicular dendritic cells in B-cell follicles, *HEV* high endothelial venules – sites of extravasation of blood lymphocytes, *CD4+25+* regulatory lymphocytes

cell infiltrates of epidermis, dermis, and subcutaneous tissue (Fig. 10.5), (4) fibrosis of the peri-lymphatic tissues and muscular fascia (Fig. 10.6), (5) growth of skin and fat tissue.

So-called primary or idiopathic lymphedema: (1) normally structured wall of lymphatic collectors, (2) acellular deposits under the endothelium narrowing, or fibrotic structures obstructing the lumen (Fig. 10.7), (3) slow fibrotic process in the subcutaneous tissue, (4) small but normally structured lymph nodes.

Remarks

In lymphedema, tissues deprived of tissue fluid and lymph drainage are the site of a continuous inflammatory process. Fluids accumulating in skin and subcutaneous tissues in lymphedema contain cytokines, chemokines, activated immune cells,

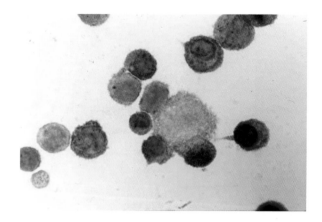

Fig. 10.2 Histological analysis of lymph cell smear from a normal human calf lymphatic vessel. The large cell in the middle is a Langerhans' cell (dendritic, veiled) with attached CD4 T-helper (*rosy*) lymphocytes forming a so-called immune cluster. Antigen (bacterial, own tissue-specific) is processed by Langerhans' cells and presented to the T-helper lymphocytes. In close vicinity are the CD8 cytotoxic lymphocytes (*brown*), which also participate in the immune prosesses. The type of cells in lymph is totally different from that of blood. Extravasation of specific cell precursors takes place in the dermal and lymph node blood capillaries. These cells further migrate to the initial lymphatics

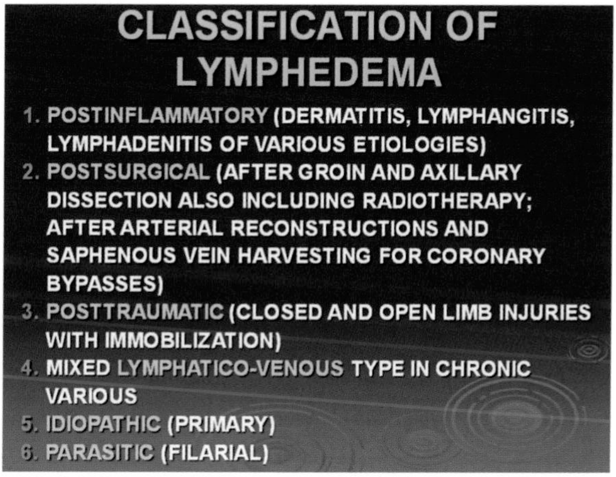

Fig. 10.3 Classification of lymphedema. Adding the causative term in front of "lymphedema" provides information necessary for a proper understanding of the mechanism, establishing the treatment protocol and formulating prognosis

CLASSIFICATION OF LYMPHEDEMA

1. POSTINFLAMMATORY (DERMATITIS, LYMPHANGITIS, LYMPHADENITIS OF VARIOUS ETIOLOGIES)
2. POSTSURGICAL (AFTER GROIN AND AXILLARY DISSECTION ALSO INCLUDING RADIOTHERAPY; AFTER ARTERIAL RECONSTRUCTIONS AND SAPHENOUS VEIN HARVESTING FOR CORONARY BYPASSES)
3. POSTTRAUMATIC (CLOSED AND OPEN LIMB INJURIES WITH IMMOBILIZATION)
4. MIXED LYMPHATICO-VENOUS TYPE IN CHRONIC VARIOUS
5. IDIOPATHIC (PRIMARY)
6. PARASITIC (FILARIAL)

and, most importantly, microorganisms. Microorganisms normally penetrate the epidermis in small numbers and are quickly eliminated by the circulating immune cells. However, in conditions of lymph stasis, they are not removed and may proliferate, evoking a host reaction. This is the reason for clinical attacks of dermato-lymphangio-adenitis (DLA) and histological changes such as infiltrates and formation of fibrous tissue.

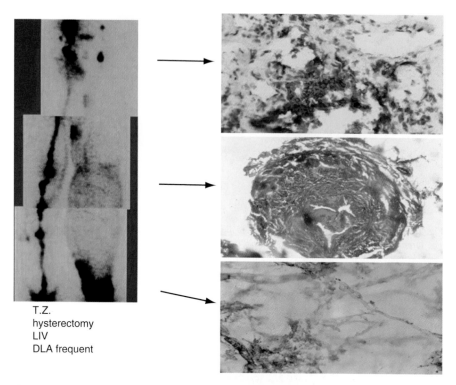

T.Z.
hysterectomy
LIV
DLA frequent

Fig. 10.4 Pathological changes in lymphatics in a patient with postsurgical, postradiation lymphedema stage IV. *Left panel* – lymphoscintigram showing lack of lymphatics in the swollen limb. *Right panel* – histological pictures from tissue at levels indicated by *arrows*. Dilated, irregular structured subepidermal lymphatic (*lower panel*), obliterated lymphatic collector (*middle panel*) and remnants of an inguinal lymph node (*upper panel*) with few remaining lymphocytes (*red*). This is a typical picture of changes in the lower limb lymphatic system in a long-lasting lymphedema

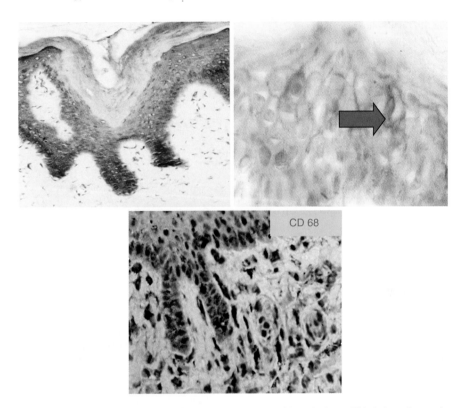

Fig. 10.5 Histological pictures of skin changes in advanced lymphedema. This is hyperkeratosis with 10–15 keratinocyte layers (normal 5–8) and protrusion of the proliferating keratinocytes toward the dermis. In the epidermis, multiple activated Langerhans' cells expressing HLADR antigens are seen. Also the adjacent keratinocytes become HLA DR-positive. In the dermis, numerous CD 68-activated macrophages (*brown*) are seen

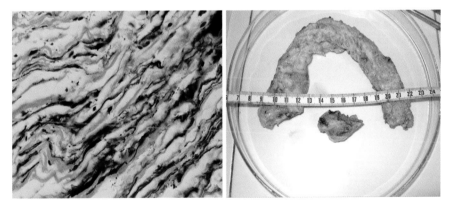

Fig. 10.6 Histological changes in lymphedema involve not only lymphatics and nodes, but also dermis, subcutaneous tissue, and fascia. Fibrosis is the main process, starting from the most distal parts of the limb and progressing to the knee. The accumulating tissue fluid deforms the subcutaneous tissue creating thousands of lakes and semi-open channels (*blue stained*). In due course these channels become closed by proliferating fibroblasts. Muscular fascia becomes totally fibrotic, attaining a thickness of 2–3 cm

Fig. 10.7 Histological
picture of a lower limb
lymphatic in so-called
"primary lymphedema".
All vessel layers are normally
developed. In the lumen
fibrotic material with
mononuclear infiltrates
partly occludes the lumen.
The etiology of changes
remains unknown; however,
an infectious factor cannot
be excluded

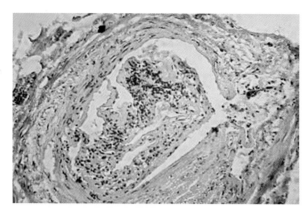

References

1. Olszewski WL, Grzelak I, Engeset A. Cells in lymph draining normal human skin. *Lymphology*. 1982;15:168-173.
2. Olszewski WL. Cells in lymph. In: Olszewski WL, ed. *Lymph Stasis: Pathophysiology, Diagnosis and Treatment*. Boca Raton, FL: CRC Press; 1991:259-283.
3. Olszewski WL, Grzelak I, Ziolkowska A, Engeset A. Immune cell traffic from blond through the normal human skin to lymphatics. *Clin Dermatol*. 1995;13:473-483.
4. Olszewski WL, Engeset A, Romaniuk A, Grzelak I, Ziolkowska A. Immune cells in peripheral lymph and skin of patients with obstructive lymphedema. *Lymphology*. 1990;23:23-33.
5. Olszewski WL, Jamal S, Manokaran G, Lukomska B, Kubicka U. Skin changes in filarial and non-filarial lymphoedema of the lower extremities. *Trop Med Parasitol*. 1993;44(1):40-44.
6. Olszewski W, Machowski Z, Sokolowski J, Sawicki Z, Zerbino D, Nielubowicz J. Primary lymphedema of lower extremities. I. Lymphangiographic and histological studies of lymphatic vessels and lymph nodes in primary lymphedema. *Pol Med J*. 1972;11:1564-1572.

Part IV
Clinical Diagnosis

Chapter 11
Clinical Diagnosis: General Overview

Mauro Andrade

General Considerations

Lymphedema, or lymphatic edema, refers to increased volume of body segments due to localized or extensive lymphatic system disturbances that cause decreased lymph transport, without regard to the primary cause. Characteristically, chronic lymph stasis promotes both fluid accumulation and tissue changes. Defective uptake of large molecules retains water within the interstitial space and, over time, lymph stasis leads to progressive tissue changes, characterized by abnormal growth of subcutaneous tissue and intercellular matrix, and increased skin thickness. It is noteworthy that, beyond tissue fluid control, lymphatics play other important roles in tissue homeostasis, which makes lymphedema unique and far more complex than edema caused by other vascular or systemic factors.

Nevertheless, lymphedema is the most striking clinical feature of lymphatic insufficiencies, although lymphedema is hardly a disease in itself. Lymphedema is best evaluated as part of a much more complex syndrome, with diverse clinical manifestations that may cause significant functional, cosmetic, and psychosocial consequences to affected individuals.[1] In addition, some features that accompany lymph stasis may actually precede edema development and are an important issue in lymphatic disorders. Immune cell trafficking,[2] and thus the local immune response,[3] are impaired in patients with deranged lymph flow. Lymph node resection in breast cancer treatment compromises normal lymphatic drainage of the upper limb and that constitutes a sufficient reason for practitioners to advise patients to avoid skin lesions, to thereby prevent infectious episodes that could trigger or worsen arm lymphedema. After axillary lymphadenectomy, some patients may display an adipose, rather than an edematous, arm,[4,5] where tissue growth, especially that of the

M. Andrade
Department of Surgery, University of São Paulo Medical School,
São Paulo, Brazil

B.-B. Lee et al. (eds.), *Lymphedema*,
DOI 10.1007/978-0-85729-567-5_11, © Springer-Verlag London Limited 2011

subcutaneous fat, is more relevant than fluid retention. This particular group of patients underscores another clinical feature of lymph stasis: tissue hypertrophy, a bigger challenge than edema for physical therapy and volume control.

In this sense, akin to other syndromic states, edema is a clinical sign with in the constellation of many others and is caused by different etiologies of lymphatic disturbance. A similar thought is given to congestive heart failure, where the clinical picture is derived from a variety of cardiac disorders and presents many clinical signs, edema among them. Cardiac valve lesions or ischemic heart disease, disorders of completely different etiologies and therapeutic approaches, may produce similar clinical symptoms because of the failure of cardiac output. Lymphatic hypoplasia and lymphatic obstruction, which are also diverse situations with regard to their etiological and structural aspects, may display similar clinical features of volume increase and tissue changes. Also, it is known that some disturbances causing cardiac insufficiency may not be accompanied by lower limb edema and that some lymphatic insufficiencies do not promote limb swelling. Neither of these facts should change our interpretation of the clinical problems, either lymphatic or cardiac.

Clearly, definition influences clinical diagnosis. If we diagnose the condition based only on edema, an opportunity to prevent volume increase may be lost in many cases. This situation applies to known lymphatic disturbances in which edema is not yet clinically evident; this is best exemplified by nodal resection operations. Also, some patients with unilateral primary lymphedema of the lower limb have structural abnormalities of the clinically normal limb.[6] To avoid such paradoxes, a Stage 0, or latent phase of lymphedema, is recognized.[1,7] Interestingly, the absence of edema can be considered to be a stage of lymphatic edema.

Clinical Diagnosis

It is common knowledge that the diagnosis of lymphedema (but not lymphatic insufficiency) is best made on clinical grounds and the following chapters will cover many different aspects of the clinical features and the best strategies for evaluating signs and symptoms of edema caused by lymphatic disturbances.

As in all medical disorders, a detailed history and clinical evaluation and a thorough physical examination are necessary, considering that edema may also be a complaint or existing sign in many diseases. In lymphedema patients, history should include age at onset, episodes of inflammatory attacks, medical treatments that could result in secondary lymphedema, and previous travels to tropical countries with endemic filariasis. Transient edema of the affected limb and a family history of limb edema should also be noted.

Regarding physical findings and complaints, the diagnosis of edema of lymphatic origin is based on a few points[8]:

1. Distribution
   In lower limbs, lymphedema is usually unilateral. If it is bilateral, it is usually asymmetric. We must bear in mind that pure lower limb lymphedema, thus not

considering the widespread lymphatic involvement in all other forms of edema, is relatively rare as a primary condition. Bilateral edema is most probably due to general conditions and unilateral edema occurs more commonly secondary to venous diseases. On the other hand, the presence of visible varicosities and venous insufficiency does not exclude simultaneous lymphedema that can be aggravated by fluid overload caused by associated venous stasis.

2. Symptoms

Lymphedema is a painless condition, unless complications have arisen (inflammation, neurological involvement or compression by tumors). Some authors concede that an acute development of edema may produce pain by tissue distention. A usual complaint is heaviness. It is easy to understand, if volume excess is considered. Surprisingly, sometimes the patients' complaint is not directly related to limb volume and it is not rare to observe patients with mild edema who are more concerned about heaviness than other subjects with longstanding advanced lymphedemas.

3. Stemmer's sign

Broadening of the skin folds at the base of toes and fingers due to excessive skin thickness, fluid accumulation or tissue overgrowth (either isolated or in combination) is considered to have a high specificity as a clinical sign for the diagnosis of lymphedema, although its sensitivity is not very high. It can be absent in cases of descending lymphedema where edema begins at the root of the limb, characteristically found in secondary lymphedemas, proximal hypoplasia or malignant compression/obstruction of the iliocaval trunks. Intriguingly, a survey among healthy German physiotherapists has shown a small percentage of positive Stemmer's sign with no visible or previous history of leg or foot edema[8] and patients with venous disorders can also show positive Stemmer's sign.[9]

4. Godet's sign

Present in most forms of edema from different etiologies, so not diagnostic of lymphedema, this sign is essential to the physical evaluation. Presence and intensity of Godet's sign in lymphedema patients is related to treatment prognosis and indirectly reflects tissue alterations. Deeper depressions caused by examination mean a high fluid content and less tissue hardening. On the other hand, shallow depressions represent a lesser amount of displaceable interstitial fluid. In these patients, fat or fibrotic tissue accounts for most of the volume increase.

Other signs of lymph stasis may be present and should be routinely sought on physical examination. Skin changes such as pinkish-red discoloration, hyperkeratosis, papillomatosis, lymph vesicles (clear or chylous), or yellow discoloration of the nails may accompany some forms of lymphedema. Not diagnostic, but of foremost importance in swollen limbs, is the identification of nail or interdigital lesions caused by fungi, a frequent and dangerous condition which must be treated and prevented before infectious episodes supervene and aggravate swelling.[10] Lymphedema does not cause chronic skin ulcers. If ulceration occurs, it is most probably related to concomitant venous insufficiency or skin cancer, which should be ruled out.

Lymphangiosarcoma may rarely arise in longstanding lymphedemas. This rare and fatal condition was initially described by Stewart and Treves as a late complication arising in secondary arm lymphedema, but it can also occur in the lower limb.[11] Purple stains in the skin, edema worsening and pain characterize this complication.

Associated Disorders

Great attention should be given to possible associated disorders at any age, for they can change diagnostic pathways and therapeutic approaches. Congenital forms of lymphatic edema may be present with malformations in other organs and systems. Later in life, cancer, neurological, pulmonary, cardiac, renal, and metabolic diseases and treatments may be concomitant with lymphatic disorders or contribute to their clinical features.

Congenital lymphedemas arise secondary to heritable features such as genetic mutations or chromosomal aneuploidies.[12] Milroy's syndrome, Meige's syndrome, lymphedema distichiasis and yellow nail syndrome are the most prevalent hereditary disorders featuring lymphedema as an important clinical sign, while the most common aneuploidy is Turner's syndrome (XO).

Cardiac defects, mental retardation and renal problems may accompany some congenital lymphedemas. Occasionally, facial defects, such as cleft palate or double eyelashes (distichiasis), can be seen. Varicosities, trunk or limb stains, nevus, disproportionate limbs, fingers or toes, genital malformations are necessarily sought.

Nutritional status and stunted growth may be related to intestinal lymphangiectasias and chylous pleural and peritoneal effusions.

Milroy's syndrome can be due to a mutation in the 5q35.3 locus, the gene that encodes VEGFR-3.[13] Usually, these patients have lower limb edemas, occasionally associated with genital edemas and seldom with upper limb edemas. The original description does not associate this form of congenital lymphedema with other general or distant anomalies. Meige's disease also affects lower limbs but appears during puberty and its causative mutation is still unknown. Again, no associated disorders are to be expected. Lymphedema distichiasis syndrome is accompanied by cardiac problems, cleft palate, ptosis, double eyelashes, and yellow nails. Interestingly, the gene responsible for this syndrome has been identified at the locus q24.3 of the chromosome 16, but a gene knockout experimental model fails to develop lymphedema, even if the hyperplastic and dilated lymph vessels observed in the animal resemble the corresponding human structural defect.[14]

Complex vascular malformations, more commonly Proteus and Klippel-Trenaunay syndromes, may present with lymphedema although hardly as the most prominent clinical feature, being part of a disseminated vascular malformation.

Turner's syndrome is promptly recognizable through its general and characteristic aspects. Lymphedema may accompany and is usually bilateral, distal and symmetrical. Sometimes, lymphangiomas are observed in these patients. Frequently, for unknown reasons, edema spontaneously subsides with the passage of time.

Older patients can present associated common diseases. Patients with lymphedema can also be hypertensive, diabetic, hypothyroid, and so on. Like patients with no lymphatic disturbances, co-morbidities must be taken into consideration and adequately treated. Affected subjects with cardiac or renal insufficiency may require changes in therapeutic planning to avoid circulatory overload and pulmonary edema, should decongestive methods be employed.

Special attention should be given to patients with lymphedema secondary to cancer. Unexpected clinical worsening of the lymphedema and pain can be signs of recurrence.

When Further Investigation Is Needed

History and clinical examination are usually sufficient to make a correct clinical diagnosis of lymphedema. Occasionally, differential diagnosis with other disorders or association of lymphatic and extra-lymphatic disturbances may not be so clear. In such circumstances, lymphoscintigraphy is the method of choice in order to depict lymphatic involvement. There is a general agreement that lymphoscintigraphy must be part of the initial evaluation of any lymphedema patient (recommendation grade 1B).[1,7] Nevertheless, it is still undecided whether lymphoscintigraphy has prognostic value or if it can dramatically change therapeutic decision-making.

Venous ultrasound is recommended for lower limb edema, especially in adults, where association with venous insufficiency may be a cause of fluid overload within a defective lymphatic system, or to unveil unsuspected venous causes of edema.

Extra caution should be taken in the case of suspected secondary lymphedemas, mainly those that predominate at the root of the limb. In these cases, occult tumors may have invaded or compressed the lymphatic pathways in the thorax or abdomen. Imaging by magnetic resonance or computed tomography is mandatory to avoid delays in obtaining a proper diagnosis before establishing a therapeutical strategy.

Genetic testing should be undertaken in familial lymphedemas,[7] even if it is not a common practice. Only a few lymphatic disorders have thus far been associated with a specific gene defect. Genetic counseling and possible future gene therapy will certainly play an important role in primary disorders of the lymph vessels and nodes.

Other controversial points regarding further investigation in lymphedema patients are medico-legal problems and health insurance coverage. It is debatable whether the practitioner should demand additional tests when clinical history and physical examination are sufficient to make a correct diagnosis and establish adequate therapeutic planning. Nevertheless, malpractice issues are more likely to arise in the absence of full clinical documentation. Initiation of typical physical therapy in a patient with active and undiagnosed underlying tumoral obstruction prior to proper and extensive investigation may cause serious problems for both the patient and the practitioner. To a lesser extent, the same applies to edema due to systemic causes not identified by the clinician. Also, health insurance companies may demand additional confirmation beyond the clinical diagnosis in order to provide the patient with treatment and compression stockings.

References

1. International Society of Lymphology. The diagnosis and treatment of peripheral lymphedema. *Lymphology*. 2009;42:51-60.
2. Olszewski WL, Engeset A, Romaniuk A, Grzelak I, Ziolkowska A. Immune cells in peripheral lymph and skin of patients with obstructive lymphedema. *Lymphology*. 1990;23:23-33.
3. Ruocco V, Brunetti G, Puca RV, Ruocco E. The immunocompromised district: a unifying concept for lymphoedematous, herpes-infected and otherwise damaged sites. *J Eur Acad Dermatol Venereol*. 2009;23:1364-1373.
4. Tassenoy A, Vermeiren K, van der Veen P, et al. Demonstration of tissue alterations by ultrasonography, magnetic resonance imaging and spectroscopy, and histology in breast cancer patients without lymphedema after axillary node dissection. *Lymphology*. 2006;39:118-126.
5. Brorson H, Ohlin K, Olsson G, Karlsson MK. Breast cancer-related chronic arm lymphedema is associated with excess adipose and muscle tissue. *Lymphat Res Biol*. 2009;7:3-10.
6. Browse NL, Stewart G. Lymphoedema: pathophysiology and classification. *J Cardiovasc Surg (Torino)*. 1985;26:91-106.
7. Lee BB, Andrade M, Piller N, et al. Consensus on primary lymphedema. *Int Angiol*. 2010; 29(5):454-470.
8. Földi E, Földi M. Lymphostatic diseases. In: Földi E, Földi M, Kübik S, eds. *Textbook of Lymphology*. Munich: Urban & Fischer; 2003:231-319.
9. Pannier F, Hoffmann B, Stang A, Jöckel KH, Rabe E. Prevalence of Stemmer's sign in the general population. Results from the Bonn Vein Study. *Phlebologie*. 2007;36:289-292.
10. Andrade M, Nishinari K, Puech-Leão P. Intertrigo in patients with lower limb lymphedema. Clinical and laboratory correlation. *Rev Hosp Clin Fac Med Sao Paulo*. 1998;53:3-5.
11. Andrade M, Lederman A, Puech-Leão P. Lymphangiosarcoma in primary lymphedema of the lower limbs. *Lymphology*. 2002;35(suppl):737-744.
12. Witte MH, Erickson RP, Reiser FA, Witte CL. Genetic alterations in lymphedema. *Phlebolymphology*. 1997;16:19-25.
13. Holberg CJ, Erickson RP, Bernas MJ, et al. Segregation analyses and a genome-wide linkage search confirm genetic heterogeneity and suggest oligogenic inheritance in some Milroy congenital primary lymphedema families. *Am J Med Genet*. 2001;98:303-312.
14. Kriederman BM, Myloyde TL, Witte MH, et al. FOXC2 haploinsufficient mice are a model for human autosomal dominant lymphedema-distichiasis syndrome. *Hum Mol Genet*. 2003;12: 1179-1185.

Chapter 12
Clinical Staging

Sandro Michelini, Marco Cardone, Alessandro Failla, and Giovann Moneta

The problem of the staging of lymphedema is a perennial topic for discussion at consensus meetings within national and international congresses. First of all, for definitions and scope of pathology to be universally accepted, the requirements of simplicity, recognizability, and worldwide utilization must be met.

Four proposals based on different clinical and instrumental aspects of pathology have been presented at the international level, yet only some of the attributes are common to all. Through the work of a special world commission, a synthesis of the different proposals will provide scientific communication with universally recognized and accepted parameters.

Primary and secondary lymphedemas have different clinical stages of evolution, in part mutually reversible, that influence affected patients differently from the physical, emotional, and psychological points of view.

Achieving common acceptance of stages of lymphedema, as in other diseases, seems to be a problem that cannot be postponed further for reasons of "scientific communication" and for the undoubted medicolegal and social impact. In more advanced clinical stages, the condition takes on the characteristics of a real "social disease," the costs of which are generated both from medical care and from loss of productive capacity.

The clinical staging, reported in the "consensus document" of the International Society of Lymphology,[1] currently includes four clinical stages (Table 12.1); it initially included three clinical stages (I, II, and III), but recently, motivated by our Italian classification,[2-5] which underscored the importance of including the "pre-clinical" aspect of the primary and secondary types of lymphedema, potentially progressive (e.g., mastectomy with coincident limbs), the pre-clinical stage, defined

S. Michelini (✉)
San Giovanni Battista Hospital, Rome, Italy

B.-B. Lee et al. (eds.), *Lymphedema*,
DOI 10.1007/978-0-85729-567-5_12, © Springer-Verlag London Limited 2011

Table 12.1 Staging according to the "consensus document" of the International Society of Lymphology

Clinical stage	Evidence
0	Subclinical with possible clinical evolution
I	Edema regressing with treatments with positive pitting test
II	Edema partially regressing with treatments with negative pitting test
III	Elephantiasis with cutaneous complications and recurrent infections

as stage 0, was included. Stage 0 refers to a latent or sub-clinical condition, where swelling is not evident despite impaired lymph transport. Stage I represents an early accumulation of fluid relatively high in protein content (in contrast to "venous edema") that subsides with limb elevation. Pitting may occur. Stage II signifies that limb elevation alone rarely reduces tissue swelling and that pitting is manifest. Stage III encompasses lymphostatic elephantiasis where pitting is absent and trophic skin changes, such as acanthosis, fat deposits, and warty overgrowths develop. The severity of the stages is based on the volume differences: minimal (<20% increase), moderate (20–40% increase), and severe (>40% increase). These stages only refer to the physical condition of the extremities.

Some healthcare workers examining disability utilize the World Health Organization's guidelines for the International Classification of Functioning, Disability, and Health (ICF). Quality of Life issues (social, emotional, physical inabilities, etc.) may also be addressed by individual clinicians and can have a favorable impact on therapy and compliance.[6]

At the recent XX World Congress of the International Society of Lymphology, held in Brazil, in a special Consensus session, a special world commission was organized to finalize a new, official staging of the International Society.[2]

In Germany, led by Prof. Ethel Foeldi, four clinical stages[11] have been introduced for the first time, adding to those reported in the actual 'consensus document' a stage 0, which represents all cases of sub-clinical lymphedema, but with a significant risk of clinical progression (e.g., lymphoscintigraphy strongly predictive; Table 12.2).

Since 1994,[2] five clinical stages have been recognized in Italy (Table 12.3). This system emphasizes the importance of pre-clinical cases at risk of evolution (in stage I) and cases of elephantiasis with major chronic inflammatory and infectious complications and risk of neoplastic tissue degeneration (stage V). Depending on the stage it is also possible to direct the therapeutic treatment toward the corresponding preventive options.[7]

In Japan, a team led by Prof. Moriji Ohkuma, a dermatologist with heightened sensitivity to infectious complications in cutaneous and subcutaneous tissues, proposed four-phase staging involving inspection and palpation of the affected areas and of assessing the frequency of the infectious episodes and inflammatory complications; based upon the developmental stage, it is possible to obtain prognostic information (Table 12.4). This is obviously a staging with a more strictly dermatological point of view; while clinical, it is conceptually valid, since it considers some clinical and inflammatory aspects, complications that are frequently found in patients with both primary and secondary forms of lymphedema.[8,9]

Table 12.2 Staging according to the German Society of Lymphology (Prof. E. Foeldi)

Clinical stage	Evidence
0	No edema, but evidence of a risk condition for evolution
I	Edema regressing with treatments with positive pitting test
II	Edema partially regressing with treatments with negative pitting test
III	Elephantiasis with cutaneous complications and recurrent infections

Table 12.3 Staging according to the Italian Society of Lymph-Angiology (Michelini–Campisi)

Clinical stage	Evidence
I	No edema in individuals at risk (pre-clinical)
II	Edema that regresses spontaneously with elevation and with night rest
III	Edema that does not regress spontaneously, only with treatments and partially
IV	Elephantiasis (abolition of tendon and bone projections)
V	Elephantiasis complicated by cutaneous and recurrent infections and impairment of deep body structures (muscles, joints)

Table 12.4 Staging according to the Japanese Society of Lymphology (Prof. M. Ohkuma)

Clinical stage	Inspection	Palpation	Acute Dermo-epidermitis	Prognosis
I	Normal	Pitting ++	Absent	Temporary
II	Thin skin	Increase in thickness, pitting +	Absent	Permanent
III	Cutaneous lichenification	Increase in thickness, pitting –	Present	Worsening
IV	Verrucosis	Pitting absent	Very often	Worsening

The staging proposed in South America, and, in particular in Brazil by Prof. Mauro Andrade, is of substantial interest because, in addition to taking into account the importance of pre-clinical cases at risk of development of infectious and degenerative complications, it also analyzes the functional effects of edema on the limb with impairment of one, two, or three major joints (Figs. 12.1–12.5). This aspect also permits better definition of the commitments of global functional rehabilitation, the degree of care needed by the patient and the impairment in "Daily Living Activities." (Table 12.5). This classification thus utilizes both clinical and functional criteria for patient assessment.[9]

It should be emphasized, however, that the new Brazilian proposal addresses deficiencies that have been recognized in other stages so far presented.

The respective positions of the "experts" at such a delicate and transitional moment for both public and private health systems in different countries also stems from the need to redefine welfare parameters for these highly prevalent diseases.[10] At more advanced stages of disease, in fact, we can identify the extremes of a true social disease for which the health system must provide incentives and normative facilitations comparable to the other diseases for which such benefits and advantages are provided.

Fig. 12.1 Lymphedema
stage 0 (pre-clinical)

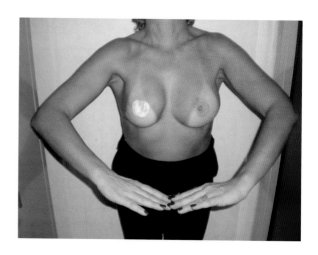

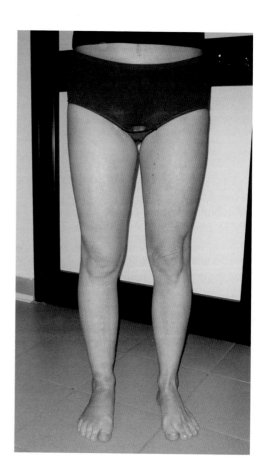

Fig. 12.2 Lymphedema stage I
(involvement of one major joint)

Fig. 12.3 Stage II (involvement of two major joints of the limb)

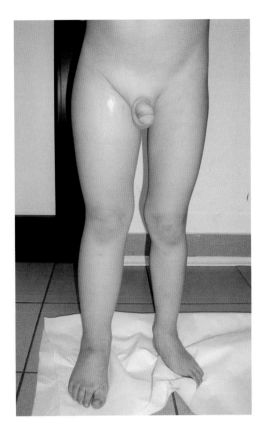

It is pointless to say that, currently, many National Healthcare Systems provide therapies to patients with both primary and secondary lymphedema in an inequitable manner, with poor distribution of healthcare resources. In most countries, the costs of materials, elastic garments and phlebo-lymph-active drugs are charged to the patient.

Thus, it is essential to solve these problems in each country at a governmental level. Epidemiological studies are still insufficient and must be updated in order to better define a problem that for too long has been totally ignored, while the number of patients affected is increasing daily.

It should also be noted that the various staging criteria examined take into account only aspects of the organic and physical involvement of the patients; yet, the variable emotional and psychological involvement, in some cases, regardless of the clinical evolution, the age, or the socio-economic and cultural condition of the patient, assumes greater functional significance. These factors that, over time, have a more profound influence on behavior, personal performance, and social relationships, and reinforce the simple physical problem, are overlooked in the staging schemes.

Fig. 12.4 Stage III (involvement of three major joints of the limb)

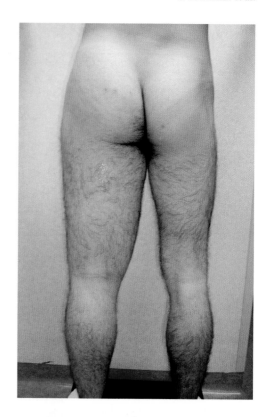

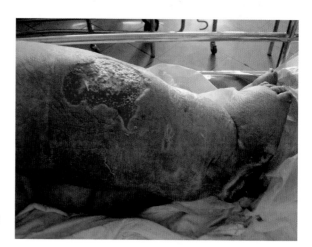

Fig. 12.5 Stage IV (cutaneous infections and inflamatory complications of the limb)

Table 12.5 Staging according to the Brazilian Society of Lymphology (Prof. M. Andrade)

Clinical stage	Evidence
0 (Fig. 12.1)	No edema in individuals at risk (pre-clinical)
I (Fig. 12.2)	Edema that regresses spontaneously with elevation, pitting ++, Stemmer +, involvement of one major joint of the limb
II (Fig. 12.3)	Edema that does not regress spontaneously, only with treatments, pitting +, Stemmer ++, involvement of at least two major joints of the limb
III (Fig. 12.4)	Edema that does not regress spontaneously, only with treatments, pitting +, Stemmer ++, involvement of three major joints of the limb
IV (Fig. 12.5)	Edema that does not regress spontaneously, only with treatments, pitting +, Stemmer ++, involvement of three major joints of the limb, with cutaneous infections

References

1. International Society of Lymphology. The diagnosis and treatment of peripheral lymphedema. Consensus document of the International Society of Lymphology. *Lymphology.* 2003;36: 84-91.
2. Michelini S, Failla A. Linfedemi: inquadramento diagnostico clinico e strumentale. *Minerva Cardioangiol.* 1997;45(6 suppl I):11-15.
3. Michelini S, Campisi C, Ricci M, et al. Linee Guida Italiane sul Linfedema. *Eur Med Phys.* 2007;43(suppl 1–3):34-41.
4. Campisi C, Michelini S, Boccardo F. Guidelines of the Società Italiana di Linfangiologia. *Lymphology.* 2004;37(4):174-179.
5. Campisi C, Michelini S, Boccardo F. Lymphology in medical and surgical practice. Italian guidelines looking towards Europe and World. *Eur J Lymphol.* 2004;14(42):26-28.
6. World Health Organization. *International Classification of Functionng, Disability and Health.* Geneva: WHO; 2001.
7. Campisi C, Michelini S, Boccardo F, Zilli A, Borrelli V. Modern stadiation of lymphedema and corresponding preventive options. *Eur J Lymphol.* 1999;7(25):27-31.
8. Ohkuma M. In lymphedema-related acute dermatitis. Abstract book of XX Congress of International Society of Lymphology. Sociedade Brasileira de Linfologia. Salvador Bahia; September 2005: 46.
9. Michelini S, Campisi C, Failla A, et al. Staging of lymphedema: comparing different proposals. *Eur J Lymphol.* 2006;16(46):7-10.
10. Tretbar LL, Morgan CL, Lee BB, Simonian SJ, Blondeau B. *Lymphedema Diagnosis and Treatment.* London: Springer; 2008.
11. Foldi M, Foldi E, Kubik S. *Foldi's Textbook of Lymphology.* Munchen: Elsevier; 2004.

Chapter 13
Combined Clinical and Laboratory (Lymphoscintigraphic) Staging

Byung-Boong Lee, James Laredo, and Richard F. Neville

Accurate assessment and clinical staging of patients with chronic lymphedema remains the most reliable objective methods of classifying patients for proper treatment and management.[1,2]

The clinical staging proposed by the International Society of Lymphology (ISL) over the last decade has remained the most popular staging system despite widespread dissatisfaction with its crude approach based on clinical, mostly physical findings alone.[3,4]

This ISL-recommended (clinical) staging system was initially proposed as part of a general consensus on the diagnosis and management of peripheral edema based on the old concept that failed to incorporate the new concept proposed during the recent update of the ISL consensus.[5,6]

Throughout the last decade, the concept of chronic lymphedema has undergone significant change; chronic lymphedema is no longer considered to be a "static" condition of simple lymph fluid stasis. It is now believed to be an ever-changing condition affecting the entire soft tissue, well beyond the lymphatic system.[7,8]

Current ISL staging is still far too simple. Appropriate staging is required to develop a complicated treatment strategy. Accurate staging of chronic lymphedema is critical when reconstructive or ablative surgical therapy is considered as a supplement in a patient who has failed to respond to complex decongestive therapy (CDT).[9,10] Appropriate timing of this surgical option is critical.[7,11]

Therefore, improved staging with new advanced diagnostic assessment is required for close monitoring of the disease process. This is especially true not only for general management of lymphedema, but also for determining the need for surgical implementation.

Various noninvasive to minimally invasive tests (e.g., radionuclide lymphoscintigraphy)[12-15] have been developed over the last decade to better assess the

B.-B. Lee (✉)
Department of Surgery, Division of Vascular Surgery,
George Washington University School of Medicine, Washington, DC, USA

B.-B. Lee et al. (eds.), *Lymphedema*,
DOI 10.1007/978-0-85729-567-5_13, © Springer-Verlag London Limited 2011

Table 13.1 Quality of life (QOL)

Excellent	No limitation or difficulty with extra activity (e.g., hobby) physically, psychologically, and/or socioeconomically in addition to daily activity
Good	Some limitation of extra activity, but occasionally, physically, psychologically, and/or socioeconomically, but with no limitation of daily activity
Fair	Significant limitation of extra activity, but no limitation of daily activity physically, psychologically and/or socioeconomically, or occasionally some limitation of both daily and extra activity
Poor	Significant limitation of both daily activity and extra activity, frequently physically, psychologically, and/or socioeconomically
Bad	Profound limitation of daily activity as well as extra activity or no daily activity feasible without assistance physically, psychologically, and/or socioeconomically

progression of the lymphedema and allow better treatment and prevention of complications associated with chronic lymphedema (e.g., infection).

Advances in diagnosis and clinical staging have allowed assessment of patient quality of life (QoL)[16,17] (Table 13.1). The ultimate goal of the contemporary management of lymphedema[7,11] is to improve the QoL by allowing better social interaction and improved functional and psychological well being.

New laboratory data have never been fully incorporated in a manner that might improve the traditional treatment approach, which is solely based on clinical judgment. Currently available staging methods for assessing treatment outcome and progression of lymphedema are still dependent on this "clinical" staging alone and fail to reflect all aspects of the chronic lymphedema.[18,19]

Therefore, we have developed a new staging system that includes laboratory data for better assessment of the dynamic, ever-changing status of chronic lymphedema beyond the limits of "clinical" staging.[1,2]

Initially, we attempted to incorporate lymphoscintigraphic data of chronic lymphedema patients into the conventional clinical–ISL–staging system. Integrating the clinical findings with those of laboratory findings (e.g., radionuclide lymphoscintigraphy) was too complicated and, in cases in which a significant mismatch between clinical and laboratory findings was observed, more confusion was added to the staging system.

We therefore proposed two separate staging systems, one clinical and the other using laboratory (lymphoscintigraphy) data. Together, these two staging systems classify the clinical manifestation and/or progress of the lymphedema more precisely based on two independent criteria (Table 13.2).

The new clinical staging classifies the clinical manifestation and progression of lymphedema using a four-stage system (clinical stages I through IV). Systemic and local clinical conditions associated with lymphedema are included along with QoL measures.

The limitations of the ISL system (three stages) based on clinical data, mostly local factors (edema and skin change), are by and large now fully compensated for by the inclusion of various systemic factors including sepsis, daily activity limitation, and QoL parameters – physical, functional, socioeconomic, and psychological, in addition to the lymphedema, making the staging system more appropriate (four stages).[20,21]

Table 13.2 Guideline criteria for the new clinical and laboratory staging system (I–IV)

Laboratory (lymphoscintigraphic) staging	Clinical staging	
Grade I (stage)	• Lymph node uptake (LN): decreased (±) • Dermal backflow (DBF): none (−) • Collateral lymphatics (CL): good visualization (+) • Main lymphatics (ML): decreased visualization (±) • Clearance of radioisotope from injection site (CR): decreased lymphatic transport (±)	• Edema (swelling): mild and/or easily reversible (+) • Skin change: none without dermatofibrosclerosis (DFS) (−) • Sepsis (systemic and/or local): none (−) • Daily activity limitation (DAL): no limitation (−) • Quality of life (QOL): good with minimal and/or occasional limitation (e.g., exercise, hobby) physically, psychologically and/or socioeconomically	Stage I

Grade II (stage)	• LN: decreased to none (−)
	• DBF: visualization (+)
	  * IIA – extent of DBF does not exceed half of each limb
	  * IIB – exceed half of each limb
	• CL: decreased visualization (±)
	• ML: poor to no visualization (±)
	• CR: more decreased (±)
		• Edema: moderate and/or reversible with effort (+)
		• Skin change: none to minimum without DFS (±)
		• Sepsis: none to occasional (±)
		• DAL: occasional and/or moderate limitation (±)
		• QOL: fair with moderate limitation physically, psychologically and/or socioeconomically
			Stage II

Grade III (stage)	• LN: no uptake (−) • DBF: visualization (+) • CL: poor visualization (−) • ML: no visualization (−) • CR: no clearance (−)	• Edema: moderate to severe and/or minimally reversible to irreversible (±) to (−) • Skin change: moderate with significant DFS (+) • Sepsis: common (+) – less than four times a year • DAL – frequent and significant (+) • QOL – poor with significant limitation	Stage III
Grade IV (stage)	• LN: none (−) • DBF: poor to no visualization (−) • CL: no visualization (−) • ML: no visualization (−) • CR: no clearance (−)	• Edema: severe and/or irreversible (−) • Skin change: severe with advanced DFS (╫) • Sepsis: very frequent (╫) – four times or more a year • DAL: constant and severe (╫) • QOL: bad with severe limitation	Stage IV

*Minimum two or more lymphoscintigraphic findings for laboratory staging and three or more clinical findings for clinical staging

Clinical stage is determined based on a total score of various clinical factors involved: edema (swelling), skin change, sepsis, daily activity limitation, and QoL (Table 13.2).

The subjective and objective findings of the local condition of the skin and subcutaneous soft tissue are assessed with the degree of skin change (dermatofibrosclerosis),[8,22] swelling, and natural reversibility.

The presence of local and/or systemic sepsis is assessed along with the presence of erysipelas and cellulitis. Functional limitation of daily activity as a result of the various subjective symptoms is assessed, including pain, uncomfortable sensory complaints (heaviness, tightness, numbness) and skin texture, feeling of the swollen limb, and difficulty wearing clothes because of the swelling (Table 13.2).

The evaluation of daily activity limitation was originally included in the QoL assessment with sepsis; however, this arrangement made interpretation of the clinical status more complicated. Therefore, both items were removed from the QoL assessment. Only a limited part of the physical condition was left for the QoL assessment, which incorporates the physical factors, including strength, movement, restriction of duties at home and work, and psychological and socioeconomical factors[1,2,20,21] (Table 13.2).

The QoL was evaluated by the impact of the lymphedema on the patient's physical, psychological, and socioeconomic limitations and well-being (Table 13.1). The physical factors for the QoL include strength of the affected limb, restriction of movement compared with the unaffected limb, as well as further additional impact on duties at home, work, and recreational activity. The psychological factors included feelings of depression, frustration, anger due to the lymphedema, and difficulty sleeping. The socioeconomic factors included difficulty with intimate relationships and social activities.[1,2]

This new clinical staging system could not separate and exclude the economic factors in the review of the QoL. We learned that patient economic issues have both social and psychological implications for overall patient well-being.

A separate laboratory staging system using four grades (stages) was developed based on lymphoscintigraphic findings of the lymphedema.[23-25]

Laboratory stage was determined by the sum total of various normal and abnormal findings on lymphoscintigraphy. These findings include the lymph node (LN) uptake status, the dermal backflow (DB) status, the collateral and main lymphatic visualization status, and the clearance of the radioisotope (CR) from the injection site as a parameter of the lymphatic transport ability[1,2] (Table 13.2).

Laboratory staging also has its limitations, although separate staging has significantly minimized the confusion associated with staging systems utilizing both clinical and laboratory data. Clinical staging combined with laboratory staging of chronic lymphedema is now useful in the treatment decision-making process, especially with regard to patients with advanced, chronic lymphedema requiring the timely addition of various reconstructive and ablative surgery where CDT has failed.[26-29]

Several revisions of the new staging systems have been made by a multidisciplinary team through the years, in order to make them more user-friendly.

Table 13.3 Demographic data of the initial clinical and laboratory stage of chronic lymphedema

Clinical (C) stage[a]		Laboratory (L) stage (grade I–IV)				
		I	II	III	IV	Unidentified[b]
I	77	53	19	1	0	4
II	98	6	66	24	1	1
III	29	0	2	15	10	2
IV	16	0	1	6	9	0
Total	220	59	88	46	20	7 (total)

220 patients, selected for a 4-year follow-up assessment (1995–2004)
[a]Based on the new four-stage system
[b]Unavailable for the comparison study

Table 13.4 Demographic data of the clinical (C) stage of chronic lymphedema in progress (deterioration or improvement)

Initial C-stage		Final (progress) C-stage				
Clinical stage		Clinical stage				
		I	II	III	IV	Further deterioration
I	77	70	6	1	0	0
II	98	3	81	11	2	1
III	29		2	14	12	1
IV	16			1	6	9

Four year follow-up evaluation of the complex decongestive physiotherapy (CDP)-based therapy results among 220 patients

Clinical Experience[1,2]

Among a total of 840 chronic lymphedema patients, 220 patients (85 primary and 135 secondary: 169 female and 51 male: mean age 41.3 years) were randomly selected during the period 1995 through 2004 to be evaluated using new clinical and laboratory staging systems (Table 13.2).

The patients underwent various combinations of standard CDT and compression therapy. Periodic clinical evaluation was made with an average interval of 6 months, but no longer than a year's interval. Lymphoscintigraphic study was performed on a annual basis, except in situations where recurrent sepsis was present. In these cases, an additional study was performed whenever feasible.

A comparison of clinical (C) stage and laboratory (L) stage during the initial diagnosis of 220 patients showed a broad overlap between the two different stagings; each group of patients with the same C stage, had various L stages, and patients with the same L stage also had a wide range of C stages. In general, a more advanced L-stage patient was more likely to have a more advanced C stage (Table 13.3).

Clinical implementation of this new staging system (Table 13.4) demonstrated reliable staging regarding both the progression of lymphedema and improvement of the clinical status following therapy.

Among 220 patients, 49 patients were appropriately classified by this new staging: 43 had deterioration and 6 showed improvement in their clinical stage. Deterioration of the clinical stage occurred despite adequate therapy in various C stages, but was more frequent among patients with advanced C stage, which was mainly related to decreased compliance.

The majority of patients who deteriorated at the same clinical stage were among the higher L-stage accompanying group: 5 out of the 7 in C-stage I who progressed had L-stage II (4/5) and III (2/5) initially, while 10 out of the 14 in C-stage II who progressed also had a higher L-stage III (9/10) and IV (1/10) from the beginning. Another 11 out of the 13 in C-stage III, who progressed, had L-stage IV or higher before treatment.

Maintenance of the initial clinical stage throughout the 4 year follow-up period was achieved in the majority of patients (171/220) with good to excellent compliance. Further improvement in the C stage was observed in a limited number of patients, particularly among the excellent compliance group with a good motivation, reversing the C stage (Table 13.4). Two out of the 3, converted from C-stage II to I, and showed a concomitant improvement in the L-stage from II to I.

This limited experience with a new, combined, clinical and laboratory staging system appears to be useful in guiding surgical therapy. Using the staging system allowed earlier determination of treatment failure in patients with minimal clinical improvement with CDT and allowed optimal timing of various surgical therapies during the appropriate stage of chronic lymphedema as a supplement to failed CDT.

Patients experiencing progression of lymphedema by C stage, despite maximum CDT, benefited from reconstructive surgery[7,11,29] when surgery was added during an earlier C stage, before a minimum of 2 years in order to become a surgical candidate when C-stage patients were also classified as having advanced L stage. The excisional surgery[26-29] was also added to the lymphedema in C-stage III and IV, based on the same principle.

The addition of laboratory staging in the development of this new clinical staging system has improved the overall predictability of treatment outcome with regard to clinical response to various therapies and progression of the lymphedema. A patient with an advanced L-stage, compared with lymphedema patients in the same C stage, demonstrated a tendency to progress faster in this study.

Therefore, L-stage has been used to help determine which lymphedema patients would benefit from different treatment modalities, particularly surgical therapy in order to prevent further disease deterioration.

Conclusion

The two separate staging systems described may be useful in establishing guidelines for the treatment of chronic lymphedema and in the decision-making process for supplemental surgical therapy. Further clinical implementation of the staging systems is still needed to prove its clinical efficacy, especially in defining the role of surgical therapy.

References

1. Lee BB, Bergan JJ. New clinical and laboratory staging systems to improve management of chronic lymphedema. *Lymphology*. 2005;38(3):122-129.
2. Lee BB. Classification and staging of lymphedema. In: Tredbar LL, Morgan CL, Lee BB, Simonian SJ, Blondeau B, eds. *Lymphedema-Diagnosis and Treatment*. London: Springer; 2008:21-30:chap 3.
3. International Society of Lymphology. The diagnosis and treatment of peripheral lymphedema. 2009 consensus document of the International Society of Lymphology. *Lymphology*. 2009; 42:51-60.
4. International Society of Lymphology Executive Committee. The diagnosis and treatment of peripheral lymphedema. *Lymphology*. 1995;28:113-117.
5. Lee BB, Villavicencio JL. Primary lymphedema and lymphatic malformation: are they the two sides of the same coin? *Eur J Vasc Endovasc Surg*. 2010;39:646-653.
6. Lee BB. Chronic lymphedema, no more stepchild to modern medicine! *Eur J Lymphology*. 2004;14(42):6-12.
7. Lee BB, Kim DI, Whang JH, Lee KW. Contemporary management of chronic lymphedema – personal experiences. *Lymphology*. 2002;35(Suppl):450-455.
8. Olszewski WL. Episodic dermatolymphangioadenitis (DLA) in patients with lymphedema of the lower extremities before and after administration of benzathine penicillin: a preliminary study. *Lymphology*. 1996;29:126-131.
9. Hwang JH, Lee KW, Chang DY, et al. Complex physical therapy for lymphedema. *J Korean Acad Rehabil Med*. 1998;22(1):224-229.
10. Szolnoky G, Lakatos B, Keskeny T, Dobozy A. Advantage of combined decongestive lymphatic therapy over manual lymph drainage: a pilot study. *Lymphology*. 2002;35(Suppl): 277-282.
11. Lee BB. Current issue in management of chronic lymphedema: personal reflection on an experience with 1065 patients. Commentary. *Lymphology*. 2005;38:28.
12. Case TC, Witte CL, Witte MH, et al. Magnetic resonance imaging in human lymphedema: comparison with lymphangioscintigraphy. *Magn Reson Imaging*. 1992;10:549-558.
13. Yeo UC, Lee ES, Lee BB. Ultrasonographic evaluation of the lymphedema. *Ann Dermatol*. 1997;9(2):126-131.
14. Ketterings C, Zeddeman S. Use of the C-scan in evaluation of peripheral lymphedema. *Lymphology*. 1997;30:49-62.
15. Szuba A, Shin WS, Strauss HW, Rockson S. The third circulation: radionuclide lymphoscintigraphy in the evaluation of lymphedema. *J Nucl Med*. 2003;44(1):43-57.
16. Azevedo WF, Boccardo F, Zilli A, et al. A reliable and valid quality of life in patients with lymphedema – version of the SF-36. *Lymphology*. 2002;35(suppl):177-180.
17. Launois R, Mègnigbêto AC, Pocquet K, Alliot F. A specific quality of life scale in upper limb lymphedema: the ULL-27 questionnaire. *Lymphology*. 2002;35(suppl):181-187.
18. Nieto S. Stages of lymphedema according to correlation among pathophysiology, clinical features, imaging and morphology of the affected limbs. *Lymphology*. 2002;35(suppl):163-167.
19. Bruna J, Miller AJ, Beninson J. The clinical grading and simple classification of lymphedema. *Lymphology*. 2002;35(suppl):160-162.
20. de Godoy JMP, Braile DM, de Godoy MF, et al. Quality of life and peripheral lymphedema. *Lymphology*. 2002;35:72.

21. Johansson K, Ohlsson K, Ingvar C, et al. Factors associate with the development of arm lymphedema following breast cancer treatment: a match pair case-control study. *Lymphology.* 2002;35:59.
22. Foldi E. Prevention of dermatolymphangioadenitis by combined physiotherapy of the swollen arm after treatment for breast cancer. *Lymphology.* 1996;29:48-49.
23. Hwang JH, Lee KW, Lee BB. Improvement of lymphatic function after complex physical therapy. *J Korean Acad Rehabil Med.* 1998;22(3):698-704.
24. Choi JY, Hwang JH, Park JM, et al. Risk assessment of dermatolymphangioadenitis by lymphoscintigraphy in patients with lower extremity lymphedema. *Korean J Nucl Med.* 1999;33(2):143-151.
25. Hwang JH, Kwon JY, Lee KW, et al. Changes in lymphatic function after complex physical therapy for lymphedema. *Lymphology.* 1999;32:15-21.
26. Kim DI, Huh S, Lee SJ, Hwang JH, Kim YI, Lee BB. Excision of subcutaneous tissue and deep muscle fascia for advanced lymphedema. *Lymphology.* 1998;31:190-194.
27. Huh SH, Kim DI, Hwang JH, Lee BB. Excisional surgery in chronic advanced lymphedema. *Surg Today.* 2003;34:434-435.
28. Lee BB. Surgical management of lymphedema. In: Tredbar LL, Morgan CL, Lee BB, Simonian SJ, Blondeau B, eds. *Lymphedema: Diagnosis and Treatment.* London: Springer; 2008:55-63:chap 6.
29. Lee BB, Kim YW, Kim DI, Hwang JH, Laredo J, Neville R. Supplemental surgical treatment to end stage (stage IV–V) of chronic lymphedema. *Int Angiol.* 2008;27(5):389-395.

Chapter 14
Early Diagnosis in Latent Phase

Leigh C. Ward

Lymphedema is typically characterized by the time of onset (staging) and the severity of the symptoms (grading). Various staging schemes have been proposed, but increasingly most use a four-stage scale: stage 0, a latent or subclinical phase when swelling is not evident, although lymphatic insufficiency is presumed; stage I, accumulation of tissue fluid that generally resolves with elevation of the affected limb with minimal swelling (<20% increase); stage II, when elevation fails to reduce a moderate amount of swelling (20–40% increase) and pitting edema is present; and stage III, irreversible, severe (>40% increase) swelling is present and the tissue is fibrotic.[1] Despite the absence of outward clinical signs of lymphedema in the latent stage, lymphoscintigraphy or lymphangiography shows disrupted lymphatic function.[2] Detection of patients in the latent phase has been recognized as important for identification of those in whom advanced lymphedema may occur.[3] This enables therapeutic intervention at the earliest opportunity, which has been shown to be more effective than intervention after lymphedema has become established,[4] but this approach is predicated on the ability to detect lymphedema in the latent phase.

A wide variety of objective methods, other than clinical examination, are available for the detection of lymphedema.[5] However, many are either technologically complex (e.g., magnetic resonance imaging [MRI] or dual energy X-ray absorptiometry [DEXA]), invasive, and involve a radiation hazard (e.g., isotopic lymphoscintigraphy) or are otherwise not suitable for routine clinical use because of cost, e.g., computed tomography (CT). The most commonly used techniques for lymphedema detection are those based on detecting an increase in volume due to the presence of edema and include water displacement, opto-electrical perometery, bioelectrical impedance and circumferential measurements. Unfortunately, because, by definition, the latent phase of lymphedema is that prior to detectable swelling, the utility of such techniques is questionable. Nevertheless, such methods are currently

L.C. Ward
School of Chemistry and Molecular Biosciences,
The University of Queensland, Queensland, Australia

B.-B. Lee et al. (eds.), *Lymphedema*,
DOI 10.1007/978-0-85729-567-5_14, © Springer-Verlag London Limited 2011

Table 14.1 Accuracy and precision of methods for assessment of lymphedema of the limbs

Method	Accuracy	Precision and reproducibility[a]	References
Impedance	<±1%	ICC>0.94 (15 Ω, ~4%)	8,9
Water displacement	±0.5%	ICC>0.94 (81 mL, ~4%)	10-13
Perometry	±2%	ICC>0.99 (81 mL, ~4%)	8,10,13
Tape measurement	±1%	ICC>0.95 (85 mL, ~4%)	8,12,13

ICC intra-class correlation coefficient
[a]Absolute values and approximate percentage of measured value

accepted as the best measurement options to detect pre-clinical lymphedema.[6] Stout Gergich and colleagues[4] defined a 3% change in volume from a baseline or pre-operative measurement in the case of secondary lymphedema as a diagnostic criterion for subclinical lymphedema. They further suggested that, in the absence of perometry, (which was used in their study), other tools that assess swelling, such as water displacement, bioimpedance or girth measurements, may be equally useful. Unfortunately, there are no universally recognized diagnostic criteria for each of these methods and equivalence between instruments has not been defined. Furthermore, assessment of lymphedema lags behind many other branches of science where standardization of measurement has long been recognized as the key to quality control and assurance. Preference should be given to methods of assessment that meet accepted standards for accuracy, precision, sensitivity, and specificity of measurement, and that are practical and applicable for routine clinical use.[7]

Accuracy can be difficult to assess because the "true" value, i.e., the smallest change in the measured parameter (volume, impedance, or girth) presumptive of lymphedema, is unknown. It is necessary to resort to using "phantoms" of precisely known characteristics, such as cylinders of known volume or electronic circuits of known impedance. Precision or reproducibility of measurement is more easily determined from repeated measurements, using either phantoms or human subjects. Published data, summarized in Table 14.1, suggests that the various methods used to assess early-stage lymphedema perform similarly with an accuracy of about ±1% and reproducibility of approximately ±4% standard error of measurement.

Of greater importance for the detection of sub-clinical lymphedema than absolute accuracy or precision is the limit of detection; the magnitude of difference for a given measurement parameter that can be reliably detected. This is calculated as the minimal detectable change (MDC) and is given by 1.96 ±2 SEM (standard error of measurement).

The MDC for volume measurements is approximately 140 mL, assuming a typical SEM of 50 mL for volumetric measurement. This can be compared with the generally accepted inter-limb difference of 200 mL used as a detection threshold for breast cancer-related lymphedema (BCRL). Czernieic et al.[8] have shown that a minimum of a 120-mL change is required to account for normal fluctuation in limb volume in the absence of lymphedema to be confident of an effect while Stout Gergich and colleagues[4] have recommended a 3% change in perometrically measured volume from a pre-lymphedema baseline measurement as a threshold for lymphedema treatment intervention. With respect to impedance measurements, similar calculations suggest a detection limit of approximately 40 Ω or an inter-limb

Table 14.2 Comparison of potential technologies for the early detection of lymphedema

	Cost	Portability	Ease of use	Time involved	Patient convenience	Operator skills
Impedance	Low to high	High	High	Low	High	Low
Perometry	Very high	None to medium	High	Low	High	Low
Tape	Very low	High	High	High	Medium to high	Low
Water displacement	Very low	Low	Medium to high	Medium	Low	Low

ratio difference of 0.04 in BCRL.[8] Again, larger change is required (a ratio of 0.08) to account for normal fluctuation of approximately 4.8%.[8] We should, however, question the relevance of this to the detection of pre-clinical lymphedema. By definition, lymphedema in the latent phase is *prior to* a detectable change in volume. On this basis, simple volumetric measurements, irrespective of how small the limit of detection, can never be used for lymphedema assessment at this early stage. Equally, bioimpedance techniques are not suitable either, since the magnitude of changes in impedance equate to changes of comparable magnitude in volume.

A more pragmatic approach is to assess promising technologies on the basis of their practicality in use and sensitivity and specificity for detection at the earliest opportunity. Surprisingly, relatively few studies have been undertaken. Despite detection thresholds such as a 200-mL volume difference being widely promulgated, the evidence base for their validity is sparse and sensitivity and specificity analyses are few in number.[7] Box et al.[14] demonstrated a 100% confirmation of BCRL in women when using a 200 mL detection threshold, but this cannot be classed as latent phase lymphedema. Hayes et al.[15] showed, again in women with BCRL, that compared with bioimpedance, set at 100%, circumferential measurements of the arm had good specificity (88–100%), but much worse sensitivity (35%). The data of Cornish et al.[16] are perhaps most persuasive that bioimpedance, at least, may be capable of detecting changes indicative of impending lymphedema at an early stage. In a prospective study, BCRL was detectable by bioimpedance up to 10 months prior to clinical confirmation. This study has yet to be confirmed and extended to other forms of lymphedema, but provides encouragement that using relatively simple non-invasive technology lymphedema may be detectable in the latent phase or at least prior to observable changes in volume. The sensitivity of impedance assessment over other diagnostic modalities is supported by the theory on which the technology is based. The impedance that is measured is solely that of the extracellular fluid, which includes the lymph.[17] In contrast, simple volume measurement, be it by water displacement, perometry or tape measure, is that of the total tissue and may be confounded by changes in tissue compartments other than lymph, e.g., adipose tissue mass.

Detection of latent phase lymphedema implies screening of at-risk individuals. It is therefore important that the instruments adopted for assessment are fit for this purpose. Ease of use and cost are important considerations in the uptake of technologies into routine clinical practice. All of the methods referred to above have their advantages and disadvantages (Table 14.2). A tape measure is inexpensive to purchase and is, undoubtedly, easy to use, but its use is time-consuming. Perometry is also easy to use and rapid to perform, but initial equipment costs are high. Water displacement is inexpensive, but may not always be suitable, for example, where there are infections or wounds. Impedance is rapid to perform, with modest cost (dependent upon instrumentation), but its utility for all forms of lymphedema has yet to be established.

In conclusion, detection of lymphedema in the latent phase poses significant challenges. The definition of latent phase or sub-clinical lymphedema that it is prior to appearance of swelling appears to preclude many of the methods currently used to detect lymphedema. Other than technologies that measure lymphatic function, such as lymphoscintigraphy, covered elsewhere in this volume, tools in current use without exception measure volume either directly or indirectly as in the case of impedance. Nonetheless, the routine use of these techniques is of clinical value, particularly where change compared with baseline measures are available, as shown by the work of Stout Gergich.[4] Maximum benefit will be gained by routine surveillance of those at risk of developing lymphedema. At present, the tool most suited for this purpose appears to be impedance in that it is suitable for home use by those at risk of or with incipient lymphedema.[18] It would be remiss, however, not to additionally acknowledge the importance of self-report by those with lymphedema. Objective assessments in current use may simply not be measuring the correct parameters that characterize the subtle early changes in tissue morphology and physiology that occur in the latent phase. These may, however, be apparent to the patient. Much additional research into the biology of the development of early-stage lymphedema is required to allow us to determine the optimal detection strategy.

References

1. International Society of Lymphology. The diagnosis and treatment of peripheral lymphedema. Consensus document of the International Society of Lymphology. *Lymphology*. 2003;36:84-91.
2. Bagheri S, Ohlin K, Olsson G, Broroson H. Tissue tonometry before and after liposuction of arm lymphedema following breast cancer. *Lymphat Res Biol*. 2005;3:66-80.
3. Campisi C, Boccardo F. Lymphedema and microsurgery. *Microsurgery*. 2002;22:74-80.
4. Stout Gergich NL, Pfalzer LA, McGarvey C, Springer B, Gerber LH, et al. Preoperative assessment enables the early detection and successful treatment of lymphedema. *Cancer*. 2008; 112:2809-2819.
5. Rockson SG. Lymphedema. *Am J Med*. 2001;110:288-295.
6. Piller N, Keeley V, Ryan T, Hayes S, Ridner S. Early detection: a strategy to reduce risk and severity? *J Lymphoedema*. 2009;4(1):89-95.
7. Ward LC. Is BIS ready for prime time as the gold standard measure? *J Lymphoedema*. 2009;4(2):52-56.
8. Czerniec SA, Ward LC, Refshauge KM, et al. Assessment of breast cancer related arm lymphedema – comparison of physical measurement methods and self-report. *Cancer Invest*. 2010;28:54-62.
9. Oldham NM. Overview of bioelectrical impedance analyzers. *Am J Clin Nutr*. 1996;64: 405S-412S.
10. Man IOW, Markland KL, Morrissey MC. The validity and reliability of the Perometer in evaluating human knee volume. *Clin Physiol Funct Imaging*. 2004;24:352-358.

11. Lette J. A simple and innovative device to measure arm volume at home for patients with lymphedema after breast cancer. *J Clin Oncol.* 2006;24:5434-5440.
12. Taylor R, Jayasinghe UW, Koelmeyer L, Ung O, Boyages J. Reliability and validity of arm volume measurements for assessment of lymphedema. *Phys Ther.* 2006;86:205-214.
13. Deltombe T, Jamart J, Recloux S, Legrand C, Vandenbroeck N, et al. Reliability and limits of agreement of circumferential, water displacement, and optoelectronic volumetry in the measurement of upper limb lymphedema. *Lymphology.* 2007;40:26-34.
14. Box RC, Reul-Hirche HM, Bullock-Saxton JE, Furnival CM. Physiotherapy after breast cancer surgery: results of a randomised controlled study to minimise lymphoedema. *Breast Cancer Res Treat.* 2002;75:51-64.
15. Hayes S, Cornish B, Newman B. Comparison of methods to diagnose lymphoedema among breast cancer survivors: 6-month follow-up. *Breast Cancer Res Treat.* 2005;89:221-226.
16. Cornish BH, Chapman M, Hirst C, Mirolo B, Bunce IH, et al. Early diagnosis of lymphedema using multiple frequency bioimpedance. *Lymphology.* 2001;34:2-11.
17. Ward LC, Kilbreath SL, Cornish BH. Bioelectrical impedance analysis for early detection of lymphoedema. In: Weissleder H, Schuchhardt C, eds. *Lymphedema Diagnosis and Therapy.* 4th ed. Essen: Viavital Verlag Gmbh Publ; 2008:502-517:chap 15.
18. Ridner SH, Dietrich MS, Deng J, Bonner CM, Kidd N. Bioelectrical impedance for detecting upper limb lymphedema in non laboratory settings. *Lymphat Res Biol.* 2009;7:11-15.

Chapter 15
Review of National and International Consensuses on Chronic Lymphedema

Michael J. Bernas

Consensus Documents

Consensus documents are produced in an effort to help move a field forward and/or to offer to patients the best evidence/expert-based treatment approaches. The results can be positive, by promoting clearly beneficial options in the face of multiple choices, but they can also be harmful by limiting therapeutic options and stifling research for future advances. Some physicians, policy-makers, and patients desire documents with clear unalterable protocols, whereas an equal cohort exists that believe that these documents confine and distort the practice of medicine. An inherent problem that will not easily be resolved is that these types of guidelines are based on studies of populations of patients and generate protocols appropriate for a range of patients. However, each patient brings his or her own individual constellation of issues and findings, rendering it impossible for a consensus to address each item. Therefore, sound clinical judgment and modification will always be required.

A pitfall of consensus or guideline documents is the delays involved in generating the documents and the rapidity of changes in the field (particularly when based on imperfect data). An analysis of large systematic reviews has shown that there is a need for frequent updating. A recent study evaluating 100 systematic reviews (a median of 13 studies with 2,633 participants each) demonstrated indications for updating of 15% in 1 year and 23% within 2 years with a median change-free survival of 5.5 years for all studies.[1] Supporting this are groups like the American College of Physicians, with strong rules for clinical practice guidelines, such as any guidelines that are not updated within 5 years are considered invalid and are withdrawn.[2] The type and quality of evidence can also be problematic in consensus or guideline documents. A recent large study from the American College of

M.J. Bernas
Department of Surgery, University of Arizona
College of Medicine, Tucson, AZ, USA

B.-B. Lee et al. (eds.), *Lymphedema*,
DOI 10.1007/978-0-85729-567-5_15, © Springer-Verlag London Limited 2011

Cardiology and American Heart Association, reviewing practice guidelines from 1984 to 2008, demonstrated that only 11% of the studies reported levels of evidence noted as level A (the highest), and of those documents with revision or update by 2008, there was a 48% increase in the number of recommendations.[3]

An additional problem is the lack of appropriate and well-designed studies. What if there is no, or very limited, high-quality evidence upon which to base these clinical decisions? Because no trial can answer all possible questions about a treatment, different experts will interpret trial results differently, and it soon becomes clear that the "evidence" is subject to "opinion."[4] The challenge is how to move beyond poor evidence-based data and opinion-based data to treating the patients in the real world. Finally, conflict of interest and expert commercial/promotional bias in the development of the specific guidelines is an increasingly troublesome problem. Some groups, such as the American College of Physicians, have very clear and detailed rules to avoid conflict and bias,[2] but this is lacking in many of the consensus or guideline documents.

Consensus Documents in the Treatment of Lymphedema

Because there are no definitive studies that have been published concerning the best treatment for patients with lymphedema, we are left with an ever-growing collection of studies with lower levels of evidence. These, combined with expert opinions, largely shape the consensus documents that have been produced.

Just as in clinical medicine, where every treatment must be evaluated on a cost–benefit ratio, consensus documents concerning lymphedema must undergo cost-benefit analysis. They can be beneficial in setting minimum standards, gathering and analyzing multiple and disparate research studies to produce treatment justification, and for education of providers, payers, and consumers. But they can also be harmful by stifling innovative research into new treatments and promoting defensive medicine, as well as creating the danger of treating patients by population-based care instead of individualized, personal care.

No double-blind controls for the physical treatments for lymphedema exist or may even be possible. Some blinding can be used for measurement personnel, but blinding of the therapist or, in most cases, of the patient, to the treatment is not feasible or possible. The field also reflects a theme common to many other clinical trials, in that the methods are tested against nothing or a placebo, and only rarely against a well-recognized, accepted standard. It is likely that such trials will never be completed because of logistical considerations and also lack of funding to support head-to-head trials of multiple currently used therapies. Despite the existence of some clinics that have treated thousands or even tens of thousands of patients over years, we have no published studies of this magnitude that would lend considerable weight regarding evaluation of methods.

We are left with informative, but inadequate data ranging from small pilot trials to larger trials that suffer from some design defects. This lack of strong evidence-based information has led us to search and pursue meta-analyses for answers (realizing that the underlying studies are inadequate), in an attempt to avoid opinion-based medicine. Unfortunately, in the field of treatment for lymphedema, we have not yet advanced to this level, and we still need to rely on the opinions of experts from around the globe. Therefore, the best documents are those that are generated by wide-reaching groups of experienced clinicians and researchers who frequently meet to review, argue, and revise their consensus opinions (mindful of conflict or bias issues) with the understanding that these guidelines are provided as the best ideas on how to treat and move forward despite the limitations in the field and the specific context of the patient.

International Society of Lymphology

The first document to examine is by far the oldest, and also has the most recent update: the Consensus Document on the Diagnosis and Treatment of Peripheral Lymphedema of the International Society of Lymphology.[5] This document represents the centerpiece of current views on diagnosis and treatment of peripheral lymphedema from the broad international perspective of leading lymphologists from the 42 nations represented by the members of the International Society of Lymphology (ISL). It has been extensively cited and used throughout the world, and it is broad in scope reflective of the ISL membership, their national origins, and also the variety of patients with lymphedema.

The document coalesced from an initial thesis prepared by Professors Michael and Etelka Földi and developed into a working document at the 1994 ISL Executive Committee meeting at the Földiklinik in Hinterzarten, Germany. Following several rounds of reviews/criticisms/edits by Executive Committee members and other ISL experts, it was developed for international publication in 1995.[6] It has been debated openly at each biennial International Congress of Lymphology meetings since, at regional and national ISL affiliate meetings and openly at Executive Committee Meetings from 2000 to 2010, resulting in major published revisions in 2001, 2003, and most recently, in 2009.[5] Thus, the ISL Consensus Document reflects the evolving global consensus underlying the theory and practice of lymphology, highlighting diagnosis and assessment, a wide range of treatments, and acknowledging and promoting areas of research and exploring uncertainties and unknowns, from which future advances will emerge. The document does list and briefly explain many therapeutic techniques utilized worldwide by multi-specialty physicians and other health care providers and proposes that in the optimal setting the combination of skin care, manual lymph drainage, compression bandaging, garments, and exercise is a strongly supported multi-modal choice. This regimen is noted as CPT-combined physiotherapy, but it is also known by related names such as complete or complex physiotherapy (CPT), complex decongestive therapy (CDT), complex decongestive physiotherapy (CDPT), lymphatic therapy (LT), or decongestive lymphatic therapy (DLT) among others.

The ISL document is a useful tool and not a set of strict protocols, algorithms, or best practice mandates with exhaustive references or meta-analyses. Such an approach would rigidly define the boundaries of quality care for specific forms or location of lymphedema without consideration of complicating features or complex syndromes and local practice conditions. This document is not perfect or ideal, but it strives to be inclusive of ISL members worldwide and looks to the future to improve assessment by combining imaging and physical examination for phenotyping; incorporate the genetic and psychosocial context of the patients; recognize and appreciate many available therapeutic options including those that may be country-/region-/resource-specific; and promote a research agenda to advance understanding, diagnosis, and treatment. Special features of this document are the recognition and statement of the need for more epidemiological studies of incidence, prevalence, and risk factors; encouragement of database registries; promotion of studies on prevention; the advancement of imaging technologies; and the promise of molecular lymphology and genomic/proteomic studies.

International Lymphedema Framework

The International Lymphedema Framework published their Best Practice guidelines in 2006[7] as the culmination of a multi-year process in the United Kingdom (UK). The document was generated by UK clinicians, therapists, researchers, industry, and patient participants and was reviewed and/or endorsed by a wide international group of experts and Societies. It is written rather as a guideline for care in a clinical setting with added depth because of a diligent research review and is also valuable for policy review in those countries that have health care systems that match the UK model. Its strength is found in the extensive literature review and grading of evidence for treatment modalities, the inclusion of references culled from a growing volume of literature, and detailed illustrations and flowcharts that may be useful in the clinic for quick reference or for policy makers for quick study. The document confirms the lack of substantial published data for many of the treatment modalities and the great need for more investigations with none of the recommendations reaching their level A (clear research evidence) support and most being noted as limited supporting research (level B) or experienced common sense judgment (level C). The framers envision that the document will be updated approximately every 5 years, and such efforts are currently underway with affiliated groups such as the American Lymphedema Framework. What these changes will bring about is unclear at this point, since each country will have a different focus to bring to the Framework. As an example, the original document described the manual massage and compression as separate treatment modalities while in the United States and many other places around the world (e.g., Germany) the most recommended treatment (as also supported by the ISL Consensus Document) is the combination of the manual massage and compression bandaging (i.e., CPT).

Italian

The guidelines from the Italian Society were published in 2004[8] following an open session at the University Master Course on the guidelines for the diagnosis and treatment of lymphedema in Genoa, Italy. The group consisted of primarily Italian physicians and healthcare professionals and also patients and a few international guests from Belgium and Korea. The guidelines have not yet been updated, and they are patterned after the ISL document with customization for the Italian Society. The guidelines are, therefore, similar to the ISL with 143 references added and recommendations for each section. The document describes CPT along with other treatment modalities (i.e., pneumatic compression and pharmacology). Here also, the lack of optimal studies is documented with only the diagnostic imaging section recommended as Level A evidence. The guidelines do include additional data concerning angiodysplasias and neonatal lymphatic dysplasias along with an expanded section on surgical treatments.

Latin American

The Latin American Consensus on the Management of Lymphedema was published in 2004 following a meeting in March 2003 in Buenos Aires specifically for the development of a consensus. Over 30 clinical experts from Latin America were in attendance, with the document undergoing final editing by J. Ciucci.[9] It has not been updated. The document is similar to the ISL document in that it does not include references or recommendations, but it does not have the same depth and is not as all-encompassing. As with the Framework document, it also does not link massage and bandaging into the more commonly accepted CPT. It includes strongly written sections on pneumatic compression and pharmacotherapy that are uniquely reflective of the Latin American consensus and also has valuable sections on multidisciplinary treatment and psychotherapy.

Australian

This document is the result of committee meetings designed to provide the government with a review of the current practices and the near future in Australia. Collected from data up to 2004, it was finalized and approved in 2005 and published in 2006.[10] It includes a detailed literature review with a wide breadth of the field including diagnosis and assessment as well as treatment options. The substantial document tends to appear overly bureaucratic, at 105 pages in length with references included. It reports that there are no Australian standards established for the treatment and reaffirms the lack of high-quality evidence or randomized controlled trials for supporting treatments. However, it does state that there is reasonable evidence to indicate that early, accurate diagnosis followed by the routine use of prescription compression garments and physical therapy can provide short-term improvements. It further describes CPT as having favorable outcomes, but that evidence from trials is inconsistent and additional data are required to define an optimal strategy.

American Cancer Society

The American Cancer Society supported a Lymphedema Workshop in 1998 focusing on breast cancer treatment-related lymphedema. One of the workgroups focused on the diagnosis and management of lymphedema and produced a document resulting from the workgroup.[11] It was a review of current opinions of experts at the meeting that is now somewhat dated and only focused on breast cancer-related lymphedema. It has not been updated. The workshop addressed the issue of treatment and supported the view that CPT is the best approach for treatment. It also mentions the issue of the various names for this treatment and suggests a more universal "decongestive lymphatic therapy" for the future. It is interesting that, despite both this and the ISL document being published early, subsequent documents have failed to combine the massage and bandaging as CPT.

National Lymphedema Network

The National Lymphedema Network based in the United States has published a series of position papers concerning various aspects of lymphedema. One such paper concerns treatment of lymphedema,[12] is produced by the Medical Advisory Committee of the organization, and has undergone revision with the current version of the document last approved in August 2006. It does include references and is without recommendations. The document is more reflective of the treatment options in the United States and is focused and concise enough to be appropriate for multiple users. The treatment focus is on CPT, which it covers well, and it does review primarily the precautions related to pneumatic compression, surgical treatments, and pharmaceutical options.

Summary

In the field of treatment for lymphedema, these multiple documents serve as proof that there does not yet exist a comprehensive treatment approach for all patients in all nations (and that likely none will ever exist). There is also clearly a need for large-scale trials and for those to compare multiple treatments (and combinations).

Until these studies are completed or until some large patient series is published, the field will struggle for solid evidence. Diligence will be needed to confront efforts to lump all relevant, but poorly randomized controlled trials into one all-encompassing database for which multiple metanalyses will be run to determine the best odds ratios for treatments. The field is striving to achieve the goal of evidence-based medicine (despite the caveats of its danger) in order to offer the best treatment to our patients while at the same time being aware of pitfalls such as *Eminence*-based medicine (opinions of senior physicians, which can sometimes be a substitute for evidence) or *Vehemence*-based medicine (where the substitution of volume for evidence clouds the issues).[13]

Concluding Thought

This is how doctors and patients make shared decisions – by considering expert guidelines, weighing why other experts may disagree with the guidelines, and then customizing the therapy to the individual. With respect to "best practices," prudent doctors think, not just follow, and informed patients consider and then choose, not just comply.

Jerome Groopman and Pamela Hartzband[14]

Disclosure

The Author is the Executive Editor of the journal *Lymphology*. He has been a member of the Executive Committee of the International Society of Lymphology, and functions as the point person responsible for collecting criticisms, comments, and suggestions for editing into revisions of the Society's Consensus Document. He is also a member of the American Lymphedema Framework Project and the National Lymphedema Network.

References

1. Shojania KG, Sampson M, Ansari MT, Ji J, Doucette S, Moher D. How quickly do systematic reviews go out of date? A survival analysis. *Ann Intern Med*. 2007;147:224-233.
2. Qaseem A, Snow V, Owens DK, Shekelle P. The development of clinical practice guidelines and guidance statements of the American College of Physicians: summary of methods. *Ann Intern Med*. 2010;153:194-199.
3. Tricoci P, Allen JM, Kramer JM, Califf RM, Smith SC. Scientific evidence underlying the ACC/AHA clinical practice guidelines. *JAMA*. 2009;301:831-841.
4. Hampton JR. Evidence-based medicine, opinion-based medicine, and real-world medicine. *Perspect Biol Med*. 2002;45:549-568.
5. International Society of Lymphology. The diagnosis and treatment of peripheral lymphedema: 2009 consensus document. *Lymphology*. 2009;42(2):51-60.

6. International Society of Lymphology Executive Committee. The diagnosis and treatment of peripheral lymphedema. *Lymphology*. 1995;28:113-117.
7. International Lymphoedema Framework Project. *Best Practice for the Management of Lymphoedema: International Consensus*. London: Medical Education Partnership Ltd; 2006.
8. Campisi C, Michelini S, Boccardo F. Guidelines of the societá italiana di linfangiologia. *Lymphology*. 2004;37:165-184.
9. Ciucci JL. 1st Latin American consensus on the management of lymphedema. *Phlebolymphology*. 2004;44:258-264.
10. Australian Health Ministers' Advisory Council Report. A review of current practices and future directions in the diagnosis, prevention and treatment of lymphoedema in Australia 2006. Available at: http://www.msac.gov.au/internet/msac/publishing.nsf/Content/Review+of+lymp hoedema+in+Australia accessed 05/11/2011.
11. Rockson SG, Miller LT, Senie R, et al. American Cancer Society lymphedema workshop. Workgroup III: diagnosis and management of lymphedema. *Cancer*. 1998;83(12):2882-2885.
12. National Lymphedema Network Medical Advisory Committee. Position statement of the treatment of lymphedema [document on the Internet]. National Lymphedema Network; 2011 [updated 2011, February]. Available at: http://www.lymphnet.org/pdfDocs/nlntreatment.pdf accessed 05/11/2011.
13. Isaacs D, Fitzgerald D. Seven alternatives to evidence based medicine. *BMJ*. 1999;319:1618.
14. Groopman J, Hartzband P. Sorting fact from fiction on health care. *The Wall Street Journal*. August 31, 2009. Available at: http://online.wsj.com/article/SB100014240529702037066045 74378542143891778.html accessed 05/11/2011.

Chapter 16
Differential Diagnosis – General Considerations

Neil B. Piller

Introduction

To gain an accurate differential diagnosis of a limb in a presenting patient, a parallel medical and lymphedema assessment should be made. There are strong benefits when the assessment/diagnosis of lymphedema is able to be established early because, currently, noninvasive bio-impedance-spectroscopy (BIS) can detect lymphedema in its "subclinical" form (International Society of Lymphology "stage 0"), enabling earlier targeted treatment and better outcomes.

Bio-impedance spectroscopy can also be used in the differential diagnosis of lymphedemas from myxedemas and lipedemas, but it has not yet shown to be able to separate primary from secondary lymphedemas, or lymphedemas from conditions exhibiting fluid changes, such as phlebedema or phlebolymphedema. Details of BIS will be presented later in this book.

This guiding chapter is intended to generate confidence in treatment selection and direction derived from an early, accurate, and differential diagnosis. It is based around a scenario of a patient who presents with a swollen limb (either in whole or in part) subsequent to surgery and radiotherapy as part of treatment for cancer, and on the frequently mistaken assumption that the swelling is lymphedema.

There are many etiologies for a swollen limb, and exploring these is crucial, not only from the point of view of an accurate diagnosis, but also because these etiologies often require differing targeting, treatment sequencing, and treatments. From the patient's perspective, knowing that the swelling is not lymphedema, and is not likely to lead to it, can provide significant relief from the fear of this manifestation as a potential sign of the return of the cancer and from the fear that the swelling may persist for life.

N.B. Piller
Lymphoedema Assessment Clinic, Department of Surgery, School of Medicine,
Flinders University and Medical Centre, Bedford Park, SA, Australia

B.-B. Lee et al. (eds.), *Lymphedema*,
DOI 10.1007/978-0-85729-567-5_16, © Springer-Verlag London Limited 2011

For those without lymphedema, but for whom the risk is present, the onset of clinically overt lymphedema is likely to be preventable through this recognition, with a targeted treatment response to the early signs, through education and through some relatively simple management options. It is in this early detection and screening that the general practitioner and specialist have an important role to play.

For those who present with a swollen limb, the first task is to determine the reason for the swelling, and to determine whether it is associated with a failure of the lymphatic system or is due to some other underlying problem. Once the lymphatic factors are determined, the next step is to explore if there are likely to be underlying primary malformations or secondary change and then to target treatment and management, all of which is dealt with in detail in later chapters.

Differential Diagnosis: Other Reasons for a Swollen Limb

The first part of the assessment should be a medical one, with the aim of excluding other causes of swelling before the nature of the lymphedema is explored.[1]

When a patient presents with a swollen arm, then it is likely to be lymphedema unless there are issues of axillary venous stenosis or vascular entrapment in scar tissue, both of which are straightforward to determine. However, there can be many reasons for a patient's presentation with a swollen leg. Ideally, these should be identified and an attempt made to treat or manage them prior to dealing with the lymphatic problems, particularly when they may be having an impact on the load upon a compromised lymphatic system.[2]

Edema can reflect generalized (but sometimes regional) accumulation of vascular pericapillary fluids associated with increased intracapillary pressure within the lower extremities, due to a dysfunctional lymphatic system caused by chronic venous insufficiency. Edema is associated with acute DVT, post-thrombotic syndrome, arthritis, Baker's cyst for unilateral swellings, and congestive heart failure, chronic venous insufficiency (CVI), stasis edema, renal or hepatic dysfunction, hypoproteinemia, hypothyroidism, medication-induced edemas and lipedemas for bilateral swellings.

Phlebedema, the excessive accumulation of fluids due to lymphatic overload that is a consequence of the additional load imposed by a failing vascular system when the lymphatic system is still healthy and capable of working optimally.[3] Examples are early-stage chronic venous insufficiency, often associated with problems of vascular fragility, inflammation of the blood vessel walls, and venous thrombosis. The term phlebo-lymphedema, perhaps represents a semantic nuance, but there may be a need to understand the pathogenesis, i.e., which came first, lymphatic (lympho-phlebedema) or vascular dysfunction (phlebo-lymphedema)?

On most occasions, the lymphatic system is structurally and functionally normal and can manage a large additional load of fluids, such as that which occurs when there is a compromised venous system; however, continuing excessive loads above the maximum transport capacity can lead to its failure.[4] If, in addition, the lymphatic system has a structural impairment of the type that occurs when the lymphatic system is malformed, the transport capacity can be significantly reduced.

If the assessment shows an underlying issue with the lymphatic system, one of the aims should be to work in concert with a lymphatic disease specialist to determine what might be done to improve lymphatic function.

Guidelines for the differential diagnosis are not yet well-defined or agreed upon. Most of our diagnostic outcome terminology, and the situations in which the term "lympho-phlebedema" might be used are based upon the status of the lymphatic system and whether or not it is able to function within its limits.[4,5]

Myxedema is associated with a dysfunctional thyroid (usually hypothyroidism), which, if uncorrected, can lead to the accumulation of mucinoid materials (proteoglycans) in the tissues. Testing of thyroid function will help confirm if it is this that contributes to the limb swelling.

Lipedema is the excessive accumulation of fatty subcutaneous tissues due to a metabolic disorder. It is easily distinguished from lymphedema by the fact that lipedema usually affects both legs with sparing of the feet, the skin on the affected limbs bruises easily, and often there is pain with externally applied pressure. In regions affected by abnormal fat deposition, there is no tendency to pit and the skin is soft and elastic. Even with apparent lipedemas there are various forms and a true lipedema must be differentiated from lipo-hypertrophy. The latter is normally distinguished by a slender trunk and symmetrical fat deposits in the hips and legs. Most concur that lipo-hypertrophy does not present in its latter stages with excessive fluid accumulation, as occurs with the later stages of lipedema – which is correctly called lipo-lymphedema. Their differential diagnosis will be dealt with in the next chapter.

Differentiating the Lymphedemas

Any recommendations concerning the screening and diagnosis of lymphedema, should take note of the recommendations of the International Lymphoedema Framework (ILF)[1] and the International Society of Lymphology (ISL),[2] as well as many regional groups (European Lymphology Society, Italian, German, and Dutch societies).[6]

As a starting point, the ISL consensus recommends using a three-stage classification system, with a growing movement toward a four-stage system that encompasses the latent or sub-clinical stage.[2] These stages refer only to the physical condition of the extremities and it is acknowledged that a more detailed and inclusive classification must be created based on our growing comprehension of the underlying pathophysiologies. Within each stage there is currently an "inadequate but functional severity assessment" based on simple volume differences, but these changes can be varying degrees of fluid, fat, and fibrous accumulation as the lymphedema progresses. Within the ISL severity assessment, "minimal" is described as less than a 20% increase (over normal limb or baseline – allowing for limb dominance), "moderate" when it is 20–40%, and "severe" when it is more than 40%.[2] Of course, it is never advisable to concentrate exclusively on the physical elements of disease: there is a range of instruments to assess disability, quality of life, etc., but, in realistic terms, these aspects will not have an impact on the accuracy of differential diagnosis and are considered in subsequent chapters.

One aspect of accurate diagnosis is lymphoscintigraphy. A lymphoscintigram can give an indication of the functional status of the lymphatic system, where and which drainage pathways are hypo- or dysfunctional, where there are areas of dermal backflow or reflux. Lymphoscintigraphic processes and techniques have yet to be well standardized, but the outcomes (both qualitative and quantitative) can provide strong evidence for a dysfunctional lymphatic system.[7] This and other diagnostic tools will be considered in subsequent chapters.

Filarial Lymphedema

Lymphedema often only manifests during the latter stage of this disease, a fact that is often overlooked. The clinical manifestation and presentation depends on the type and feeding preferences of the mosquito carrying the filarial parasite. The major diagnostic confirmation is achieved through sero-conversion and through examination of a peripheral blood sample taken in the late evening or early morning. A thoroughly conducted medical history will help to determine if the patient has lived in areas where the parasite is endemic.

Malignant Lymphedema

Usually associated with a rapid onset and a location that is more proximal/central than the more commonly encountered forms of iatrogenic lymphedema, this variant occurs through reduction of lymph transport as a consequence of external obstruction of nodes or collectors, or through invasion and proliferation of neoplastic tissues. In addition to the differential diagnostic points already considered, there can be significant pain, as well as abnormalities of the skin, which can often be shiny and sometimes cyanotic as well.

Factitious Lymphedema

This may occur in patients who seek attention for an illness initiation or exacerbation. A good differential diagnosis is best gained through a detailed medical/surgical history.

Primary Lymphedema

In all tests, primary lymphedemas resemble the secondary form. This differential diagnosis is generally best established through a review of the patient's family, medical, and surgical history. Approximately 3–10% of lymphedemas are primary in nature and caused by some heritable malformation (generally hypoplasia, but sometimes hyperplasia) of the lymphatic system, which can become apparent at birth (Nonne–Milroy), puberty (Meige or praecox) or in later life (tarda). Some patients may be surprised at the onset of the lymphedema after an apparently minor surgical intervention, but an exploration of family history may expose genetic predisposition.

When a Patient Might First Present

A person who has a damaged lymphatic system has a lifetime risk of developing lymphedema, although the risk level may vary with time. It is the responsibility of both patient and physician to keep the risk as low as possible by recognizing and managing all of the factors that can increase the lymphatic load.

Risk Factors to Consider at Presentation

Some risk factors, such as body mass, skin integrity, activity levels (inactivity seeming to be the worst), constrictive clothing (particularly underwear that has elastic across the line of the groin) and bras (those that are under-wired and have narrow straps) are under a patient's control.

Some factors, such as patient age, the extent of axillary or groin clearance, the area of radiotherapy, whether the surgery/radiotherapy was on the dominant arm, seroma duration, the number of drains, and wound infection, are beyond the patient's control.

Signs to Look for at Presentation

Even if there is no obvious swelling, it is worth testing whether the distal part of the limb shows signs of pitting or considering the use of one of the more objective instruments to detect subtle fluid differences through bio-impedance spectroscopy.[8] These are dealt with in other chapters of this book.

It is important to be aware that lymphedema progresses in a different fashion than hydrostatic edema. There is no epi-fascial fatty tissue deposition in edema, but this is characteristic of lymphedema as it progresses (ISL stage II and III).

There may also be signs of tissue changes associated with the accumulation of fibrotic tissue (ISL stage III). These changes can often be detected through conducting a "pinch and roll test," by holding the affected tissues between the thumb and forefinger and gently rolling the tissues between them (generally referred to as a Stemmer sign when used at the base of the digits of the hand or foot). While not always useful in early lymphedema, the Stemmer sign is common in the middle and late stages. The Stemmer sign is useful to distinguish lipedema and other forms of tissue swelling from lymphedema, although the Stemmer sign is best used in combination with other diagnostics. A positive Stemmer sign reflects the inability to pick up a fold of skin at the base of the big toe or fingers; more objective correlates can be detected through tissue tonometry, ultrasound or some other measure of epifascial tissue change.[9]

To determine if the limb is swollen, a circumference measurement can be performed at fixed points in the fore/upper arms or calf and thigh. Unfortunately, this is only useful if the problem is a unilateral one, where a comparison can be made with the contra-lateral (normal) limb and the progression assessed against this baseline. If the problem is bilateral, then, at best, the measurements can be used as a baseline, acknowledging that this baseline may not be the beginning of the lymphedema. There are international best practice guidelines for this.[1,9]

References

1. Framework L. *Best Practice for the Management of Lymphoedema. International Consensus.* London: MEP Ltd; 2006.
2. International Society of Lymphology. The diagnosis and treatment of peripheral lymphoedema. 2009 consensus document of the International Society of Lymphology. *Lymphology.* 2009;42(1):51-60.
3. Cavezzi A, Michelini S. *Phlebolymphoedema from Diagnosis to Therapy.* Bologna: Edizioni PR; 1998.
4. Foeldi M, Foeldi E. Sufficiency and insufficiency of the lymphatic system. In: Foeldi M, Foeldi E, Kubik S. *Textbook of Lymphology for Physicians and Lymphoedema Therapists.* Munich: Urban and Fisher; 2003.
5. Lee BB, Piller NB. Lymphoedema and lymphatic malformation consensus group report. Union Internationale de Phlebologie; August 2009; Monaco.
6. Damstra R, Kaandorp C. Multidisciplinary guidelines for early diagnosis and management. *J Lymphoedema.* 2007;2(1):57-61.
7. Keeley V. The use of lymphoscintigraphy in the management of chronic lymphoedema. *J Lymphoedema.* 2006;1:42-57.
8. Rockson S. Bioimpedance analysis in the assessment of lymphoedema diagnosis and management. *J Lymphoedema.* 2007;2:44-48.
9. Piller NB. To measure or not to measure? What and where is the question. *J Lymphoedema.* 2007;2:39-45.

Chapter 17
Differential Diagnosis – Lipedema

Győző Szolnoky

Introduction

Lipedema is an infrequently recognized and often neglected clinical entity that nearly always affects women. It poses a diagnostic challenge as one of the common disorders that is easily confused with lymphedema.[1-4]

Definition

Lipedema is disproportional obesity characterized by bilateral, symmetrical, biker's hosiery-shaped fatty swelling of the legs; arms are also commonly involved.[1-4] Various synonyms are found in the literature (adiposalgia, adipositas dolorosa, adipositas spongiosa, adipositas edematosa, thick leg of healthy woman, fat leg, fatty edema, lipidosis, lipomatosis dolorosa, rider's hosiery disorder, column leg, stove pipe leg, jelly leg, areal adiposity, lipohypertrophia corporis inferioris, segmental adiposity, inferior obesity). This abundance of terminology and unclear definitions have resulted in some confusion about lipedema, causing under-diagnosis and misdirected treatment.[5]

Manifestations of lipedema typically appear after puberty.[2-4] Women are affected almost exclusively. Men usually develop lipedema on the basis of hormonal disturbance; however, there is one published case report in which a healthy man was diagnosed with lipedema.[6] The general incidence of lipedema among women is reported to be as high as 11%.[2] Ten to 18% of all patients referred to lymphedema clinics are diagnosed with lipedema. It has been suggested that among all women with increased fat deposits of the lower extremities, 60% are caused by obesity, 20% by lipedema, and 20% by a combination of both.[3]

G. Szolnoky
Department of Dermatology and Allergology, University of Szeged, Szeged, Hungary

B.-B. Lee et al. (eds.), *Lymphedema*,
DOI 10.1007/978-0-85729-567-5_17, © Springer-Verlag London Limited 2011

Lipedema presumably occurs against an endocrinological and genetic background.[2,7,8] Two leading hallmarks are the frequent appearance of ecchymosis and hematomas, even after minor traumatic injuries, and spontaneous or palpation-induced pain.[1-4] Lipedema, especially in advanced stages, occurs quite frequently in association with lymphatic or venous insufficiency. The comorbidities may substantially modify the original limb shape and obscure the diagnosis.[2-4]

Clinical Diagnosis

In most cases the diagnosis of lipedema can be established by the patient's history and clinical examination.[2-4] There is no absolutely unambiguous pathognomonic diagnostic test for lipedema.

Classification

At stage I, the skin looks flat, but the subcutis is already enlarged and on palpation feels like "styrofoam balls in a plastic bag" (see Fig. 17.1). At stage II (see Fig. 17.2), walnut- to apple-sized indurations develop and the overlying skin has an irregular surface ("mattress phenomenon"). Stage III shows larger indurations and deforming-to-lobular fat deposits (see Fig. 17.3).

A classification scheme has been proposed on the basis of the location of the fat deposits: mainly buttocks (type I), buttocks to knees (type II), buttocks to ankles (type III), mainly arms (type IV), and mainly lower legs (type V).[9]

Differential Diagnosis

The most notable differential diagnosis of lipedema (see Tables 17.1–17.3) embraces obesity, various forms of lipohypertrophy and venous edema or lymphedema.

Unilateral or bilateral venous edema is a hallmark of chronic venous insufficiency. Pitting edema usually disappears or is minimal after bed rest. In contrast to lymphedema, Stemmer sign is typically negative.[2]

In obesity, the distribution of subcutaneous fat deposits is usually generalized. Simple obesity may equally affect men and women. Furthermore, the typical sparing of the feet and the pain of lipedema are lacking. Unlike lipedema, simple obesity efficiently responds to restricted diet and increased exercise. Lipedema is frequently combined with obesity and altered body structure may misdirect the clinician, resulting in an inaccurate diagnosis. Early lipedema may be associated with normal weight.[2,10]

Fig. 17.1 Stage I lipedema

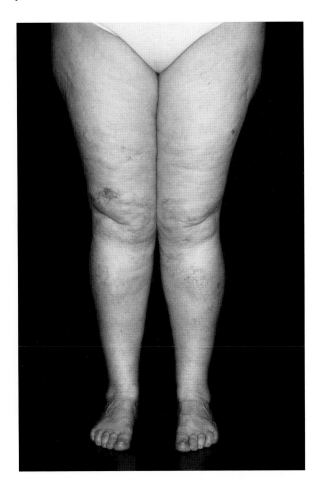

Lipohypertrophy is described as increased symmetrical subcutaneous fat deposits, mostly on the legs and arms in women.[11] Lipedema is preceded by lipohypertrophy. The basic difference between lipohypertrophy and lipedema resides in the absence of edema and pain in lipohypertrophy. However, there are also painful subtypes of lipohypertrophy. One widely used categorization identifies *lipomatosis indolens simplex* (multiple lipomas without relevant symptoms), *lipomatosis dolorosa* (painful fat deposition), *lipomatosis atrophicans* (accompanying fat atrophy), and *lipomatosis gigantea* (overgrowing fatty parts).

The term "lipodystrophy" is usually reserved for local damaged subcutaneous fat.[12] Acquired partial lipodystrophy is called Barraquer–Simons syndrome, in which adipose tissue loss is noted primarily in the neck, face, arms, thorax, and upper abdomen. The clinical onset is during childhood or adolescence, predominantly among women. These women are frequently subject to hirsutism, amenorrhea or polycystic ovary syndrome.

Fig. 17.2 Stage II lipedema

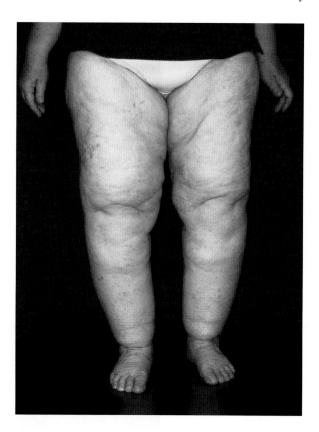

Dercum's disease (*lipomatosis dolorosa*) is a rare, symmetrical disorder involving the inner side of upper arms, elbows, stomach wall, buttocks, inner and outer surfaces of thighs and knees with painful subcutaneous adipose tissue deposits.[13] Severe hyperalgesia is triggered by even light pressure. It is 5–30 times more frequent in women than in men and usually results in a number of psychosocial problems that may partially be attributed to the context of chronic pain syndrome. Other characteristic symptoms are swollen hands and fingers with accompanying paresthesias, numbness, joint stiffness, dryness of eyes and mouth, and teleangiectasia with increased fragility of vessels causing ecchymoses. It may first occur in menopause and is not associated with edema.

Benign symmetric lipomatosis (Madelung's disease or Launois–Bensaude syndrome) is a rare, benign disorder of unknown etiology.[14,15] This syndrome is characterized by multiple, symmetric, non-encapsulated fatty accumulation diffusely involving the neck and upper trunk areas. It uncommonly involves the lower limbs and lower trunk. Madelung's disease can be divided into three major forms according to location: type I (neck), type II (shoulders, interscapular region, and upper arms), and type III (lower trunk). In other classifications, there are proximal (neck, shoulders, scapular region), central (backs, thighs), and distal (knees, hands, and

Fig. 17.3 Stage III lipedema

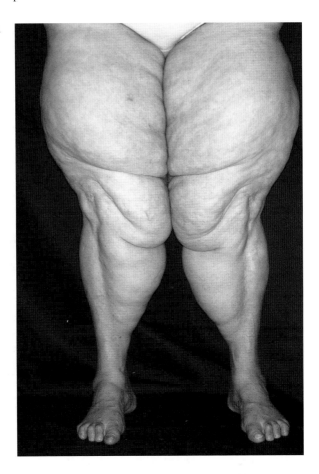

feet) forms. Postulated etiologies include abnormal proliferation of brown fat cells and mitochondrial mutations. It predominantly affects middle-aged men of Mediterranean origin with a history of alcohol abuse. It is usually asymptomatic; however, in advanced forms, dysphagia, diminished cervical range of motion, hoarseness and respiratory complications may appear. Glucose intolerance and increased serum insulin level are commonly found. There are signs of primary neuropathy and neurogenic muscular atrophy.

Steatopygia is characterized by protrusion and excessive adipose deposition localized solely to the buttock region.[16]

Fibro-fatty syndrome (*juxta-articular adiposis dolorosa*) shares some similarities with lipedema in having enlarged fatty mass on the thighs and the inner side of the knee joints; however, some experts consider this disorder to be an early form of Dercum's disease.[17] In half of the cases there are additional foot deformities and varicosities. Compromised lymphatic and venous circulation are believed to play a significant role in the maintenance and further progression of this disorder. It is sometimes combined with arterial hypertension.

Table 17.1 Differential diagnosis

	Gender	Family history	Onset	Location	Symmetry	Excess fat	Pain at pressure
Lipedema	Female	Possible	Puberty	Leg, arm	Yes	Yes	Yes
Lipo-hypertrophy	Female	Possible	Conva-lescent, adult	Hip	Yes	Yes	Rarely
Primary lymphedema	Female > male	Yes	From birth to third decade	Buttock, leg, arm	Uni- or bilateral	Possible	No
Phlebedema	Both	No	Adult	Leg	Uni- or bilateral	No	No
Morbus Dercum	Female	No	Menopause	Neck	Yes	Yes	Yes
Morbus Madelung	Male	No	Adult	Arms, trunk, legs	Yes	Yes	No
Obesity	Both	No	Adults	General	Yes	Yes	No

Table 17.2 Differential diagnosis

	Edema	Foot affected	Arm affected	Dietary effect	Effect of elevation	Stemmer sign
Lipedema	Yes	No	Yes	No	Minimal	No
Lipohypertrophy	No	No	Yes	No	No	No
Primary lymphedema	Yes	Yes	Possible	No	Minimal	Yes
Phlebedema	Yes	Possible	No	No	Efficient	No
Morbus Dercum	No	No	No	No	No	No
Morbus Madelung	No	No	Possible	No	No	No
Obesity	Rarely	No	Yes	Yes	No	No

Table 17.3 Differential diagnosis

	Ankle fat pad	Consistency	Pitting edema	History of cellulitis	Progression	Hereditary factor
Lipedema	Yes	Soft-to-firm	No	No	Yes	Probable
Lipo-hypertrophy	No	Soft	No	No	Possible	No
Primary lymphedema	No	Firm	Yes	Yes	Yes	Yes
Phlebedema	No	Soft-to-firm	No	No	Yes	Possible
Morbus Dercum	No	Soft-to-firm	No	No	Yes	No
Morbus Madelung	No	Soft-to-firm	No	No	Yes	No
Obesity	No	Soft	No	No	Yes	No

Laboratory Diagnosis

Waist-to-Height Ratio

Of the anthropometric measurements the waist-to-height ratio may give the most reasonable results in lipedema.[10]

Streeten Test

If cardiac, renal, and venous insufficiencies are excluded, the patient can be subjected to examination. The patient drinks 20 ml water/kg of body weight and remains in an upright position for 4 h. During this period of observation, urine is collected. The leg volume is measured prior and subsequent to the test. Normal healthy individuals excrete more than 60% of the ingested water and the leg volume does not increase by more than 350 ml/kg. Pathological results indicate the existence of increased permeability of blood capillaries.[18]

Capillary Fragility Assessment

Bruising is attributed to increased capillary fragility in lipedema.[2-4,19] Capillary fragility measurement is accomplished with a vacuum suction chamber (Parrot's angiosterrometer) exerting an adjustable suction on the skin. Determination of capillary fragility is based on the quantified petechiae. Uncomplicated simple obesity was compared with uncomplicated lipedema from the perspective of capillary fragility (unreported study). The vacuum suction method (−30 mmHg pressure for 1 min) revealed that the number of induced petechiae was significantly higher in the lipedema group, emphasizing the possible role of angiosterrometry, or other methods of capillary fragility measurement, as a potential tool for discrimination of disease.

Assessment of Aortic Distensibility and Stiffness in Lipedema

In an unreported clinical trial where women with uncomplicated lipedema were compared with healthy age- and BMI-matched individuals, lipedema was associated with notably higher aortic stiffness and lower distensibility.[20]

Pain Perception Assessment

The pinch test is the simplest method of pain detection.[2] Lipedematous pain is difficult to describe; therefore, a 30-item questionnaire was designed to characterize the most typical adjectives.[21] A four-grade scale was assigned to each item and adjectives with the highest grades referred to the most characteristic descriptions. In a comparative clinical trial the top ten items, as well as a special numerical analog scale (from 0 to 10) called the Pain Rating Scale[22] and the Wong Baker Faces scale were applied for pain assessment.[23]

Ultrasound Examination

High-resolution duplex ultrasound is a method that can distinguish lipedema from venous edema or lymphedema with a high level of sensitivity.[24,25]

Lipedematous subcutaneous tissue is definitely enlarged and has substantially higher echogenicity ("snowfall sign") without hypoechoic spaces or channels. Subcutaneous septae are thickened and have increased echogenicity. Lymphedema has thickened subcutaneous tissue with enhanced echogenicity with associated small, <1-mm hypoechoic spaces (initial dilated lymphatic vessels) and larger, longer hypoechoic spaces and channels with echo-rich margins (congested lymphatic collectors). Beyond venous stasis and dilated veins, often varicose, no specific duplex ultrasound features are described in venous edema.

CT and MRI Examination

Computed tomography[26] and MRI[27] are typically indicated for scientific purposes or subtle cases, and show that the objective edema is minimal and that limb swelling can mostly be attributed to bilateral homogeneous enlargement of the subcutaneous compartment in the early stages of lipedema.

These examinations provide the possibility of volumetry, the evaluation of various tissue components, and the simultaneous display of blood or lymphatic vessels with high precision.[28]

Lymphoscintigraphy and Fluorescent Microlymphography

The peculiar enlargement of subcutaneous fat is presumably linked with microangiopathy and altered microcirculation, leading to increased permeability and protein-rich fluid extravasation that further enhances the amount of interstitial fluid. Therefore, in less advanced forms of lipedema, increased lymph flow may be visualized by lymphoscintigraphy. Lymph vessels must raise their transport capacity, because of augmented capillary filtration and increasing volume of interstitial fluid. In later stages the lymphatics may become exhausted.[29,30] Fluorescent microlymphography displays lymphatic microaneurysms and dilated vessels of the uppermost lymphatic network, indicating that lymph vessels are also involved.[31]

Clinical Management

The conservative approach corresponds to complex decongestive physiotherapy (CDP) consisting of manual lymph drainage (MLD) and, optionally, intermittent pneumatic compression (IPC), physical exercise, multilayered compression bandaging, and meticulous skin care.[2] The first observational study on the effect of CDP in lipedema showed that the maximally achieved reduction was nearly 10% of the original leg girth.[32] In a clinical study, MLD-based CDP was compared with MLD plus IPC-based CDP. Each treatment modality resulted in significant limb volume reduction; however, no significant difference was observed between the two regimens.[33] In other controlled trials MLD+IPC-based CDP drastically decreased capillary fragility and pain perception of lipedema patients.[19]

Various forms of surgical lipoaspiration give more reliable benefit to lipedema patients without proven damage of the lymphatics.[34]

Prognosis

Early diagnosis and treatment are mandatory for this disorder; otherwise, gradual enlargement of fatty deposition causes impaired mobility, debilitation, and further co-morbidities like arthrosis and lymphatic insufficiency. Interlobar areas may become susceptible to fungal and, especially, bacterial infections that may further progress to cellulitis or septicemia especially when lymphedema coexists. Lipedema has a remarkable psychological impact, ranging from mild upset to severe anxiety, depression or even anorexia.[2-4]

References

1. Allen EV, Hines EA. Lipedema of the legs: a syndrome characterized by fat legs and orthostatic edema. *Proc Staff Meet Mayo Clin.* 1940;15:184-187.
2. Földi E, Földi M. Das Lipödem. In: Földi M, Kubik S, eds. *Lehrbuch der Lymphologie.* 5th ed. München-Jena: Gustav Fischer; 2002:449-458.
3. Langendoen SI, Habbema L, Nijsten TE, Neumann HA. Lipoedema: from clinical presentation to therapy. A review of the literature. *Br J Dermatol.* 2009;161:980-986.
4. Todd M. Lipoedema: presentation and management. *Br J Community Nurs.* 2010;15:S10-S16.
5. Meier-Vollrath I, Schneider W, Schmeller W. Lipödem: Verbesserte Lebensqualität durch Therapiekombination. *Dtsch Ärtzteblatt.* 2005;102:1061-1067.
6. Chen S, Hsu SD, Chen TM, Wang HJ. Painful fat syndrome in a male patient. *Br J Plast Surg.* 2004;57:282-286.
7. Child AH, Gordon KD, Sharpe P, et al. Lipedema: an inherited condition. *Am J Med Genet A.* 2010;152A:970-976.
8. Szolnoky G, Kemeny L. Lipoedema: from clinical presentation to therapy: further aspects. *Br J Dermatol.* 2010;162:889.
9. Meier-Vollrath I, Schneider W, Schmeller W. Das Lipödem: neue Möglichkeiten der Therapie. *Schweiz Med Forum.* 2007;7:150-155.
10. Herpertz U. Adipositas-Diagnostik in der Lymphologie. *LymphForsch.* 2009;13:90-93.
11. Herpertz U. Das Lipödem. *Z Lymphol.* 1995;19:1-11.
12. Capeau J, Magré J, Caron-Debarle M, et al. Human lipodystrophies: genetic and acquired diseases of adipose tissue. *Endocr Dev.* 2010;19:1-20.
13. Lange U, Oelzner P, Uhlemann C. Dercum's disease (Lipomatosis dolorosa): successful therapy with pregabalin and manual lymphatic drainage and a current overview. *Rheumatol Int.* 2008;29:17-22.
14. Alameda YA, Torres L, Perez-Mitchell C, Riera A. Madelung disease: a clinical diagnosis. *Otolaryngol Head Neck Surg.* 2009;141:418-419.
15. Verna G, Kefalas N, Boriani F, Carlucci S, Choc I, Bocchiotti M. Launois-Bensaude syndrome: an unusual localization of obesity disease. *Obes Surg.* 2008;18:1313-1317.
16. Ersek RA, Bell HN. Serial and superficial suction for steatopygia (Hottentot bustle). *Aesthetic Plast Surg.* 1994;18:279-282.
17. Eisman JM, Swezey RL. Juxta-articular adiposis dolorosa. What is it? Report of 2 cases. *Ann Rheum Dis.* 1979;38:479-482.
18. Streeten DH. Idiopathic edema pathogenesis, clinical features, and treatment. *Endocrinol Metab Clin North Am.* 1995;24:531-547.
19. Szolnoky G, Nagy N, Kovács RK, et al. Complex decongestive physiotherapy decreases capillary fragility in lipedema. *Lymphology.* 2008;41:161-166.

20. Nemes A, Gavallér H, Csajbók É, Forster T, Csanády M. Obesity is associated with aortic enlargement and increased stiffness: an echocardiographic study. *Int J Cardiovasc Imaging.* 2008;24:165-171.
21. Schmeller W, Meier-Vollrath I. Schmerzen beim Lipödem: Versuch einer Annäherung. *LymphForsch.* 2008;12:7-11.
22. Hamner JB, Fleming MD. Lymphedema therapy reduces the volume of edema and pain in patients with breast cancer. *Ann Surg Oncol.* 2007;14:1904-1908.
23. Wong DL, Baker CM. Smiling faces as anchor for pain intensity scales. *Pain.* 2001;89: 295-300.
24. Marshall M, Schwahn-Schreiber C. Lymph-, Lip- und Phlebödem. Differenzialdiagnostische Abklärung mittels hochauflösender Duplexsonographie. *Gefässchirurgie.* 2008;13:204-212.
25. Naouri M, Samimi M, Atlan M, et al. High resolution cutaneous ultrasonography to differentiate lipoedema from lymphoedema. *Br J Dermatol.* 2010;163:296-301.
26. Vaughan BF. CT of swollen legs. *Clin Radiol.* 1990;41:24-30.
27. Dimakakos PB, Stefanopoulos T, Antoniades P. MRI and ultrasonographic findings in the investigation of lymphedema and lipedema. *Int Surg.* 1997;82:411-416.
28. Lohrmann C, Foeldi E, Langer M. MR imaging of the lymphatic system in patients with lipedema and lipo-lymphedema. *Microvasc Res.* 2009;77:335-339.
29. Brauer WJ. Altersbezogene Funktionslymphszintigraphie beim Lipödem und Lipolymphödem. *LymphForsch.* 2000;4:74-77.
30. Harwood CA, Bull RH, Evans J, Mortimer PS. Lymphatic and venous function in lipedema. *Br J Dermatol.* 1996;134:1-6.
31. Amann-Vesti BR, Franzeck UK, Bollinger A. Microlymphatic aneurysms in patients with lipedema. *Lymphology.* 2000;134:170-175.
32. Deri G, Weissleder H. Vergleichende prä- und posttherapeutische Volumenmessungen in Beinsegmenten beim Lipödem. *LymphForsch.* 1997;1:35-37.
33. Szolnoky G, Borsos B, Bársony K, Balogh M, Kemény L. Complete decongestive physiotherapy of lipedema with or without pneumatic compression: a pilot study. *Lymphology.* 2008;41:50-52.
34. Schmeller W, Meier-Vollrath I. Tumescent liposuction: a new and successful therapy for lipedema. *J Cutan Med Surg.* 2006;10:7-10.

Part V
Laboratory/Imaging Diagnosis

Chapter 18
Laboratory/Imaging Diagnosis: General Guidelines

Mauro Andrade

General Considerations

The perfect diagnostic method employed for any disease evaluation should provide good anatomical definition, relevant pathophysiological information, be non-invasive, and must be reproducible, offering reliable data on evolution and treatment. As for most human diseases, there are many different diagnostic methods to study lymphatic insufficiency, all of them with their advantages and disadvantages, all of them fulfilling specific aspects regarding investigation of lymphatic disorders, but none of them possessing all of the required features to be considered ideal.

Historically, direct oil lymphography, developed by Kinmonth in the 1950s, was a cornerstone in the field of lymphology.[1] This diagnostic method provided most of the basis for our current knowledge and systematization about lymphatic diseases, but, even if lymphography must be honored for its significance, it is no longer a useful test for routine lymphatic examination, because it is not a practical method and complications may be severe.[2] Radiological lymphography, currently reserved for exceptional clinical situations, like chylous reflux and thoracic duct injuries, has been largely replaced by less invasive diagnostic explorations, even though its anatomical definition remains unparalleled.

Almost simultaneously, the first reports regarding functional studies of the lymphatic system through measurements of peripheral uptake of injected radioactive particles and their appearance in regional lymph nodes[3] established the foundation of the current use and techniques of lymphoscintigraphy for exploration of lymphatic disorders.

As outlined in the Clinical Diagnosis chapter (Part 6), lymphedema is a result of deranged lymph flow secondary to abnormalities in lymph absorption and/or

M. Andrade
Department of Surgery,
University of São Paulo Medical School,
São Paulo, Brazil

B.-B. Lee et al. (eds.), *Lymphedema*,
DOI 10.1007/978-0-85729-567-5_18, © Springer-Verlag London Limited 2011

transport, leading to edema and tissue changes. Selected diagnostic methods can be aimed at the structure and function of lymph vessels and lymph nodes and can provide estimation of tissue alterations caused by lymph stasis.

When Clinical Examination Should Be Complemented by Imaging

Not considering differential diagnosis, medicolegal issues, and research protocols, which may require supplementary studies, a decision about whether any additional investigation should be undertaken for an individual patient, and which one(s), depends mostly on clinical judgment. Clearly, history and physical examination are usually sufficient to make a correct diagnosis of the subjacent lymphatic disorder and to choose the initial therapeutic approach. Only occasionally will diagnostic methods change the initial clinical impression or offer a reliable prognosis tool better than careful clinical evaluation and close follow-up.

Imaging methods to further explore affected limbs are mandatory whenever the diagnosis of lymphedema is not clear or other associated diseases may mask the relevance or concomitance of lymphatic involvement.[2]

The preferred imaging method to depict lymphatic abnormalities is lymphoscintigraphy or radionuclide lymphography.[2,4] In fact, lymphoscintigraphy is considered to be an essential part of the primary evaluation of any lymphedema patient (level of evidence 1B),[4] even though its usefulness regarding etiological diagnosis (primary or secondary),[5] initial therapeutic choice or prognostic value may be controversial in most cases.

In lower limb lymphedemas, duplex ultrasound examination of the venous system is advisable.[2,4] Beyond differential diagnosis, unsuspected venous insufficiency may aggravate lymphatic load and once diagnosed, may change proposed treatments.

Methods to Evaluate Lymph Flow, Lymphatic Vessels, and Lymph Nodes

Lymphochromy or the blue dye test, examination of initial uptake and lymphatic transport, consists of subdermal or intradermal injection of a vital dye and is an essential step for direct oil lymphography. Along with Landis' test, its elegant functional radionuclide successor, lymphochromy may be used to assess local lymph flow, but has little relevance in daily clinical practice for the evaluation of lymphedemas.

Peritumoral injection of patent blue, either alone or coupled with radioactive tracers, is another method derived from classical lymphochromy. This anatomical test is very useful for identifying sentinel lymph nodes, most commonly in breast cancer and melanoma operations. Interestingly, a method developed in the past to explore lymphedemas is currently essential to avoid unnecessary lymphadenecto- mies, thus playing an important role in preventing lymphedema development.

Quantitative and semi-quantitative analysis of lymphatic drainage are best achieved with lymphoscintigraphy. Quantitative studies are obtained by quantitative nuclear imaging in selected regions of interest using a time curve graphic. By assigning predetermined grades to some observed morphological characteristics analyzed by visual interpretation, the semi-quantitative evaluation[6] avoids unneces- sary problems related to physical properties of the radiotracer. In clinical practice, lymphatic transport and structure are more often estimated by qualitative analysis. This is a reliable method to evaluate the lymphatic system and, even if qualitative evaluation always relies upon subjective interpretation, it fulfills most diagnostic needs. Qualitative lymphoscintigraphy uses detailed description of many character- istics that may be observed: local spread of the radiotracer, dermal flow in the absence of patent collector vessels, and dermal back flow in proximal obstructions; appearance, quantity, and location of the lymph collectors; number, location, and time of appearance of lymph nodes. Either way, an important concept to keep in mind is that images obtained in lymphoscintigraphy will only represent the lym- phatic drainage of the injection site and not the entire lymphatic system of the affected limb. Injection in the interdigital spaces of the feet will preferentially show the greater saphenous pathway, which is the normal drainage for that region. If, for instance, the collectors accompanying the lesser saphenous vein and popliteal nodes are visible, deranged lymph drainage of the superficial system is diagnosed, as this deviation to the deep system of the popliteal area is not the expected pathway emerg- ing from the injection point. Patients with leg swelling may display completely different patterns of lymph vessels and lymph flow if injection is performed between the toes or in the medial aspect of the knee. As a corollary, lack of patent lymphatic collectors after interdigital injection of radiotracer does not always mean that no collectors are patent. Additionally, there is no direct relationship between qualita- tive or quantitative lymphoscintigraphy and the clinical severity of lymphedema.

Lymphoscintigraphy also has its drawbacks: lack of standardization regarding various radiotracers with variable radioactivity and volumes, choice of subcutane- ous or intradermal injection sites, exercise protocols that vary according to the diag- nostic center, different imaging times, dynamic or static acquisition of the images.[2] All these variables prevent this useful examination from being a universal language for defining lymphatic function.

Chylous disorders or thoracic duct fistulas require a more accurate anatomical definition than the one that can be provided by lymphoscintigraphy and are best demonstrated by conventional oil contrast lymphangiography,[7] especially if coupled with CT. Special techniques of lymphoscintigraphy, e.g., unilateral injection and demonstration of reflux to the contralateral side, may be useful for chylous reflux patients.[8] Since these challenging problems are rare in clinical practice and should be managed by experienced lymphatic disease specialists, it is unlikely that a gen- eral practitioner will even request a conventional lymphography during routine clinical activity.

Imaging of enlarged lymph nodes (or tumoral masses, as part of a complete diagnostic evaluation of lymph stasis) can be very important in lymphedema patients, especially when malignant lymphedema is suspected. For this purpose, ultrasound or, more usefully, MRI and CT, may unveil subjacent obstruction or compression of the lymphatic pathways.

Excisional lymph node biopsy, except for sentinel node biopsy in the groin or axilla for staging malignancy, should be avoided in peripheral lymphedema patients, for it risks aggravating distal swelling.[2] Moreover, histological information is seldom helpful. Where pathological specimens are judged necessary, fine needle aspiration can be diagnostic if malignancy is suspected.

Methods of Evaluating Tissue Changes

Chronic lymph stasis leads to several modifications in the affected limb that may be variable in their severity, but are unique in aggregate, as they are not seen in any other cause of edema.

Skin thickening, fibrosis, fat changes, and fluid retention, together and in various proportions, account for the volume change observed in these patients. Mostly, lymphedema interferes with suprafascial tissues and the muscular compartment remains unchanged. Due to overuse or disuse of the affected limb, muscular hypertrophy or atrophy can be respectively observed in some patients.

Evaluation of suprafascial tissues includes magnetic resonance imaging, computed tomography, ultrasound, DEXA, or bi-photonic absorptiometry, among other possible but less useful methods. MRI and CT offer remarkable insight into tissue fibrosis, fluid accumulation, skin thickness, and cross-sectional area. The "honeycomb" pattern observed in the subcutaneous tissue is specific to lymphedema.[9] Both can also be used to evaluate volumetric and tissue density reduction after treatment.[10]

Although still investigational, technological development of MRI will offer the possibility to evaluate lymphatic collectors, lymph nodes, and tissue changes at the same time.[11] This would seem to be a promising and complete method of studying most lymphatic disorders in the future.

Considering the recent and growing interest in the relationship of lymph stasis to fat formation, dual-energy X-ray absorptiometry (DEXA), or bi-photonic absorptiometry, has great potential for use in estimating the contribution of the fat component to the overall volumetric increase.[12] Such knowledge may prove to be useful for therapeutic purposes[13] or prognosis.

References

1. Kinmonth JB, Taylor G, Tracy C, Marsh J. Primary lymphedema clinical and lymphographic studies of a series of 107 patients in which he lower limbs were affected. *Br J Surg*. 1957;45:1-11.

2. International Society of Lymphology. The diagnosis and treatment of peripheral lymphedema. *Lymphology.* 2009;42:51-60.
3. Sherman AI, Ter-Pogassian M. Lymph node concentration of radioactive colloidal gold following interstitial injection. *Cancer.* 1953;6:1238-1240.
4. Lee BB, Andrade M, Bergan J, et al. Diagnosis and treatment of primary lymphedema. Consensus Document of the International Union of Phlebology (IUP)-2009. *Int Angiol.* 2010;29:454-470.
5. Weissleder H, Weissleder R. Lymphedema: evaluation of qualitative and quantitative lymphoscintigraphy in 238 patients. *Radiology.* 1988;167:729-735.
6. Cambria RA, Gloviczki P, Naessens JM, Waher HW. Noninvasive evaluation of the lymphatic system with lymphoscintigraphy: a prospective, semiquantitative analysisin 386 extremities. *J Vasc Surg.* 1993;18:775-782.
7. Campisi C, Bellini C, Eretta C, et al. Diagnosis and management of primary chylous ascites. *J Vasc Surg.* 2006;43:1244-1248.
8. Andrade M, Puech-Leao P. Surgical treatment of primary chylous reflux to the lower limbs. In: Jamal S, Shenoy J, Manokaran G, eds. XVII International Congress of Lymphology; 1999; Chennai – India. 36.
9. Hadjis NS, Carr DH, Banks L, Pflug JJ. The role of CT in the diagnosis of primary lymphedema of the lower limb. *AJR.* 1985;144:361-363.
10. Andrade M, Almeida MT, Puech-Leão P. Standard CT assessment of lymphedematous limbs. Radiological pattern change after conservative treatment. *Lymphology.* 1996;29(suppl): 97-100.
11. Dimakakos E, Koureas A, Koutoulidis V, et al. Interstitial magnetic resonance lymphography: the clinical effectiveness of a new method. *Lymphology.* 2008;41:116-125.
12. Brorson H, Ohlin K, Olsson G, Karlsson MK. Breast cancer-related chronic arm lymphedema is associated with excess adipose and muscle tissue. *Lymphat Res Biol.* 2009;7:3-10.
13. Brorson H, Svensson H, Norrgren K, Thorsson O. Liposuction reduces arm lymphedema without significantly altering the already impaired lymph transport. *Lymphology.* 1998;31: 156-172.

Chapter 19
Radionuclide Lymphoscintigraphy

Walter H. Williams, Magdalene Ochart, Michael J. Bernas,
Charles L. Witte, and Marlys H. Witte

Brief Historical Note

After McMaster[1] used intracutaneous injection of vital dyes to visualize streamers and to follow lymph flow in patients with heart failure and other edematous conditions, Kinmonth et al.[2] developed conventional lymphography by incising skin over the blue-stained streamers seen on the dorsum of the foot or hand and exposing tiny skin lymphatics. Subsequent cannulation of the larger lymphatic draining collectors was followed by pump-controlled infusion of oily contrast. Kaindl and Servelle[3] directly cannulated pathologically dilated, often delicate fragile peripheral and central lymphatics and those associated with the viscera and injected them with iodinated contrast material.

For the next 40 years, conventional lymphography was the gold standard for the definitive delineation of the lymphatic system – both peripheral and central channels – and nodes. This time-consuming, tedious procedure requires an incision for visualization, and the cannulation of often tiny lymphatics is challenging and commonly unsuccessful. Moreover, iodinated contrast material is irritating to the lymphatic endothelial lining, and this contrast agent remains in the lymphatics, particularly in the lymph nodes, for an extended period of time. Uptake in the lung, heart, liver, and spleen obscures the upper abdominal and mediastinal lymphatics. Conventional lymphography may also cause symptomatic oil (fat) embolism, particularly to the lungs, and local wound infection at the injection site.[4] This procedure is now rarely used in everyday practice, except when specifically indicated (Fig. 19.1).

M.H. Witte (✉)
Department of Surgery, University of Arizona College of Medicine, Tucson, AZ, USA

B.-B. Lee et al. (eds.), *Lymphedema*,
DOI 10.1007/978-0-85729-567-5_19, © Springer-Verlag London Limited 2011

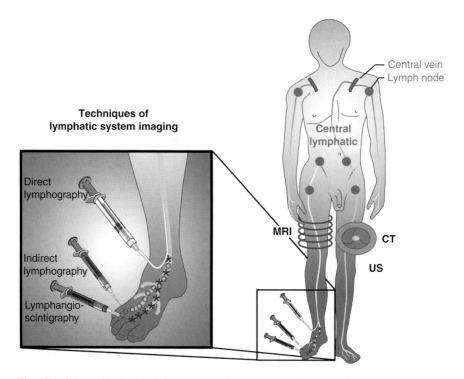

Fig. 19.1 Scheme illustrating different approaches to imaging the lymphatic system

Sherman and Ter-Pogossian[5] first showed radioisotopic colloidal uptake in lymph nodes. The improvement in isotope lymphography (also called lymphangio-scintigraphy [LAS]) with whole-body modification (WB-LAS) using technetium 99m-labeled macromolecules, such as albumin[6] or colloid as the radioactive tracer, has transformed the field.

Materials and Methods

A large molecule, such as sulfur colloid, dextran, hetastarch, or preferably human serum albumin (HSA), is linked to radioactive technetium (Tc)-99m. Tc-99m is nearly completely decayed with gamma radiation in 24 h (half-life 6 h).

We have found the following protocol optimal for obtaining clear, comprehensive, and consistent LAS images. Tc-99m HSA and Tc-99m sulfur colloid have been evaluated using dynamic LAS. 550 uCi (18.5 MBq) Tc-99m labeled colloid or human serum albumin is instilled intradermally to create a wheal in the second web space of the hand or foot for upper or lower extremity studies respectively (single injection per limb). Both arms and legs are examined to provide a normal control in unilateral lymphedema. After mild exercise (flexion of the hands or feet [often walking]), the patient returns for WB-LAS at 3–4 h post-injection.

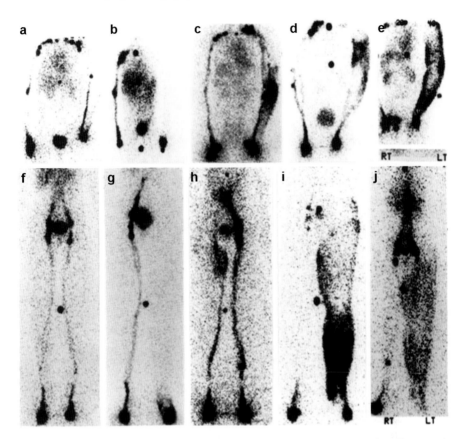

Fig. 19.2 Common patterns of lymphangioscintigrams of arms (*upper row*) and legs (*lower row*). (**a**, and **f**), Normal lymphatics and regional nodes. (**c–e**, **h**, and **i**) Unilateral limb lymphatic obstruction (radical mastectomy or groin dissection). (**b**, **g**, and **j**) Left limb primary lymphedema. (**j**) A tracer (technetium-99m-labeled human serum albumin) was injected only into the right foot and refluxes into the left leg. Round midline markers denote sternal notch, xiphoid, pubis, and knees (superior to inferior) (Reprinted with permission from Witte et al.[7])

Interpretation and Comments

Lymphangioscintigraphy is a safe, single, non-invasive, and rapidly repeatable technique. WB-LAS provides clear dynamic images of lymphatic transport and peripheral and central lymphatic structures and function, often in complex settings (Fig. 19.2a, f). A variety of structural and functional changes in lymphatic flow dynamics can be visualized. Delayed imaging with Tc-99m HSA or sulfur colloid shows lymph node uptake, albeit without detailed structural features seen on conventional lymphography. HSA migrates more rapidly from the distal limb injection sites and shows better defined deep lymphatic trunks than observed with colloids. Axillary or inguinal lymph nodes are typically visualized within 15–25 min.

The transport index score (TIS)[8] allows semi-quantification of peripheral lymphatic radiotracer transport by means of a relative value score (0–9) for each marker. The scores are added together to arrive at an overall numeric index derived from objective and subjective criteria based on lymphatic and nodal temporal and spatial distribution of the radionuclide and its rate of appearance in regional lymph nodes (groin or axilla). The TIS ranges from 0 to severely pathological (45) and is calculated as follows:

$$TIS = K + D + 0.04\,T + N + V$$

where K = lymphatic transport kinetics (degree of transport delay); D = radionuclide distribution pattern (degree of dermal extravasation), T = timing of radionuclide appearance in regional lymph nodes (in minutes normalized for 200 min, the maximum delay accepted for lymph node appearance), N = demonstration and intensity of lymph nodes, and V = demonstration and intensity of lymphatic collectors.[8] Although variable, a high TIS supports either congenital or acquired lymphatic disease. Retarded lymph transport or faint or absent nodal visualization typically contribute to the abnormally high TIS.[9,10]

Whole-body lymphangioscintigraphy (WB-LAS) is a reliable screening technique to evaluate the etiology and pathophysiology of upper and lower extremity edema. For example, confinement to a wheelchair or other sedentary conditions causing disuse may be associated with peripheral swelling. WB-LAS demonstrates sluggish flow, but eventual clearance of the radiotracer because the lymphatic vessels are intact and not the primary cause of edema. Morbid obesity, and specifically lipedema, is a condition worthy of special consideration. Affected patients often present with large, heavy legs, corpulent buttocks and bulky upper arms. The feet show no definite abnormality and may even be small, and there is no dorsal hump. WB-LAS usually shows normal deep lymphatic trunks without obstruction, and tracer transport may be within normal limits (Fig. 19.3). Occasionally, however, repeated cellulitis and trauma may lead to areas of lipolymphedema with corresponding WB-LAS alterations.

Most importantly, WB-LAS is a rapid, non-invasive, dynamic, and definitive means of assessing the nature and distribution and pinpointing the specific anatomical and functional features of pure or mixed lymphatic disorders (as indicated in the following sections). In addition, lymphatic abnormalities may be revealed before edema becomes manifest, allowing early preventive or precautionary measures to be undertaken.

Primary Lymphedema

An intrinsic inborn abnormality in the lymphatic conducting pathways underlies primary lymphedema (Fig. 19.2b, g, j). Most patients with this condition have unilateral or bilateral lower limb swelling, but less commonly, arms, viscera, face, or

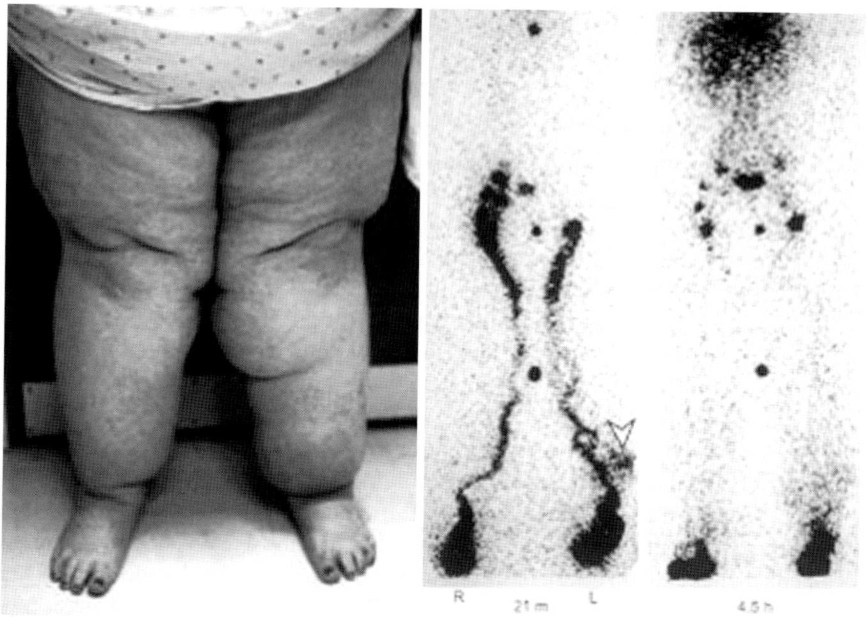

Fig. 19.3 Obesity with distal lymphatic dysfunction in a 34-year-old woman. (**a**) Clinical photograph demonstrates marked enlargement of the legs. (**b**) Lymphangioscintigrams obtained 21 min (*left*) and 4.5 h (*right*) after injection of radiotracer show bilateral intact, but tortuous lymphatic trunks corresponding to rolls of fat. Slight dermal backflow is seen in the lower left leg (*arrowhead*). These findings, along with MRI with fat subtraction, demonstrate that morbid obesity is the primary contributor to marked enlargement of the legs in this patient, with lymphedema being a minor component

other parts of the body may be affected. Patients whose case histories are consistent with either congenital lymphedema (at birth, early childhood, lymphedema praecox at puberty or up to approximately age 25, and some lymphedema tarda with even later onset) fall into this category. Hereditary/familial forms are relatively rare (estimated ~ 5–10% of primary lymphedema case presentations).

On WB-LAS, images in primary lymphedema often show absent or very delayed tracer transport from the injection site(s) and lack of lymph collectors with progressive dermal diffusion into the superficial lymphatics of the limb progressively outlining its contours. Paradoxically, a smaller group of patients show delayed transport, but with intact and even enlarged and more numerous collectors (i.e., lymphatic hyperplasia as in lymphedema–distichiasis syndrome) typically also refluxing (through incompetent valves) into the superficial lymphatic system. In primary lymphedema, regional lymph nodes may not be visualized or alternatively are small and reduced in number and occasionally resemble "grape clusters" of small nodes. In addition, there may be coexistent abnormalities in the retroperitoneal lymphatics or central structures such as the cisterna chyli and its tributaries and the thoracic duct associated with chylous and non-chylous reflux syndromes (see below).

Secondary Lymphedema

Secondary lymphatic dysplasia (Fig. 19.2c–e, h, i) has a multitude of causes with the underlying abnormality being obstruction or obliteration of lymph flow from an acquired source. In developed countries, the most common antecedent is cancer treatment. Regional axillary, inguinal, or retroperitoneal lymph nodes are excised, irradiated, or otherwise destroyed along with surrounding lymphatic vessels, e.g., for staging and/or treatment of breast cancer, melanoma, or gynecological malignancies. Lower extremity lymphedema can result from radical hysterectomy or groin or abdominal node dissections that disrupt regional lymph drainage. A variety of other surgical procedures adjacent to or involving lymphatic structures directly can also interfere with peripheral or central lymph drainage resulting in non-chylous and chylous fluid collections, lymphoceles, cysts, and even ascites and pleural effusions.

Infection, trauma, insect bites, and chronic venous disease are other causes of secondary lymphedema. The occurrence of lymphedema positively correlates with the increased number of resected nodes and irradiation as well as the extent of the operative procedure or tissue damage from other inciting agents. Appearance time of lymphedema is highly variable from months, years, to even decades later. This prolonged delay in appearance probably reflects vigorous lymphatic collateral formation, which gradually succumbs to progressive valve incompetence associated with lymphatic hypertension and fibrotic changes in the obstructed trunks along with associated soft tissue alterations. Lymphatic pumping gradually fails over time because of unremitting or escalating resistance to lymphatic flow.[11]

Chylous Reflux Syndromes

Among the rarer lymphatic disorders are chylous reflux syndromes (Fig. 19.2j), where intestinal lymph flows retrograde through incompetent lymphatic valves and accumulates in various organs, other body parts, and tissues or leaks to the outside. There are congenital forms, which may be generalized as in neonatal chyledema, from defective lymphatic growth and valve formation, or acquired from functional or anatomical obstruction (e.g., lymphatic filariasis) or traumatic disruption of the thoracic duct, cisterna chyli, or their tributaries; or indeterminate (as in lymphangioleiomyomatosis).

Both congenital and acquired forms most typically manifest as chylous effusions in the peritoneal, pleural, or pericardial cavity, chylous vesicles on the skin or genitalia, or leakage into the urinary tract (chyluria) or even the tracheo-bronchial tree (chyloptysis).

Chylous syndromes often present substantial challenges in defining the nature and location of the structural or functional abnormalities. Understanding the lymphodynamic events and treating the condition through non-operative and operative means is imperative. Radionuclide WB-LAS represents a major advance in non-invasively documenting the structural and lymphodynamic aspects of chylous reflux syndromes and providing documentation of the effectiveness of therapeutic interventions designed to reduce, divert, or eliminate the chylous reflux.

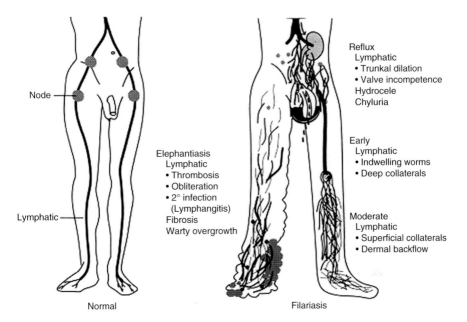

Fig. 19.4 Schematic diagram summarizing filarial lymphatic dysfunction. The normal functioning lymphatic system is depicted on the left. On the right, impedance of lymph transport develops early with dermal lymphatic collateralization and backflow. Lymph transport is preserved until repeated infections and lymphadenitis ensue. Later, lymph reflux (eg., chyluria and hydrocele) may develop even without peripheral lymphedema. (Modified with permission, Witte et al.[7])

Lymphatic Filariasis

In contrast to secondary lymphedema in developed countries, acquired lymphedema in less developed or third-world countries is often caused by filariasis or other infectious processes. Transmitted in larval form by insect vectors, the adult filarial nematode takes up residence in the peripheral lymphatic vessels and nodes. Seemingly impervious to the host defense mechanisms (lymph nodes, lymphocytes, circulating lymph) or else confounding them by molecular mimicry, the active adult worms interfere with lymph flow, and in extreme cases, the involved limbs or genitalia take on an elephantine or pachyderm appearance. Some patients have predominant or concomitant visceral lymphatic involvement, which may culminate in conditions such as chyluria, hydrocele, chylous reflux (chylometrorrhagia or chylous vesicles), genital edema, or even massive breast engorgement.[7] Because many patients in endemic areas often walk barefoot, it is thought that overt or subclinical bacterial infection contributes to the grotesque deformities often associated with these parasitic conditions. WB-LAS vividly depicts a full range of lymphatic structural and functional abnormalities in this condition (Fig. 19.4).

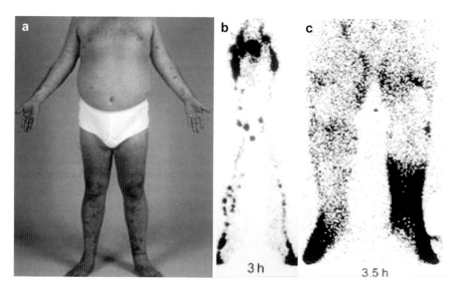

Fig. 19.5 Progressive lymphedema in a 47-year-old man with Kaposi sarcoma and AIDS. (**a**) Clinical photograph demonstrates Kaposi lesions on the extremities. (**b**) Lymphangioscintigram obtained at the time the clinical photograph was taken (3 h after injection of radiotracer) shows minimal edema with uninterrupted lymph flow and intact lymphatic vessels, but with cutaneous "hot spots" corresponding to Kaposi lesions (see **a**). (**c**) Lymphangioscintigram obtained 5 years later (3.5 h after the injection of radiotracer) when the patient had considerably more leg edema with Kaposi skin lesions that had progressed to confluence shows marked dermal extravasation

Kaposi Sarcoma

Kaposi sarcoma is a proliferative "tumor" of the microvasculature, specifically the lymphatic endothelium. Lymphedema in AIDS-related and non-AIDS-related Kaposi sarcoma ranges from mild and limited to woody and severely disabling, extending well beyond the limbs to the trunk, genitalia, face, and viscera. WB-LAS may show typical features of secondary lymphedema with delayed tracer transport, sluggish to absent lymph flow or markedly ectatic dysplastic refluxing lymphatic trunks with filling of Kaposi skin lesions. If spreading lesions and dermal lymphatic obliteration are present, longitudinal WB-LAS studies can document progressive lymphatic dysfunction (Fig. 19.5).[9,12]

Klippel–Trenaunay and Other Lymphangiodysplastic/Mixed Syndromes

The Klippel–Trenaunay (KT) vascular birthmarks syndrome is often associated with venous Klippel–Trenaunay–Servelle syndrome. Lymphatic abnormalities occasionally coexist with arterial disturbances in KT-Weber, which is thought to be caused by a somatic mutation in utero. Clinically, and for guidance in therapy, the structural and functional aspects of these complex disturbances can be unraveled in part using WB-LAS when combined with other imaging modalities, such as vascular scintigraphy (whole-body blood pool analysis), MRI, contrast venography and arteriography, and ultrasound techniques.

The Future

Lymphangio/adenoscintigraphy (by an analogous protocol applied to the peritumoral site rather than the peripheral limb) is much more commonly performed today for sentinel lymph node delineation preparatory to determination of cancer staging. With improved sensitivity and reliability, radiolabeled immunoconjugates or monoclonal antibodies could be directed against tumor-associated antigens and identification of tumor deposits accomplished by immunoscintigraphy. Immunoscintigraphy may also permit tumoricidal drugs to be selectively targeted.

On the other hand, multimodal simultaneous or asynchronous imaging incorporating refined LAS as one element further delineates the structure and function of the peripheral and central lymphatic system providing better resolution and definition of perplexing peripheral and central lymphatic disorders along with specific molecular or other diagnostic, theranostic, and therapeutic implications.

Conclusions

Peripheral lymphatic vessels can be visualized as easily as arteries and veins. Dynamic lymphangioscintigraphy is safe and repeatable and can be performed before and after treatment and is an important adjunct to the patient's history and physical examination. The efficacy of drugs, surgery and physical methods designed to facilitate lymph movement or reduce lymph formation can be assessed.

Diagnostic WB-LAS appropriately combined with MRI can be used to verify the accuracy of the diagnosis of lymphedema, pinpoint the specific abnormality and provide a framework for subsequent therapy. That the subfascial compartment in peripheral lymphedema, both acquired and congenital, has been shown to be intact supports the conclusion that lymphedema is primarily a disorder of the skin and subcutaneous tissue (epifascial) compartment.

In summary, LAS is non-invasive, repeatable, easy to perform, and harmless to the lymphatic endothelial lining. Clear images of truncal lymph transport and draining nodes are routinely obtained. Follow-up studies can be used to document functional changes in lymphatic dynamics.

References

1. McMaster PD. The lymphatics and lymph flow in the edematous skin of human beings with cardiac and renal disease. *J Exp Med.* 1937;65:373-377.
2. Kinmonth JB. Lymphangiography in man; a method of outlining lymphatic trunks at operation. *Clin Sci (Lond).* 1952;11:13-20.
3. Servelle M. Klippel and Trenaunay's Syndrome: 768 operated cases. *Ann Surg.* 1985;210: 365-373.
4. Steckei RJ, Furumanski S, Dunam R, et al. Radionuclide perfusion lymphangiography: an experimental technique to compliment the lymphangiogram. *Am J Roentgenol.* 1975;124: 600-609.
5. Sherman AI, Ter-Pogossian M. Lymph node concentration of radioactive gold following interstitial injection. *Cancer.* 1953;6:1238.
6. McNeill GC, Witte MH, Witte CL, et al. Whole-body lymphangioscintigraphy: preferred method for initial assessment of the peripheral lymphatic system. *Radiology.* 1989;172: 495-502.
7. Witte MH, Jamal S, Williams W, et al. Lymphatic abnormalities in human filariasis as depicted by lymphangioscintigraphy. *Arch Intern Med.* 1993;153:737-744.
8. Baumeister RG, Siuda S, Bull U, Moser E. Evaluation of transport kinetics in lymphoscintigraphy: follow-up study in patients with transplanted lymphatic vessels. *Eur J Nucl Med.* 1985;10:349-352.
9. Witte CL, Witte MH, Unger E, Williams WH, McNeill GC, Stazzone A. Advances in imaging of lymph flow disorders. *Radiographics.* 2000;20:1697-1719.
10. Williams W, Bernas M, NcNeill G, Witte C, Witte M. Lymphatic Transport Index in peripheral lymphedema syndromes. *Lymphology.* 1996;29:134-136.
11. Olszewski W. On the pathomechanism of development of post-surgical lymphedema. *Lymphology.* 1973;6:35-51.
12. Witte MH, Fiala M, McNeill GC, Witte CL, Williams WH, Szabo J. Lymphangioscintigraphy in AIDS-associated Kaposi's sarcoma. *Am J Roentgenol.* 1990;155:311-315.

Chapter 20
Duplex Ultrasonography

Attilio Cavezzi

Diagnosis of lymphedema (LYM) of upper and lower limbs currently relies upon the clinical assessment and upon lymphoscintigraphy in most cases. Color-duplex ultrasound (CDU) is an extremely reliable diagnostic technology for arterial and venous investigation, and the application of ultrasound investigation in LYM diagnostics has been reported since 1986,[1,2] to complement these imaging modalities. The exploitation of this safe, easily repeatable, quite reproducible, and relatively inexpensive technology for lymphatic disorders has resulted in the possibility of collecting some useful information before, during, and after any LYM treatment.

High-frequency (10–20 MHz) ultrasound probes allow a fine study of the more superficial tissues,[3] including the LYM sites, with regard to both qualitative and quantitative findings on the accumulation of fluid in supra- and subfascial planes, and elucidating the architecture. Similarly, ectatic lymphatic vessels,[4-7] with some degree of complexity, alterations in lymph node morphology/vascularization in particular, and venous or arterial hemodynamics may be visualized (Fig. 20.1); any concomitant anatomical abnormality, such as nodules or cysts that appear in a lymphedematous limb, will be easily imaged with CDU as well. Since the early 1990s,[8-12] an ultrasound semiology has been proposed to exploit the CDU diagnostic proprieties in this new field. More recently, comparison of ultrasound imaging, magnetic resonance imaging, computed tomography, spectroscopy, and histology in LYM cases has revealed a good intercorrelation of the diagnostic findings,[13,14] confirming the usefulness of this inexpensive technology.

By means of repeatable measurements it is possible to monitor the LYM evolution and the therapeutic results. CDU examination may equally detect any venous concomitant disorder with great accuracy and is necessary and sufficient for most of the differential diagnoses of the swollen limb (e.g., deep venous thrombosis, [DVT],

A. Cavezzi
Vascular Unit, Poliambulatorio Hippocrates and Clinica Stella Maris,
San Benedetto del Tronto (AP), Italy

B.-B. Lee et al. (eds.), *Lymphedema*,
DOI 10.1007/978-0-85729-567-5_20, © Springer-Verlag London Limited 2011

156   A. Cavezzi

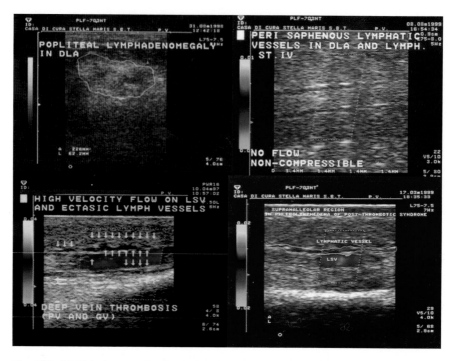

Fig. 20.1 Multiple images of color-duplex ultrasound (CDU) imaging of lymph vessels and nodes

angiodysplasia, postthrombotic syndrome [PTS]). In consideration of the possible role of CDU in identifying venous changes in lymphedematous limbs, a few authors[15] have described the possible dilation of the major deep and superficial venous structures as a consequence of the impaired lymphatic drainage in lymphedematous limbs, with or without acute dermato-lymphangioadenitis. In contrast, several publications have highlighted the possible participation of reduced venous drainage in many cases of "apparently" pure LYM. In fact, impaired subclavian–axillary venous drainage is often present in the edematous arm after mastectomy (in up to 31% of the cases),[16] and some degree of obstruction, or occlusion, of the deep veins has been demonstrated.[17,18] The phlebolymphedema, which may characterize these patients with breast cancer-related arm edema, results in an aggregate of the typical ultrasound findings of LYM (e.g., the so-called lymphatic "lakes," edematous/fibrotic tissues, etc.) and of CDU signs of a PTS and pathological patterns within the subclavian–axillary veins (Fig. 20.2).

The lower-limb PTS may, of course, represent a concomitant disease in any case of LYM of the lower extremity as well, and the CDU investigation of deep, superficial, and perforating veins in these mixed cases of phlebo-lymphedema of the lower limbs is commonly undertaken and is of great benefit for a more precise diagnostic and therapeutic approach.

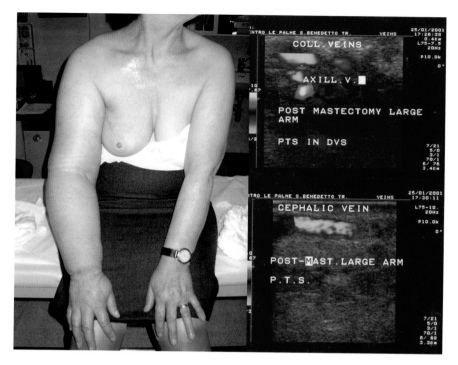

Fig. 20.2 Clinical and CDU pictures of post-mastectomy phlebolymphedema (lymphedema and post-thrombotic syndrome of the upper extremity)

On the arterial side, in 1994, Svensson et al.[19] used CDU to demonstrate increased arterial inflow in arm edema after mastectomy, possibly as a result of altered vasoconstrictor innervations.

Another CDU application relates to vascular malformations involving the lymphatic system. In fact, most "apparently" pure venous angiodysplasias exhibit a relevant lymphatic dysplastic component, and the opposite is also true. Safe and accurate use of CDU in vascular malformations has been proposed by most experts as first-line diagnostic technology, and detection of lymphatic abnormalities may be of help to focus on a proper treatment for these complex diseases.

In cases of posttraumatic or postoperative lymph stasis, CDU once more plays a decisive role: to screen for deep venous thrombosis and to image any serum and blood accumulation and other pathological findings.

With reference to the use of CDU in the investigation of lymphadenomegalias (enlarged lymph node[s]) in the groin or, more rarely, in the popliteal or axillary area, b-mode imaging is usually complemented by color-flow Doppler to highlight possible altered vascularization of the nodes, which usually represent a negative prognostic sign because of its association with neoplasms/metastases.[20] Other possible, quite common findings in CDU imaging of lymphedematous limbs include the ruptured or intact popliteal cyst and/or fluid collection in the knee joint.

The use of CDU investigation was proposed several years ago in specific LYM cases related to filariasis, and a few specific diagnostic markers (such as "the worm dance sign") have been reported.[21-23] Ultrasound imaging may help address local/regional pharmacomechanical treatment for filiariae removal. Monitoring of the infection is facilitated through repeated ultrasound scanning.

It can be argued that the complexity of differential diagnosis and of the therapeutic options available in cases of a swollen limb fully justifies extensive and systematic use of CDU, especially in expert hands.[24]

Specific Details in Ultrasound Investigation of Lymphedema

Ultrasound anatomy of normal skin and deeper layers is generally characterized by:

(a) A first, superficial hyperechogenic layer (the epidermis).
(b) The usually low-echogenicity layer of "papillary" dermis and hyperechogenicity of the deeper reticular dermis.
(c) The mixed-echogenicity of the subcutaneous layer, which is characterized by connective bands and nodule-like (adipose component) images.

At greater depths, the hyperechogenic muscular fascia is easily recognized, and the muscular layer ultrasound image is well defined.

In the case of LYM of the lower or upper limb, several possible modifications may occur in the architecture, echogenicity, and imaging characteristics within the epifascial and subfascial layers. Strict comparison of the same areas in the two limbs, especially in cases of unilateral LYM, and multiplanar transverse and longitudinal scans, together with a bimodal investigation (in the standing and supine positions), are of great help for proper CDU imaging.

A few basic features and findings can be observed through careful technique and proper ultrasound probes. A summary is proposed below.

- The presence of "lymphatic lakes," hypo-echogenic images of fluid collections, which can be located mostly in the epifascial compartment and in the subcutaneous layer, but also, in more advanced cases, in sub-fascial tissues; these fluid extravasations can be distinguished from the collectors because of their "anarchic" disposition, and their abundance and size, although some misinterpretation is always possible; the ultrasound image of the fluid collections, resembling bands of various width, gives the tissues a stratified conformation (Fig. 20.3).
- A dilation of the lymphatic main trunks/collectors is potentially imaged through high-frequency probes (ideally 18 MHz) (Fig. 20.1, 20.4, 20.5); usually the dilated lymphatic vessels are visible in the subcutaneous tissues, mostly along the greater saphenous vein axis for the leg region (where they predominantly lie in normal subjects), or in close proximity to the major lymph nodes (pre-post-lymph node collectors). The visualization of the lymphatic trunks may be more frequent in secondary LYM, because, in primary LYM, the lymphatic vessels may be atretic, hypo-functioning or totally absent; similarly, in cases of acute

Fig. 20.3 CDU imaging in lymphedema; note the lymph movement in proximity to an arteriole, beside the great saphenous vein (GSV)

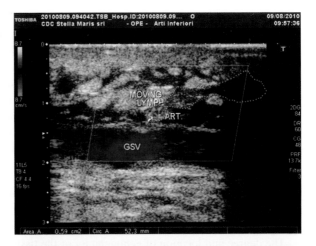

Fig. 20.4 Ectatic lymphatic vessels along the GSV at the malleolar site

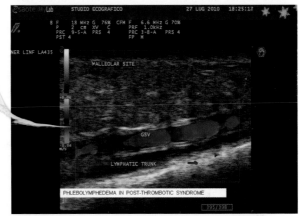

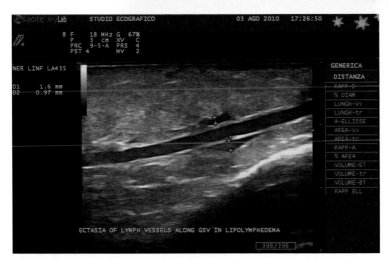

Fig. 20.5 Visible lymphatic vessels in lipolymphedema

dermato-lymphangioadenitis or lymphocele, the lymph collectors tend to dilate functionally and are more visible on ultrasound images. The ultrasound appearance of the lymphatic channel is that of a double hyperechogenic walled tube and sometimes even valves, or thrombi[7] are highlighted inside the largest trunks. Because of the extremely small caliber of these vessels and the extremely slow lymphatic flow, CDU cannot objectively detect any "colored" fluid movement and cannot always distinguish these structures from fluid collections (the so-called "lymphatic lakes") that are visible in any edematous condition.[25] Immediately before Duplex ultrasound (DUS) investigation, an injection of (diluted) liquid albumin,[26] a mini-trauma,[7] or even a tourniquet above the edematous region,[7] may enhance the ultrasound visualization of the lymphatic vessels in lymphedematous limbs or, especially, in normal limbs. Matter et al.[7] also confirmed lymph vessel ultrasound imaging through lymphatic fluid aspiration in the detected channel and through the injection of a radiopaque contrast agent within the same structure.

- The degree and location of echogenicity of the tissues, which strictly correlates with the degree of the fibrosis in the affected areas[27]; in greater detail, minimally pitting or non-pitting LYM correlates with the presence of a higher degree of fibrosis or, better, fibroadiposis, which commonly occurs in the late stages of LYM; long-lasting LYM may result in a DUS pattern that is characterized by a lack of fluid collections and by a hyperechogenicity and anarchy of the supra-sub-fascial tissues, with nodule-like images. However, the early stages of LYM, such as the non-swollen upper extremity after breast cancer surgery (which is clinically comparable to the contralateral limb), may also exhibit a pattern of deterioration of the architecture and an increased thickness and/or echogenicity of the epi-fascial layers, not necessarily showing any lymphatic lakes.[28]
- Lymph node visualization, measurement, and investigation with color-Doppler flow, or power Doppler flow, should complement the ultrasound investigation in LYM cases, to differentiate abnormalities of lymph nodes related to infections, neoplasms (metastases), functional overloading, etc.
- The increase in thickness of the dermis (especially in breast cancer-related LYM)[29] and/or of the subcutaneous layer and/or of the subfascial layer is a constant finding; it involves especially the subcutaneous space until LYM frankly deteriorates, then it involves all layers at the later stages.
- The compressibility of the tissues under the ultrasound probe pressure seems to be well-correlated with the degree of fibrosis/echogenicity, at least in the upper extremity.[30,31]

A few authors[4,25,32,33] have described several rules to differentiate pure venous edema (phlebedema), from pure LYM and especially from lipedema (lipodystrophy of the lower limbs with fat deposition and interstitial fluid retention). In the presence of phlebedema most hypo-echogenic collections are visible in the dermal layers, while in cases of lymphostasis, the fluid collections are located in the subcutaneous region and/or in the sub-fascial space. More advanced LYM cases show bands of hyper-echogenic reflection (which represent perilymphangiosclerosis in advanced cases). Finally, lipedema is usually characterized by diffused echoes along the whole

Fig. 20.6 Ultrasound images of lipedema (*left side*) and lipolymphedema (*right side*), with low-echogenicity findings in the latter condition

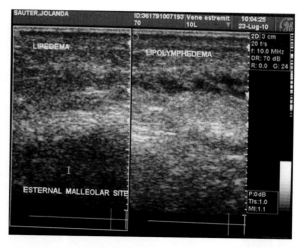

thickness of the suprafascial tissue, with no noticeable areas of low-reflection intensity (no "lymphatic lakes" are visualized) and no increase in dermal thickness (which, on the contrary, happens in LYM). During the late stages of lipedema, lymphostasis may secondarily intervene because of the progressive deterioration of the lymphatic vessels/nodes within the fat tissues and worsening fibrosis. Thus, CDU highlights the typical low-echogenicity spaces in the areas affected by lipolymphedema (Fig. 20.6).

It should be recalled that whenever edema reflects impaired (overloaded or organically pathological) lymphatic drainage and the common CDU findings pattern of hypoechogenic areas will be seen in several of the non-vascular clinical entities, such as heart/renal/liver failure or hypo-disprotidemia.

The largest lymphatic trunk, i.e., the thoracic duct, may also be the object of investigation through CDU. Franceschi[34] first published on B/W ultrasound imaging of a thrombotic obstruction of the thoracic duct and the corresponding intra-operative findings.

Ultrasound usage during LYM treatment can be based on repeated measurements at fixed locations and different measures can be highlighted (Fig. 20.7):

(a) The thickness of the suprafascial tissue (having the muscular fascia as the basal marker).

(b) The skin-to-bone thickness, in particular at the level of the ankle, the foot, and, above all, the retromalleolar regions for the lower limb and the forearm for the upper limb.

If one of the main superficial veins is included in the picture/measurements, or in the case of inclusion of one or two skin markers, such as nevi or spider veins, CDU imaging reproducibility can be improved; similarly, the inclusion of abundant gel on the skin will, on the one hand, minimize the possibility of interference with the images through unwanted pressure on the skin, while, on the other hand, it will improve imaging of the most superficial layers (Fig. 20.8). A holistic, integrated

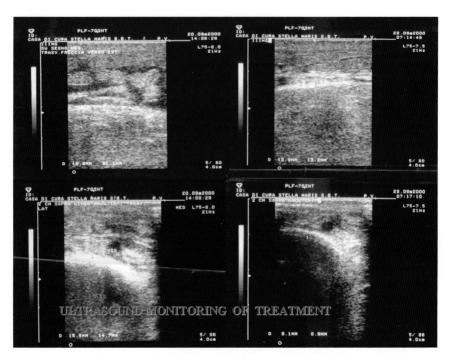

Fig. 20.7 Lymphedema treatment and CDU monitoring of the outcomes

Fig. 20.8 Optimisation of
CDU measurement in
lymphedema follow-up

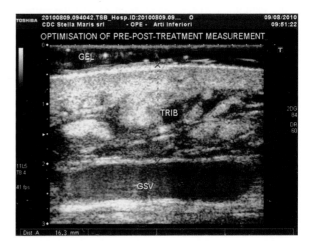

therapeutic approach to LYM is often capable of producing results after a few days
and this results in a reduction (or disappearance) of extravascular layers of liquid, as
well in a decrease in the echogenicity of the tissues, together with a reduction in size
of the lymphatic collectors. A further method of applying CDU investigation to
LYM is by using the probe to bring out some pitting in the edematous areas,[30]

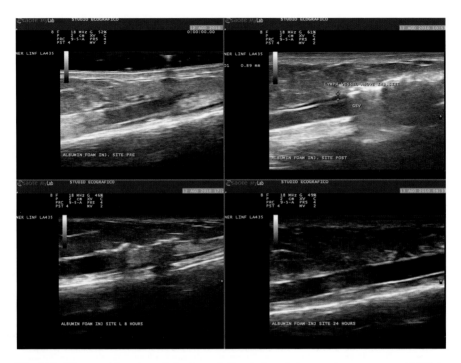

Fig. 20.9 Ultrasound imaging of injections of albumin-based ultrasound contrast agent (UCA) in a normal subject and ultrasound monitoring of UCA distribution within 24 h

highlighting the nature of the edema and its fibrotic component, as well as monitoring the treatment outcomes.

After the introduction of ultrasound contrast agents (UCA) for echocardiography in 1969,[35] the inclusion of albumin or other organic macromolecules in the chemical structure of these agents, led us to investigate the possible usage of UCA in LYM diagnostics.[26] The possibilities and limitations of albumin-based UCA, or of foamy albumin in CDU investigation of LYM, have never been assessed in depth and the few pertinent scientific data that were available from experiments in 2000[26] were not, in fact, conclusive. Several limitations of the older, preliminary experimental studies can be possibly overcome by modern technologies and by the improved knowledge of UCA and of CDU; hence, a reappraisal of those investigations has been undertaken by our group (Fig. 20.9) and some interesting (unpublished) data have been collected in the last few months.

In conclusion, the use of CDU in the field of lymphatic diseases seems to be still in the early stages, but further technological and methodological advancements hopefully will facilitate a broader usage of ultrasound in lymphatic diagnostics and therapeutics. The technical limitations, the dependence of the accuracy on the operator, together with the lack of high-level scientific evidence for CDU investigation in LYM can be counterbalanced by the non-invasive nature and low expense of this diagnostic tool, an approach that is still in its infancy.

Acknowledgments Thanks to Dr. E. Concettina for her contribution and to Prof. B.B. Lee for his patience and continuous stimulus to our scientific work.

References

1. Franceschi C, Franco G, Luizy F, Tanitte M. *Precis d'echotomographie vasculaire*. Paris: Ed.Vigot; 1986.
2. Tsyb AF, Mukhamedzhanov IKh. Ultrasound tomography of soft tissues and venous vessels in secondary edema of the upper limbs. *Vestn Rentgenol Radiol*. 1989;1:52-57.
3. Cammarota T et al. Current uses of diagnostic high-frequency US in dermatology. *Eur J Radiol*. 1998;27:215-223.
4. Schadeck M, Cavezzi A, Michelini S. Limb oedema ultrasonographic diagnostics in *Phlebolymphoedema, from diagnosis to therapy*. Bologna P.R. Communications, 1998;47-53. ISBN 88-900300-1-1.
5. Cavezzi A. Echo-colour-Doppler diagnostics in lymphedema of extremities. UIP World Congress. 1998; Sydney. Abstract Book p. 213.
6. Gallenkemper G. Visualisation of lymph vessels by high resolution colour-coded duplex sonography. UIP World Congress of Dermatology. 1998; Sydney. Abstract Book p. 246.
7. Matter D, Grosshans E, Muller J, et al. Apport de l'échographie à l'imagerie des vaisseaux lymphatiques par rapport aux autres méthodes. *J Radiol*. 2002;83:599-609.
8. Franco A, N'Guyen Khac G. Comment explorer les lymphoedemes des membres: intérêt de l'écographie-Doppler. *Sang*. 1990;2:213-216.
9. Passariello F, Carbone R, Mancini A. Semeiotica ultrasonografica delle alterazioni linfatiche nell' arto inferiore. *Min Angiol*. 1991;16(suppl 1 al n. 2):453-457.
10. Vettorello GF, Gasbarro V, et al. L'ecotomografia dei tessuti molli degli arti inferiori nella diagnostica non invasiva del linfedema. *Minerva Angiol*. 1992;17:23-25.
11. Doldi SB, Lattuada E, Zappa MA, Pieri G, Favara A, Micheletto G. Ultrasonography of extremity lymphedema. *Lymphology*. 1992;25(3):129-133.
12. Schadeck M. *Duplex and Phlebology*. Naples: Ed. Gnocchi; 1994:73-76.
13. Fumiere E, Leduc O, Fourcade S, et al. MR imaging, proton MR spectroscopy, ultrasonographic, histologic findings in patients with chronic lymphedema. *Lymphology*. 2007;40(4):157-162.
14. Tassenoy A, Vermeiren K, van der Veen P, et al. Demonstration of tissue alterations by ultrasonography, magnetic resonance imaging and spectroscopy, and histology in breast cancer patients without lymphedema after axillary node dissection. *Lymphology*. 2006;39(3):118-126.
15. Cavezzi A, Schadeck M. Venous system changes in lymphedema of lower limbs. *Eur J Lymphol Relat Probl*. 1996;6(Sp. Co. I):13.
16. Gruffaz J. Venous component in lymphedema of the upper extremity after radio-surgical therapy of cancer of the breast. *Phlebologie*. 1986;39(3):517-525.
17. Pain SJ, Vowler S, Purushotham AD. Axillary vein abnormalities contribute to development of lymphoedema after surgery for breast cancer. *Br J Surg*. 2005;92(3):311-315.
18. Svensson WE, Mortimer PS, Tohno E, Cosgrove DO. Colour Doppler demonstrates venous flow abnormalities in breast cancer patients with chronic arm swelling. *Eur J Cancer*. 1994;30A(5):657-660.
19. Svensson WE, Mortimer PS, Tohno E, Cosgrove DO. Increased arterial inflow demonstrated by Doppler ultrasound in arm swelling following breast cancer treatment. *Eur J Cancer*. 1994;30A(5):661-664.
20. Tschammler A, Wirkner H, Ott G, Hahn D. Vascular patterns in reactive and malignant lymphadenopathy. *Eur Radiol*. 1996;6(4):473-480.
21. Amaral F, Dreyer G, Figueredo-Silva J, et al. Live adult worms detected by ultrasonography in human Bancroftian filariasis. *Am J Trop Med Hyg*. 1994;50(6):753-757.

22. Dreyer G, Santos A, Noroes J, Addiss D. Proposed panel of diagnostic criteria, including the use of ultrasound, to refine the concept of 'endemic normals' in lymphatic filariasis. *Trop Med Int Health*. 1999;4(8):575-579.
23. Shenoy RK, Suma TK, Kumaraswami V, et al. Doppler ultrasonography reveals adult-worm nests in the lymph vessels of children with brugian filariasis. *Ann Trop Med Parasitol*. 2007;101(2):173-180.
24. Wheatley DC, Wastie ML, Whitaker SC, Perkins AC, Hopkinson BR. Lymphoscintigraphy and colour Doppler sonography in the assessment of leg oedema of unknown cause. *Br J Radiol*. 1996;69(828):1117-1124.
25. Gniadecka M. Localization of dermal edema in lipodermatosclerosis, lymphedema and cardiac insufficiency: high-frequency ultrasound examination of intradermal echogenicity. *J Am Acad Dermatol*. 1996;35:37-41.
26. Cavezzi A. Have ultrasonographic contrast agents a future in lymphedema investigation? *Eur J Lymphology Relat Probl*. 2000;8(31):62.
27. Balzarini A, Milella M, Civelli E, Sigari C, De Conno F. Ultrasonography of arm edema after axillary dissection for breast cancer: a preliminary study. *Lymphology*. 2001;34(4):152-155.
28. International Society of Lymphology. The diagnosis and treatment of peripheral lymphedema. 2009 Consensus Document of the International Society of Lymphology. *Lymphology*. 2009;42:51-60.
29. Mellor RH, Bush NL, Stanton AW, Bamber JC, Levick JR, Mortimer PS. Dual-frequency ultrasound examination of skin and subcutis thickness in breast cancer-related lymphedema. *Breast J*. 2004;10(6):496-503.
30. Kim W, Chung SG, Kim TW, Seo KS. Measurement of soft tissue compliance with pressure using ultrasonography. *Lymphology*. 2008;41(4):167-177.
31. Tsubai M, Fukuda O, Ueno N, Horie T, Muraki S. Development of an ultrasound system for measuring tissue strain of lymphedema. *Conf Proc IEEE Eng Med Biol Soc*. 2008;2008:5294-5297.
32. Marshall M, Wagner AD. Nichtinvasive Diagnostik des Lymph- und Lipodems. *Perfusion*. 1995;9:17-22.
33. Naouri M, Samimi M, Atlan M, et al. High-resolution cutaneous ultrasonography to differentiate lipoedema from lymphoedema. *Br J Dermatol*. 2010;163(2):296-301. Epub 2010 Apr 16.
34. Franceschi C. Pathologie du canal thoracique: intérêt de l'échographie Doppler. *Sang Thrombose Vaiss*. 2004;16(1):61-63.
35. Gramiak R, Shah PM, Kramer DH. Ultrasound cardiography contrast studies in anatomy and function. *Radiology*. 1969;92:939.

Chapter 21
Combined Role of Lymphoscintigraphy, X-Ray Computed Tomography, Magnetic Resonance Imaging, and Positron Emission Tomography in the Management of Lymphedematous Disease

Pierre Bourgeois

Introduction

Various imaging options exist for the evaluation of lymphedematous diseases. Although each imaging technique can be considered separately according to its principles and technical methodologies, the interface among these techniques has become indistinct in practice. Indeed, most of the apparatuses used today for lymphoscintigraphic (LySc) investigations utilize a combination of single photon emission computed tomography dual-headed devices (SPECT) with an X-ray computed tomography machine (CT or SPECT-CT). When positron emission tomography (PET) systems are considered, these are nearly always combined with CT devices. Although these CT scans may not conform to high radiological diagnostic standards, they allow easy fusion of the SPECT or PET images with other high-quality and high-resolution X-ray CT or magnetic resonance images, thus providing additional diagnostic data. The techniques can then be used in an orderly fashion.

The choice of technique, either alone or in combination, must be made by taking into account the clinical presentation and the diagnostic and/or therapeutic questions being addressed (Table 21.1). In the present chapter, we will review the use and contributions of these techniques in the management (e.g., diagnosis and treatment) of the following lymphedematous disorders: primary lymphedemas, secondary lymphedemas, genital lymphedemas, lymphedemas with chylous reflux, phlebo- and lipo-lymphedemas, and the lymphangiomatous diseases.

P. Bourgeois
Service of Nuclear Medicine, Institute Jules Bordet,
Université Libre de Bruxelles,
Brussels, Belgium

B.-B. Lee et al. (eds.), *Lymphedema*,
DOI 10.1007/978-0-85729-567-5_21, © Springer-Verlag London Limited 2011

Table 21.1 Respective contributions of the various imaging techniques in the management of lymphedematous diseases

	Lymphoscintigraphy		Lympho-SPECT-CT		CT		PET-CT		MRI	
	Diagnosis	Treatments	Diagnosis	Treatments	Diagnosis	Treatments	Diagnosis	Treatments	Diagnosis	Treatments
Upper Limb Edema(s) (ULE)										
Primary	++++	++++[a]	++++	++++[a]					++[b]	V
Secondary "Oncological"	++	++++[a]	+++	++++[a]	+/++	+	++	V	++[b]	++++[b]
Others	++++	++	++++	V	+++	V	?			
Lower Limb Edema(s) (LLE)										
Primary "Congenital"	++	++++[a]	+	++++[a]	+				+[b]	++++[b]
"Praecox"	+++	++++[a]	++	++++[a]	++	+	?		++[b]	++++[b]
"Tarda"	++++	++++[a]	+++	++++[a]	+++	++	+		+++[b]	++++[b]
Secondary "Oncological"	++	++++[a]	++	V	+/++	+	++	V	?	++++[b]
Others	+++	++	++++	V	+++	V	++	V	?	?
Lipo(lymph)edema	++	+/++	+++	+	++				?	?
"Phlebolymphedemas"	+++	+/++	++	+?	++		+		?	?
Lymphangioma	+		++		++++	V			++++[b]	++[b]
Lymphangiomatosis	+		+		++++	V			++++[b]	+++[b]
Chylous reflux disorders	++	+/++	'++++	+++	++				++++[b]	++++[b]
Genital Lymphedema Males	++	+/++	'++++	'++	+		?		++[b]	++++[b]
Females	++	+/++	'++++	'++	+		?		++[b]	+++

[a] With additional injections at the root of the limbs
[b] With injection of contrast medium

Lymphoscintigraphy and/or SPECT-CT Lymphoscintigraphy

Lymphoscintigraphic investigations are of proven value in the diagnosis and management of diseases of the lymphatic system.[1-4]

Lymphoscintigraphy or SPECT-CT Lymphoscintigraphy in Relation to the Clinical Presentation of the "Simple" Lymphedematous Situations

Lymphoscintigraphy and/or SPECT-CT lymphoscintigraphy can be used and interpreted by taking into account the origin of the lymphedema and the clinical stage of the disease.

In Primary Lower Limb Lymphedemas

In primary lower limb lymphedemas (praecox and, especially, tarda) in the early clinical stage (latent, intermittent, and/or spontaneously reversible, orthostatic, etc.), the classical planar lymphoscintigraphic acquisitions (instead of SPECT-CT) are adequate to assess lymphatic functional insufficiency. In such situations, the investigational protocol will evaluate the function of the lymphatic system of the limbs in standardized conditions, i.e., resting, during exercise, and after 1 h of normal activity.[5] In patients with lymphatic dysfunction, conservative management, such as massage therapy, use of compression garments, and limb elevation, should be recommended initially.

In other kinds of primary lower limb lymphedemas, such as congenital disorders, clinically more severe disease (staged II to IV), and, in particular, the descending forms (extending from the root of the limb toward the foot and suggesting lymph nodal obstructions or lymphadenodysplasias), SPECT-CT maybe useful in addition to the planar investigations to precisely evaluate the intra-abdominal lymph node status, especially among obese patients.

In Secondary Lymphedemas

In secondary lymphedemas, SPECT-CT, in addition to planar investigation, is beneficial for the following applications:

- In lower limb edema, for evaluation of intra-abdominal lymph node status, particularly among obese patients.
- In upper limb edema, for localization of various lymph nodes of potential importance (humeral, axillary, apical, retro, or supraclavicular).

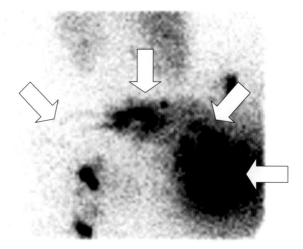

Fig. 21.1 Posterior view centered on the pelvis obtained in one woman with congenital right lower limb primary lymphedema. Peripheral injection showed no lymph nodes on the right side and only inguinal nodes on the left side. Intradermal injection of the 99mTc-HAS-nanocolloid was then performed in the external and lateral part of the right buttock (*horizontal arrow*). With manual lymphatic drainage, the tracer was shown to flow posteriorly through superficial dermal collateralization toward the right costo-lumbar area (*right to left oblique arrow*), to reach and cross the midline (*vertical arrow*), and from there to reach the left inguinal nodes through normal right-sided lymphatic vessels (*left to right oblique arrow*)

Lymphoscintigraphy to Demonstrate the Collateralization Pathways

When no lymph nodes are visualised in the inguinal and/or iliac regions after peripheral subcutaneous injections of the radiolabeled colloid in the feet, and when no lymph nodes are visualized in the axillary and/or clavicular areas after peripheral subcutaneous injections of the radiolabeled colloid in the hands, it may be necessary to perform intradermal injections of the same tracer in the external part of the root of the edematous limb(s) to demonstrate lymphatic collateralization pathways[6] (Figs. 21.1, 21.2). The results of such injections will be of the utmost importance for physical therapists, so that they can be informed of the possible collaterals requiring stimulation.

SPECT-CT Lymphoscintigraphy for the Lymphedematous Disorders Complicated by Chylous Reflux and/or Leakage

SPECT-CT lymphoscintigraphy (after conventional three-phase planar acquisitions) is particularly useful in patients with chylous reflux or/and leakage, either clinically obvious[7-10] or suspected. According to our experience, abdominal SPECT-CT should be performed in the following situations:

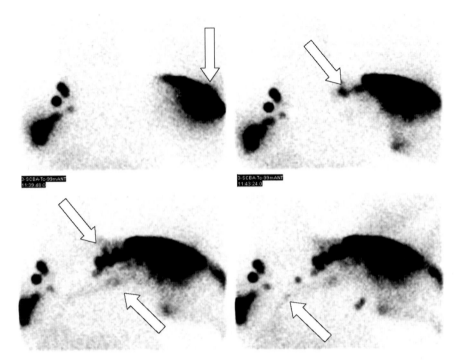

Fig. 21.2 From left to right and from top to bottom, anterior views centered on the axilla in a woman with post-therapeutic left upper limb lymphedema where the subcutaneous injection of 99mTc-HAS nanocolloid in the first interdigital space of the hands showed normal right axillary nodes, but no node in the left axilla. Intradermal injection was then performed at the level of the upper and external part of the left arm (*vertical arrow*) and the tracer was shown to spontaneously flow toward the retro-clavicular lymph nodes (*left to right oblique arrows*) and also toward the left anterior chest wall, to cross the midline to reach the opposite axillary lymph nodes (*right to left oblique arrows*)

- In any patient in whom activity is observed in the abdomen that does not correspond with classical anatomical localization of infra-diaphragmatic lymph nodes (Figs. 21.3, 21.4).
- When lymphatic reflux and dermal backflow are observed in the genital organs and/or at the level of the abdominal wall (Figs. 21.5, 21.6).

Lymphoscintigraphy, Lymphoceles, and Lymphangiomas?

Identification of lymphangioma by lymphoscintigraphy is rarely reported.[11-14] In these patients, as in some patients with lymphoceles, SPECT-CT lymphoscintigraphy will be of clinical utility in order to demonstrate the exact anatomical connections and relationships between the lymphatic collection and the lymphatic vessels or nodes.

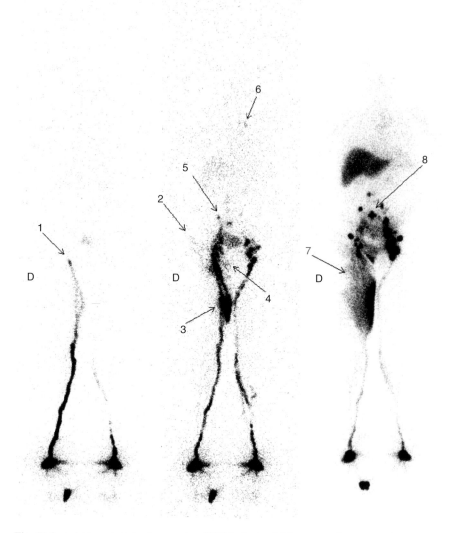

Fig. 21.3 Anterior whole-body scanning (WBS) obtained (after one subcutaneous injection of 99mTc-labeled HAS nanosized colloid in the first interdigital space of each foot, the patient lying on the examination table), from right to left, after 30 min without movement, after 5 min of tiptoe-ing, and after 1 h of walking. This man was sent for evaluation of right lower limb lymphedema (he also had pre-pubic edema on clinical examination) secondary to surgery and radiotherapy for prostatic carcinoma. After 30 min without movement, the tracer has reached the first inferior ingui-nal node on the right side (*arrow 1*), but progressed only to the level of the knee on the left side. After 5 min of tiptoeing, lymphatic reflux is seen in collaterals toward the external part of the right buttock (*arrow 2*), up to and in the mid internal part of the thigh (*arrow 3*), and in the right pre-pubic area (*arrow 4*). One right common iliac lymph node is observed (*arrow 5*) as well as – faintly – two left retro-clavicular lymph nodes (*arrow 6*), proving that the thoracic duct is pervious. After 1 h of walking, the reflux of lymph in the superficial collateralization lymphatics extends to the upper and inner half of the right thigh (*arrow 7*), but one abnormal zone of activity is also demon-strated in the mid supra-pubic part of the abdomen (*arrow 8*)

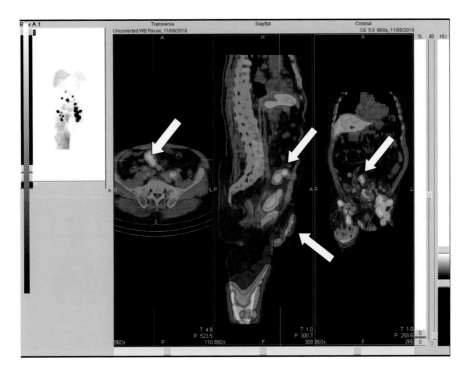

Fig. 21.4 From left to right, selected transverse, sagittal, and coronal/frontal fused slides from the SPECT-CT across the abdomen and pelvis showing nicely (1) (*top to bottom oblique arrows*) that the abnormal zone of activity seen on the planar WBS image in the mid supra-pubic part of the abdomen corresponds, in fact, to lymph flowing back from lumbar aortic nodes in the digestive tract and (2) (*bottom to top oblique arrow*) dermal back flow in the right pre-pubic area

X-Ray Computed Tomography?

Computed tomography is rarely necessary for the diagnosis of simple lymphedema-tous disorders, but may be useful for the pre-treatment evaluation and initial work-up, because it provides an objective depiction of anatomical abnormalities.[15]

Computed tomography will be of greater clinical utility, and is particularly useful, in patients with lymphangiectasia, lymphangioma, or lymphangiomatosis. In these patients, CT can be used to assess both the nature and distribution of lesions[16] or to facilitate their catheter-guided percutaneous sclerosis or obliteration.[17]

Positron Emission Tomography or Positron Emission Tomography Combined with X-Ray Computed Tomography?

As mentioned in the Introduction, the use of PET alone is becoming progressively less prevalent in the Nuclear Medicine department, being replaced by hybrid devices combining PET and CT.

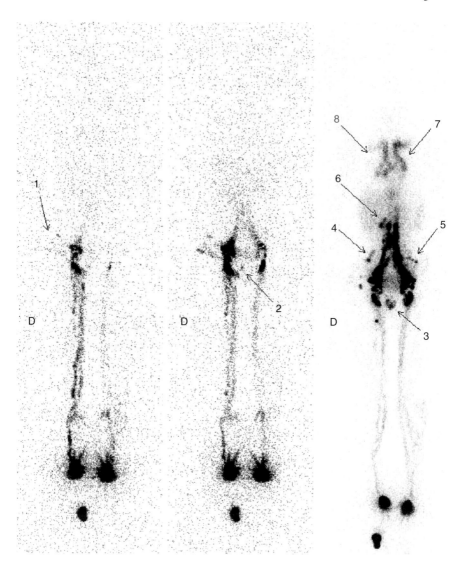

Fig. 21.5 Anterior WBS obtained (after one subcutaneous injection of 99mTc-labeled HAS nano-sized colloid in the first interdigital space of each foot, the patient lying on the examination table), from right to left, after 30 min without movement, after 5 min of tiptoeing, and after 1 h of walking. This young woman did not complain of lower limb edema, but was referred for evaluation of intermittent lymph leakage at the level of her right labium majorum. After 30 min without movement, the tracer reached the first inferior inguinal node on the left side and all the inguinal nodes on the right side, but with lymphatic collaterals appearing from the inguinal nodes toward the external part of the buttock (*arrow 1*). After 5 min of tiptoeing, infra-diaphragmatic lymph nodes are now seen on both sides (and right collaterals are confirmed); the beginning of lymphatic reflux in the right labium majorum can also be observed (*arrow 2*). After 1 h of walking, the reflux of lymph in the right magna labia is now obvious (see *arrow 3*), but abnormal zones of activity are also demonstrated in the right and left lateral part of the abdomen (*arrows 4* and *5*) as well as at least two right para-renal lymph nodes (*arrow 6*) and, at the supradiaphragmatic level, there is a completely abnormal presentation of the great lymphatic thoracic duct with right and left components persisting (*arrows 7* and *8*). For more information on these anomalies, see Bourgeois et al.[33]

Fig. 21.6 Coronal/frontal slide from the SPECT across the chest, the lumbar aortic nodes and the ilioinguinal nodes showing nicely, in the mediastinum, serpentine channels forming the thoracic duct and, in the abdomen, the lake of lymphatic activity in the right and left digestive tract

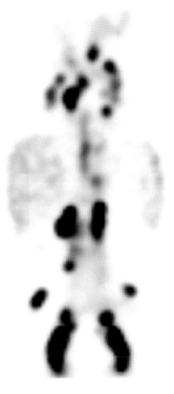

In the management of secondary upper and/or lower lymphedemas, PET-CT imaging using an appropriate tracer (18F-DG, 11C-Choline, etc.) is useful, for instance, when serum tumor markers are increasing or when lymphedemas become treatment-resistant. Focusing on the use of CA 15-3 in breast carcinoma and CA 125 in ovarian carcinoma, Pecking et al.[18] found the sensitivity and predictive value of PET-CT with 18F-FG to be nearly 100%. An additional application of PET-CT in such patients is to exclude and/or demonstrate distant (non-nodal) metastases.

As shown by Figs. 21.7, 21.8, this can also be useful in some patients in a first time classified as with primary lymphedemas.

Magnetic Resonance Imaging and/or Lymphangio-MRI with Injection of Contrast Enhancement?

Magnetic Resonance Imaging in the Diagnosis of Pathologically Positive Lymph Nodes?

With regard to the possible use of MRI to evaluate malignant involvement of lymph nodes (sometimes responsible for the development, aggravation, and/or resistance of lymphedema to treatment), Klerckx et al. performed a systematic

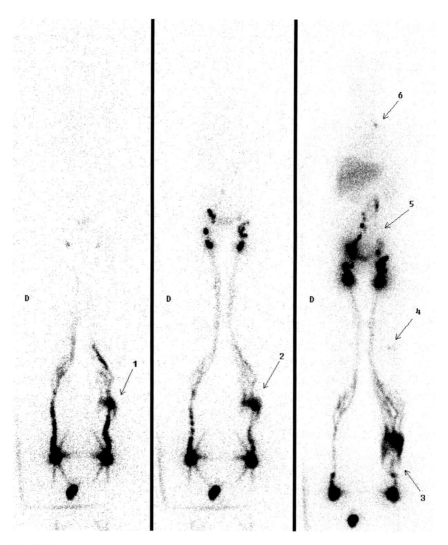

Fig. 21.7 Anterior whole-body scanning (WBS) obtained (after one subcutaneous injection of 99mTc-labeled HAS nanosized colloid in the first interdigital space of each foot, the patient lying on the table of examination), from right to left, after 30 min without movement, after 5 min of tiptoeing, and after 1 h of walking. This woman was sent for evaluation of left lower limb lymphedema. After 30 min without movement, the tracer has reached the first inferior inguinal node on both sides, but the beginning of lymphatic reflux is seen at the level of the distal part of the left calf (*arrow 1*). After 5 min of tiptoeing, lymphatic reflux in the left calf is more obvious (*arrow 2*). After 1 h of walking, the reflux of lymph in the superficial collateralization lymphatics is obviously extended to the left ankle (*arrow 3*), one left popliteal lymph node (*arrow 4*), and one left retro-clavicular lymph node (*arrow 6*), but not the left common iliac nodes (*arrow 5*). On the basis of this lymphoscintigraphic examination, the diagnosis of primary lymphedema tarda was proposed

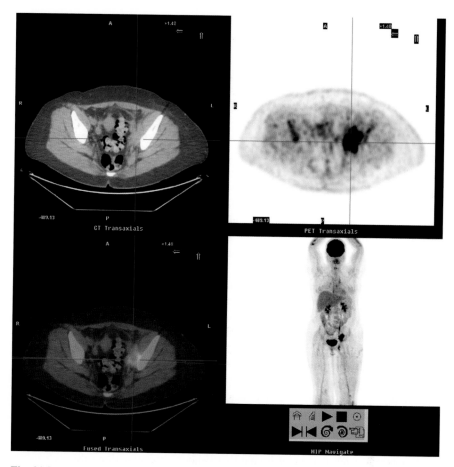

Fig. 21.8 The patient later developed left sciatica and blockage of the common iliac vein was suspected. PET-CT after IV injection of 18F-DG was performed and demonstrated (on the selected transverse PET-CT slides) a hypermetabolic process later histologically proven to represent metastatic tumor of uterine cervix origin

review and meta-analysis of existing data on the accuracy of gadolinium-enhanced MRI for staging lymph node metastases.[19] The weighted estimates of sensitivity and specificity for all studies combined were 0.72 (95% confidence interval [CI] = 0.66–0.79) and 0.87 (95% CI = 0.82–0.91) respectively. Estimates of sensitivity and specificity were essentially unchanged for studies that used a single malignancy criterion (n = 11 studies) or multiple malignancy criteria without contrast enhancement (n = 6 studies). The sensitivity increased to 0.84 (95% CI = 0.70–0.92), with a specificity of 0.82 (95% CI = 0.72–0.89), for the nine studies that incorporated contrast enhancement in their multiple malignancy criteria.

Heavily T2-Weighted Imaging or Magnetic Resonance Lymphangiography for Lymphedemas?

According to Lu et al.,[20] heavily T2-weighted imaging has greater sensitivity and the MRL image has higher legibility for the detection of the pathologically modified lymphatic vessels and accompanying complications.

MRI or MRL in Lymphedemas?

In a series of 39 patients (27 male and 12 female) with lower extremity lymphedema and/or skin lymphorrhea of the abdominal wall or external genitalia with peripheral and central lymphatic malformations, Liu et al.[21] reported that non-contrast 3D MRI provided extensive information on the anatomy of the dysfunctional vasculature as well as on the effects of lymphatic dysfunction on local structures and tissue composition.

With the intracutaneous injection of gadobenate dimeglumine into the interdigital webs of the dorsal foot of 27 patients with primary lymphedema, the same authors[22] reported, more recently, that contrast MR lymphangiography was capable of visualizing the precise anatomy of lymphatic vessels and lymph nodes in lymphedematous limbs and also provided information concerning the functional status of lymph flow in the lymphatic vessels and lymph nodes.

Notohamiprodjo et al. reported on the use of intracutaneous injection of gadolinium-diethylene-triamine-pentaacetic-acid in 16 patients,[23] concluding that MRL at 3.0 T provides very high spatial resolution and anatomical detail of normal and abnormal peripheral lymph vessels. However, they also stated that the examination was non-diagnostic in one case where contrast medium was injected subcutaneously instead of intracutaneously and that venous contamination (always present) was diagnostically problematic in another patient.

In a small series of patients, Lohrmann et al.[24,25] also demonstrated the efficacy of MRI in lipo-lymphedemas and in post-traumatic edemas of the lower extremities.

MRI in Chylous Reflux?

Magnetic resonance imaging permits visualization of deep-lying, ordinarily inaccessible lymphatic vessels, such as those of the retroperitoneum in chylous reflux syndromes.[26] Combined transaxial and coronal imaging allows visualization of these lymphatic vessels and provides visual guidance for the injection of sclerosing agents for the obliteration of external lymph leakage (e.g., skin, vagina) or bulky lymphangiomas.[26] Non-enhanced MRI is also a feasible option for locating and depicting the morphological features of the thoracic duct[27] and, thus, might be of interest in chylothorax situations.

MRI and Lymphangiomatosis?

Lohrmann et al.[28] confirmed the utility of MRI in 15 patients with diffuse lymphangiomatosis, using magnetic resonance lymphangiography with T1-weighted 3D spoiled gradient-echo and a T2-weighted 3D-TSE sequence.

MRI and Lymphangiomas?

Because MRI accurately predicts subsequent intraoperative findings and accurately demonstrates lymphatic architecture at different tissue levels, Liu et al.[21] consider MRI the diagnostic modality of choice in lymphangioma. In contrast, Dubois et al.[29] suggest that Doppler ultrasound should be the initial imaging technique, and that MRI can be used to evaluate the extent of the lesion(s) prior to treatment. Kuhlmann et al.[30] preferred MR imaging when intravenous contrast material cannot be given for CT.

Lymphoscintigraphy and/or MRI?

Our estimation of the relative advantages and drawbacks of lymphoscintigraphic and MRI imaging techniques is presented in Table 21.2. To summarize, MRI techniques offer good anatomical resolution, but are more expensive and up until now, have been used in only relatively small series of patients. Additionally, the potential renal toxicity of the imaging contrast agent must be considered. On the other hand, lymphoscintigraphic techniques have been evaluated on very large series of patients and are (relatively) less expensive, but require radiation exposure and offer reduced anatomical resolution. Because MRI lymphangiography requires intradermal injections, we considered its functional contributions lower than those of the lymphoscintigraphic techniques where the tracer is injected subcutaneously,[1,31] which may be more useful in stage 0–2 lymphedema.

Table 21.2 Lymphoscintigraphic and MRI techniques: the pros and cons

	LySc	SPECT CT LySc	MRI	Lymphangio MRI
Overall anatomical contribution	+	++	+++	++++
Functional imaging of the lymphatic system	+++	+++	+?	++?
Value established in large series?	++++	+	++	+?
Potential limitations	Pregnant?		Obese, claustrophobia, pace-maker, metallic prosthesis...availability of the imaging agent?	
Irradiation	+	++	/–/	/–/
Potential toxicity of the imaging agent	/–/	/–/	/–/	+? (kidneys?)
Cost	+	++	+++	++++

Conclusions

Conventional oil-contrast lymphography has, in the past, been the mainstay for lymphatic imaging. Lymphoscintigraphy now more easily permits imaging of peripheral lymphatic vessels and provides insight into lymph flow dynamics. It is indispensable for patients with known or suspected lymphatic circulatory disorders to confirm the diagnosis and to delineate the pathogenesis and evolution of lymphedema. In several cases, the injection of radiolabeled colloids at the root of the edematous limbs will demonstrate lymphatic collateralization pathways and provide useful information for the physical therapists. In patients with lymhadenodysplasia, with reflux and/or leakage of lymph and/or chyle and with suspected abnormalities at the level of the thoracic duct, SPECT-CT lymphoscintigraphy is useful in providing detailed anatomy of the abnormalities. PET-CT after injection of 18F-DG is efficacious in patients with secondary lymphedema and/or increased serum tumor markers. Patients with a provisional diagnosis of peripheral lymphatic dysfunction or idiopathic edema after lymphoscintigraphy should undergo, in select cases, MR imaging to verify diagnostic accuracy, pinpoint the specific abnormality, and help guide subsequent therapy, especially surgery.[32] MR imaging will also complement lymphoscintigraphy in the monitoring and treatment of more complex lymphatic circulatory disorders, whereas CT will facilitate catheter-guided percutaneous sclerosis or obliteration of specific lymphangiectasia or lymphangioma syndromes. The choice of technique, either alone or in combination, must be made by taking into account the clinical presentation and the diagnostic and/or therapeutic questions being addressed (Table 21.1).

References

1. Bourgeois P. Critical analysis of the literature on the lymphoscintigraphic investigations of the limb edemas. *Eur J Lymphology Relat Probl.* 1996;6:1-9.
2. Szuba A, Shin WS, Strauss HW, Rockson S. The third circulation: radionuclide lymphoscintigraphy in the evaluation of lymphedema. *J Nucl Med.* 2003;44:43-57.
3. Scarsbrook AF, Ganeshan A, Bradley KM. Pearls and pitfalls of radionuclide imaging of the lymphatic system. Part 2: evaluation of extremity lymphoedema. *Br J Radiol.* 2007;80:219-226.
4. Pecking AP, Albérini JL, Wartski M, Edeline V, Cluzan RV. Relationship between lymphoscintigraphy and clinical findings in lower limb lymphedema: towards a comprehensive staging. *Lymphology.* 2008;41:1-10.
5. Bourgeois P, Munck D, Becker C, Leduc O, Leduc A. Reevaluation of a three-phase lymphoscintigraphic investigation protocol for the lower limb-edemas. *Eur J Lymphology Relat Probl.* 1996;6:10-21.
6. Bourgeois P, Belgrado JP. Interest of lymphoscintigraphic investigations in the post-therapeutic upper limb edemas [abstract]. *Eur J Nucl Med Mol Imaging.* 2009;36:S215.
7. Li LY, Zhao QX, Luo WC. An analysis of 30 cases of chylothorax and chyloperitoneum [Article in Chinese]. *Zhonghua Nei Ke Za Zhi.* 1991;30:347-349, 382.
8. Howarth D, Gloviczki P. Lymphoscintigraphy and lymphangiography of lymphangiectasia. *J Nucl Med.* 1998;39:1635-1638.

 9. Nishiyama Y, Yamamoto Y, Mori Y, et al. Usefulness of Technetium-99m human serum albumin lymphoscintigraphy in chyluria. *Clin Nucl Med.* 1998;23:429-431.
10. Pui MH, Yueh TC. Lymphoscintigraphy in chyluria, chyloperitoneum and chylothorax. *J Nucl Med.* 1998;39:1292-1296.
11. Wells RG, Ruskin JA, Sty JR. Lymphoscintigraphy: lower extremity lymphangioma. *Clin Nucl Med.* 1986;11:523.
12. Boxen I, Zhang ZM, Filler RM. Lymphoscintigraphy for cystic hygroma. *J Nucl Med.* 1990;31:516-518.
13. Okizaki A, Shuke N, Yamamoto W, et al. Protein-loss into retroperitoneal lymphangioma: demonstration by lymphoscintigraphy and blood-pool scintigraphy with Tc-99m-human serum albumin. *Ann Nucl Med.* 2000;14:131-134.
14. Kuang-Tao Y. Detection of chylothorax and cervical cystic hygroma in hydrops fetalis using lymphoscintigraphy. *Clin Nucl Med.* 2006;31:205-206.
15. Marotel M, Cluzan R, Pascot M, Ghabboun S, Alliot F, Lasry JL. CT findings in 150 cases of lower extremity lymphedema. *J Radiol.* 1998;79:1373-1378.
16. Wunderbaldinger P, Paya K, Partik B, et al. CT and MR imaging of generalized cystic lymphangiomatosis in pediatric patients. *AJR Am J Roentgenol.* 2000;174:827-832.
17. Witte CL, Witte MH, Unger EC, et al. Advances in imaging of lymph flow disorders. *Radiographics.* 2000;20:1697-1719.
18. Pecking AP, Mechelany-Corone C, Pichon MF. 1959–1999: from serum markers to 18-FDG in oncology: the experience of the René-Huguenin Center [Article in French]. *Pathol Biol (Paris).* 2000;48:819-824.
19. Klerkx WM, Bax L, Veldhuis WB, et al. Detection of lymph node metastases by gadolinium-enhanced magnetic resonance imaging: systematic review and meta-analysis. *J Natl Cancer Inst.* 2010;102:244-253.
20. Lu Q, Xu J, Liu N. Chronic lower extremity lymphedema: a comparative study of high-resolution interstitial MR lymphangiography and heavily T2-weighted MRI. *Eur J Radiol.* 2010;73:365-373.
21. Liu N, Wang C, Sun M. Noncontrast three-dimensional magnetic resonance imaging vs lymphoscintigraphy in the evaluation of lymph circulation disorders: a comparative study. *J Vasc Surg.* 2005;41:69-75.
22. Liu NF, Lu Q, Jiang ZH, Wang CG, Zhou JG. Anatomic and functional evaluation of the lymphatics and lymph nodes in diagnosis of lymphatic circulation disorders with contrast magnetic resonance lymphangiography. *J Vasc Surg.* 2009;49:980-987.
23. Notohamiprodjo M, Baumeister RG, Jakobs TF, et al. MR-lymphangiography at 3.0 T – a feasibility study. *Eur Radiol.* 2009;19:2771-2778.
24. Lohrmann C, Foeldi E, Langer M. MR imaging of the lymphatic system in patients with lipedema and lipo-lymphedema. *Microvasc Res.* 2009;77:335-339.
25. Lohrmann C, Pache G, Felmerer G, Foeldi E, Schaefer O, Langer M. Post-traumatic edema of the lower extremities: evaluation of the lymphatic vessels with magnetic resonance lymphangiography. *J Vasc Surg.* 2009;49:417-423.
26. Molitch H, Unger E, Witte C, vanSonnenberg E. Percutaneous sclerotherapy of lymphangiomas. *Radiology.* 1995;194:343-347.
27. Yu DX, Ma XX, Zhang XM, Wang Q, Li CF. Morphological features and clinical feasibility of thoracic duct: detection with nonenhanced magnetic resonance imaging at 3.0 T. *J Magn Reson Imaging.* 2010;32:94-100.
28. Lohrmann C, Foeldi E, Langer M. Assessment of the lymphatic system in patients with diffuse lymphangiomatosis by magnetic resonance imaging. *Eur J Radiol.* 2009 Nov 11. [Epub ahead of print].
29. Dubois J, Garel L. Imaging and therapeutic approach of hemangiomas and vascular malformations in the pediatric age group. *Pediatr Radiol.* 1999;29:879-893.
30. Kuhlman JE, Bouchardy L, Fishman EK, Zerhouni EA. CT and MR imaging evaluation of chest wall disorders. *Radiographics.* 1994;14:571-595.

31. Bourgeois P, Leduc O, Belgrado JP, Leduc A. Scintigraphic investigations of the superficial lymphatic system: quantitative differences between intradermal and subcutaneous injections. *Nucl Med Commun.* 2009;30:270-274.
32. Lohrmann C, Felmerer G, Foeldi E, Bartholomä JP, Langer M. MR lymphangiography for the assessment of the lymphatic system in patients undergoing microsurgical reconstructions of lymphatic vessels. *Microvasc Res.* 2008;76:42-45.
33. Bourgeois P, Munck D, Sales F. Anomalies of thoracic lymph duct drainage demonstrated by lymphoscintigraphy and review of the literature about these anomalies. *Eur J Surg Oncol.* 2008;34:553-555.

Chapter 22
Oil Contrast Lymphangiography

J. Leonel Villavicencio

Ever since the lymphatic vessels were discovered incidentally in 1622 by Gasparo Asselius, Professor of Anatomy at Pavia University in Italy,[1] the anatomy and physiological functions of these tiny structures have posed a challenge to the investigators because of their small size and the difficulties involved in visualization. Contrary to what happens in the arterial and venous systems, where visualization is relatively easy, visualization of the lymphatic system has been technically challenging. After Asselius's description, the lymphatics were the focus of attention of many investigators who used injections of mercury into cadavers to gain as much knowledge as possible about these intriguing little vessels. At the Medical–Surgical Military Academy of Austria, founded in 1785 by Joseph II, 1,192 beautiful anatomical wax models, crafted in Florence at the end of the eighteenth century, are on public display. Here, unique models of whole-body dissections of the lymphatic system created by the Italian artists can be admired.

The complex network of small lymphatic capillaries that absorb fluid from the interstitial space was described by Casley-Smith, who called them "initial lymphatics."[2] They are formed by a single layer of 10 to 60 μm endothelial cells. These lymphatic capillaries drain into larger valved channels of the dermis and subcutaneous tissues that run along the veins above the muscular fascia. Visualization of the initial lymphatics was the subject of the 1984 International Symposium in Zurich, Switzerland, and a publication edited by A. Bollinger, J. Partsch, and J.H.N. Wolfe[3] in which demonstration and functional evaluation of superficial lymphatics was explored using fluorescence microlymphography[4] and Iotasul (indirect lymphography).[5] Of course, all of these efforts came after the pioneering work of Professor John B. Kinmonth of Saint Thomas Hospital in London, of whose life the lymphatic system, its visualization by lymphography, its classification, and its function became

J.L. Villavicencio
Distinguished Professor of Surgery, Department of Surgery,
Uniformed Services, University School of Medicine,
Director Emeritus Venous and Lymphatic Teaching Clinics,
Walter Reed Army and National Naval Medical Centers,
Washington DC and Bethesda, MD, USA

B.-B. Lee et al. (eds.), *Lymphedema*,
DOI 10.1007/978-0-85729-567-5_22, © Springer-Verlag London Limited 2011

the focus. In the introduction to the first edition of his book in 1972, it is compelling to read the following citation:

> The chief author had the good fortune to work in the years after the war with Professor Sir James Patterson Ross at St Bartholomew's Hospital. At that time there was no satisfactory clinical method of investigating lymphatic function. Pure speculation reigned. One eminent authority on vascular diseases even stated that "he doubted if the lymphatics existed, and if they did they were of no importance." Another said that such research was valueless: "you won't find anything out and if you do, no-one will believe you." But Sir James was encouraging. When on a ward round at Bart's he saw a picture of one of the first successful deep lymphangiograms and he said, "don't lose that slide it is going to be very important." Much of our early studies were on patients with lymphedema with aplasia or hypoplasia of the lymphatics. We did not know it but we had chosen the most difficult subjects for lymphography. Often we felt like the poet W.B. Yeats, "the fascination of what is difficult has dried the sap out of my veins."[6]

After the groundbreaking investigations of Hudack and McMaster, who injected patent blue dye intradermally and demonstrated small lymphatics in the skin,[7] Servelle in 1944,[8] and Kinmonth in 1952[9] explored the use of patent blue in the experimental and clinical visualization of the lymphatic vessels. This pioneering work culminated with the description of the technique of lymphography as a preliminary step to the visualization of the dermal and subcutaneous lymphatics. Cannulation of these vessels and injection of contrast materials produced some of the first radiological imaging of the lymphatic vessels. Kinmonth devoted the following 25 years of his life to the study of the lymphatic system and the development of techniques of lymphatic visualization that produced the first lymphangiographic and clinical classification of lymphedemas. By the time he published his book, he had performed more than 2,000 direct lymphographies. This author had the privilege to have met Professor Kinmonth and to have worked with him in 1957 during a visit to his close friend, and my mentor, Professor Richard Warren of the Peter Bent Brigham Hospital in Boston. Professor Kinmonth gave me a small bag containing several grams of patent blue violet powder (also known as Patent Blue V, Alphazurine 2G) with detailed instructions on how to prepare an 11% sterile aqueous solution of the vital dye whose capacity to diffuse into the tissues and be absorbed by the lymphatics was higher than that of other vital dyes. Professor Kinmonth's visit sparked my life-long interest in the lymphatic system and my efforts to study the lymphatic system in different edema-producing conditions. An apparatus of my own design to measure the intra-lymphatic pressure (lymphomanometer) and perform direct visual and radiological lymphography was constructed and used in different types of lymphedema (Fig. 22.1). The results of my investigations on lymphatic pressure are beyond the scope of this chapter.

Visual Lymphography and Radiological Lymphography

Visual lymphography is performed by injecting 0.1–0.3 mL of patent blue dye through a fine needle (27-gauge) into two to three interdigital spaces of the foot or hand. Gentle massage and active movements of the foot/hand are recommended to

Fig. 22.1 (**a**) Direct lymphography after lymphomanometry. This photograph shows a lymphatic vessel cannulation on the dorsum of the foot after injection of 0.2 mL of aqueous solution of patent blue violet into each of three interdigital spaces of the foot. (**b**) A 1-mm ID diameter micro-pipette attached by one end to a plastic tube connected to a syringe and a U water manometer and by the other to a 30-gauge needle. After the lymphatic pressure determination, a slow injection of ultrafluid lipiodol was performed by gradual turning of the metal piston on the syringe plunger

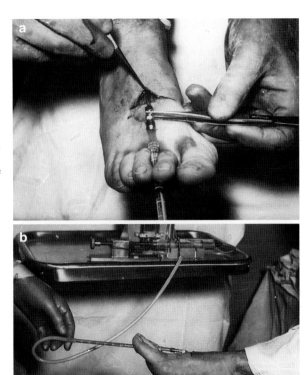

facilitate dye absorption and proximal progression. In patients with lymphatic truncal or nodal obstruction, a fine reticular cutaneous pattern (dermal backflow) may appear 5–15 cm proximal to the site of injection (Fig. 22.2). In addition to the detection of dermal backflow, visual lymphography is widely used intra operatively to facilitate the surgical identification of the lymphatic trunks travelling next to the greater saphenous vein or the superficial veins of the upper extremity in patients subjected to lymphovenous anastomosis or other lymphatic/node reconstruction procedures. The injection of patent blue can be performed in other areas of the body, such as the neck, testes (lymphocele, hydrocele), axilla, pelvis, etc., to visualize nodes or lymph trunks.

Radiological Lymphography

After the dye injection has been absorbed by the lymphatics, one often may detect the blue lymph channels through the skin. A small transverse incision on the dorsum of the foot or hand is carefully performed using gentle strokes of the scalpel.

Fig. 22.2 (**a**) Reflux of the
dye to the skin is called
"dermal backflow" and is
strongly suggestive of
lymphatic obstruction.
(**b**) Visual lymphography.
The interdigital injection of
0.2 mL of an 11% aqueous
solution of patent blue violet
into three to four web spaces
produced this image

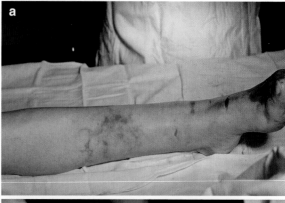

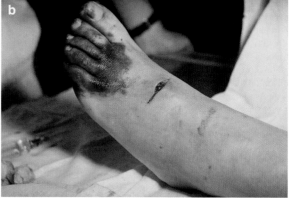

Magnification using 4+ surgical loupes or a 6+ surgical microscope is of great value
in identifying the lymphatic trunks and distinguishing them from the neighboring
veins. The lymphatic trunks appear stained in beautiful blue against the yellowish
contrast of the fatty tissue. Dissection of the lymphatic is done carefully, freeing its
anterior and lateral aspects and leaving the posterior segment intact to serve as a
support for the cannulation. We used a # 30-gauge hypodermic needle with four
small side holes in its distal 5 mm. The lateral holes drilled by a watchmaker
decrease the resistance to the injection of the contrast material.

Oil Contrast Lymphography

Oil soluble contrast materials such as ultrafluid lipiodol were used extensively in
direct lymphography. Lipiodol contains 38% of iodine and is more viscous than its
aqueous counterpart, "Conray" 280 or 420. The injection must be performed very
slowly, using automatic injectors (1 mL every 6–7 min). A total of no more that
10 mL of lipiodol should be injected. The progress of the dye is monitored by serial

radiographs. The calf and thigh are massaged to assist the oil in its centripetal flow and further radiographs are taken at intervals of several hours. The contrast material has the disadvantage of producing inflammation of the vessels and, often, obstruction of the lymphatics. The latter complication is responsible for possible obstruction and lack of visualization of surgical lymphovenous anastomosis and thus, difficulty in assessing the patency and benefits of the procedure. Oil lymphography may also produce allergies and, on occasion, oil embolization, manifested by dyspnea, pyrexia, and slight hemoptysis. In spite of its risks, the procedure was extensively used throughout the world and was instrumental in the development of a lymphedema classification. The Kinmonth classification was based on clinical, lymphangiographic and histopathological studies. He described:

(a) The normal lymphatic system
(b) Hypoplasia of the lymphatic trunks
(c) Aplasia of the trunks and lymph nodes
(d) Hyperplasia or varicose dilatations of the lymph trunks

Primary lymphedemas have aplasia or hypoplasia of trunks with or without node aplasia. Secondary lymphedemas have abnormal patterns of lymph transport secondary to damage to the lymph trunks or to the nodes, such as in lymphadenectomy for malignancy and/or radiation.

Lymphography, as described, provided useful information on anatomy and morphology of the lymphatics. However, the procedure was tedious and time-consuming and requires exquisite patience and skill. It did not provide dynamic information and its use has been practically abandoned. Like many advances in science, lymphography has been a stepping-stone in the progress toward better technological procedures. Lymphoscintigraphy was the next step in the effort to obtain visualization and better information on flow dynamics and transport of fluids.[10-13] With the introduction of technetium-99m human serum albumin and advances in the digital gamma camera, improved resolution of the entire body lymphatic system was obtained.[14,15]

The lymphoscintigraphy technique as utilized in our department[15] requires the injection of 1 mc of Tc-$Sb_2 S_3$ mixed with 0.3–0.5 mL of normal saline, subcutaneously, into three interdigital web spaces of each foot. Before injecting the isotope, the patient exercises by walking for 5 min. Images are obtained in a gamma camera at 10 min intervals with a large field of view. Inguinal nodes are usually observed at or before 30 min. A normal lymphoscintigraphic pattern consists of symmetrical, bilateral transit of the tracer to the inguinal nodes within 1 h. Abnormal lymphoscintigraphic patterns include dermal backflow, complete obstruction, lymphoceles, reflux, and lateral channels. Because the tracer enters the lymphatics by diffusion rather than direct endolymphatic injection, lymphoscintigraphy accurately and reliably depicts the anatomy and function of the lymphatic system.[16]

Magnetic resonance imaging (MRI) has shown its value in congenital vascular anomalies. It has been used in the differential diagnosis of lipedema, venous edema, and lymphedema. Patients with lymphedema show a typical honeycomb pattern of the subcutaneous tissue. An advantage of the method is that it is possible to visualize the lymphatic trunks or nodes proximal to lymphatic obstruction, something that lymphoscintigraphy cannot do.[17]

There is no doubt in my mind that the field of lymphatic imaging continues to evolve with the development of newer imaging methods such as positron emission tomography (PET), dynamic contrast-enhanced MRI (DCE-MRI), and color Doppler ultrasound (CDUS). These techniques provide structural and functional information using minimally invasive interstitial imaging techniques with new contrast agents. As occurs in the field of congenital vascular malformations, multi-modal techniques might be more appropriate for diagnosing and studying lymphatic diseases.[18]

The poor resolution of the conventional diagnostic method of radionuclide-based imaging has served as the incentive to investigate MRI and new contrast agents in the anatomical and functional evaluation of the lymphatics and lymph nodes in the diagnosis of lymphatic circulatory disorders, particularly in primary lymphedema. In a recent study, contrast-enhanced lymphangiography was performed with a 3.0-T MR unit after intracutaneous injection of gadobenate dimeglumine into the inter-digital webs of the foot. This study demonstrated the possibility of visualizing the precise anatomy of lymphatic vessels and lymphatic nodes in patients with lym-phedema, as well as functional data regarding lymph flow transport in the lymphatic vessels and nodes.[19]

From the direct lymphography of Kinmonth to the current wave of novel radiological techniques and newer contrast materials, many years of clinical and experimental investigations have elapsed, always in search of better methods and tech-niques to discover the true significance of the challenging and elusive lymphatics.

References

1. Asselius G. *De Lattibus Sine Lacteis Venis*. Mediolani, Apud lo B Bidellium;1927.
2. Casley-Smith JR. The fine structure and functioning of tissue channels and lymphatics. *Lymphology*. 1980;12:177.
3. Bollinger A, Partsch H, Wolfe JHN eds. The Initial Lymphatics. New Methods and Findings. *International Symposium Zurich*. Pub Georg Thieme Verlag, Stuttgart, New York, 1985; 117-130.
4. Bollinger A, Jaeger K, Sgier F, Seglias J. Fluorescence microlymphography. *Circulation*. 1981;64:1195.
5. Partsch H, Wenzel Hora BI, Urbanek H. Differential diagnosis of lymphedema after indirect lymphography with Iotasul. *Lymphology*. 1983;16:12.
6. Kinmonth JB. *The Lymphatics: Surgery, Lymphography and Diseases of the Chyle and Lymph Systems*. 2nd ed. London: Edward Arnold; 1982:1-17.
7. Hudack SS, McMaster PD. The lymphatic participation in human cutaneous phenomena. *J Exp Med*. 1933;57:751.
8. Servelle M. A propos de la Lymphographie experimentale et Clinique. *J Radiol Electro Med Nucl*. 1944;26:165.
9. Kinmonth JB. Lymphangiography in man. *Clin Sci*. 1952;11:13.
10. Sherman AI, Ter-Porgassian M. Lymph node concentration of radioactive colloidal gold following interstitial injection. *Cancer*. 1953;6:1238-1240.
11. Kaplan WD. Iliopelvic lymphoscintigraphy. *Semin Nucl Med*. 1983;13:42-53.

12. Cambria RA, Bender CE, Hauser MF. Lymphoscintigraphy and lymphangiography. In: Gloviczki P, Yao JST, eds. *Handbook of Venous Disorders. Guidelines of the American Venous Forum.* New York: Chapman and Hall Medical; 1996:580-599.
13. Collins PS, Villavicencio JL, Abreu SH. Abnormalities of lymphatic drainage in lower extremities. A lymphoscintigraphic study. *J Vasc Surg.* 1989;9:145-152.
14. Witte CL. Lymphatic imaging. *Lymphology.* 1993;26:109-111.
15. Villavicencio JL, Pikoulis E. Lymphedema. In: Raju S, Villavicencio JL, eds. *Surgical Management of Venous Disease.* Baltimore: Williams & Wilkins; 1997:163-164.
16. Weissleder H, Weissleder R. Lymphedema evaluation of qualitative and quantitative lymphoscintigraphy in 238 patients. *Radiology.* 1988;167:729-735.
17. Weissleder R, Elizondo G, Wittenburg J. Ultrasmall superparamagnetic iron oxide: an intravenous contrast agent for assessing lymph nodes with MR imaging. *Radiology.* 1990;175:494-498.
18. Barret T, Choyke PL, Kobayashi H. Imaging of the lymphatic system: new horizons. *Contrast Media Mol Imaging.* 2006;1(6):230-245.
19. Liu NF, Lu Q, Jiang ZH, Wang CG, Zhou JG. Anatomic and functional evaluation of the lymphatics and lymph nodes in diagnosis of lymphatic circulation disorders with contrast magnetic resonance lymphangiography. *J Vasc Surg.* 2009;49(4):980-987.

Chapter 23
Fluorescent Microlymphangiography

Claudio Allegra, Michelangelo Bartolo, and Anita Carlizza

Like the blood capillaries, the lymphatic microvessels are formed by a thin layer of endothelial cells resting on a delicate basal membrane. This structure, particularly at the initial segment, is widely fenestrated. The cells are anchored to filaments which, as interstitial pressure increases, are believed to open the fenestrations and allow the lymph to enter the lymphatic microvessel.[1,2] The cutaneous microlymphatic circulation is formed by two superficial networks joined by small perpendicular vessels through which the lymph drains from the superficial into the deep network. This deep network is connected by channels that run in a perpendicular direction from the skin downward to the lymphatic precollectors.[1-3] The lymphatic system is currently conceptualized as an integral component of a drainage network originating from the venous end of microcirculation. Together with the venous portion of the capillary circulation and the interstitium, it constitutes a single system that may be defined as a functional microcirculatory unit.[2-6] The venous and the lymphatic systems work together; they are connected by tiny lymphovenous anastomoses that activate when the pressure in the lymphatic system rises.[7-9] Persistent venous stasis will lead to functional overload in the lymphatic system that may result in dynamic insufficiency because the fluid overload exceeds the transport capacity of the lymphatics. In these conditions, lymphangiopathy develops and, in turn exacerbating edema, which is no longer only of venous, but also of lymphatic, origin.[3,10-15]

With today's technologies, the initial lymphatics in any body compartment can be visualized to study microlymphatic vessel morphology, diameter, and permeability; number of microlymphatic loops; and extension of the contrast halo from the injection site. Contrast enhancement of microlymphatics is obtained by injecting 0.01 mL of fluorescein isothiocyanate dextran 150,000 into the subderma under fluorescence videomicroscopy using a microsyringe (approximately 0.2 mm).[1,16-18] The images are recorded on a videocassette and then processed by computer to visualize the data.

C. Allegra (✉)
Angiology Department, San Giovanni Hospital, Rome, Italy

B.-B. Lee et al. (eds.), *Lymphedema*,
DOI 10.1007/978-0-85729-567-5_23, © Springer-Verlag London Limited 2011

Microlymphography in Healthy Individuals, in Chronic Venous Disease, and in Lymphedema (Table 23.1)

Because microlymphography permits the visualization and study of microlymphatic vessels, it can be employed to study lymphatic pathophysiology in common micro- and macrocirculatory diseases. In healthy individuals, few microlymphatics are ordinarily visualized because there is good drainage of contrast material into the deep lymphatic circulation[16] (Fig. 23.1). Involvement of the microlymphatics in chronic venous disease (CVD) offers a characteristic microlymphatic pattern, displaying an increased number of loops and typical fragmentation[1,19,20] (Fig. 23.2).

In early-stage lymphedema, the number of microlymphatic loops is particularly high and the microlymphatic pressure is much higher than the normal range. This finding can be interpreted as a mechanism of initial insufficiency (Fig. 23.3).[1,21,22]

In long-standing lymphedema, the microlymphatics cannot be seen because of the presence of fibrosis[1,23] (Fig. 23.4).

Microlymphography calculates the following parameters:

1. Number of open or available lymphatic vessels
2. Morphology of open or available lymphatic vessels
3. Permeability of available lymphatic vessels
4. Superficial diffusion of contrast material from the injection site (mm)
5. Diameter of available lymphatic vessels (micron)
6. Intralymphatic pressure (mmHg)
7. Interstitial pressure

When the data from dynamic capillaroscopy and capillary blood velocity (CBV) are combined with microlymphography, a more complete picture can be obtained for understanding the pathophysiology of a microcirculatory unit.[1-3,5,8,16,17]

Measurement of Microlymphatic Pressure

During the 1960s microcirculatory pressure was measured directly using micropipettes (at least 15 µm in diameter). With this passive method, the time needed to measure pressure was about 10 s.[24] The large micropipettes altered the delicate pressure balance inside the microlymphatics, rendering measurement extremely difficult. A significant advance in measuring intramicrolymphatic pressure came in the 1970s when Marcos Intaglietta created the Servo Nulling System, a device that permitted active pressure measurement with real-time response (0.05 s).[25] The micropipettes in this system were less than half the diameter of the old ones (about 7 µm). With later refinements to the Servo Nulling System (Model 5a created in 1990) and positioning of a preamplifier near the micropipette, the pressure could be measured with much smaller micropipettes (about 1 µm in diameter).[26] The use of micropipettes of only 1 micron in diameter led the way to detailed study of intramicrolymphatic

Table 23.1 Microlymphography in chronic venous disease, in lymphedema and in healthy controls

	No. of open or available lymphatics	Morphology interrupted, broken	Permeability	Superficial diffusion of contrast material from injection site (mm)	Lymphatic capillary diameter (micron)	Lymphatic capillary pressure in human skin (mmHg)	Interstitial pressure (mmHg)	Capillary blood velocity
Controls	6.6±5	–	–	7.8±2.6	62.3±7.4	4.19±1	0.65±1.6	0.38±0.7
CEAP 2–3	16.8±8.2	+	+	n.a.	72.77±17.3	6.7±2.6	1.47±1.7	0.34±0.1
CEAP 4–6	13.8±8	++	++	n.a.	88.5±19.6	5.51±2.4		0.29±0.1
Lymphedema	>30	–	+	22.1±13.1	>100	n.a.	4.33±1.7	n.a.
Lymphedema in fibrosis	n.d.	n.d.	+++++	n.a.	n.d.	n.d.	n.d.	n.a.

+ present, – absent, *n.d.* not determinable, n.a. not available, *CVD* chronic venous disease, plus or minus values are the means ± SD

Fig. 23.1 Microlym-
phography in a healthy
subject

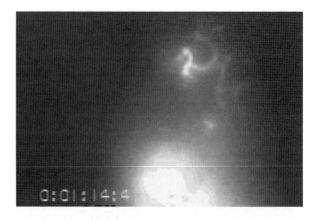

Fig. 23.2 Microlym-
phography in chronic venous
disease, CEAP 2–3

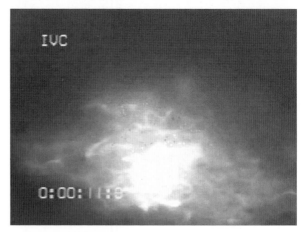

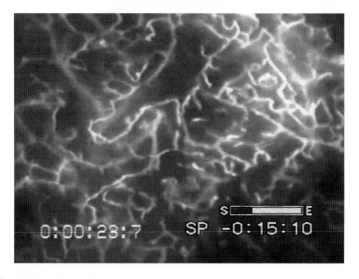

Fig. 23.3 Microlymphography in lymphedema

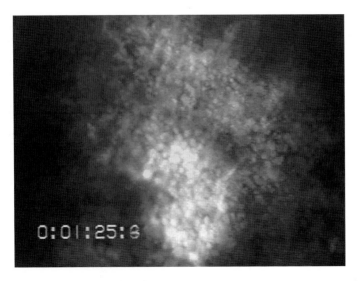

0:01:25:3

Fig. 23.4 Microlymphography in fibrosis

pressure. Pressure is measured for at least 1 min at baseline conditions with the patient supine and having rested for at least 30 min beforehand.

Studies by Allegra et al. using the system have improved our knowledge of the pathophysiology of the lymphatic circulation in healthy subjects and in patients with chronic venous disease, lymphedema, and other vascular conditions.[19,20,22,23] Besides intramicrolymphatic pressure, this method can be used to measure interstitial pressure in healthy individuals and in those with chronic venous disease and lymphedema.

Lymphatic Vasomotion and Lymphatic Flow Motion

Several important findings were discovered by chance. After having recorded thousands of microlymphographs and fast-forwarded several images, we noticed that it was sometimes possible to recognize, even with the naked eye, flow movement inside the microlymphatics. We digitized several microlymphographs and observed and measured lymphatic flow. For the first time, the velocity of lymphatic flow was visualized and measured in vivo in a human. We noted two different types of intramicrolymphatic flow: a very slow granular flow, which we termed "lymphatic flow motion" (about 10 ± 4 µ/s), and a pulsating, "stop and go" flow pattern, faster than the former (about 91 ± 58 µ/s), with periodic accelerations, which we termed "lymphatic vasomotion." The periodicity of the flow accelerations was about 1 min ± 25 s.

We were unable to visualize either type of flow pattern in healthy subjects; however, in patients with CVD (CEAP 2,3) we sometimes found a pulsating flow (lymphatic vasomotion) in the proximity of the precollectors, but never granular flow (lymphatic flow motion). In patients with soft edema, we more often found a granular flow pattern, but rarely a periodic flow pattern in the proximity of the precollectors[19,20,22,23] That granular flow pattern is visible only in a setting of soft lymphedema, but not in patients with CVD or healthy subjects; it may be linked to an increase in the superficial flow that compensates for obstruction of normal deep flow.

In the setting of lymphedema, the presence of a pulsating flow (lymphatic vasomotion) is related to deep drainage because of the opening of the precollectors, probably resulting from critical pressure levels. As regards CVD, the pulsating flow pattern is related to similar dynamics, even if the underlying pathophysiological mechanism is failure of the microlymphatic system and increased interstitial pressure due to capillary stasis.[19,20,22,23] In healthy subjects, neither flow pattern is detected since the lymph flows not in the superficial, but, rather, in the deep network through the collectors and therefore cannot be visualized. Recent developments in monitoring and studying lymphatic flow have provided insights into the pathophysiology of lymphatic circulation (Table 23.1).

References

1. Bollinger A, Fagrell B. *Clinical Capillaroscopy*. Toronto: Hogrefe & Huber Publishers; 1990.
2. Pratesi F. Sistema microvasculotessutale:morfologia funzionale. In: *Microcircolazione e Microangiologia*. Torino: Ed.Min. Med; 1990:17-30.
3. Allegra C, Carlizza A. Oedema in chronic venous insufficiency: physiopathology and investigation. *Phlebology*. 2000;15:122-125.
4. Allegra C. *Endotelio Come Organo*. Milano: Pragma Ed.; 1991.
5. Allegra C, Carioti B. Diffusione endoteliale capillare in vivo. *Minerva Angiol*. 1993;18 (1 suppl 1):245-251.
6. Allegra C, Carlizza A. Rheopletysmography and laser-Doppler velocimetry in the study of microcirculatory flow variability. In: Allegra C, Intaglietta M, Messmer K, eds. *Vasomotion and Flowmotion. Progress in Applied Microcirculation*, vol. 20. Basel: Karger; 1991.
7. Allegra C. *Appunti di Flebologia*. Arti Grafiche Istaco Ed.1991;15-19.
8. Allegra C, Carlizza A. Constitutional functional venopathy. *Adv. Vasc Pathol*. Int Congress Series 1150. 1997;123-129.
9. Spiegel M, Vesti B, Shore A, Franzeck UK, Bollinger A. Pressure of lymphatic capillaries in human skin. *Am J Physiol*. 1992;262:H1208-H1210.
10. Speicer DE, Bollinger A. Microangiopathy in mild chronic venous incompetence: morphological alterations and increased transcapillary diffusion detected by fluorescence videomicroscopy. *Int J Microcirc Clin Exp*. 1991;10:55-66.
11. Allegra C. The role of the microcirculation in venous ulcers. *Phlebolymphology*. 1994;2:3.
12. Husmann MJ, Barton M, Vesti BR, Franzeck UK. Postural effects on interstitial fluid pressure in humans. *J Vasc Res*. 2006;43(4):321-326.
13. Agus GB, Allegra C. Guidelines for diagnosis and therapy of diseases of the veins and lymphatic vessels. *Int Ang*. 2001;2(suppl. 2):53-64.
14. Gretener SB, Lauchli S, Franzeck UK. Effect of venous and lymphatic congestion on lymph capillary pressure of the skin in healthy volunteers and patients with lymphedema. *J Vasc Res*. 2000;37(1):61-67.
15. Guyton AC. Interstitial fluid pressure. *Physiol Rev*. 1971;51:527-532.

16. Bartolo M Jr, Allegra C. Image: can we see lymphatics? *Int J Microcirc Clin Exp*. 1994;14 (suppl 1):191.
17. Allegra C. Microcirculatory techniques and assessment of chronic venous insufficiency. *Medicographia*. 1996;18:30.
18. Lauchli S, Haldimann L, Leu AJ, Franzeck UK. Fluorescence microlymphography of the upper extremities. Evaluation with a new computer programme. *Int Angiol*. 1999;18(2): 145-148.
19. Bartolo M Jr, Carioti B, Cassiani D, Allegra C. Lymphatic capillary pressure in human skin of patients with chronic venous insufficiency. *Int J Microcirc Clin Exp*. 1994;14(suppl 1):191.
20. Allegra C, Bartolo M Jr. Haemodynamic modifications induced by elastic compression therapy in CVI evaluated. by microlymphography. *Phlebology '95*. 1995;1:9-17.
21. Fischer M, Costanzo U, Hoffmann U, Bollinger A, Franzeck UK. Flow velocity of cutaneous lymphatic capillaries in patients with primary lymphedema. *Int J Microcirc Clin Exp*. 1997;17(3):143-149.
22. Allegra C. Lymphatics of the skin in primary lymphoedemas. *Int J Microcirc Clin Exp*. 1996;16(suppl 1):114.
23. Allegra C, Bartolo M Jr, Sarcinella R. Morphologic and functional changes of the microlymphatic network in patients with advanced stages of primary lymphedema. *Lymphology*. 2002;35:114-120.
24. Wunderlich P, Scherman J. Continuous recording of hydrostatic pressure in renal tubules and blood capillaries by use of a new pressure transducer. *Pflugers Arch*. 1969;313:89-94.
25. Intaglietta M. Pressure measurements in the microcirculation with active and passive transducers. *Microvasc Res*. 1973;5:317-323.
26. Intaglietta M, Tompkins WR. Simplified micropressure measurements via bridge current feedback. *Microvasc Res*. 1990;39:386-389.

Chapter 24
Alternative Assessment and Measurement Tools

Neil B. Piller

The stage and status of any lymphedematous limb (or other part of the body) and the impact of treatment on it can be measured objectively and accurately,[1] yet, very few health professionals (and even fewer patients) ever make any attempt to make even the most basic measurements to obtain a complete assessment of the limb, few bother to compare the at-risk or affected limb with the contralateral one, and even fewer have the opportunity to measure a high-risk limb prior to an intervention.

Why is this so? Time is certainly an issue, but is not an excuse because a good understanding of the limb and its current presentation should help target and sequence treatment and thus gain a better outcome for the patient (and a better reputation for the treating clinician or therapist). The lack of enthusiasm for measuring is also another issue. This is often perceived as another chore, which can be bad news for the practitioner. Accurate information will certainly help the patient, but it can also help protect the practitioner should a legal claim be made against him or her.

A number of simple and easily used alternate tools and strategies can detect early changes in the tissues before the clinician or the patient might otherwise notice them (as a change in the size of a limb) and indicate how the treatment is progressing.

I strongly believe that we must all make every attempt to detect lymphedema before it manifests clinically; this means easier treatment, a greater chance of patient involvement, better outcomes, and, from the perspective of the health care system, a better cost-benefit analysis.

The alternative tools and techniques that are available to help us better understand and react to changes in limb structure (fibrotic tissue build-up) and function (shown as changes in levels of extracellular fluids) will be described.

N.B. Piller
Lymphoedema Assessment Clinic, Department of Surgery, School of Medicine,
Flinders University and Medical Centre, Bedford Park, SA, Australia

B.-B. Lee et al. (eds.), *Lymphedema*,
DOI 10.1007/978-0-85729-567-5_24, © Springer-Verlag London Limited 2011

Measurement of Fibrotic Induration

Perhaps one of the first noticeable sequelae of surgery and radiotherapy is the formation of local or diffuse fibrous tissue. This is part of the tissue repair process, but also can be associated with a wound infection. Scarring associated with the surgical or radiotherapeutical sites at the root of the extremity may significantly reduce the ability of new lymph capillaries and collectors to grow or existing ones to regenerate.

In addition, as lymphedema progresses, so too does the extent and distribution of fibrotic tissue, with fluids being replaced by fatty and then fibrous tissues. The rate of this progression varies greatly. Tonometry, which measures the resistance of the tissues to compression, is an indicator of the extent of underlying fibrosis.[2] It has been used since 1976 and, when used over the major lymphatic territories or at the watersheds, can indicate the extent of induration and of the impact of treatment. Tonometry is quickly and easily performed and can be used by individuals with minimal training. It does not measure the actual amount of fibrous tissues but, rather, the tissue resistance to compression by measuring the depth of compression of the tissues when a standard weight is placed on them. With current tonometers (made by BME at Flinders Medical Centre) accuracy to 1 mm is possible.

Variations in fibrotic tissue can be cross-confirmed with ultrasound (or CT if necessary initially) when this is performed at the same site as tonometry. When fibrotic induration is detected, strategies such as low-level laser or frictional massage or special MLD can be used to target it. There are perhaps more accurate ways of measuring scarring and its location (e.g., ultrasound, MRI), but they take longer and are expensive.

Measurement of Fluid Content

One of the early signs of a failure of the lymphatic system is the accumulation of small amounts of extra-cellular fluids in the affected lymphatic territory or the whole limb. Fluid accumulation is a sign that, regionally, the lymphatic system is failing. The patient or clinician may not be able to detect or measure this subtle indication of lymphatic system failure. As there is no detectable increase in limb volume or circumference when measured by the more traditional techniques of tape measurement, the early detection of fluids is possible using multi-frequency bio-impedance.[3] Current equipment is claimed to detect differences and changes in limb extra-cellular fluids as small as 5 mL. There is a large range of bio-impedance devices available at the moment, but not all have been clinically tested. At this time, the SFB7 is best suited for office use (Impedimed Queensland); for larger, more complex clinical care settings, Multi frequency (which measures the whole body composition) Inbody Bio-space (South Korea) will be useful for multipurpose applications. There is also a radio frequency-based unit that can detect local area fluids, marketed under the name of Bio-impedance and Radio-frequency (Delfin, Finland). Alone or in combination with tonometry, these devices can provide valuable information about subtle changes in the latent phase (non-clinically manifest) of lymphedema and of the impact of treatment on the lymphedema once it becomes clinically apparent. Importantly, these techniques facilitate early treatment, presumably reducing the risk and severity of clinically manifest stage 1 (ISL classification) lymphedema.

Measurement of Limb Volume and Circumference

While limb volume and circumference are often seen as traditional measures of limb change, often their full value is not exploited, nor their accuracy utilized.

There are a number of ways to measure these variables. Perometry[4] is suited to larger clinics, while water displacement and/or determination of segmental or whole limb volume by calculation following the use of a tape measure[5] is often easier for smaller ones. All can be equally accurate and reliable, but accuracy is dependent on their correct use.

Perometry, for instance, can discriminate at 1 mm for circumferences and to the nearest 10 mL for volume. Similar accuracy is possible with water displacement. Both can be used to assess segmental changes in limb volumes, but water displacement needs additional circumference measurements to be made, which facilitate cross-checking.

When tape measurement at specified positions is used, care must be taken to minimize errors in the tension on the tape, the placement of the tape, the distance between measurement sites, and the side of measurement. Excel or other statistical programs can be used to calculate volume. Tape measurement is able to discriminate to 1 mm, but due to the variables identified, 5 mm is more realistic. The Australasian Lymphology Association has defined a program to ensure accuracy and repeatability in measurement (www.lymphology.asn.au). Such strategies can be used to add accuracy to the measurement for garment selection (in addition to manufacturers' recommendations regarding intervals and limb position for measurement) and can reduce the rate of patient rejection of garments, reduce the potential for a tourniquet effect of garments and improve patient compliance.

Measurement of Functional Status of the Lymphatic System

While lymphoscintigraphy might also be regarded as a traditional technique, it is often used inappropriately or inaccurately.

While initially expensive, in reality it can be a cost-effective technique for determining lymphatic system status. It is best used in patients in whom the treatment outcome has been poor because of case complexity. The initial cost can be worthwhile in terms of the range of information it can provide, including the functional status of the lymphatic system, the location of functional (and dysfunctional collectors), relationships between the deep and superficial lymphatics and areas of dermal backflow. Importantly, the information can be used to help the health professional direct flow to functional pathways.[6,7] There are quantitative aspects to lymphoscintigraphy, in the interpretation of the location of the radiotracer and its density and distribution, but also quantitative aspects in terms of the rate and time of arrival at specified regions of interest, such as the groin or axilla. Graphs of these events can help determine functional status and repeat measures can show the effect of any intervention. Accuracy is possible at the level of millimeters per minute of travel of the tracer, although most often graphs are compared for slope and tracer counts at specific times within a region of interest.

Measurement of the Structural Status of the Lymphatic System and of the Limb

If the "gold standard" of structural information is sought, the most effective method would seem to be ultrasound and, perhaps, its fractal analysis. Ultrasound is useful for informing us about changes in the thickness of the deep and superficial fascias, and of the thickness of fibrotic or other changes in the epifascial compartment. Again there are qualitative and quantitative aspects to these analyses, with the measurement of thicknesses and depths able to be undertaken to an accuracy of 1 mm. Even if this is only done once (at tonometry points described above), for reassessments, only tonometry will need to be undertaken. Of course MRI and other, similar techniques offer greater accuracy and discrimination, but cost often precludes their use.

Measurement of the Status of the Vascular System

It is clear that there are often significant changes to the vascular inflow and outflow patterns. Laser Doppler and other strategies such as fractal ultrasound allow these changes to be determined and interventions to be undertaken. Recent studies indicate that we should be paying more attention to changes in the vascular system inflow and outflow loads[8] and patterns, as well as to the lymphatic pumping mechanisms,[9] not only in a limb with lymphedema, but also limbs at risk.

Measurement of the Subjective Parameters

Lymphedema is more than just a swelling of the tissues.[10,11] Its symptoms, even in the early stages, include heaviness, tension, aches and pains, significant impacts on quality of life and on the ability to undertake the activities of daily living. For some patients it is these that are important, even more so than the size of the limb or its range of movement.

If we are going to help a patient deal with his problem from a holistic perspective, then we must also undertake measurement of these variables and other subjective parameters, using visual analog and other scales. There is a range of simple and validated test instruments, some specific, such as the LBCQ, and others more general, such as the SF –12 or –36.

Treatment Outcomes

Often, in lymphedema, treatment impacts how the limb feels, followed by softening and then, perhaps, by subtle changes in the volume of extracellular fluids, and, finally, by a change in volume or circumference. Detection and response to these changes can not only help the health professional to determine the impact of treatment, but can also be used to indicate to the patient that change is occurring and that the treatment from the professional is working or that the patient's self-management strategies are effective. Patients often suffer treatment fatigue and so it is important to give them continuing feedback. Some or all of the described alternate assessment and measurement methods would seem to provide effective opportunities to accomplish this goal.

References

1. Hayes S et al. Comparison of the methods to diagnose lymphoedema among breast cancer survivors: 6 month follow-up. *Breast Cancer Res Treat*. 2005;89:221.
2. Bates D et al. Quantification of the rate and depth of pitting in human oedema using an electronic tonometer. *Lymphology*. 1994;27(4):159.
3. Cornish BH, Chapman M, Hirst C, et al. Early diagnosis of lymphedema using multifrequency bioimpedance. *Lymphology*. 2001;34(1):2-11.
4. Stanton A et al. Validation of an optoelectronic limb volumeter (perometer). *Lymphology*. 1997;30(2):77.
5. Meijer RS et al. Validity and intra/inter observer reliability of an indirect volume measurement in upper limb lymphoedema. *Lymphology*. 2004;37(3):127.
6. Brautigam R et al. Analysis of lymphatic drainage in leg lymphoedema using two compartment lymphoscintigraphy. *Lymphology*. 1998;31(2):43.
7. Piller NB, Goodear M, Peter D. Lymphoscintigraphic evidence supports the evidence of axillo-inguinal anastomotic pathways in a patient with chronic secondary lymphoedema. *Eur J Lymphol*. 1998;6(24):97-100.
8. Dennis R. Haemodynamics of lymphoedema. *J Lymphoedema*. 2008;3(2):45-49.
9. Modi S, Stanton AWB, Svensson W, Peters A, Mortimer P, Levick J. Human lymphatic pumping measured in healthy and lymphoedematous arms by lymphatic congestion lymphoscintigraphy. *J Physiol*. 2007;583:271-285.
10. Amer M, Ramati A. Post traumatic symptoms, emotional distress and quality of life in long term survivors of breast cancer. *J Anxiety Disord*. 2002;16:195-206.
11. Amer MA, Stewart R. A comparison of 4 diagnostic criteria for lymphoedema in a post breast cancer population. *Lymphat Res Biol*. 2005;3(4):208-217.

Part VI
Infection

Chapter 25
Infection

Waldemar L. Olszewski

General Overview

Infections and inflammation of the skin and soft tissues of the lower and upper limbs are more common than those of other cutaneous regions because of exposure to the environment. The hands and feet have direct contact with surrounding matter, which is covered in micro-organisms and chemical substances. Readily acquired damage to the epidermis, such as abrasions, cuts, pricks, and closed injuries, create portals of entry for environmental bacteria.[1,2] The skin surface, and appendices such as sweat, sebaceous glands, and hair follicles, are inhabited by commensal bacteria, mostly *Staphylococcus epidermidis* and coagulase-negative strains. *Staphylococcus aureus* and corynebacteria are also present. In addition, the feet and calves may be colonized by pathogenic microbes originating from the perineal region, such as *Enterococcus*, *Enterobacter*, *Acinetobacter*, *Proteus*, *Escherichia coli*, and *Pseudomonas*. These microbes float down from the perineum on desquamated epidermal scales.

The commensal microbes are not pathogenic as long as they remain in their physiological niche. Once they have penetrated the epidermis the local host defense response is initiated. This response depends on the mass of penetrating microbes. A mass of 10^5 of bacteria per gram of tissue is the threshold value. Interestingly, the skin-colonizing bacterial strains are sensitive to most antibiotics.

W.L. Olszewski
Department of Surgical Research and Transplantology,
Medical Research Centre, Warsaw, Poland

B.-B. Lee et al. (eds.), *Lymphedema*,
DOI 10.1007/978-0-85729-567-5_25, © Springer-Verlag London Limited 2011

Primary and Secondary Infections

Primary Infections

These include lymphangitis, erysipelas, necrotizing fasciitis, and other rare conditions. The predisposing conditions are lymph stasis in the form of latent or overt lymphedema and chronic venous insufficiency.

Lymphangitis is characterized by the occurrence of an inflammatory streak (red, warm, and painful), the topography of which is that of the superficial lymphatic vessels. It is accompanied by fever. There is a non-inflammatory spreading lesion.

Erysipelas is a non necrotizing bacterial subdermal inflammation usually associated with streptococcal infection.[3-5] Group A beta-hemolytic *Streptococcus* (*S. pyogenes*) is the usual etiological agent. It may sometimes be a complication of chronic lymphedema.[6] Erysipelas is often of sudden onset, marked by frank systemic signs – fever >38° C, chills – and general malaise. Local signs develop within a few hours; a red, warm, painful, inflammatory spreading lesion with centrifugal extension develops within a few days. Inflammatory, satellite adenopathy and lymphangitis are associated with erysipelas.

Necrotizing dermal–subdermal bacterial infection, or necrotizing fasciitis, is characterized by necrosis of the fascia and myositis, resulting in a presentation of infectious gangrene. Diffuse, indurated edema extends beyond the margins of the erythematous and sometimes slightly inflammatory spreading lesion. Deep necrosis may be manifest in the initial stage solely as a cyanotic, grayish-blue, poorly demarcated swelling with a geographical map-like presentation. Fever is a usual finding, but it can be mild or absent. A septic syndrome (with hemodynamic signs, hypoxia, and thrombocytopenia) subsequently develops. This should prompt emergency hospitalization of the patient.

Other acute forms of dermal–subdermal bacterial infection are caused by *Erysipelotrix rhusiopathiae* (Rouget's swine erysipelas), *Haemophilus influenzae*, *Pasteurella multocida*, and *Borrelia burgdorferi*.

Secondary Infections: Dermato-Lymphangio-Adenitis

Chronic Dermatolymphangioadenitis

Each case of lymphedema is predisposed to infections and chronic dermatolymphangioadenitis (DLA).[7] This is due to impairment of bacterial elimination via lymphatics. Lymphedema is complicated by infection of the skin and deep tissues in approximately 40% of cases, irrespective of what is the primary etiological factor for the development of this condition. In the upper extremities after mastectomy and local irradiation, infection of the swollen limb, expressed as acute and later as chronic inflammation, ranges between 20% and 40%.[4] The recurrence rate of acute attacks of DLA is higher in subjects with a long duration of edema. It is followed by a rapid increase in limb volume. In the lower extremities, infection with inflammation is estimated to affect 50% of patients.[8] It is most common in the post-inflammatory type of lymphedema, followed by the post-traumatic and post-surgical types. Lower limbs are particularly exposed to the environmental microbial flora. Bacterial, fungal, and viral infection are more common there than in other skin regions. In advanced stages of lower limb lymphedema, systemic septic accidents requiring hospitalization and intensive antibiotic therapy are common, especially in tropical countries.

Acute DLA

Severe systemic symptoms during attacks of DLA resemble those of septicemia. The clinical characteristics are local tenderness and erythema of the skin, sometimes red streaks along the distribution of the superficial lymphatics, and enlarged inguinal lymph nodes. Systemic symptoms include malaise, fever, and chills. In its subacute or latent form, only skin involvement is observed. Each episode of DLA is commonly followed by worsening of limb swelling. Patients with acute episodes of DLA reveal bacteremia in a high percentage of cases.[8] Blood bacterial isolates were found in 21% of acute cases and 26% of subacute cases. The diversity of blood and tissue bacterial isolates in these patients points to a breakdown of the skin immune barrier in lymphedema and subsequently indiscriminate bacterial colonization of deep tissues and spread to blood circulation. Fatal cases have been observed.

Differential Diagnosis of Lymphangitis, Erysipelas and Dermato-Lymphangio-Adenitis

There is a lot of misunderstanding concerning the differences among these three conditions, which has implications for treatment decisions:

(a) Lymphangitis is a primary, local, non-systemic, non-spreading change in the skin and subcutaneous tissue caused by the patient's own skin flora, with a mild clinical course. It may lead to the development of lymphedema.
(b) Erysipelas is a primary, acute, local, spreading condition in the skin with systemic reaction. It is caused by streptococci. It may be contagious. It either develops in lymphedematous tissues or is the primary factor for lymphedema development.
(c) Dermato-lymphangioadenitis is a secondary condition complicating lymphedema of the soft tissues in the limb, caused by colonizing staphylococci, but not streptococci (which cause erysipelas). It is non-contagious and has a tendency to recur. In the United States, DLA is commonly referred to as cellulitis, which is the accepted non-European term for soft tissue bacterial infection. Cellulitis must not be confused with "cellulite," a cosmetic term that describes the presence of fatty deposits that cause a dimpled or uneven appearance, typically of thighs and/or buttocks.

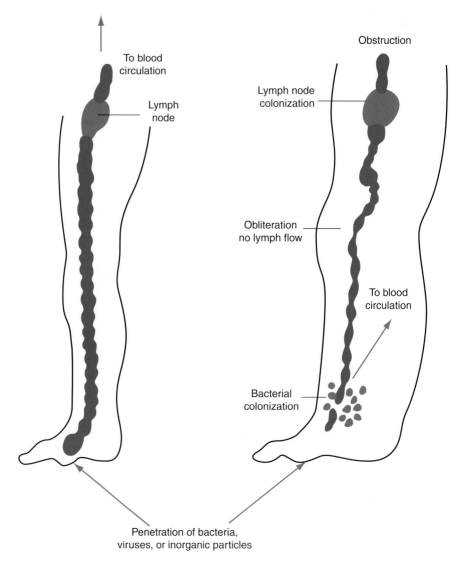

Fig. 25.1 Schematic presentation of the pathways of the spread of skin bacteria in deep tissues and penetration to blood circulation in lower limb lymphedema

Pathogenesis of Tissue Infection and Inflammation in Lymphedema

Under normal conditions, microbes that penetrate the glabrous skin of the palm or sole are transported away from the tissue via lymphatics and eliminated in the regional lymph nodes (Fig. 25.1). These are the strains that reside permanently on the skin and are acquired from the environment. The bacterial load is low and there is no clinically detectable reaction. In lymphedema, lymphatic transport is mildly to

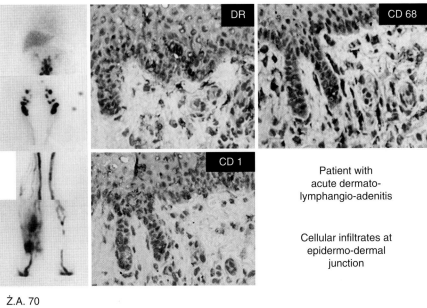

Ż.A. 70
RIII 5y DLA 5x/y
acute DLA

Fig. 25.2 A lymphoscintigram and skin histology in a patient with acute recurrent attack of DLA in the right lower limb. Lymphoscintigraphy depicts focal accumulation of isotope in the calf with dilatation of lymphatics below the knee. On histology, cellular infiltrates of DR-positive, brown-stained activated migrating immune cells, CD68-positive cells (macrophages) and CD1-positive cells (Langerhans' cells). Under normal conditions CD1 cells normally reside only in the epidermis. In DLA they are also seen in dermis being attracted, presumably, by bacterial antigens

severely restricted. The penetrating microbes colonize tissues, proliferate, and evoke a local inflammatory reaction with recruitment of host immune cells. Frequently, bacteria begin to proliferate rapidly and inflammation of all of the soft tissues of the limb develops, as well as systemic septic symptoms with bacteremia (Fig. 25.1). On histology, infiltration of the dermis and epidermis by mononuclear cells and granulocytes, macrophages, and Langerhans' cells is seen (Fig. 25.2).

Bacteriology of Lower Limb Skin

Bacterial Flora of Normal Foot and Calf Skin

Swabs taken from the surface of the foot and calf skin reveal the presence of microbes in 100% (Table 25.1). The dominant species are cocci (60%). Among them, *S. epidermidis* and other coagulase-negative strains account for 90% of all isolates. The other, less frequent strains are *E. coli*, *Citrobacter*, *Corynebacterium*, *Acinetobacter*, *Proteus*, and *Bacillus cereus*. These strains originate from the patient's perineum and anal skin.

Table 25.1 Prevalence of bacterial isolates from specimens obtained from lower limb tissues, lymph, and lymph nodes of 54 European patients with secondary lymphedema. The values from 30 healthy volunteers are given in parentheses

Specimen	Number of specimens		Percentage of positive culture
	Total	Positive	
Toe-web swab	52	52	100 (100)
Calf skin swab	52	52	100 (100)
Calf surgical incision swab	41	4	10 (7)
Leg lymph	20	12	60* (7)
Inguinal lymph node	20	6	33* (0)

$*p < 0.05$

Table 25.2 Numerical prevalence of bacterial strains in tissues and fluid specimens from lymphedematous legs of 54 European patients

	Toeweb swab	Calf skin swab	Surgical wound swab	Lymph	Lymph node
Number of specimens	52	52	41	20	20
Enterococcus					
E. durans		2			
E. faecium	2	2			
Citrobacter	3	2			
Coryneforms					
Group 2	2				
ANF	3	11			
Pseudo	1				
Minutissimus	1				
Group F	1				
Xerosus	3				
Klebsiella					
K. oxytoca	1				
K. pneumoniae	1	1	1		
Acinetobacter	5	6			
Escherichia coli	2				
Proprionibacterium	1				
Neisseria flava	1	1			
Bacillus subtilis	2	4			

Bacterial Flora of Normal Leg Lymph

Staphylococcus epidermidis was detected in 12% of samples collected in volunteers in studies of lymphatic lipid transport.

Bacterial Flora of Lymphedematous Leg Lymph

Cocci were isolated in 60% of samples from European populations, with *S. epidermidis* and occasionally *S. aureus* predominating (Tables 25.2, 25.3). In the Indian

Table 25.3 Numerical prevalence of microorganisms isolated from specimens obtained from lymphedematous legs of 54 European patients

	Toeweb swab	Calf skin swab	Surgical wound swab	Lymph	Lymph node
Number of specimens	52	52	41	20	20
Micrococcus					
species	31	28			
M. luteus	6	11		2	2
Staphylococcus					
S. aureus	4	9			
S. capitis	2	4		2	
S. cohni	11	7			
S. epidermidis	24	15			
S. hemolyticus	4	6	2		4
S. hominis	20	18		6	
S. lentus	2	1			
S. simulans	1		1		
S. sciuri	3			2	
S. saprophyticus	6	4			
S. warneri	6	2			
S. xylosus	6	3			
Streptococcus					
S. milleri		2			
S. mitis		1			
S. faecium	3	2			

population, with high-risk exposure to environmental infections, the values were higher and reached 70% of isolates, mostly cocci, in lymph and lymph nodes.[9]

Sensitivity of Isolates to Antibiotics

The skin, subcutaneous tissue, lymph, and lymph node isolates, from both patients with lymphedema and normal subjects, were sensitive to most antibiotics (Tables 25.4, 25.5).[10] Surprisingly, microbes showed the least sensitivity to penicillin, although this antibiotic proved to be very effective in the prevention of DLA attacks in a long-term administration protocol.[11,12] The high level sensitivity of most strains suggests their environmental, but not hospital, origin.

Prophylaxis of Recurrent DLA

Chronic DLA

Dermato-lymphangio-adenitis is of bacterial etiology and has a tendency toward recurrence. Chronic bacterial propxhylaxis is therefore necessary. It should be of

Table 25.4 Sensitivity to antibiotics of bacterial isolates from skin surface, surgical skin incision, lymph and lymph nodes in 54 European patients with lymphedema of lower limbs and 30 normal controls (in %)

| | Gram-negative *cocci, bacilli, coryneforms* | | | |
| | Lymphedema | | Normals | |
	+++	+	+++	+
Penicillin	67[a]	0	27	5
Cefotaxime	100	0	80	25
Kanamycin	67	0	100	0
Tobramycin	83	0	100	0
Amikacin	67	0	100	0
Gentamycin	86	14	100	0
Tetracyclin	71	0	80	0
Quinolones	83	17	100	0
Cotrimoxazole	67	0	80	0

[a]Percentage of isolates

Table 25.5 Sensitivity to antibiotics of bacterial isolates from skin surface, surgical skin incisions, lymph and lymph nodes of 54 European patients with secondary lymphedema of lower limbs and 30 normal controls

| | *Cocci* | | | |
| | Lymphedema | | Normals | |
	+++	+	+++	+
Penicillin	24[a]	0	28	2
Oxacillin	72	0	73	0
Meticillin	80	0	80	0
Kanamycin	68	6	44	8
Tobramycin	74	5	75	15
Gentamycin	79	3	85	4
Tetracyclin	49	0	61	2
Minocyclin	96	4	100	0
Erythromycin	49	4	59	8
Lincomycin	60	14	69	6
Pristinamycin	92	1	100	0
Fosfomycin	57	6	45	8
Nitrofurantoin	85	6	54	25
Quinolons	72	18	62	12
Rifampicin	91	6	91	9
Fusidic acid	81	11	77	18
Yancomycin	92	0	88	2
Teicomycin	92	0	79	0
Clotrimoxazole	78	4	80	0

[a]Percentage of isolates

long duration, or even permanent, since the effect of acute treatment is only temporary. It requires the use of penicillin: intramuscular benzathine penicillin 1.2–2.4 million units every 2–3 weeks, or oral penicillin V 2–4 million units in 2–3 doses a day.[10-12] The intramuscular route with local anesthetic ensures better compliance and has proven effective. The alternative, although less effective, is oral 2 g amoxicillin with clavulanic acid for 3 days every 2–3 weeks. Longer breaks between antibiotic administration had a tendency to increase the DLA recurrence rate. In the case of ß-lactam allergy, it is advisable to prescribe a macrolide, such as, for example, roxithromycin.

We investigated the clinical course of lymphedema with respect to the prevalence of DLA in patients receiving injections of long-acting penicillin (benzathine penicillin). Recurrent episodes of DLA over 1 year of follow-up decreased from 100% to 9% in the PCN-treated group ($p<0.002$).[11] There was increased prevalence of cocci and gram-positive bacilli, with a concomitant decrease in Gram-negative bacilli on the foot and calf skin surface. Simultaneously, decreased prevalence of Gram-positive cocci and Gram-negative bacilli isolates was seen in the deep tissues of the limb and in lymph. No resistance to penicillin and other tested antibiotics developed in isolates from the skin surface, deep tissues or lymph.

Treatment of Acute DLA Attacks

All wide-spectrum antibiotics are effective in controlling acute DLA. We recommend oral 2 g amoxicillin with clavulanic acid for 3–5 days. It should be followed by administration of benzanthine penicillin in a regimen analogous to that for chronic DLA.

References

1. Dreyer G, Addiss D, Gadelha P, et al. Interdigital skin lesions of the lower limbs among patients with lymphoedema in an area endemic for bancroftian filariasis. *Trop Med Int Health*. 2006;11:1475-1481.
2. McPherson T, Persaud S, Singh S, et al. Interdigital lesions and frequency of acute dermatolymphangioadenitis in lymphoedema in a filariasis-endemic area. *Br J Dermatol*. 2006;154:933-941.
3. Damstra RJ, van Steensel MA, Boomsma JH, et al. Erysipelas as a sign of subclinical primary lymphoedema: a prospective quantitative scintigraphic study of 40 patients with unilateral erysipelas of the leg. *Br J Dermatol*. 2008;158:1210-1215.
4. Vaillant L, Gironet N. Complications infectieuses des lymphoedèmes. *Rev Méd Interne*. 2002;23(suppl):403-407.
5. Vaillant L. Critères diagnostiques de l'érysipèle. *Ann Dermatol Vénéréol*. 2001;128:326-333.
6. Woo PC, Lum PN, Wong SS, et al. Cellulitis complicating lymphedema. *Eur J Clin Microbiol Infect Dis*. 2000;4:294-297.

7. Dreyer G, Medeiros Z, Netto MJ, et al. Acute attacks in the extremities of persons living in an area endemic for bancroftian filariasis: differentiation of two syndromes. *Trans R Soc Trop Med Hyg*. 1999;93:413-417.

8. Olszewski WL, Jamal S, Manokaran G, et al. Bacteriological studies of blood, tissue fluid, lymph and lymph nodes in patients with acute dermatolymphangioadenitis (DLA) in course of 'filarial' lymphedema. *Acta Trop*. 1999;73:217-224.

9. Olszewski WL, Jamal S, Manokaran G, et al. Bacteriologic studies of skin, tissue fluid, lymph, and lymph nodes in patients with filarial lymphedema. *J Trop Med Hyg*. 1997;57:7-15.

10. Olszewski WL. Episodic dermatolymphangioadenitis (DLA) in patients with lymphedema of the lower extremities before and after administration of benzathine penicillin: a preliminary study. *Lymphology*. 1996;29:126-131.

11. Olszewski WL, Jamal S, Manokaran G, et al. The effectiveness of long-acting penicillin (penidur) in preventing recurrences of dermatolymphangioadenitis(DLA) and controlling skin, deep tissues, and lymph bacterial flora in patients with "filarial" lymphedema. *Lymphology*. 2005;38:66-80.

12. Badger C, Seers K, Preston N, Mortimer P. Antibiotics/anti-inflammatories for reducing acute inflammatory episodes in lymphedema of the limbs. *Cochrane Database Syst Rev*. 2004; 2:CD003143.

Part VII
Physical and Medical Management

Chapter 26
Physiological Principles of Physiotherapy

Waldemar L. Olszewski

Introduction

Lymphedema of the extremities is caused by insufficient transport of tissue fluid via the lymphatics. The inadequacy of the lymphatic conduits is most commonly caused: (a) by their obliteration after infectious inflammation and subsequent scarring, (b) by their interruption during lymphadenectomy, and (c) after local irradiation and trauma. Impairment of transport capacity is the consequence of anatomical lesions caused by destruction of valves, degeneration of muscle cells, and obstruction of lumen by clot and external fibrous scarring. In advanced lymphedema most collecting lymphatics are closed.[1] Tissue fluid water, proteins, migrating immune cells, and cellular debris accumulate in the interstitial space. Identifying the location of mobile tissue fluid accumulation in the extremity and the nature of the morphological changes that develop in skin and subcutaneous tissue, muscular fascia, and muscles are prerequisite to rational manual or pneumatic compression therapy.[2]

Sites of Accumulation of Lymph and Tissue Fluid in Lymphedema

Only approximately 5% of tissue fluid enters the sub epidermal lymphatics to become lymph, whereas 80% accumulates in the interstitial space of the subcutaneous tissue between the collagen bundles and around small veins. The remaining 15% is located above and below the muscular fascia and in the muscles.[2] Obstruction of the deep lymphatic system always causes fluid accumulation in the muscular compartment. This applies to the lower as well as the upper extremities.

W.L. Olszewski
Department of Surgical Research and Transplantology,
Medical Research Centre, Warsaw, Poland

B.-B. Lee et al. (eds.), *Lymphedema*,
DOI 10.1007/978-0-85729-567-5_26, © Springer-Verlag London Limited 2011

Morphological Changes in the Lymphedematous Skin and Subcutis

These are (a) hyperkeratosis, (b) thickening of the dermis with an increase in the collagen content and mononuclear infiltrates, (c) deposition of collagen in the subcutaneous tissue with formation of multiple fibrous septa, (d) growth of fat tissue, and (e) fibrosis and depletion of lymphocytes in lymph nodes deprived of lymph flow and afferent stimulatory signal from the drained regions. Generally, not only the water content, but also the dry mass of the soft tissues steadily increases. The processes of hyperkeratosis and fibrosis change the mechanical properties of the tissues; consequently, this brings about the requirement for application of high compression forces to propel fluid during massage.

Hydraulic Conditions in the Subcutaneous Tissue

The bulk of stagnant tissue fluid is contained in the subcutaneous tissue. Massaging of this tissue requires knowledge of local hydraulics. Until recently, human experimental data on lymph and tissue fluid physics have not been available in the pertinent literature. We undertook the task of measuring lymph and tissue fluid pressures in normal and lymphedematous human lower and upper limbs and, below, we present the recent data. These may differ from what has thus far been presumed. The lymph and tissue fluid pressure and flow values presented here may be useful for rational physiotherapy, including manual or pneumatic massage and elastic support. Lymph pressures were measured in cannulated leg lymphatic collectors, tissue fluid was recorded using subcutaneously implanted sensors and fluid flow was calculated from changes in limb circumference continuously measured with a strain gauge plethysmograph.

Pressures

Under normal conditions, lymph flows only during spontaneous rhythmic contractions of the lymph vessel wall at pressures from 0 to 10 mmHg, independently of body position. There is no hydrostatic component even in an upright position because, under normal conditions, collecting lymphatics contain only a few microliters of lymph in lymphangions separated by valves. There is no flow during the non-contraction (diastolic) period[3] In lymphedema, in the few non-obliterated lymphatic collecting vessels, the lymphatic pump is largely ineffective and there is a to-and-fro movement of lymph during limb muscle contractions.[4] Backflow is caused by valve insufficiency. Lymph pressures may reach levels above 100 mmHg in the upright position (the hydrostatic component not present in normal lymphatics) and during limb muscular activity.[4] Tissue fluid: mobile tissue fluid, even in very

Fig. 26.1 A recently designed deep tissue tonometer recommended for measuring tissue compliance. The length of the plunger is 10 mm and its cross surface area is 1 cm². Force is expressed in g/cm². The tonometer is pressed against the skin at a depth of 10 mm. Wings protect against pushing the plunger into the tissue deeper than 10 mm. The data obtained are helpful for setting proper pressure in the pneumatic compression devices (see Fig. 26.2)

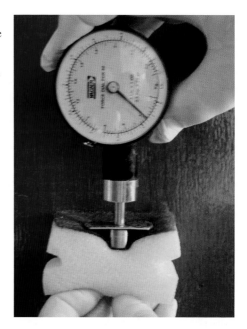

advanced stages of lymphedema, reveals low pressures ranging from 0 to 10 mmHg.[4] Subcutaneous tissue acquires the anatomical structure of a sponge with thousands of fluid "lakes". Its anatomical structure creates hydraulic resistance to flow. To overcome this resistance, minimum fluid pressure of above 30 mmHg is required.[4,5]

Pressure Gradient Across Skin and Subcutaneous Tissue

It is expected that the external force applied to the lymphedematous tissues will partly dissipate in the fibrotic skin and subcutis as the rigidity of these tissues in lymphedema is significantly higher than that of normal tissues. Thus, the tissue fluid pressure during massage should be lower than that exerted by the massaging hand or the pneumatic sleeve. In order to measure the rigidity of soft tissues of the limbs, special tonometers have been designed by us. They measure the force required to create a standard 10-mm deep soft tissue indentation (Fig. 26.1). The readings of the force applied to tissues correlate with tissue fluid pressures created by the pressing tonometer (Fig. 26.2). For example, the tonometer was pressed into the swollen tissue at a depth of 10 mm and the force was 1,000 g/cm². The simultaneously measured tissue fluid pressure achieved 50 mmHg. In another subject with fibrous skin, a force of 1,500 g was needed to obtain fluid pressure of 50 mmHg. To move tissue fluid in the subcutaneous space the minimum pressure of 30 mmHg is required.[4] We plotted the applied force values against the generated tissue fluid pressures at various levels of the lower limb. A curve was drawn that allowed us, knowing the tonometer values, to predict the pneumatic sleeve

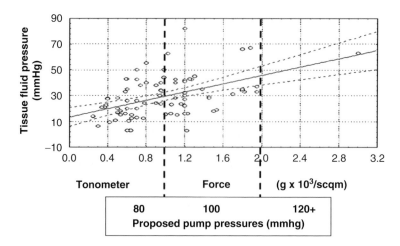

Fig. 26.2 Correlation between tonometer applied force and tissue fluid pressure in lymphedematous calves (stages I–IV). Measurements were carried out at six levels of the limb (above the ankle, at mid-calf, below and above the knee, at mid-thigh, and below the inguinal fossa). For the application of the tonometer see the text. In each case the tonometer was pressed 10 mm deep. With increasing skin and subcutaneous rigidity (depending on the stage of lymphedema), more force had to be applied to obtain fluid pressures between 30 and 70 mmHg. The minimum fluid pressure to move tissue fluid is 30 mmHg. A tonometer force of 1,000 g/cm^2 would give the recommendation for 50–80 mmHg in the pneumatic sleeve. Tonometer values of 1,500 g/cm^2 and 2,000 g/cm^2 would be a hint to set sleeve pressures of 100 and 120 mmHg respectively (80 tests, $X = 13.534 + 16.140 * Y$, corr. coeff. $= 0.48389$ CI95%)

pressures necessary for obtaining fluid pressures above 30 mmHg and initiating flow (Fig. 26.2). A tonometer value of 1.0 kg/cm^2 would give the recommendation for 50–80 mmHg in the pneumatic sleeve. Tonometer values of 1.5 and 2.0 kg/cm^2 would be a hint to set sleeve pressures of 100 and 120 mmHg respectively (Fig. 26.2).

Conditions for Creating Centripetal Tissue Fluid Flow

The tissue fluid flow should be directed proximally and there should not be any backflow. To obtain efficient flow, high external pressures should be applied, overcoming the natural hydraulic resistance of the tissues. They depend on mechanical compliance of the skin. We believe that applying compression pressure close to 100 mmHg, or above, is not harmful to the tissues because the compression force is acting in a perpendicular and not horizontal direction. Also, as tissue fluid flow is extremely slow, there is no shear stress. To avoid backflow after manual massage, immediate distal bandaging of the limb (minimum pressure 40 mmHg) should be carried out, and, during sequential pneumatic massage, the distal sleeve chambers should not be deflated.

Manual Massage

Indications

Manual lymphatic drainage has been reported to be effective when used in combination with other anti-edema modalities, such as complex decongestive therapies, as well as in combination with intermittent compression pumping.[6-8] Manual massage has been very effective in subjects with segmental disfigurement of the limb (e.g., excessive swelling at the ankle level), at sites where the pneumatic sleeve cannot be adjusted to the shape of the extremity.

Advantages and Shortcomings

Advantages: (a) "softening" of fibrotic tissues especially in patients with very hard skin, (b) local mobilization of stagnant tissue fluid at sites of highest accumulation, and (c) moving fluid from disfigured parts of the limb not suitable for pneumatic massage. There are also some shortcomings. External pressures exerted upon a small massaged area (masseur's hand area) not embracing the entire limb do not build up fluid pressures high enough to initiate centripetal flow. Short time intervals of hand compression are not sufficient for effective centripetal tissue fluid flow to be generated and, upon hand release, the fluid backflow occurs. Manual compression does not stimulate intrinsic lymph and tissue fluid flow.[9] Massaging should be followed by immediate bandaging of the distal segments of the limb.

Manual Massage Hydraulics

In tissue fluid pressures generated by hand massage, the therapist does not know how much pressure he generates at various tissue depths. Based on the results of our studies, these pressures range from 40 to 120 mmHg and are disseminated radially at a distance of only 3 cm (Fig. 26.3).[4,5] Removal of the massaging hand brings about an immediate drop in tissue fluid pressure and, as a consequence, a cessation of flow (Fig. 26.4).

Pneumatic Massage

Indications

Every case of lymphedema of the lower or upper extremity is suitable for pneumatic massage.[10] The contraindications are: active dermatitis, skin ulcer, and recent venous thrombosis.

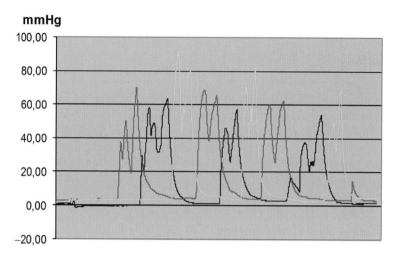

Fig. 26.3 Tissue fluid pressures in the subcutaneous tissue of a lymphedematous calf during manual massage. The therapist's hand was placed at three levels: above the ankle, in the mid-calf, and below the knee. There were three consecutive hand compressions at each level. The hand force generated pressures of 40–90 mmHg, although the therapist tried to use the same force. Cessation of hand compression caused a rapid drop in pressure, allowing fluid backflow

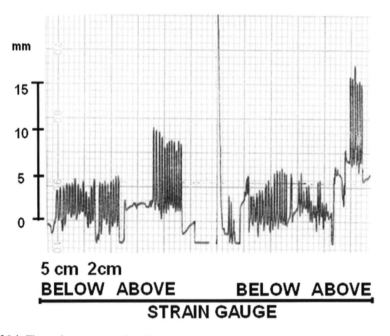

Fig. 26.4 The strain gauge was placed in the mid-calf during manual massage for continuous measuring of the increase in circumference. Each hand compression produced a short-lasting increase in the circumference proximal to the compression site, to decrease suddenly after the release of hand pressure. This was followed by fluid backflow to the tissue pit. It proves that there is a lack of fluid proximal flow. Scale 15 mm = 5 mm circumference increase = 10–15 ml tissue flow

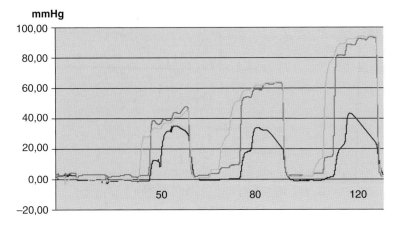

Fig. 26.5 Tissue fluid pressures measured subcutaneously during sequential pneumatic compression at pressures 50, 80, and 120 mmHg of a lymphedematous calf. Pressure sensors were placed at a depth of 5–7 mm above the ankle, in the mid-calf and below the knee. During first inflation, the pressure curve above the ankle increased to 25 mmHg although the sleeve chamber pressure was 50 mmHg. The second curve in the mid-calf rose to 40 mmHg only. The third curve was low as fluid easily flowed to the popliteal fossa with loose tissue. Similarly, tissue fluid pressures were lower than in sleeves at the inflation pressure of 80 and 120 mmHg. A high gradient between the inflated sleeve chamber and tissue fluid was due to hard fibrotic skin

Advantages and Shortcomings

The advantages are: (a) tissue fluid is moved proximally in the whole compressed fragment of the limb embraced by the sleeve; (b) sequential compression creates unidirectional fluid stream reaching the groin or arm region during one cycle, (c) it keeps distal chambers non-deflated, during sequential inflation of the proximal ones, which protects against fluid backflow; (d) the procedure is easily performed by the patient, can be repeated several times per day, and does not engage additional care labor; (e) it can be applied in large cohorts of patients. The shortcomings are: (a) it has little effect in very advanced stages of lymphedema with hard skin, and (b) its high cost.

Pneumatic Compression Hydraulics

The sleeve pressures that we recommend, based upon the tissue fluid pressure that we have measured during pneumatic massage, range between 50 and 120 mmHg.[4,5] The level of applied sleeve pressure depends on the rigidity of the soft tissues. We believe that, the higher the rigidity, the higher the applied pressures should be. Soft tissue tonometry helps to set an effective sleeve pressure. Note that tissue fluid pressures are, in each case, lower than those in the sleeve (Fig. 26.5).[4,5] The time needed

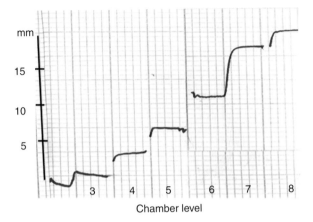

Fig. 26.6 A strain gauge was put around the limb at six levels and changes in the circumference generated by proximal fluid flow during sequential pneumatic compression were recorded. Inflation of consecutive sleeve chambers moved fluid in the proximal direction from 3 to 8. Changes in circumference were recalculated into volume. Inflation time 55 s, sleeve pressure 120 mmHg. This method allows the tissue fluid flow to be quantitated and the effectiveness of the compression device to be evaluated[4]

for inflation of the sleeve chambers should be long enough to reach an effective tissue fluid pressure (above 30 mmHg) and initiate flow. Data originating from debulking surgery, when the surgeon uses the fingers to squeeze fluid from the incised tissue to facilitate the excision procedure, indicate that 50–90 s is a minimum time period necessary to mobilize tissue fluid. Contemporary pumps are set at only 5–20 s. The distal chambers of the sleeve should be kept inflated to prevent fluid backflow and blood inflow with subsequent stasis in the superficial venous system of the limb. Deflation should occur simultaneously in all chambers. Continuous measuring of circumference changes during the sequential compression cycle provides insight into the moved fluid volume (Fig. 26.6).[4,5]

Remarks for Users of Compression Devices

We predict that high tissue fluid pressures are necessary to propel fluid proximally because of the rigidity of the skin and subcutaneous tissue, the low hydraulic conductivity of tissues (collagen excess, fibrosis), and the flow hindrance at the groin and axilla level. The fluid pressure head is always lower than that in the sleeve. Pressure is low in areas with loose connective tissue (popliteal, groin, arm pit), and padding of these regions is helpful for prevention of fluid accumulation. Tissue fluid channels are formed during long-term pneumatic massage taking over the fluid transportation burden from the obliterated lymphatics.[11] Groin tissue and the inguinal crease as well as the arm pit are the main anatomical barriers for the massaged tissue fluid to flow to the non-edematous tissues of the hypogastrium and hip or shoulder.

References

1. Rijke AM, Croft BY, Johnson RA, de Jongste AB, Camps JA. Lymphoscintigraphy and lymphedema of the lower extremities. *J Nucl Med*. 1990;31:990-998.
2. Olszewski WL, Jain P, Ambujam G, Zaleska M, Cakala M. Where do lymph and tissue fluid accumulate in lymphedema of lower limbs caused by obliteration of lymphatic collectors. *Lymphology*. 2009;42:105-111.
3. Olszewski WL. Contractility patterns of human leg lymphatic in various stages of obstructive lymphedema. *Ann NY Acad Sci*. 2008;1131:110-118.
4. Olszewski WL, Jain P, Ambujam G, Zaleska M, Cakala M, Gradalski T. Tissue fluid pressure and flow in the subcutaneous tissue in lymphedema – hints for manual and pneumatic compression therapy. *Phlebolymphology*. 2010;17:144-148.
5. Olszewski WL, Jain P, Ambujam G, Zaleska M, Cakala M, Gradalski T. Tissue fluid pressure and flow during pneumatic compression in lymphedema of lower limbs. *Lymph Res Biol*. 2010; (in press).
6. Szolnoky G, Lakatos B, Keskeny T, Varga E, Varga M, Dobozy A, Kemeny L. Intermittent pneumatic compression acts synergistically with manual lymphatic drainage in complex decongestive physiotherapy for breast cancer treatment-related lymphedema. *Lymphology*. 2009;42:188-194.
7. Andersen L, Højris I, Erlandsen M, Andersen J. Treatment of breast-cancer-related lymphedema with or without manual lymphatic drainage – a randomized study. *Act Oncol*. 2000;39:399-405.
8. Vignes S. Management of following breast cancer lymphedema. *Bull Cancer*. 2007;94: 669-674.
9. Olszewski WL, Engeset A. Intrinsic contractility of prenodal lymph vessels and lymph flow in human leg. *Am J Physiol*. 1980;239:H775-H783.
10. Brennan MJ, Miller LT. Overview of treatment options and review of the current role and use of compression garments, intermittent pumps, and exercise in the management of lymphedema. *Cancer*. 1998;83(12 suppl):2821-2827.
11. Olszewski WL, Jain P, Ambujam G, Zaleska M. Newly formed tissue fluid channels take over the fluid flow burden in long-lasting lymphedema of lower limbs. *Lymph Res Biol*. 2010; (in press).

Chapter 27
Complete Decongestive Therapy

Etelka Földi and Martha Földi

Introduction

Lymphedema is a chronic condition; therefore, in clinical practice, therapies try to reduce the disease to its latent state (a condition relatively free from edema, despite the limited function of the lymphatic drainage system) and thereby attain a prolonged alleviation of the affliction. As early as 1892, Winiwarter recognized physiotherapy as the most effective form of therapy. In his book *"Krankheiten der Haut und des Zellgewebes"* ("Skin and Cellular-Tissue Disorders,"[1]) he describes a "new" therapy concept that would coordinate various kinds of physical measures like massage, methodical compression, exercise, and skin care. He was already emphasizing the need for "comprehensive medical care."

In recent decades, physiotherapy for lymphedema has experienced a revival and has developed into "complete decongestive physiotherapy" (CDP). Its objectives are:

- To improve the function of lymph vessels
- To soften the fibrosclerotic indurations
- To reduce increased connective tissue
- To sanitize the skin to prevent opportunistic infections

In addition, attaining a quality of life that is individual, active, and suited to age is just as essential as performing self-treatment procedures.

The adequate administration of CDP enables patients to integrate into their social surroundings and to secure their schooling and professional education. Among geriatric patients, we are able to delay the imminent need for high-maintenance care for many years. The quality of life of patients of all ages can be improved. The goals of therapy should be set by both the doctor and patient, in a shared decision-making process.

E. Földi (✉)
Clinic for Lymphology, Földiklinik,
Hinterzarten, Baden-Württemberg, Germany

B.-B. Lee et al. (eds.), *Lymphedema*,
DOI 10.1007/978-0-85729-567-5_27, © Springer-Verlag London Limited 2011

Complete Decongestive Physiotherapy

CDP is the basic therapy for limb lymphedema, even if any possibility of a surgical procedure is given. Its components are:

1. Manual lymph drainage[2,3]: a massage technique that is described extensively in Chap. 28.
2. Compression therapy[4]: this form of therapy generally is carried out with medical compression bandages in phase 1 of CDP (see below), and with made-to-measure compression garments in phase 2. Short-stretch bandages of various widths are used with appropriate padding. The effects of compression therapy are as follows[5-7]:

- Displacement of fluid in the interstitium and reduction in venous pressure; these, in turn, have an anti-edematous effect
- Normalization of a pathologically raised ultra-filtration, i.e., a reduction of the lymphatic water load
- Accelerated inflow of tissue fluid into the lymph capillaries, i.e., an increase in lymph formation
- Increase in lymph flow in the lymph vessels that are still functioning, particularly when combined with exercise

Medical compression bandages are required:

- To give an optimal, even distribution of pressure, whilst taking into consideration the condition of the skin
- Not to restrict movement
- To have firm application without slipping or hurting

Composition of medical compression bandages[8,24]:

According to the appropriate curative and protective skin-care procedure, a tubular dressing made from cotton wool is wrapped around the skin to protect it. Padding materials are applied over this cylindrical bandage: a padding bandage made of synthetic fibers or thin layers of foam for an even distribution of pressure. Uneven foam padding materials can be used, too, in order to achieve a micro-massage effect during movement. Compression pressure is finally secured with short stretch elastic bandages. It should be taken into account that as well as the layer of protective padding material, skin wrinkles and indentations must be filled with made-to-measure pieces of foam. Fingers and toes are wrapped with double layers of elastic bandages. Table 27.1 shows the desired compression, the type of protective padding material and the wearing time of the medical compression bandage, according to the age of the patient.

The medical compression stockings are custom-made,[9] flat-knitted garments, which are meant to prevent re-accumulation of edema fluid. Their stretchability should match that of the elastic bandages. Patients with chronic lymphedema must wear medical compression stockings their whole life, even if the lymphedema can be successfully reduced to its latent state with therapy. The type of compression stockings a patient requires (Table 27.2) can change over the course of his life, relative to the receding of the lymphedema or the occurrence of new illnesses (orthopedic, neurological, etc.).

Table 27.1 Compression bandaging depends on the age of the patient and the stage of the lymphedema

		Pressure	Padding		Maximum application time
Children	6 months–2 years	10–20 mmHg	Smooth (padding bandages/ foam)		12–16 h
	2 years–6 years	20–30 mmHg	Smooth Uneven	Padding bandage Foam	16–20
	6 years–12 years	20–30 mmHg	Smooth Uneven	Padding bandage Foam	16–20 h
Adults	Stage I	20–30 mmHg	Smooth Smooth	Padding bandage Foam	12–16 h
	Stage II	30–46 mmHg	Smooth Uneven	Padding bandage Foam	18–22 h
	Stage III	46 mmHg and stronger	Smooth Uneven	Padding bandage Foam	18–22 h
	Lymphedema combination forms	Individual	Individual		Individual
Geriatric	60–70 years	30–46 mmHg	Smooth Uneven	Padding bandage Foam	18–22 h
	Over 70 years	20–30 mmHg	Smooth	Padding bandage	12–16 h

Table 27.2 Compression stockings depend on the stage and localisation of the lymphedema

Location	Stage I	Stage II	Stage III
Toes/foot	Toe caps CCl. I Socks CCl. I	Toe caps CCl. I Socks CCl. II	Toe caps CCl. I Socks CCl. III
Lower leg + toes/ foot	Toe caps CCl. I Knee stockings CCl. II	Toe caps CCl. I Knee stockings CCl. II	Toe caps CCl. I Knee stockings CCl. IV
Whole leg + toes/ foot	Toe caps CCl. I Groinal stocking CCl. II	Toe caps CCl. I Groinal stocking CCl. III	Toe caps CCl. I Groinal stocking CCl. IV
Truncal quadrant, + whole leg + toes/foot	Toe caps CCl. I Tights with one leg CCl. II	Toe caps CCl. I Tights with one leg CCl. III Truncal garment CCl. II	Toe caps CCl. I Tights with one leg of CCl. IV Truncal garment CCl. II
Truncal quadrant, + both legs + toes/foot	Toe caps CCl. I Tights CCl. II	Toe caps CCl. (a) Knee stockings CCl. III (b) Half-hose CCl. II	Toe caps CCl. I (a) Knee stockings CCl. IV (b) Half-hose CCl. II/III
Lower arm + hand	Long glove CCl. I	Long glove CCl. II	Long glove CCl. II or III
Whole arm + hand	Sleeve CCl. I Glove CCl. I	Sleeve CCl. II Glove CCl. II	Sleeve CCl. II or III Glove CCl. II

3. Decongestive kinesiotherapy and respiratory therapy[10,11]: the positive effects of kinesiotherapy on venous hemodynamics and lymph flow are experimentally and clinically proven. The contraction and relaxation of the skeletal muscles lead to an increase in pressure in the interstitium, which transfers to the lymphatic wall, resulting in an increase in the pulsation of the lymphangions. Depending on the position of the body, intensive abdominal breathing can have a similar effect on the central part of the veins and lymphatic trunks. Decongestive kinesiotherapy and respiratory therapy can be performed as a single treatment or as group therapy. In addition to this, the patient should learn an individual training program, devised according to his age and profession, which would then be continued as long-term therapy. Walking – Nordic walking, cycling – treadmill, stationary cycling, swimming, i.e., endurance sports, are specifically suitable.

4. Dry, itchy skin is often a part of chronic lymphedema. Due to the disturbance in the physiological balance between the moisture and lipid content of the skin, bacterial and mycotic infections, inclusive congestive dermatitis, frequently occur.[12,13] The application of disinfectant and antimycotic agents is indicated as the therapy for infections. Antihistamine agents are shown to be effective against congestive dermatitis, cortisone cream can be temporarily indicated, too. Urea, ceramides and cholesterol-containing moisturizers have proved themselves capable of restoring the physiological balance between moisture and lipid content. Since skin maceration and intertrigo can occur in deep wrinkles, we would recommend powder and, if necessary, padding, to give the skin a dry disposition after disinfecting it.

The Use of CDP

Complete decongestive therapy is a two-phase therapy[14-17]:

Phase 1 is aimed at mobilizing the congested protein-enriched fluid and, if present, initiates a reduction in increased connective tissue. The instructions and information about self treatment procedures and a suitable life style are given during this phase.

Phase 2 involves optimizing and preserving the success already achieved by the therapy in phase 1. The dose of therapy procedures to be undertaken (Table 27.3) depends on the stage of disease in which lymphedema therapy is commenced.

The long-term success of complete decongestive physiotherapy depends on the comprehensive medical care of the patient. Notoriously, the extent of the restriction in function of the lymphovascular system is only a part of the pathophysiology of lymphedema. The clinical picture and also the therapy requirements are influenced by several co-morbidities that lead to an increase in the amount of fluid to be transported. Diseases that influence the function of the arteries, blood capillaries, veins, and the ground substance impede lymph formation or increase lymphatic loads. Such pathophysiological processes can aggravate both primary and secondary lymphedema. Patients who suffer from chronic limb lymphedema require a complete medical assessment before complete decongestive physiotherapy is begun, and later, as is often the case with chronic illnesses, a regular medical check-up. Adequate treatment of diseases that aggravate lymphedema is essential if complete decongestive physiotherapy is to succeed.

Table 27.3 Prevention and two-phase treatment of lymphedema with CDT

Stage	Symptoms	Phase I decongestion	Phase II optimization	Phase III preservation
Stage 0	No swelling, pathological lymphoscintigram	Prevention when lymphedema risk factors present		
Stage I	Edema of soft consistency, raising of the limb reduces swelling	MLD: 1 × per day, compression bandaging, exercise, duration 14–21 days		MLD: in series compression garments as required or consistent in the long-term
Stage II	Edema with secondary tissue alterations, raising of the limb without effect	MLD: 2 × per day, compression bandaging, exercise, duration 24–28 days	MLD: 1–2 × per week for the duration of 2–5 years, compression garments and bandaging, exercise, repetition of phase I	MLD: in series or 1 × per week, compression garments worn consistently in the long-term, exercise
Stage III	Elephantiasic hard swelling, often of lobular form with typical skin alterations	MLD: 2–3 × per day, compression bandaging, exercise, duration 28–35 days	MLD: 2–3 × per week for the duration of 5–10 years, compression garments and bandaging, exercise, repetition of phase I	MLD: in series or 1–2 × per week, compression stockings worn consistently in the long-term, exercise

Indications, Contraindications and Modification of CDP

In order to prevent any side-effects of CDP, awareness of the indications, contraindications, and the forms of its modification is mandatory.[18] There are many diseases that require an individual adaptation of the application of complex decongestive physiotherapy to the condition of the patient. The most commons include:

- Hypertension
- Coronary heart disease
- Heart failure
- Diabetes mellitus
- Chronic venous insufficiency
- Malignancies
- Rheumatic disorders
- Peripheral artery occlusive disease
- Peripheral polyneuropathy

  Contraindications of CDP are:

- Acute erysipelas
- Acute thrombophlebitis
- Phlebothrombosis
- Decompensated heart failure
- Stage IV peripheral artery occlusive disease

Treatment of head lymphedema and genital lymphedema with complete decongestive physiotherapy demands a large amount of experience in this area and should only be carried out under specialized clinical conditions.

Quality of life and patient satisfaction during treatment by complete decongestive physiotherapy depends to a large extent on realistic therapy goals and their achievement. Many patients can only achieve their therapy goals by keeping psychosocial support in mind and using it. Professional therapy and assistance are essential. Even the diagnosis of lymphedema and the implementation of the necessary self-treatment procedures call for a great psychosocial effort on the part of the patient and his family to adjust to the diagnosis and its implications. Psychotherapy is usually required to help with this.[19-21]

Long-Term Therapy Results

Long-term results of conservative treatment of lymphedema with complete decongestive physiotherapy depend not only on the stage of lymphedema, during which treatment is begun, but also on the compliance of the patient, as well as the presence of comorbidities that aggravate edema as well on the skill of the therapist.

As a rule, primary lymphedema in infancy presents without concomitant diseases. A clinical trial including 452 children that lasted 12 years showed that in 85% of cases the success of therapy after phase I of CDP could not only be preserved, but could be further improved. Furthermore, it shows equal possibilities in education and professional life compared with unaffected children.[22]

A second clinical trial concerning the long-term success of the treatment was carried out with 512 adult patients. It showed that there was a strong correlation between the prevalence of comorbidities and edema relapses: in patients with lymphedema of the lower limb without concomitant diseases, therapy success after phase I of CDP can be maintained for 15 years. In patients with combination forms of lymphedema, 91% of cases repeated phase I of CDP due to edema relapses over the same length of time.[23]

In geriatric patients, long-term success and goals of therapy not only depend on comorbidities, but also on the mental state of the patient. On the other hand, it is precisely the improvement in the mobility of lymphedema sufferers that is a distinct measure against mental afflictions.

References

1. Winiwarter A. In Billroth & Luecke (Hrsg) *Die Krankheiten der Haut und des Zellgewebes.* Stuttgart: Ferdinand Enke; 1892.
2. Vodder E. *Die manuelle Lymphdrainage und ihre medizinischen Anwendungsgebiete.* Erfahrungsheilkunde 16; 1966.
3. Földi M, Strößenreuther R. *Grundlagen der manuellen Lymphdrainage.* 4th ed. München: Elsevier; 2007.
4. Földi E, Földi M, Weissleder H. Conservative treatment of lymphedema of the limbs. *Angiology.* 1985;36:171-180.
5. Schneider W, Fischer H. Grundlagen und Technik der Kompressionsbehandlung. *Internist.* 1967;8:383.
6. Jünger M et al. Einfluss einer Kompressionstherapie bei Patienten mit chronischer venöser Insuffizienz auf die kutane Mikrozirkulation. In: Weissler H, ed. *Kompressionsbestrumpfung bei Extremitätenlymphödemen.* Köln: Viavital Verlag; 1999:21-30.
7. Bollinger A. Fließgeschwindigkeit in der Vena saphena magna und der Vena femoralis mit und ohne Kompressionsverbände. *Swiss Med.* 1980;2:61.
8. Thoma H, Schneider B, Strößenreuther R. Application of compression bandages. In: Foeldi M, Foeldi E, eds. *Foeldi's Textbook of Lymphology.* München: Elsevier/Urban-Fischer; 2006.
9. Wienert V, Hansen R. Anmessen von medizinischen Kompressionsstrümpfen am liegenden oder stehenden Patienten? *Phlebologie.* 1992;21:236-238.
10. Strößenreuther R. Entstauende Bewegungs- und Atemtherapie, Krankengymnastik sowie weitere Maßnahmen der physikalischen Therapie. In: *Lehrbuch der Lymphologie.* 6th ed. Stuttgart: Elsevier; 2005.
11. Partsch H. Verbesserte Förderleistung der Wadenmuskelpumpe unter Kompressionsstrümpfen bei Varizen und venöser Insuffizienz. *Phlebol U Proktol.* 1958;7:58-66.
12. Asmussen P. Hautpflege beim Lymphödem. In: Földi M, Földi E, eds. *Das Lymphödem und verwandte Krankheiten.* 8th ed. München: Urban & Fischer; 2003.
13. Földi E. Prevention of dermatolymphangioadenitis by combined physiotherapy of the swollen arm after treatment for breast cancer. *Lymphology.* 1996;29:48-49.

14. Brunner U, Frei-Fleischlin C. Gegenwärtiger Stand der kombinierten physikalischen Entstauungstherapie beim primären und sekundären Lymphödem der Beine. VASA 1993; Band 22(1).
15. Földi E. The treatment of lymphedema. *Cancer.* 1998;83(suppl 12):2833-2834.
16. Földi E, Baumeister R, Bräutigam P, Tiedjen K. Zur Diagnostik und Therapie des Lymphödems. *Sonderdruck Deutsches Ärzteblatt.* 1998;13,S.: A-740–747, B-610–614, C-561–565.
17. Bernas M, Witte MH. Consensus and dissent on the ISL consensus document on the diagnosis and treatment of peripheral lymphedema. *Lymphology.* 2004;37:165-167.
18. AWMF-Leitlinien online. Diagnostik und Therapie der Lymphödeme. www.uni-duesseldorf.de/AWMF, Stand 04/2009.
19. Williams AF, Moffatt CJ, Franks PJ. A phenomenological study of the lived experiences of people with lymphoedema. *Int J Palliat Nurs.* 2004;10(6):279-286.
20. Flaggl F, Döller W, Jäger G, Apich G. Prävalenz komorbider psychischer Störungen bei Lymphödempatienten in der medizinischen Rehabilitation. *Praxis Klinische Verhaltensmedizin und Rehabilitation.* 2006;71:75-82.
21. Jäger G, Döller W, Roth R. Quality of life and body image impairments in patients with lymphedema. *Lymphology.* 2006;39:193-200.
22. Schöhl J. *Das primäre Lymphödem des Kindes: Langzeittherapieverlauf und Lebensqualität.* [Inaugural-Dissertation, University Freiburg]. 2010.
23. Földi, E. Results and failures of conservative treatment (CDT) of lymphedema. Lecture during 22. ISL-Congress, Sydney, Australia; 2009.
24. Földi M, Földi E, Kubik S (eds): *Textbook of Lymphology.* Elsevier GmbH, München: Urban & Fischer Verlag.

Chapter 28
Manual Lymph Drainage (Földi Method)

Etelka Földi and Martha Földi

Introduction

Manual lymph drainage is a massage technique that is one of the components of complete decongestive physiotherapy (CDP) (described intensively in Chap. 27). Manual lymph drainage[1,2] is used in the treatment of all forms of lymphedema, but in stages II and III it has to be combined with additional manual techniques to soften and reduce fibrosclerotic connective tissue alteration. The effectiveness of manual lymphedema treatment depends on anatomical and pathophysiological insights of the physiotherapist performing the therapy within the field of microcirculation, as well as the therapist's knowledge about the clinical stages of lymphedema (Figs. 28.1–28.3).

Manual Lymph Drainage (MLD/Vodder I)[1]

The basic Vodder stroke consists of four techniques[1]:

- Stationary circle
- Rotary stroke
- Pump stroke
- Scoop stroke

The application of these four strokes is based on a common fundamental schema. The characteristics of these four techniques are a gentle pressure phase followed by

---

[1]Manual Lymph Drainage according to Dr. E. Vodder

E. Földi (✉)
Clinic for Lymphology, Földiklinik,
Hinterzarten, Baden-Württemberg, Germany

B.-B. Lee et al. (eds.), *Lymphedema*,
DOI 10.1007/978-0-85729-567-5_28, © Springer-Verlag London Limited 2011

Fig. 28.1 Stage I

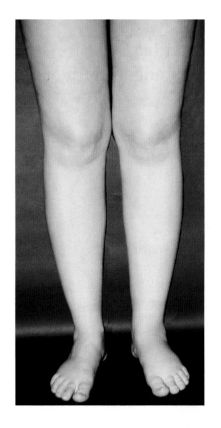

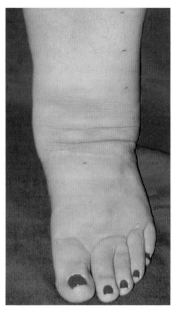

Fig. 28.2 Stage II

Fig. 28.3 Stage III

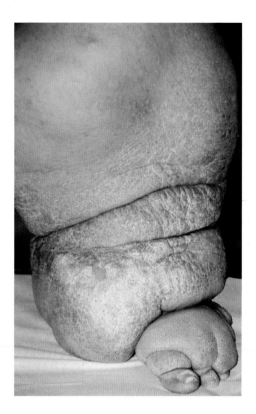

relaxation. Further aspects play an important role as well, such as the direction of the movement (the thrust and the rhythm). The stretching of the skin has an effect on suprafascial lymph vessels; it causes an increase in the lymphangion pulsation.[3,4] The raise in interstitial pressure promotes lymph formation.[2,5-8] During the relaxation phase, where contact with the skin is barely maintained, the fluid is carried passively out of the tissue so that the vessels can again be filled distally ("suction effect"). The rhythm of the thrust and relaxation must gradually become the so-called 1-sec movement, with five to seven repetitions in one place. The therapist must understand that the diameter of the lymph vessels is small – it can be less than a millimeter. The movement of the hand, therefore, has to be slow and gentle, to not overtax the vessels. The basic strokes of MLD/Vodder I are adjusted depending on the area of the body being treated. The effect of MLD/Vodder I is dependent upon the precondition that functional lymph vessels are present within the treated area. Therefore the basic Vodder strokes are indicated as a lymphedema prophylactic measure to treat lymphedema at stage I, and as a proximal pre-treatment in the trunk region bordering the edematous area in all stages of lymphedema.

Detailed Characterization of MLD
According to Dr. E. Vodder

Stationary Circle

The stationary circle consists of an active (pressure) phase and a passive (relaxation) phase. During the active semicircle, the skin is stretched maximally in the direction of drainage (avoiding slipping of the hand). During the passive phase, the release of pressure on the stretched skin leads to the completion of the circle, and the starting position of the circle is reached again.

Rotary Stroke

In the starting position only the fingertips are in contact with the skin. During the next phase the whole hand is in contact with the skin while the thumb gradually abducts. Fingers 2–5 point toward the drainage direction. During the subsequent phase, the palm exerts pressure in the direction of the fingers while the thumb is adducted. The technique ends with the relaxation phase, and a new starting position is reached by moving fingers 2–5 forward.

Pump Stroke

This technique can be applied either with one hand (small areas) or with both hands (large areas). It may be applied in combination with (i.e., alternating with) stationary circles. If one works with both hands, the hands will alternate. One must make sure that the stroke of the first hand is completed before the second hand starts a new stroke (each stroke ends with the relaxation phase). In the starting position of the pump technique, the wrist is palmar flexed, and the thumb and index finger are in contact with the skin. With extension of the wrist, the palm comes into full contact with the skin as well. A flat shearing force toward the drainage direction results. During the subsequent relaxation phase, the distention of the tissue passively pulls the therapist's hand. To reach the starting position again, the wrist is palmar flexed again and the hand moves proximally (the strokes should overlap).

Scoop Technique

The scoop technique is characterized by a continuous movement of the therapist's hand without a clear separation between the pressure and the relaxation phases. As with the pump technique, this stroke starts with the wrist in palmar flexion while the thumb and index finger touch the lateral surface of the extremity. During extension of the wrist the hand slides to the back surface of the extremity, where the whole hand establishes contact with the skin. Eventually, the palm and the fingers become parallel with the longitudinal axis of the extremity (perpendicular stretching of the lymph vessels occurs). At the conclusion of this phase the longitudinal pressure is increased and, thus, further sliding is impossible (emptying of the lymph vessels). To reach the starting position again, the wrist is flexed without losing contact with the skin, so that the thumb and index finger automatically reach the next position.

Manual Lymph Drainage (MLD/Vodder II)[2]

In cases in which the treatment of lymphedema starts at stage II or III a modification of the basic Vodder strokes is necessary. The pressure that is applied is higher and the rhythm is slower. The stretching must not only have an effect on the skin, it must extend deeper in to the area of the fascia. In addition to the therapeutic goals of MLD/Vodder I to increase lymph flow and lymph formation, the aim of the treatment is to soften and reduce fibrosclerotic tissue. One must consider that the resistance to lymph flow is higher, the function of the existing lymph vessels is hampered because of the tissue alteration, and the prelymphatic channels are partially closed in stages II and III of lymphedema. Therefore, the stroke must be calibrated to the degree of the fibrosclerotic alteration of the connective tissue.

Additive Manual Techniques

The additive manual techniques can be indicated already in stage II of lymphedema treatment. The manual treatment of lymphedema of the extremities at stages II and III requires substantial experience from the therapists. Because it is not technically feasible to measure massage pressure, it is not possible to prescribe an optimal treatment pressure. However, elevated stroke pressure in manual lymph drainage, as well as other types of massage technique, are indicated for the treatment of fibrosclerotic tissue. In addition to the "classic massage," we use length and crossway friction, petrissage, and kneading.

These types of techniques can generally be used for treatment of myogeloses and contractures of tendons. The application of these additional strokes is permitted

---

[2]Manual lymph drainage according to Dr. E. Vodder: higher pressure, slower rhythm

Table 28.1 Manual treatment of lymphedema

Stage	Location	MLD/Vodder I and Vodder II	Additive manual measures
0		MLD Vodder I – if lymphedema risk factors are present	
I	Extremities	MLD/Vodder I	–
	Trunk region	MLD/Vodder I	–
II	Extremities	MLD/Vodder II	Length and crossway friction
		+ →	Petrissage
			Kneading
	Trunk region	MLD/Vodder I	–
III	Extremities	MLD/Vodder II	Length and crossway friction
		+ →	Petrissage
			Kneading
			Joint mobilization techniques
	Trunk region	MLD/Vodder I	–

only in the area of pronounced fibrosclerotic tissue alteration. To optimize the therapeutic results, especially in the treatment of lymphedema stage III, joint mobilization techniques may be necessary (Figs. 28.1–28.3).

Indication and Contraindication

Manual lymph drainage (MLD/Vodder I) is indicated (Table 28.1):

- In fluid retention syndrome
- Severe cases of premenstrual syndrome
- Polycystic ovary syndrome
- After lymph node dissection to prevent lymphedema
- Lipedema
- Lymphedema in stage I
- As a proximal pretreatment generally

Manual lymph drainage (MLD/Vodder II) and additional strokes are indicated in the treatment of chronic lymphedema at stages II and III.

General contraindications for manual lymph drainage/combined manual lymphedema treatment:

- Decompensated cardiac insufficiency
- Acute inflammation caused by pathogenetic germs (bacteria fungi, viruses, the germs could be spread by the manual lymph drainage with resulting sepsis)
- Acute deep venous thrombosis
- Severe untreated cardiac arrhythmia

Relative contraindication:

• Sudeck syndrome (sympathic reflex dystrophy)
• Lymphedema caused by malignancy
• Acute episode of severe dermatological disease

References

1. Vodder E. Die manuelle Lymphdrainage und ihre medizinsichen Anwendungsbeite. *Erfahrungsheilkunder.* 1966;16:7.
2. Földi M, Földi E, Kubik S (eds). *Textbook of Lymphology*, Elsevier, GmBH; 2006.
3. Mislin H. Die Motorik der Lymphgefäße und Regulation der Lymphherzen. In: Altmann H-W et al. Hrsg. *Handbuch der allgemeinen Pathologie.* 3 Band, 6. Teil. Heidelberg: Springer; 1972.
4. Mislin H. The lymphangion. In: Földi M, Casley-Smith R, eds. *Lymphangiology.* Stuttgart: Schattauer; 1983:165-175.
5. B. Kriederman, T. Myloyde, M. Bernas, L. Lee-Donaldson, S. Preciado, et al., "Limb volume reduction after physical treatment by compression and/or massage in a rodent model of peripheral lymphedema," *Lymphology.* 2002 March;35(1):23-27.
6. Földi M, Strößenreuther R. *Grundlagen der manuellen Lymphdrainage.* 4 Aufl., München: Elsevier; 2007.
7. Brunner U, Frei-Fleischlin C. Gegenwärtiger Stand der kombinierten physikalischen Entstauungstherapie beim primären und sekundären Lymphödem der Beine. *VASA.* 1993; Band 22(Heft 1):8-14.
8. Franzeck UK et al. Combined physical therapy for lymphedema evaluated by fluorescence microlymphography and lymph capillary pressure measurements. *J Vasc Res.* 1997;34:306-311.

Chapter 29
Manual Lymph Drainage (Leduc Method)

Olivier Leduc and Albert Leduc

Introduction

The International Society of Lymphology has published a consensus for edema treatment since 1995.[1] Some countries have elaborated a more locally adapted consensus.[2,3] Nevertheless, the basic techniques mentioned in the different proposals are the same: manual lymphatic massage (or manual lymphatic drainage [MLD]), intermittent sequential pneumatic compression therapy (ISPT), and multilayer bandages (MLB). Some other techniques, such as ultrasound, endermology, and thermalism, can be utilized in addition to these basic physical techniques, but they are considered to be adjunctive.

Edema results from an excess of filtration and/or a decrease in lymphatic transport. Excessive filtration induces an accumulation of fluid, and a deficit of drainage also increases the content of macromolecules.

We propose to analyze the efficacy of the different physical techniques through their effect upon two parameters, excess fluid and macromolecules, which can lead to chronic inflammation and fibrosis.[4-6] Adipose content of the tissues increases through stimulation of lipogenesis when edema becomes chronic.[7,8]

Investigations

The influence of MLD, according to our concept (Leduc method®), was initially investigated in animals[9] and, afterward, in human beings. To evaluate the influence of MLD on the resorption of macromolecules we performed lymphoscintigraphy on

O. Leduc (✉)
Department of Physical Therapy, Unité de lympho-phlébologie, Haute Ecole P.H. Spaak, 91, Avenue Schaller, 1160 Brussels, Belgium
e-mail: oleduc@skynet.be

B.-B. Lee et al. (eds.), *Lymphedema*,
DOI 10.1007/978-0-85729-567-5_29, © Springer-Verlag London Limited 2011

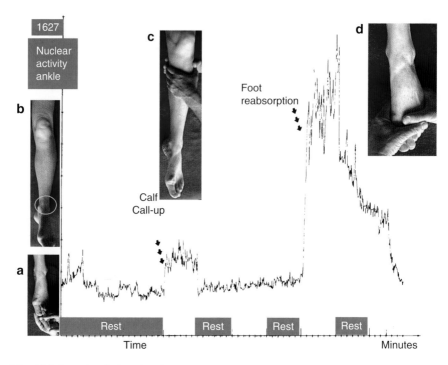

Fig. 29.1 Lymphoscintigraphy of the lower extremity by healthy human. Injection of radiola-belled colloids in the first interdigital space (**a**). The camera is centrated on the ankle (**b**). MLD (*call-up*) of the calf (**c**) increases the passage of the colloids. MLD (*reabsorption*) on the injected area (**d**)

the lower limbs of 12 healthy subjects (Fig. 29.1) and those of patients.[10,11] The injected radio-labeled colloids assimilated within the local protein-rich edema.

The MLD inciting (call-up) increases lymph flow. The MLD reabsorption is more efficient than the call-up technique, but the use of call-up before the reabsorption technique significantly increases the effect of reabsorption.

To estimate the influence of MLD on the fluid component of edema, we used echo-Doppler on nine patients hospitalized in a coronary unit.

We measured and calculated the following parameters: Mitral E wave (m/s), Mitral A wave (m/s), Mitral E/A ratio, Mitral E' wave (m/s), Mitral E/E' ratio, Ratio dP/dT, VTI aortic (cm), Cardiac rate (beats/min), cardiac output (cm³/min), maximal tricuspid insufficiency gradient (mmHg), Tricuspid E wave (m/s), Tricuspid A wave (m/s), Tricuspid E/A ratio, Tricuspid E' wave (m/s), Tricuspid E/E' ratio, max Ø Inf Vena Cava – min Ø Inf Vena Cava (cm), Mean perimeter of the leg (cm).

All patients had significant left ventricular dysfunction. During MLD, the heart rate and the mean perimeter of the leg decreased significantly (Table 29.1), in contrast to all of the hemodynamic parameters.

To conclude, the influence of MLD on fluid reabsorption is not significant and MLD may be prescribed to patients with heart insufficiency.

Table 29.1 Mean ± SD values expressed as percentages for the different parameters

Parameter (mean in %)	T0	T1	T2	P value (ANOVA)
Heart rate (beats/min)	100	104.14	86.70	0.02
SD	0	7.13	33.64	
Mean perimeter of the leg (cm)	100	98.11		0.0004
SD	0	0.82		

T0 baseline measurements, *T1* measurements after 5 min MLD, *T2* measurements after 15 min MLD

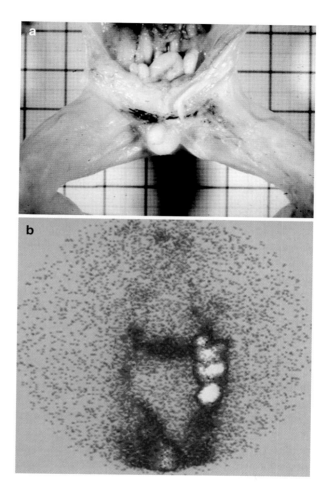

Fig. 29.2 (**a**) Inguino-inguinal lymphatic pathway on a human cadaver. (**b**) Inguino-inguinal lymphatic pathway on a patient during lymphoscintigraphy

When lymph node excision is performed, the normal lymphatic pathway is disrupted and it is possible for lymph to flow along substitution pathways,[12] crossing the midline defined by Sappey.[13] MLD must be performed according to these theoretical principles (Fig. 29.2a, b).

ISPT was evaluated by lymphoscintigraphy. We evaluated the influence of two different ISPT devices. One has five compartments and the other has only one. The population comprised nine healthy subjects and five patients who had undergone breast cancer surgery. The intensity of the pressure we applied was 80 mmHg for 20 min.[14,15] The conclusion of this investigation is that there was no effect on the resorption of colloids during ISPT.

The influence of ISPT on the fluid component was measured on 12 patients hospitalized in a coronary unit.[16] The measurements were registered by means of a Swan–Ganz catheter.

Intermittent sequential pneumatic compression therapy was applied on both lower limbs. After 2 min, the mean right atrial pressure increased from 4 to 8 mmHg. The mean wedge pressure increased to 17 mmHg. In two patients, the wedge pressure was increased to 28 and 32 mmHg respectively.

We conclude that ISPT facilitates very significantly the reabsorption of fluid and that the use of ISPT is contra-indicated for patients with cardiac insufficiency. We finally also conclude that physical treatment of lymphedema limited to ISPT alone is contra-indicated because this technique concentrates macro-molecules in the edematous tissue.

The influence of MLB on macromolecules was investigated by means of lymphoscintigraphy in a healthy population.[17,18]

Multilayer bandage is applied to the forearm and the nano-colloids are injected subdermally in the middle of the anterior side of the forearm. Muscle contractions, through flexing of the wrist against 30% of maximal resistance (one contraction every 3 s), are required over 10 min. Two minutes after wrist flexion begins, the appearance of nano-colloids in the axillary lymph nodes increases. During the rest period, after exercising, the arrival of the nano-colloids is still maintained for more than 20 min, showing the marked influence of muscle activity on the resorption of the proteins when the limb is wrapped with MLB.

The influence of MLB on the fluid part of the edema was evaluated by measuring the hemodynamic parameters during muscle activity of individuals subjected to MLB on the lower limb.[19] This investigation was performed on five patients hospitalized in a coronary unit.

The hemodynamic parameters were quantitated by means of echo-Doppler.

During muscle activity limited to flexion and extension of the ankle, the pressure in the right atrium, in the pulmonary artery and the wedge pressure increased very significantly in all patients.

The heart rate was stable because, in these patients with cardiac insufficiency, the heart is not able to react when the pre-load increases.

To conclude, MLB increases fluid resorption during muscle activity. Another conclusion is that MLB is not to be applied to the lower limbs in patients with heart failure.

References

1. International Society of Lymphology. Diagnosis and treatment of peripheral lymphedema. Consensus document of the International Society of Lymphology. *Lymphology*. 2003;36:84-91.

2. Leduc O. Rehabilitation after breast cancer treatment. European consensus. *Eur J Lymphology Relat Probl.* 2008;19(55).

3. Ciucci JL. *Consenso latinoamericano para el tratamiento del linfedema* Linfologia Nayarit. ed. 1 Edn. Argentina;2008.

4. Doldi SB, Latuada E, et al. Ultrasonography of extremity lymphedema. *Lymphology.* 1992; 25:129-133.

5. Szuba A, Rockson SG. Lymphedema: anatomy, physiology and pathogenesis. *Vasc Med.* 1997;2(4):321-326.

6. Vaughan BF. CT of swollen legs. *Clin Radiol.* 1990;41(1):24-30.

7. Idy-Peretti I, Bittoun J, et al. Lymphedematous skin and subcutis: in vivo high resolution magnetic resonance imaging evaluation. *J Invest Dermatol.* 1998;110(5):782-787.

8. Fumière E, Leduc O, et al. MR imaging, proton MR spectroscopy, ultrasonography, histologic findings in patients with chronic lymphedema. *Lymphology.* 2007;40(4):157-162.

9. Leduc A, Lievens P. Les anastomoses lympho-lymphatiques: incidences thérapeutiques. *Trav Soc Sci Belge Kinésithérapie.* 1976;IV(1):7-11.

10. Leduc O, Bourgeois P, et al. Manual lymphatic drainage: scintigraphic demonstration of its efficacy on colloidal protein reabsorption. In: Partsh H, ed. *Progress in Lymphology XI.* Amsterdam: Excerpta Medica; 1988:551-554.

11. Kafajan-Haddad AP, Janeiro Perez MC, et al. Lymphoscintigraphic evaluation of MLD for lower extremity lymphedema. *Lymphology.* 2006;39(1):41-48.

12. Leduc A, Caplan I, Leduc O. Lymphatic drainage of the upper limb. Substitution lymphatic pathways. *Eur J Lymphology Relat Probl.* 1993-1994;4(13):11-18.

13. Sappey C. *Anatomie. Physiologie. Pathologie des vaisseaux lymphatiques de l'homme et des vertébrés.* V. A Delahaye et Cie Ed. Paris;1874.

14. Leduc A, Bastin R. *Experimentele bijdrage tot de invloed van druktherapie op de lymfestroom.* Werkem B.W.V.K.; 1985.

15. Partsch H, Mostbeck G et al. Experimental investigation on the effect of a pressure wave massage apparatus (Lympho Press®) in lymphedema. *Phlebologie und Proctologie.* 1980;9: 124-128.

16. Dereppe H, Hoeylaert M et al. Répercussions hémodynamiques de la pressothérapie. *J Mal Vasc.* Paris, Masson,1990; 15:267-269.

17. Leduc O, Peeters A, et al. Approche expérimentale de l'influence de la contraction musculaire par méthode isotopique. *Kinés Scient.* 1991;300:43-45.

18. Leduc O, Bourgeois P, et al. Scintigraphic demonstration of its efficacy on colloïdal protein reabsorption during muscle activity. In: Nishi M, Uchino S, Yabuki S, eds. *Progress in Lymphology.* Amsterdam: Elsevier Science Publishers B.V.; 1990:421-423. Congress Book Tokyo 1989.

19. Wilputte F, Renard M, et al. Hemodynamic response to multilayered bandages dressed on a lower limb of patients with heart failure. *Eur J Lymphol Relat Probl.* 2005;15(45):1-4.

Chapter 30
Compression Therapy

Stanley G. Rockson

Intermittent pneumatic compression has been employed in the medical approach to vascular diseases for more than 80 years.[1] Multilayered bandage compression and elastic graduated compression garments are now both considered mainstays in the management of lymphedema, forming two of the elements of complex decongestive therapy for this condition.[2-4] These represent two of the many varieties of compression devices that are available.

Graduated Compression Garments

Standardized manufacture of stockings and sleeves has permitted the assignment of a standard grade of compression. This is calculated by creating a maximal value at the apex (i.e., the ankle or wrist) and a minimal value at the base (thigh or upper arm). Compression is commercially available in four distinct classes: I, with an applied pressure of 20–30 mmHg; II, 30–40 mmHg; III, 40–50 mmHg; and IV, more than 60+ mmHg. In patients with lymphedema, it is typically recommended that chronic compression be administered at a minimal value of 30–40 mmHg (Class II). Sleeves generally extend to the upper reaches of the arm and end below the axilla, although shoulder attachments and anchoring devices are also available. For the legs, though knee-length stockings can be purchased, either thigh-length garments or a panty hose–style garment, is recommended for use by patients with lymphedema.

Once a level of compression is selected, the garment is carefully fitted on the basis of meticulous limb measurements. Such garments lose their compressive capabilities after 3–6 months and must be replaced.

S.G. Rockson
Division of Cardiovascular Medicine, Stanford University School of Medicine,
Falk Cardiovascular Research Center, Stanford, CA, USA

B.-B. Lee et al. (eds.), *Lymphedema*,
DOI 10.1007/978-0-85729-567-5_30, © Springer-Verlag London Limited 2011

Perhaps the greatest impediment to the chronic utilization of maintenance compression is the difficulty that patients encounter when donning the garments. While class II compression does not pose extraordinary difficulties for the average patient, higher degrees of compression become limiting,[5] especially in the settings of advanced age, obesity, or arthritis.[1] Fortunately, many manufacturers provide assistive devices that partially combat this problem.[1]

For those patients who cannot successfully utilize the elasticized stockings and sleeves, a variety of devices have been devised to serve as alternative forms of maintenance compression. In addition, these devices, which include, but are not limited to, the Circ-Aid, the Reid sleeve, and the Jovi-Pak, can be used to augment the baseline compression achieved with the standard garments, particularly during nocturnal use. Analogous forms of compression devices have also been marketed for the nonappendicular forms of lymphedema (chest wall, breast, genitalia, head, and neck).

The efficacy of graduated compression garments has been quantitated and validated in various contexts.[6-9] During the maintenance phase of lymphedema therapy, it often is recommended that patients utilize the garments for up to 20 h/day; statistically significant reductions in edema volume have been demonstrated after use of the garment for 6 h consecutively per day.[10] The garments are typically removed during nocturnal recumbency.

Multilayered Bandage Compression

The use of repetitive, sequential, multilayered bandaging represents a mainstay of the acute approach to lymphedema of the limb.[3,11] These bandages behave as a nonelastic envelope. As muscle contraction evokes pressure in the limb, there is a variable response of the pressure within the bandaged part in relation to the contraction intensity.[12] The bandaging materials affect the quality of the treatment response: use of non-elastic, low-stretch bandaging materials will result in a resistance to stretching that will maximize the pressure generated during muscle contraction. The efficacy of this therapy in the clearance of macromolecules from the interstitium has been demonstrated through lymphoscintigraphic imaging.[13]

Daily sequential treatment in this manner results in a progressive decline in limb volume (Fig. 30.1). The most significant reduction in volume typically occurs during the first week of treatment.

Intermittent Pneumatic Compression

Intermittent pneumatic pump devices can also be used to deliver the desired external compression to lymphedematous limbs.[14] While at times employed as stand-alone therapy, they are generally recommended to be used adjunctively; the use of sequential

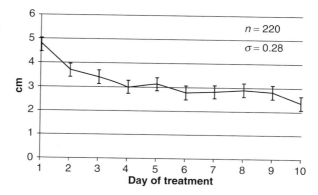

Fig. 30.1 The impact of daily multilayered bandaging upon edema volume in lymphedema (Reproduced with permission from Leduc et al.[12])

gradient pumps should be avoided in the absence of a multidisciplinary treatment program.[11] This subject is addressed in more detail in Chap. 31.

Impact of Compression Therapy upon Lymphedema Outcomes

Taken together, the use of multilayer bandage compression in the first phase of lymphedema treatment and of compression garments in the maintenance phase, represents the core of the complex physiotherapeutic intervention for lymphedema.[4,11] As such, the efficacy of intensive, short-term decongestive lymphatic therapy has been prospectively documented.[15,16] It has been demonstrated that the appropriate therapeutic use of these elements can effectively promote acute limb volume reductions in patients with various causes of lymphedema and, with the use chronic compression therapy in the form of garments, as one of the elements of self care, long-term control of lymphedema is achievable (Fig. 30.2).[16]

The individual contribution of multilayer bandaging to the overall treatment response has also been prospectively studied. In a study of 90 women with unilateral lymphedema of the upper or lower limbs, a 24-week treatment regimen was undertaken, using either a garment alone, or a garment coupled with 18 days of multilayer bandaging.[3] The study revealed that the reduction in limb volume by multilayer bandaging followed by garment use was approximately double that of using the garment alone, and was sustained throughout the period of prospective observation.

Lymphedema is a chronic condition that mandates life-long treatment. The judicious application of compression is efficacious and has proven benefit, both in the reduction of limb volume and in the maintenance of the achieved benefits over time.

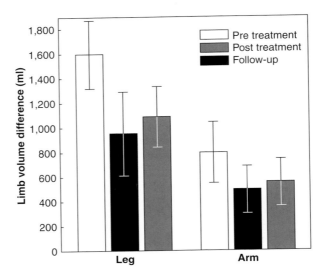

Fig. 30.2 Efficacy of the treatment intervention. Differences in limb volume (affected – unaffected limb) before treatment, after decongestive treatment, and at follow-up after self-management, which features the chronic use of compression garments. The pre – post treatment differences in volume were significant ($P<0.0001$ for the arm, $P<0.005$ for the leg), as were the differences from baseline to follow-up ($P<0.0001$ for arm, $P<0.005$ for leg) (Reproduced with permission from Szuba et al.[16])

References

1. Choucair M, Phillips TJ. Compression therapy. *Dermatol Surg.* 1998;24(1):141-148.
2. Rockson SG. Precipitating factors in lymphedema: myths and realities. *Cancer.* 1998; 83(12 suppl American):2814-2816.
3. Badger CM, Peacock JL, Mortimer PS. A randomized, controlled, parallel-group clinical trial comparing multilayer bandaging followed by hosiery versus hosiery alone in the treatment of patients with lymphedema of the limb. *Cancer.* 2000;88(12):2832-2837.
4. Rockson SG. Diagnosis and management of lymphatic vascular disease. *J Am Coll Cardiol.* 2008;52(10):799-806.
5. Szuba A, Rockson SG. Lymphedema: classification, diagnosis and therapy. *Vasc Med.* 1998;3(2):145-156.
6. Horner J, Fernandes J, Fernandes E, Nicolaides AN. Value of graduated compression stockings in deep venous insufficiency. *Br Med J.* 1980;280(6217):820-821.
7. Horner J, Lowth LC, Nicolaides AN. A pressure profile for elastic stockings. *Br Med J.* 1980;280(6217):818-820.
8. Christopoulos DG, Nicolaides AN, Szendro G, Irvine AT, Bull ML, Eastcott HH. Airplethysmography and the effect of elastic compression on venous hemodynamics of the leg. *J Vasc Surg.* 1987;5(1):148-159.
9. Partsch H. Compression therapy of the legs. A review. *J Dermatol Surg Oncol.* 1991;17(10): 799-805.
10. Bertelli G, Venturini M, Forno G, Macchiavello F, Dini D. An analysis of prognostic factors in response to conservative treatment of postmastectomy lymphedema. *Surg Gynecol Obstet.* 1992;175(5):455-460.

11. Rockson SG, Miller LT, Senie R, et al. American cancer society lymphedema workshop. Workgroup III: diagnosis and management of lymphedema. *Cancer.* 1998;83(12 suppl American):2882-2885.

12. Leduc O, Leduc A, Bourgeois P, Belgrado JP. The physical treatment of upper limb edema. *Cancer.* 1998;83(12 suppl American):2835-2839.

13. Leduc O, Bourgeois P, Leduc A. Manual lymphatic drainage: scintigraphic demonstration of its efficacy on colloidal protein reabsorption. In: Partsch H, ed. *Progress in Lymphology.* Amsterdam: Elsevier Science Publishers B.V.; 1988:551-554.

14. Brennan MJ, Miller LT. Overview of treatment options and review of the current role and use of compression garments, intermittent pumps, and exercise in the management of lymphedema. *Cancer.* 1998;83(12 suppl American):2821-2827.

15. Ko DS, Lerner R, Klose G, Cosimi AB. Effective treatment of lymphedema of the extremities. *Arch Surg.* 1998;133(4):452-458.

16. Szuba A, Cooke JP, Yousuf S, Rockson SG. Decongestive lymphatic therapy for patients with cancer-related or primary lymphedema. *Am J Med.* 2000;109(4):296-300.

Chapter 31
Intermittent Pneumatic Compression Therapy

Stanley G. Rockson

The use of intermittent pneumatic compression (IPC) devices in the therapeutic approach to lymphedema is perhaps the most controversial element of what is traditionally termed complex decongestive physiotherapy. In the United States, historically, pneumatic compression has been the mainstay of lymphatic therapy for decades.[1] IPC, preferably accomplished with multi-chamber pumps, effectively removes excess fluid from the extremity.[2-9]

Early enthusiasm for the benefits of IPC have been tempered by the theoretical concern that the pressures generated by these devices might damage skin lymphatics.[10,11] When used in lower extremity lymphedema, generation of genital edema is also a theoretical concern.[12] Development of a ring of fibrous tissue above the proximal margin of the device's sleeve has also been reported.[13]

Although IPC has this history of controversy surrounding its use, with the threat of incurred complications, the American Cancer Society Working Group on the Diagnosis and Management of Lymphedema designated intermittent compression pumps as a potential adjunctive component of decongestive lymphatic physiotherapy when used as an adjunct to the other components. Recognizing that pneumatic compression with lower pressures (≤ 40 mm Hg) had been suggested to be effective and to potentially court a lower risk of complications,[14] we undertook a prospective, randomized study to investigate the safety and relative efficacy of pneumatic compression therapy for the treatment of patients with breast carcinoma-associated upper extremity lymphedema when used adjunctively with compression bandaging and manual lymphatic massage.[15] Twenty-three previously untreated, patients were randomized to receive either decongestive lymphatic therapy (DLT) alone or decongestive therapy with daily adjunctive IPC. The addition of IPC to standard

S.G. Rockson
Division of Cardiovascular Medicine, Stanford University School of Medicine,
Falk Cardiovascular Research Center,
Stanford, CA, USA

B.-B. Lee et al. (eds.), *Lymphedema*,
DOI 10.1007/978-0-85729-567-5_31, © Springer-Verlag London Limited 2011

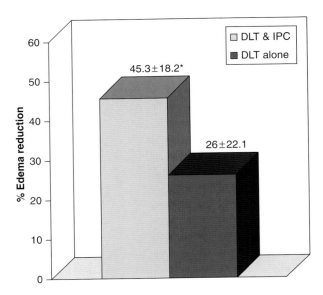

Fig. 31.1 The effect of adjunctive, intermittent pneumatic compression (*IPC*) on initial decongestive lymphatic therapy (*DLT*) in patients with breast carcinoma-associated lymphedema. The data
depict the percentage reduction in volume of the limb attained after 10 days of daily therapy with
either (1) DLT plus IPC or (2) DLT alone. The data are provided as the mean ± standard deviation
for each group. The *asterisk* denotes a statistically significant difference ($p < 0.05$)

DLT yielded additional mean volume reduction (Fig. 31.1). In 27 additional patients
assessed during the maintenance phase of therapy, the addition of IPC to DLT
enhanced the therapeutic response. In both the acute and maintenance phases of the
study, IPC was tolerated well without detectable adverse effects on skin elasticity
or joint range of motion.

Although the use of IPC in lymphedema has been hampered by individual reports
of complications and lack of efficacy,[16] focused attempts to document the adverse
effects, such as the study cited, do not seem to support the pejorative implications of
IPC, particularly when the treatment modality is utilized in an *adjunctive* manner.
The ostensible benefits of IPC correlate well with experimental physiological observations, in which the promotion of lymph formation by tissue compression is related
to the number of compressions applied and the time interval between each compression. Thus, it would seem that the benefit accrues through centripetal emptying of the
terminal lymphatics, such that the vessels refill after each compression is released.[17]

It is likely that continued refinement in the bioengineering and programmability
of the pneumatic compression devices will enhance their efficacy in translating the
physiological effects of intermittent compression to the therapeutics of lymphedema.
As an example, quite recently, an adaptation of IPC has been introduced that
purports to mechanically simulate the effects of manual lymphatic drainage. This
device, the Flexitouch® System, delivers minimal, phasic external compression to
both the affected limb(s) and the trunk in a programmable fashion. When prospectively examined for its role in patient self-management, the device has demonstrated

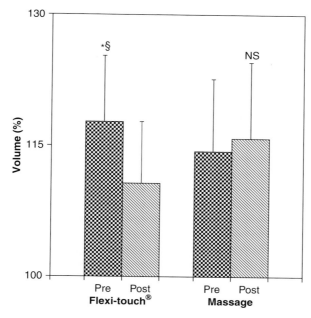

Fig. 31.2 A prospective, randomized, crossover study of maintenance therapy (Flexitouch® vs. Manual Lymphatic Drainage [MLD]) was performed in 10 patients with unilateral breast cancer-associated lymphedema of the arm. Excess volume of the affected arm is expressed as a percentage of the volume of the contralateral, normal arm. The effect of treatment on the percentage excess volume compared with the contra-lateral arm, was significant for Flexitouch™, but not for MLD (mean ± SD; *p = 0.0005 compared with the pretreatment value; §p = 0.003 compared with response to MLD)

objectively demonstrable outcome benefits (Fig. 31.2).[18] Furthermore, in 155 lymphedema patients (93 with cancer-related lymphedema), before and after treatment assessment with the 12-item Short-Form Health Survey demonstrated significant improvement in all areas of perceived physical and emotional health.[19] Clearly, further evaluation of the role of such devices is warranted.

It has been advocated that IPC can be incorporated into a multidisciplinary, therapeutic program,[1,15,20,21] but the guidelines for patient and device selection continue to evolve. Several factors are involved in these therapeutic decisions, including simple versus advanced devices (the latter offering the option, in various combinations, of multi-chamber design, programmability, and advanced technologies to permit individual, lymphedema-specific therapeutics).[16] In addition, patient selection factors must determine not only the desirability of adding IPC to the treatment regimen, but also the choice of the specific device. These patient factors include severity of lymphedema; response to conservative therapies; lymphedematous involvement of the trunk, breast, or genitalia; presence of pain or open wounds; heterogeneous, regional variability in the severity of the edema; and/or the presence of complications that contraindicate the use of simple, non-programmable devices (Table 31.1).

Table 31.1 Intermittent pneumatic compression device selection

Patient considerations
- Severity of lymphedema
- Responsiveness to conservative therapies
- Lymphedematous involvement of the trunk, breast, or genitalia
- Pain
- Open wounds
- Complications that contraindicate the use of simple, non-programmable devices

Simple versus advanced design
- Multi-chamber design
- Programmability
- Advanced technologies to permit individuated, lymphedema-specific therapeutics

References

1. Brennan MJ, Miller LT. Overview of treatment options and review of the current role and use of compression garments, intermittent pumps, and exercise in the management of lymphedema. *Cancer*. 1998;83(12 suppl American):2821-2827.
2. Zelikovski A, Haddad M, Reiss R. The "Lympha-press" intermittent sequential pneumatic device for the treatment of lymphoedema: five years of clinical experience. *J Cardiovasc Surg (Torino)*. 1986;27(3):288-290.
3. Dittmar A, Krause D. A comparison of intermittent compression with single and multi-chamber systems in treatment of secondary arm lymphedema following mastectomy. *Z Lymphol*. 1990;14(1):27-31.
4. Walby R. Treatment of lymphedema in institutions. Two weeks of in-hospital intensive lymphatic drainage followed by maintenance treatment with a pulsator. *Tidsskr Nor Laegeforen*. 1990;110(24):3125-3126.
5. Wozniewski M. Value of intermittent pneumatic massage in the treatment of upper extremity lymphedema. *Pol Tyg Lek*. 1991;46(30-31):550-552.
6. Pappas CJ, O'Donnell TF Jr. Long-term results of compression treatment for lymphedema. *J Vasc Surg*. 1992;16(4):555-562; discussion 62-64.
7. Brunner U, Frei-Fleischlin C. Current status of combined physical decompression therapy in primary and secondary lymphedema of the legs. *Vasa*. 1993;22(1):8-14.
8. Bunce IH, Mirolo BR, Hennessy JM, Ward LC, Jones LC. Post-mastectomy lymphoedema treatment and measurement. *Med J Aust*. 1994;161(2):125-128.
9. Szuba A, Rockson SG. Lymphedema: classification, diagnosis and therapy. *Vasc Med*. 1998;3(2):145-156.
10. Eliska O, Eliskova M. Are peripheral lymphatics damaged by high pressure manual massage? *Lymphology*. 1995;28(1):21-30.
11. Foldi E. Massage and damage to lymphatics. *Lymphology*. 1995;28(1):1-3.
12. Boris M, Weindorf S, Lasinski BB. The risk of genital edema after external pump compression for lower limb lymphedema. *Lymphology*. 1998;31(1):15-20.
13. Casley-Smith J, Casley-Smith J. Other physical therapy for lymphedema: pumps; heating; etc. In: Casley-Smith J, Casley-Smith J, eds. *Lymphedema*. Adelaide: The Lymphedema Association of Australia; 1991:155-159.
14. Balzarini A, Pirovano C, Diazzi G, et al. Ultrasound therapy of chronic arm lymphedema after surgical treatment of breast cancer. *Lymphology*. 1993;26(3):128-134.
15. Szuba A, Achalu R, Rockson SG. Decongestive lymphatic therapy for patients with breast carcinoma-associated lymphedema. A randomized, prospective study of a role for adjunctive intermittent pneumatic compression. *Cancer*. 2002;95(11):2260-2267.

16. Rockson SG. Current concepts and future directions in the diagnosis and management of lymphatic vascular disease. *Vasc Med*. 2010;15(3):223-231.
17. McGeown JG, McHale NG, Thornbury KD. Effects of varying patterns of external compression on lymph flow in the hindlimb of the anaesthetized sheep. *J Physiol*. 1988;397:449-457.
18. Wilburn O, Wilburn P, Rockson SG. A pilot, prospective evaluation of a novel alternative for maintenance therapy of breast cancer-associated lymphedema [ISRCTN76522412]. *BMC Cancer*. 2006;6:84.
19. Ridner SH, McMahon E, Dietrich MS, Hoy S. Home-based lymphedema treatment in patients with cancer-related lymphedema or noncancer-related lymphedema. *Oncol Nurs Forum*. 2008;35(4):671-680.
20. Rockson SG, Miller LT, Senie R, et al. American Cancer Society lymphedema workshop. Workgroup III: diagnosis and management of lymphedema. *Cancer*. 1998;83(12 suppl American):2882-2885.
21. Leduc O, Bourgeois P, Leduc A. Manual lymphatic drainage: scintigraphic demonstration of its efficacy on colloidal protein reabsorption. In: Partsch H, ed. *Progress in Lymphology*. Amsterdam: Elsevier; 1988:551-554.

Chapter 32
Other Contemporary Treatment Modalities

Neil B. Piller

Conservative Therapies for Secondary Lymph Edema

We have a plethora of treatments and strategies for dealing with lymphedema. Some show scant evidence of their effectiveness and often little rationale for their use. We must advance our knowledge in the breadth of treatments with an open mind, but must provide evidence for their efficacy so that patients and practitioners know what to expect. For many new treatments, the trials are often small, but some are well designed and are objective with rigorous evaluation, so we can have confidence in the outcomes.

Contemporary Treatments

Patients may seek contemporary treatments from others or the internet. It i'is important for therapists to be aware of these contemporary options, just as it is important to be aware of any comparative benefits of this range of therapies.

The Groupings of Contemporary Treatments

Some are patient-based with no therapist input and some are administered by a therapist or clinician. They can be broadly categorized into those that vibrate the

N.B. Piller
Lymphoedema Assessment Clinic, Department of Surgery, School of Medicine, Flinders University and Medical Centre, Bedford Park, SA, Australia

B.-B. Lee et al. (eds.), *Lymphedema*,
DOI 10.1007/978-0-85729-567-5_32, © Springer-Verlag London Limited 2011

tissues (encompassing a range of frequencies and amplitudes), those involving a pharmacological agent that induces or promotes a biological event, those that electrically stimulate the lymphatics, those that vary tissue pressures including exercise, those that encourage diet change, and those that are a result of the placebo effect.

Methods

This overview is limited to patient populations with clinically-diagnosed limb lymphedema secondary to cancer treatment and to articles written in English. Online health databases, lymphatic societies and lymphology journals were searched, with the primary study outcomes to include: a change in limb volume (generally measured by perometry, water displacement or calculated via circumference measurement), subjective symptoms and/or quality of life/activities of daily living. The quality of each article was assessed according to Mulrow and Oxman.[1] Reviews that match the above criteria are also included.

Pharmacogenomics and Medications Targeting the Lymphatic System

There have been a range of treatments that have targeted the lymphatic system or its components pharmacologically, the best known of which are the flavonoid/benzopyrone groups. Studies included those of Pecking et al.,[2,3] who first investigated Daflon, and Cluzan et al., who studied Cyclofort,[4] both of whom had significant objective improvements for the patient group tested. Lodema provided good outcomes for patients in terms of reducing their lymphedema according to one report,[5] but another showed it to have little objective effect.[6] Anecdotal information suggested excellent outcomes. The use of coumarin (5-6 benzo-α- pyrone) for the treatment of lymphedema, had hepatotoxic effects for some, but we now know that this was a consequence of a genetic metabolic problem relating to the breakdown of coumarin.[7] Developing genetic and genomic knowledge will mean that in the future we will be able to determine who will respond well (and who may not) and overcome the above adverse outcomes.

Low-Level Scanning and Hand-Held Laser

The first trials of the low-level laser in lymphedema were reported in 1995,[8] although the general benefits were first reported in the late 1960s.[9] Of key importance is the dose and delivery. Double blinded, cross-over placebo controlled trials have been conducted using laser with good subjective and objective outcomes.[10] One of the issues of general lymphedema treatment and perhaps an explanation for less than expected outcomes at times may have been the faulty decision-making process used for its sequencing. Trials[8,10] of scanning and the hand-held laser have shown that its application is particularly beneficial when there is fibrotic induration of the tissues (associated with surgical or radiation-induced scarring), in reducing swelling, softening the tissues, improving scars, and improving how the limb feels.[11,12] The low-level laser has a role to play in the early phases of treatment of lymphedema as well as in its later management (when fibrotic induration has spread through the lymphatic territories), both from the perspectives of the health professional and the patient. Optimal treatment time is generally short with gaps between treatments.[13]

Lymphatic Drainage Massage Delivered by Partners/Carers and Mechanically

Massage aimed at improving lymphatic drainage administered by trained lymph therapists possesses a body of evidence supporting its effectiveness,[14] but it is far from complete. However, it is very important that therapists, clinicians, and patients are aware of what can be expected when using tools that also can improve lymphatic drainage by mimicking therapist massage and from partner/caregiver massage.

Massage, in general terms, is known to encourage the entry of fluids into the initial lymphatics, to facilitate transport along lymph collectors and to open anastomoses between adjacent collectors or lymph territories. It does this by means of changes in tissue pressures.

Piller et al.[15] showed that when partners/caregivers were trained by lymphedema therapists, the objective and subjective results were similar to those of professional treatment programs. Perhaps the partner/caregiver knows the patient's body better and when the limb is responding and when it is not. Such programs need further research because they can empower the patient, reduce costs and travel time, and re-establish a touching relationship.

While there is a plethora of massage pads/units only a few have been subjected to a formal trial in lymphedemas and trial sizes are often small. A trial[42] of a massage pad on leg lymphedema showed that, in order to gain a good outcome, the pad had to be used so that it facilitated clearance of the lymph territories, just as in professional lymphatic drainage massage programs. Patients gained and maintained good reductions in their limb volume, with 1 h of pad use per day. Improvement also occurred in tissue softness, and how the limb felt. Patients felt more in control of the medical condition and felt better able to undertake activities of daily living. In a trial of a hand-held massage unit[16] in a moderate secondary arm lymphedema used for 25 min each evening for 1 month, there were significant volume reductions and improvements in the perception of limb size and range of movement. Again, patient control and use in their own time and at their own pace were important.

Another strategy that varies tissue pressures by tissue movement revolves around "wobbling" the limbs from side to side. It is, in fact, a form of vibration, albeit slow. In this trial patients used the equipment while supine with the legs elevated on the unit, for periods of from 3 to 12 min twice per day for 3 weeks. The results[17] were similar to the massage pad trial in that the limbs reduced in size, volume, they softened, and the limbs felt better.

Patients felt more in control and were better able to undertake their activities of daily living, a common theme with home-based management.

Mild Exercise (Tai Chi)

Tai Chi and Qi Gong can easily be performed by the patient. These actions vary tissue pressures more effectively and, when combined with variations in intra-thoracic and intra-abdominal pressures, help lymphatic system loading and flow. Patients with arm lymphedema who used Tai Chi 10 min daily achieved reductions within the same range as more demanding treatments and were able to maintain them.[18] A water-based version of this type is used in the Encore program operated in Australia and around the world, but the outcomes are yet to be published.

Moderate Exercise (In and Out of Water)

A common question is: how much exercise can I do? Most studies[19,20] indicate that mild exercise is good for the lymphatic loading and transport because of variation in tissue pressures. However, as we go up the scale of exercise intensity, we must know the capacity of the damaged lymphatic system to handle an augmented lymph load. Getting the balance right is very important.

One good way to undertake exercise, but at the same time to have tissue support through external pressure, is through the range of water-based programs. Some studies provide good evidence for this.[21-23] The temperature of the water is important, but it is physiologically sensible to have temperatures within the range of normal skin temperature: 28°C has been suggested.[21]

There are specific exercise classes available to patients with arm and leg lymphedemas. Casley-Smith[24] suggested gentle movement, deep breathing and slow rhythmic exercise of the proximal and distal muscles melded with self massage routines. Bracha and Jacob[25] showed this program to reduce limb volume and improve quality of life in some participants.

More strenuous exercise programs using weights have also been reported.[26,27] In one trial, patients with arm lymphedema were asked to undertake increasing levels of weight-lifting while performing a series of pre-determined exercises to evaluate the maximal exercise points without worsening the lymphedema. In most cases, while there was a slight increase in limb volume immediately after the exercise, the effect was short-lived as long as patients resumed their activities of normal daily living.[28] This study indicated that patients can undertake significant and even strenuous amounts of exercise/activity without worsening their lymphoedema, but obviously, it is crucial that the patient know the limit of exercise and stay below it. The impact of exercise and significant activity has been reviewed and shows an overall positive impact (varying in magnitude among studies) on limb size, range of movement, muscle strength, subjective limb symptoms, and quality of life.[19] In all studies, a cooling-down period is essential. The question of when to begin an exercise program after surgery seems to have been answered by Todd et al.,[28] who indicated that a delay of 1 week for any full shoulder mobilization reduced lymphedema incidence.

Electro-Stimulation

Lymphatics pulsate between 6 and 10 times per minute and are myogenically and neurogenically regulated. Anecdotal evidence indicates that mild electro-stimulation has an effect on lymphedema, and can reduce size and volume. A study of secondary leg lymphedema[29] indicated that electrical stimulation has such benefits over current best practice self-management. Pain, heaviness, tightness and perceived leg size also improved. Truncal fluid was also reduced, indicating a possible additional clearance of major lymphatic trunks. Other units similar in function and principle to a TENS unit have also been shown anecdotally to reduce lymphedemas, but trials are still in progress.

Tissue Manipulation

A technique originating in France, called *"endermologie"*, has generated evidence for the treatment of cellulite and obesity. Given the similarities among, mid-stage lymphedema, cellulite, lipedema, and obesity (the adipose connection), it is likely to be beneficial in the treatment of lymphedema. A single, blinded, randomized study of arm lymphedema comparing *endermologie* with traditional manual lymphatic drainage (MLD) over a 4-week period demonstrated the greatest reduction in limb volume and circumference in the first week, but showed benefit to continue over the 4 weeks of the trial.[30] Results were similar to MLD, although achieved in a shorter time. There were improvements in tissue hardness and subjective indicators. Better outcomes were achieved when combined with bandaging and with more time spent on clearance of the trunk and axillary area,[30] as is well known in CPT programs.

Kinesio-Taping

Kinesio-taping is believed to improve lymph drainage by lifting the skin away from the underlying fascial planes of the musculature, perhaps reducing interstitial pressures there, and facilitating blood and, particularly, lymph flow along these lower pressure areas. It can do this because of the puckering effect of the tape. It is widely used in sports injuries, but has recent been applied in treating lymphedemas[31,32] and seems likely to be useful in hot and/or humid climates. In an audit of the use of kinesio-tape for breast and other edemas, Finnerty et al.[33] showed that kinesio-tape was being used in lymphedema management, particularly in the more challenging areas (breast, chest) where traditional bandaging and garments are difficult to use. Good quality trials are lacking. One trial of seroma following axillary clearance for breast cancer treatment showed significant benefits of kinesio-taping in reducing the severity and duration of the seroma, as well as subjective indicators.[34]

Diet (Mid-Chain Triglycerides) and Abdominal Issues

Long-chain triglycerides are absorbed (as chylomicrons) via the mesenteric lymphatics, adding to the lymphatic load. If their structure or function is compromised, this absorbed load of fats may find its way into other organs/structures by retrograde flow.[35] Replacing long-chain triglycerides with mid- and short-chain ones is believed to reduce the incidence of this retrograde flow (chylous reflux). There are a number of suggested diets revolving around medium-chain triglycerides (MCT). The evidence is poor in the scientific literature, but is strongly represented in the "gray" literature. Other issues of diet[43], gastro-intestinal bloating, and constipation also appear in the "gray" literature and make sense empirically if the potential exists to create significant external pressure on the abdominal lymphatic collectors.

Placebo

The placebo effect is linked with the release of brain endorphins[36] associated with the anticipation of receiving active treatment. Placebos have a benefit in studies with continuous subjective outcomes measurement,[37] a phenomenon that is relevant to studies on lymphedema therapeutics.

Some of the studies cited in this chapter have used placebo groups in which patients have responded to placebo treatment, generally reporting symptomatic improvement (not usually accompanied by significant changes in limb volume). The trial investigating the effects of 5-6 benzo-α pyrone by Loprinzi et al.[6] showed that, despite an arm volume increase in both groups, there were similar positive responses to perceived arm swelling, tightness, heaviness, and arm mobility in the active treatment and the placebo groups and, even after 12 months, there was a slight preference for the placebo over the active intervention! Similar results arose in a study by Pecking et al.,[2,3] who investigated Daflon. Both the placebo and the active group reported statistically significant reductions in arm discomfort and an improvement in the perception of constant heaviness. There were no objective changes in the placebo group. Cluzan et al.[4] investigated Cyclo-fort versus placebo and found that while quantifiable edema volume increased in the placebo group patients, they nevertheless reported improvements in both arm heaviness and mobility. Casley-Smith et al.[5] investigated the effect of coumarin and found a similar improvement in patient perceptions.

Box et al.[38] studied the effects of hydrotherapy compared with a control group who did not receive any active treatment. Although the control group demonstrated an increased arm volume after 7 weeks, they reported improvements in aching, limb appearance, heaviness, tightness, and work/leisure activities. A handheld laser study by Carati et al.[10] involved a placebo group receiving sham laser with 1 and 3 months' follow-up. At 3 months, the placebo group experienced an increase in arm volume, but reported significant improvements in the overall mean perceptual score and activities of daily living.

The placebo effect may be used to the advantage of both the therapist and the patient. The patient's expectations, the therapist's belief in the treatment being offered, and the patient–therapist relationship[39-41] can accentuate the placebo effect. Being aware of these influences may help the therapist to initiate improvements in subjective symptoms, even if this is not necessarily followed by changes in more objective parameters.

Every treatment and management program needs to be balanced in terms of cost and benefit and linked to any contraindications. Treatment complacency must be avoided and perhaps changing therapy is one way around this. The overarching effect of even placebo on the patient's quality of life and frame of mind may encourage them to undertake other treatments that will have an impact on limb size, composition, and volume.

References

1. Mulrow C, Oxman A. *How to Conduct a Cochrane Systematic Review*. 3rd ed. London: BMJ Publishing Group; 1996.
2. Moseley A, Piller NB, Douglass J, Esplin M. Comparison of the effectiveness of MLD and LPG. *J Lymphoedema*. 2007;2(2):3036.
3. Pecking AP, Fevrier B, Wargon C, Pillion G. Efficacy of Daflon 500 mg in the treatment of lymphedema (secondary to conventional therapy of breast cancer). *Angiology*. 1997;48(1):93-98.
4. Cluzan RV, Alliot F, Ghabboun S, Pascot M. Treatment of secondary lymphedema of the upper limb with cyclo 3 fort. *Lymphology*. 1996;29:29-35.
5. Casley-Smith JR, Morgan RG, Piller NB. Treatment of lymphedema of the arms and legs with 5,6-BENZO-[á]-PYRONE. *N Engl J Med*. 1993;329(16):1158-1163.
6. Loprinzi CL, Kugler JW, Sloan JA, et al. Lack of effect of Coumarin in women with lymphedema after treatment for breast cancer. *N Engl J Med*. 1999;340(5):346-350.

7. Farinola N, Piller N. Pharmaco-genomics—its role in re-establishing coumarin as treatment for lymphoedema. *Lymphat Res Biol.* 2005;3(2):81.
8. Piller N, Thelander A. Treatment of chronic lymphoedema with low level laser therapy: a 2.5 year follow-up. *Lymphology.* 1998;31(2):74.
9. Carney SA, Lauwrence JC, Ricketts CR. The effect of light from a ruby laser on mesothelium of skin in tissue culture. *Biochem Biophys Acta.* 1967;148(2):525-530.
10. Carati CJ, Anderson SN, Gannon BJ, Piller NB. Treatment of postmastectomy lymphedema with low-level laser therapy. *Cancer.* 2003;98(6):1114-1122.
11. Maiya A, Olivia E, Dibya A. Effect of low energy laser therapy in the management of post mastectomy lymphoedema. *Singapore J Physiother.* 2008;11(1):2-5.
12. Wigg J. Use and response to treatment using low level laser therapy. *J Lymphoedema.* 2009;4(2):7376.
13. Tilley S. Use of laser therapy in the management of lymphoedema. *J Lymphoedema.* 2009;4(1):39-72.
14. Williams A. Manual lymphatic drainage: exploring the history and evidence base. *Br J Community Nurs.* 2010;15:S18-S24.
15. Piller NB, Rice J, Heddle R, Miller A. Partner training as an effective means of managing chronic arm lymphoedema subsequent to breast cancer surgery. *Proceedings of the XV Lymphology Congress Lymphology.* 2000;33(suppl):261.
16. Moseley A, Piller NB, Heidenreich B, Douglkass J. Pilot study of hand-held massage unit. *J Lymphoedema.* 2009;4(1):23-27.
17. Moseley A et al. A new patient focused, home based therapy for people with chronic lymphoedema. *Lymphology.* 2004;37(1):53.
18. Moseley A, Piller NB. The effect of gentle arm exercise and deep breathing on secondary arm lymphoedema. *Lymphology.* 2005;38(4):229.
19. Moseley A, Piller NB. Exercise for limb lymphoedema: evidence that it is beneficial. *J Lymphoedema.* 2008;3(1):51-56.
20. Moseley AL, Carati C, Piller NB. A systematic review of common conservative therapies for arm lymphoedema secondary to breast cancer treatment. *Ann Oncol.* 2003. doi:10.1093/annonc/md182.
21. Johansson K, Tibe K, Kanne L, Skantz H. Controlled physical training for arm lymphoedema patients. *Lymphology.* 2004;37(suppl):37-39.
22. Box R, Marnes T, Robertson V. Aquatic physiotherapy and breast cancer related lymphoedema. *5th Australasian Lymphology Association Congress Proceedings;* 2004:37-42.
23. Tidar D, Katz-Leurer M. Aqua lymphatic therapy in patients who suffer from breast cancer related lymphoedema: a randomized controlled study. *Support Care Cancer.* 2010;18(3):383-392.
24. Casley-Smith JR, Casley-Smith JR. *Modern Treatment for Lymph Edema.* 5th edn. Lymph Edema Association of Australia; 1997.
25. Bracha J, Jacob T. Using exercise classes to reduce lymphoedema. *J Lymphoedema.* 2010;5(1):46-55.
26. Johanssen K, Piller NB. Exercises with heavy weights for patients with breast cancer related lymphoedema 2005: *XXth International Congress Lymphology, Salvador, Brazil, Proceedings;* 2005.
27. Johansson K. Weight bearing exercise and its impact on arm lymphoedema. *J Lymphoedema.* 2007;2(2):115-122.
28. Todd J, Scally A, Dodwell D, Horgan K, Topping A. A randomized controlled trial of two programs of shoulder exercise following axillary node dissection for invasive breast cancer. *Physiotherapy.* 2008;94:265-273.
29. Piller NB, Douglass J, Heidenreich B, Moseley A. Placebo controlled trial of mild electrical stimulation. *J Lymphoedema.* 2010;5(1):15-25.

30. Moseley A, Esplin M, Piller NB, Douglass J. Endermoligie (with and without compression bandaging) a new treatment option for secondary arm lymphoedema. *Lymphology.* 2007;40: 128-137.

31. Rock-Stockheimer K. *Kinesiotaping for Lymph Edema and Chronic Swelling.* Kinesio, USA; 2006.

32. Kinesio UK Kinesio Taping for Lymph edema. Available online at: www.kinseiotaping.co.uk. Accessed May 13, 2009.

33. Finnerty S, Thomason S, Woods M. Audit of the use of kinesiology tape for breast oedema. *J Lymphoedema.* 2010;5(1):38-44.

34. Bosman J, Piller NB. A randomized clinical trial of lymph taping in seroma formation after breast cancer surgery. *J Lymphoedema.* 2010; 5(2): 12-23.

35. Foeldi M, Foeldi E, Kubik S. Lymphatic diseases (Chylous Reflux) In: *Textbook of Lymphology.* Urban and Fisher. 2003;311.

36. Haour F. Mechanisms of placebo effect and of conditioning: neurobiological data in human and animals. *Med Sci.* 2005;21(3):315-319.

37. Hrobjartsson A, Gotzsche PC. Is the placebo powerless? An analysis of clinical trials comparing placebo with no treatment. *N Engl J Med.* 2001;344(21):1594-1602.

38. Box R, Marnes T, Robertson V. Aquatic physiotherapy and breast cancer related lymphoedema. *5th Australasian Lymphology Association Conference Proceedings;* 2004:47-49.

39. Benson H, Friedman R. Harnessing the power of the placebo effect and renaming it "remembered wellness". *Annu Rev Med.* 1996;47:193-199.

40. Kaptchuk TJ. The placebo effect in alternative medicine: Can the performance of healing ritual have clinical significance? *Ann Intern Med.* 2002;136(11):817-825.

41. Papakostas YG, Daras MD. Placebos, placebo effect, and the response to the healing situation: the evolution of a concept. *Epilepsia.* 2001;42(12):1614-1625.

42. Piller N. Home use of massage pads for secondary leg lymphoedema. *Lymphology.* 2003; 37(suppl):213.

43. Dawson R, Piller N. Diet and BCRL: Facts and Falacies on the Web. J *Lymphoedema* 2011; 6(1):36-43.

Chapter 33
Medical Treatment

Stanley G. Rockson

In strict terms, medical treatment implies that the treating physician will venture beyond the potential physiotherapeutic and surgical options and seek to embrace the benefits of pharmacotherapy. Here, unfortunately, there is still a paucity of options that have any proven benefit for the lymphedema patient.

In 1998, the American Cancer Society convened a working group to consider the problem of lymphedema and breast cancer. When delivering its recommendations for the diagnosis and management of lymphedema,[1] the workgroup touched upon three categories of pharmacotherapy: *benzopyrones*, such as coumarin,[2] are not available for use in all parts of the world (coumarin has not been approved by the Food and Drug Administration for use in the United States); *bioflavenoids*,[3] for which efficacy outcome data are still largely lacking; and systemic *antibiotic* prophylaxis. *Diuretics* play little, if any, role in the management of isolated lymphatic vascular insufficiency[4] because the pathogenesis of the edema relies upon the elevated interstitial oncotic pressures conferred by macromolecules rather than upon inappropriate retention of water and electrolytes. However, in cases in which hydrostatic pressure is also elevated, such as, for example, the post-phlebitic syndrome with secondary hypertension, low-dose thiazide-induced diuresis may play a beneficial complementary role in the primary indicated intervention, which is compression.

Benzopyrones and Bioflavonoids

Benzopyrones are derived from naturally-occurring substances. Preparations of benzopyrones can, however, be either wholly or partially synthetic.[5] The α-benzopyrones include coumarin derivatives and the γ-benzopyrones are flavonoids, including flavones and flavonals, such as diosmin, and flavanes, such as hesperidin.

S.G. Rockson
Division of Cardiovascular Medicine, Stanford University School of Medicine,
Falk Cardiovascular Research Center, Stanford, CA, USA

B.-B. Lee et al. (eds.), *Lymphedema*,
DOI 10.1007/978-0-85729-567-5_33, © Springer-Verlag London Limited 2011

The purported mechanism of action of this drug class is to reduce vascular permeability[5] and, thereby, the lymphatic load. It is further suggested that benzopyrones might increase tissue macrophage activity,[6] thereby encouraging proteolysis and degradation of interstitial proteins, with an implied favorable effect on fluid clearance and tissue composition.[7]

In 2004, Badger et al.[7] undertook a focused review of the available prospective studies of benzopyrone efficacy in lymphedema. Of the 63 available publications, 47 were considered to be ineligible for further analysis. The authors concluded that it is impossible to judge the effectiveness of benzopyrones on the basis of these trials. On an individual basis, patients may report an improvement in symptoms such as heaviness, tightness or aching when taking these preparations but any improvement should be weighed against the lack of objective validation. Furthermore, caution is warranted in the use of systemic coumarin, in the face of the reported risk of hepatotoxicity.

Antibiotics

One common context for medical therapy in lymphedema is the recognized frequent occurrence of soft-tissue infection in these patients.[4] Four randomized controlled trials, reflecting the outcomes in 364 randomized patients, are available in the literature for analysis of this approach. Two of the trials investigated the use of intensive physical therapy with randomization to the addition of selenium (as an anti-inflammatory) versus placebo. These trials are not considered to be properly conducted randomized controlled trials[8] and, therefore, the results are inconclusive. Two additional studies have examined the effects of anti-filarials combined with penicillin as prophylaxis. In these two studies, penicillin reduced the mean number of inflammatory episodes, when combined with suitable foot care. While this is an encouraging result, it is clear that the paucity of properly conducted trials significantly hampers the ability to draw any conclusions.[8]

Conclusion

In summary, based upon the extant medical literature, there is little, if any, support for the role of pharmacology in the standard approach to lymphedema patients. It is the fervent hope of the author that advances in mechanistic insights, coupled with the design and execution of suitable, well-designed, multi-center, randomized clinical trials, will provide evidence-based efficacious options for this difficult patient population in the near future.

References

1. Rockson SG, Miller LT, Senie R, et al. American Cancer Society lymphedema workshop. Workgroup III: diagnosis and management of lymphedema. *Cancer.* 1998;83(12 suppl American):2882-2885.
2. Casley-Smith JR, Morgan RG, Piller NB. Treatment of lymphedema of the arms and legs with 5,6-benzo-[a]-pyrone. *N Engl J Med.* 1993;329(16):1158-1163.
3. Piller NB, Morgan RG, Casley-Smith JR. A double-blind, cross-over trial of O-(beta-hydroxyethyl)-rutosides (benzo-pyrones) in the treatment of lymphoedema of the arms and legs. *Br J Plast Surg.* 1988;41(1):20-27.
4. Rockson SG. Diagnosis and management of lymphatic vascular disease. *J Am Coll Cardiol.* 2008;52(10):799-806.
5. Ramelet AA. Pharmacologic aspects of a phlebotropic drug in CVI-associated edema. *Angiology.* 2000;51(1):19-23.
6. Hoult JR, Paya M. Pharmacological and biochemical actions of simple coumarins: natural products with therapeutic potential. *Gen Pharmacol.* 1996;27(4):713-722.
7. Badger C, Preston N, Seers K, Mortimer P. Benzo-pyrones for reducing and controlling lymphoedema of the limbs. *Cochrane Database Syst Rev.* 2004;(2):CD003140.
8. Badger C, Seers K, Preston N, Mortimer P. Antibiotics/anti-inflammatories for reducing acute inflammatory episodes in lymphoedema of the limbs. *Cochrane Database Syst Rev.* 2004;(2):CD003143.

Part VIII
Practical Issues in Physical Therapy

Chapter 34
Lower Limb Lymphedema

Győző Szolnoky

Introduction

Lower extremity lymphedema accounts for the majority of all lymphedema cases. Therefore, its treatment deserves more attention than treatment of any other part of the body.

Lymphedema is rarely found in its pure form because underlying pathophysiology (e.g., ischemic heart disease, diabetes, chronic venous insufficiency, etc.) and accompanying factors (e.g., administration of calcium channel blockers) may further affect the Starling equation. Chronicity is reached when the lymphatic drainage trying to overcome the increased load of extravasated fluid decompensates. The associated circulatory, lymphatic, and soft tissue changes therefore require a comprehensive management including the treatment of comorbidities.[1]

Basically, both primary and secondary lymphatic insufficiencies are incurable conditions that historically have been defied by predominantly compression- and physiotherapy-based therapeutic interventions against its progressive nature. Hence, the difference in their characteristics and behavior often influence the elements of treatment approaches.[2-4]

General Considerations

Manual lymph drainage (MLD)–based complex decongestive physiotherapy (CDP) is now the mainstay of the lower limb lymphedema treatment regimen. It consists of three different phases: intensive, transition, and maintenance phases. Each phase plays a unique role and has distinctly different aims to improve the condition; these were thoroughly reviewed in Chap. 27.

G. Szolnoky
Department of Dermatology and Allergology, University of Szeged, Szeged, Hungary

B.-B. Lee et al. (eds.), *Lymphedema*,
DOI 10.1007/978-0-85729-567-5_34, © Springer-Verlag London Limited 2011

However, MLD as the first and major component of CDP still fails to clear lingering doubt regarding its real value; despite strong empirical evidence advocating the benefits of the MLD, there are few research data to wholeheartedly support MLD, and recent clinical studies doubt its decongestive effects.[5,6]

Nevertheless, MLD is now known to increase blood flow in arterioles and capillaries; has peripheral analgesic, central sedative, antiserotonin, and antihistamine effects; evokes vagotonic reaction[7]; and improves muscular recovery after physical exercise.[8]

Hence, proper application of MLD in various forms of leg lymphedema is worthy of a revisit to emphasize its unique efficacy. Indeed, different conditions of uni- or bilateral primary or secondary lymphedema significantly influence the proper application of MLD to lower limb lymphedema.

The treatment of "unilateral" primary leg lymphedema[5] should follow the appropriate steps of central treatment, either in the supine or prone position, followed by leg treatment, also in the supine position or prone position, with the correct regimen, which were also thoroughly reviewed in Chap. 28 and 29.

However, precise application of every step of each treatment in the right sequence, either in a supine or prone position, cannot be overemphasized. Leg treatment steps should be repeated so as to treat all regions several times.

Treatment of "bilateral" primary leg lymphedema[5] is also no exception. It is consistent with unilateral primary leg lymphedema treatment, but there is an exception regarding the following steps: central treatment in the supine position should include the axillary lymph nodes of both sides, and both lower edematous body quadrants should be decongested in the direction of the axillary lymph nodes of identical sides.

In the prone position, the treatment of inguino-axillary anastomoses on both sides should be incorporated, and the gluteal region should be decongested in the direction of the axillary lymph nodes of identical sides.

Treatment of "unilateral" secondary leg lymphedema[5] would follow the same rule as for the central treatment, either in the supine or the prone position, as well as the leg treatment, which is consistent with primary lymphedema care.

However, there are some exceptions in the treatment of "bilateral" secondary leg lymphedema,[5] which is generally consistent with unilateral secondary leg lymphedema treatment as follows: in central treatment in the supine position of axillary lymph nodes of both sides should be treated together, in addition to the decongestion of both lower edematous body quadrants in the direction of the axillary lymph nodes of identical sides. In the prone position, the treatment should include inguino-axillary anastomoses on both sides and also the decongestion of the gluteal region in the direction of the axillary lymph nodes of identical sides.

Intermittent Pneumatic Compression

In accordance with the International Compression Club (ICC) Consensus, a high level of evidence supports the use of intermittent pneumatic compression (IPC) in lymphedema (Grade 1B).[9]

Intermittent pneumatic compression is assumed to reduce edema by decreasing capillary filtration, rather than by accelerating lymph return. IPC alone is particularly effective in non-obstructive edema, while MLD is strongly recommended before IPC to stimulate lymphatic flow in obstructive edema. Clinical trials prefer the utilization of multichambered pumps to single-chambered ones,[10,11] but the pressures should be adjusted according to individual response. In general, pressures of 30–60 mmHg are mostly applied. However, higher pressures also improve limb edema and lower pressures (20–30 mmHg) are advised in palliative care. Duration of 30 min to 2 h daily is recommended.[12] IPC is very efficacious in the edema treatment of immobile patients.[13] It squeezes the water content of a lymphedematous extremity, without improving the lymphatic drainage. However, it would reduce to an adequate amount, leading to an increase in the oncotic tissue pressure, necessitating a continuation of compression therapy.[14] IPC may exacerbate or cause congestion at the non-compressed root of a treated limb and also in the adjacent genital region.[15]

Compression

Compression therapy has been thoroughly reviewed through Chap. 30.

Nevertheless, the fact that compression therapy is the most effective treatment modality among the CDP components, cannot be overemphasized. However, until recently, evidence of its efficacy was based mostly on empirical studies and experimental data concerning the effect of conventional compression therapy on lymphedema have been sparse. Lately, though, the International Union of Phlebology (IUP) guideline as well as the American Venous Forum (AVF) guideline for lymphedema management has endorsed this mode of the therapy with a strong recommendation fitting to Evidence 1A.[16] A meta-analysis of the ICC found that a high of level of evidence could be attributed to the application of bandages in lymphedema (Grade 1B).[9]

Patients with lower limb lymphedema with a reduced ankle–brachial pressure index (ABPI) of 0.5–0.8 should not receive sustained compression exceeding 25 mmHg. Patients with ABPI < 0.5 can receive only intermittent compression.[17]

The most common tools of compression are bandages, stockings, and Circ-Aid. Typical lymphedema compression with bandages is performed in a multilayer fashion.[4] To achieve optimal volume reduction, high initial interface pressures are necessary to compensate for the pressure decrease. The pressure drop is already significant after 2 h and mainly caused by volume reduction, explaining the need for a more frequent bandage change in the beginning of lymphedema therapy compared with current practice where a change of bandage is recommended once a day in the initial phase.[18]

In general, inelastic compression can be worn overnight without major influence on microcirculation; hence, sub-bandage pressure does not significantly interfere with capillary function in the supine position.

Unlike inelastic compression, elastic bandages are normally not prescribed for overnight wear because in a supine position interface pressure remains high, the influence of gravity is excluded, and in the case of diminished arterial influx, serious side effects can occur.

Multilayer bandage systems may behave as inelastic systems even though the individual layers act as elastic materials due to the friction generated between bandage layers. Therefore, it is proposed that in the case of multilayer bandage systems and kits, the terms "high or low stiffness" should be used to characterize the behavior of the final bandage. Stiffness may be characterized by the increase of interface pressure measured in the gaiter area when standing up from the supine position. A pressure increase of more than 10 mmHg measured in the gaiter area is characteristic of a stiff bandage system.[16]

Use of Elastic Bandages

In some situations (ineffective calf muscle pump, phlebolymphedema, large volume loss is predicted), the inelastic bandages may be replaced with elastic ones. The stiffness produced by multiple layers produces high working pressure. However, the resting pressure is higher than with inelastic systems.

Special Compression Material

Inelastic adjustable compression enhancing comfort and patient compliance is an effective alternative to compression garments.[19]

Medical Compression Stockings

The main areas of compression garment utilization comprise long-term management of lymphedema in the maintenance phase, prophylaxis, initial treatment or may serve the only form of compression used in time-consuming controlled compression therapy, where interstitial fluid is gradually squeezed out from the affected limb by garment size reduction using a sewing machine or in a steady-state condition by ordering new stockings in decreasing sizes.[20] In general, most patients wear garments during waking hours, including exercise.

Prophylactic use of medical compression stockings for breast cancer related-lymphedema prevention seems to be of invaluably practical importance[21] and this concept has been partially extrapolated to legs as vulvar cancer treatment-related lymphatic impairment was successfully prevented with the use of graduated compression stockings.[22] Limbs with a relatively normal shape require round-knitted stockings, while flat-knitted stockings better fit limbs with an unusual shape or remarkable distorsion than round-knitted ones.

In general, compression stockings have a lower stiffness index than inelastic bandages, especially when these bandages are worn in a multilayered fashion. Superimposition of medical compression stockings (MCSs) has an increasing impact on practical lymphology. While upper limb lymphedema often requires interface pressure no more than 40 mmHg, in the case of leg lymphedema, particularly in primary lymphatic insufficiency, "subgarment" pressure measured at a medial gaiter area may even exceed 60–80 mmHg, corresponding to the superposition of two to even four medical compression stockings with various compression classes, properly retaining edema and maintaining reduced volume. MCSs drop their pressure to a much lower degree compared with compression bandages.[20,23,24]

Exercise

Exercise/movement should be tailored to the patient's needs, ability, and disease status. Compression should be worn during exercise whenever possible. Walking, swimming, cycling, and low impact aerobics are recommended. Exercise varies interstitial tissue pressure and influences both lymph propulsion and clearance, helping to transport fluid and inflammatory causing proteins from the site of formation and from the swollen limb or affected area.[25] Studies demonstrated that both mechanical limb elevation plus passive exercise[26] or 5 min of instructed deep breathing plus self massage followed by 30 min of isotonic and isometric limb exercises[27] can produce a reduction in limb volume and subjective improvements in symptoms. In aqua-lymphatic therapy the selection of the optimal water temperature is mandatory; hence, exercises at 28°C produce volume reduction, but a temperature of 34°C results in a slight increase in volume.[28] Underwater leg exercises proved to significantly enhance the efficacy of decongestive physiotherapy, especially from the perspective of patient's own perception.[29,30]

Lymphedema Severity-Adapted Forms of CDP

Initial management of leg lymphedema implements psychosocial support, education, skin care, exercise/movement, elevation, and management of any concomitant medical conditions, pain or discomfort and the utilization of various forms of compression.

Stage I Lymphedema

The pressure used should be guided by the patient's vascular status and their ability to tolerate compression and manage the garment. Skin care, exercise/movement, elevation and self-drainage should be taught alongside self monitoring and proper application, removal and care of hosiery. Patients should be examined 4–6 weeks after the initial fitting, and then after 3–6 months if the response is satisfactory. The patient should be examined at each stocking order (every 3–6 months).

Stages II and III Lymphedema

Intensive treatment comprises the standard elements of CDP and can be tailored to patient ability and comorbidity status.

Standard intensive therapy (>45 mmHg) is undertaken daily with a sub-bandage pressure >45 mmHg.

Intensive therapy with reduced pressure (15–25 mmHg) corresponds to the previous therapeutics regimen. Patients are selected for this treatment when high levels of compression are either unsafe or difficult to tolerate (moderate peripheral arterial occlusive disease [ABPI 0.5–0.8], mild neuropathy, lipedema, cancer under palliative treatment, co-morbidities requiring less aggressive reduction in swelling).

References

1. Ely JW, Osheroff JA, Chambliss ML, Ebell MH. Approach to leg edema of unclear etiology. *J Am Board Fam Med*. 2006;19:148-160.
2. Papendieck C. Lymphatic dysplasia in pediatrics. A new classification. *Int Angiol*. 1999;18: 6-9.
3. Wozniewski M, Jasinski R, Pilch U, Dabrowska G. Complex physical therapy for lymphoedema of the limbs. *Physiotherapy*. 2001;87:252-256.
4. Lymphoedema Framework. *Best Practice for the Management of Lymphoedema*, International Consensus. London: MEP Ltd; 2006:3-52.
5. Strössenreuther RHK. Hinweise zur Durchführung der ML/KPE bei primären und sekundären Lymphödemen sowie weiteren ausgewahlten Krankheitsbildern. In: Földi M, Kubik S, eds. *Lehrbuch der Lymphologie*, vol. 5. München-Jena: Gustav Fischer; 2002:621-658: Chap. 19.
6. Badger C, Preston N, Seers K, Mortimer P. Physical therapies for reducing and controlling lymphoedema of the limbs. *Cochrane Database Syst Rev*. 2004;4:CD003141.
7. Hutzschenreuter P, Brümmer H, Ebberfeld K. Experimental and clinical studies of the mechanism of effect of manual lymph drainage therapy. *Z Lymphol*. 1989;13:62-64.
8. Schillinger A, Koenig D, Haefele C, et al. Effect of manual lymph drainage on the course of serum levels of muscle enzymes after treadmill exercise. *Am J Phys Med Rehabil*. 2006;85: 516-520.
9. Partsch H, Flour M, Coleridge-Smith P, et al. Indications for compression therapy in venous and lymphatic disease. Consensus based on experimental data and scientific evidence under the auspices of the IUP. *Int Angiol*. 2008;27:193-219.
10. International Society of Lymphology. The diagnosis and treatment of peripheral lymphedema. Consensus document of the International Society of Lymphology. *Lymphology*. 2009;42: 51-60.
11. Bergan JJ, Sparks S, Angle N. A comparison of compression pumps in the treatment of lymphedema. *J Vasc Surg*. 1998;32:455-462.
12. Szuba A, Achalu R, Rockson SG. Decongestive lymphatic therapy for patients with breast carcinoma-associated lymphedema. A randomised, prospective study of a role of adjunctive pneumatic compression. *Cancer*. 2002;95:2260-2267.

13. Partsch H. Intermittent pneumatic compression in immobile patients. *Int Wound J.* 2008;5: 389-397.
14. Miranda F Jr, Perez MC, Castiglioni ML, et al. Effect of sequential intermittent pneumatic compression. *Lymphology.* 2001;34:135-141.
15. Boris M, Weindorf S, Lasinski BB. The risk of genital edema after external pump compression for lower limb lymphedema. *Lymphology.* 1998;31:15-20.
16. Partsch H, Clark M, Mosti G, et al. Classification of compression bandages: practical aspects. *Dermatol Surg.* 2008;34:600-609.
17. Marston W, Vowden K. Compression therapy: a guide to safe practice. In: European Wound Management Association (EWMA), ed. *Position Document: Understanding Compression Therapy.* London: MEP Ltd; 2003:11-17.
18. Damstra RJ, Brouwer E, Partsch H. Controlled, comparative study of relation between volume changes and interface pressure under short-stretch bandages in leg lymphedema patients. *Dermatol Surg.* 2008;34:773-778.
19. Lund E. Exploring the use of CircAid legging in the management of lymphoedema. *Int J Palliat Nurs.* 2000;6:383-391.
20. Brorson H, Ohlin K, Olsson G, Svensson B, Svensson H. Controlled compression and liposuction treatment for lower extremity lymphedema. *Lymphology.* 2008;41:52-63.
21. Stout Gergich NL, Pfalzer LA, McGarvey C, et al. Preoperative assessment enables the early diagnosis and successful treatment of lymphedema. *Cancer.* 2008;112:2809-2819.
22. Sawan S, Mugnai R, de Barros Lopes A, Hughes A, Edmondson R. Lower-limb lymphedema and vulval cancer: feasibility of prophylactic compression garments and validation of leg volume measurement. *Int J Gynecol Cancer.* 2009;19:1649-1654.
23. Partsch H, Partsch B, Braun W. Interface pressure and stiffness of ready made compression stockings: comparison of in vivo and in vitro measurements. *J Vasc Surg.* 2006;44:809-814.
24. Larsen AM, Futtrup I. Watch the pressure – it drops! *EWMA J.* 2004;4:8-12.
25. Havas E, Parviainen T, Vuorela J, Toivanen J, Nikula T, Vihko V. Lymph flow dynamics in exercising human skeletal muscle as detected by scintigraphy. *J Physiol.* 1997;504:233-239.
26. Moseley A, Piller N, Carati C, Esterman A. The impact of the Sun AnconChi Machine Aerobic Exerciser on chronic oedema of the legs. *Aust N Z J Phlebology.* 2003;7:5-10.
27. Buckley G, Piller N, Moseley A. Can exercise improve lymphatic flow? A pilot trial of the objective measurement of fluid movement in subjects with mild secondary lymphoedema. *5th Australasian Lymphology Association Conference Proceedings*; 2004:37-42.
28. Johansson K, Tibe K, Weibull A, Newton RC. Low intensity resistance exercise for breast cancer patients with arm lymphedema with or without compression sleeve. *Lymphology.* 2005;38:167-180.
29. Tidhar D, Drouin J, Shimony A. Aqua lymphatic therapy in managing lower extremity lymphedema. *J Support Oncol.* 2007;5:179-183.
30. Carpentier PH, Satger B. Randomized trial of balneotherapy associated with patient education in patients with advanced chronic venous insufficiency. *J Vasc Surg.* 2009;49:163-170.

Chapter 35
Upper Limb Lymphedema

Robert J. Damstra

Introduction

Within the realm of lymphatic disease treatment, there are many therapeutic interventions available, as highlighted in previous chapters. Treatment of lymphedema (LE) is very challenging. Therapeutic options in LE include conservative and operative modalities and should be individualized with regard to the circumstances of the patient and the lymphedema by a multidisciplinary approach. These circumstances include age, comorbidities, prognosis of (malignant) disease, psychosocial aspects, and physical potential. The goals for conservative treatment are to eliminate edema by reducing interstitial fluid accumulation and to stimulate lymphatic propulsion by compression.

Traditionally, many modalities are performed in combination. The contribution of each individual treatment modality to the outcome is, therefore, still under discussion. In this chapter we will focus on the timing of treatment, the combination of various modalities of treatment, and the phases of intervention.

Many terms are used to describe lymphatic treatments: complex decongestive therapy/treatment, complex physical therapy, or complex decongestive physiotherapy. These terms are confusing because it cannot be seen that the lymphatics are involved, "physiotherapy" is a terms used too generally, and the word "complex" is unclear.

Therefore, in 1998, the term *decongestive lymphatic therapy (DLT)* was advocated to achieve uniformity of nomenclature and foster communication among the health care professionals who administer therapy for lymphedema. DLT comprises a number of interrelated treatment modalities that are most efficacious when utilized in an interdependent fashion, as mentioned in Chap. 9.

R.J. Damstra
Department of Dermatology, Phlebology and Lympho-Vascular Medicine,
Nij Smellinghe Hospital, Drachten, The Netherlands

B.-B. Lee et al. (eds.), *Lymphedema*,
DOI 10.1007/978-0-85729-567-5_35, © Springer-Verlag London Limited 2011

Table 35.1 Useful lymphedema interventions

Therapeutic option	Initial treatment phase	Maintenance phase
Manual lymph drainage	X	
Bandaging	X	
Garments/hosiery		X
Pneumatic compression	X	X
Physiotherapy	X	
Decongestive lymphatic therapy	X	
Exercise	X	X
Weight control	X	X
Skin care	X	X
Awareness	X	X
Self-management		X
Reconstructive surgery	X	
Reductive surgery	X	

Treatment of lymphedema consists of two phases: the initial treatment phase and the maintenance phase. The first phase gradually merges into the maintenance phase. The goal of treatment is to reduce lymphedema during the treatment phase and make the patient independent from the professional health care worker. This provides the patient with as much knowledge as possible and with self-management skills to maintain the result with a good quality of life. The patient plays an active role in the maintenance of the therapeutic result. The role of the therapist during the second phase is more hands-off, monitoring and guiding the patient. The various therapeutic options are listed in Table 35.1.

Physical treatment of lymphedema should not be considered as a single therapeutic modality, but as a continuum that begins with informing and educating the patient, advocating awareness and self-management, objective early diagnostics by volumetry, and, at the end of the spectrum, individual specialized lymphedema treatments. A multidisciplinary approach, as suggested in many guidelines,[1-3] is mandatory to the success of the treatment of upper limb lymphedema.

Lymphedema of the Arm

Lymphedema of the arm is, in most cases, due to treatment of breast cancer. Many factors influence the development of breast cancer–related lymphedema (BCRL), including obesity,[4] hypertension,[5] infection, type of cancer treatment,[6] and individual impaired lymphatic drainage.[7]

Lymphedema frequently develops slowly, often with pre-clinical symptoms and signs, such as heaviness, transient swelling, and slight volume changes compared with preoperative values. Early detection is essential for a treatment program during the initial stages of lymphedema.

The practical issues in the approach to lymphedema in general, and to physical therapy in particular, are centered upon the organization and availability of care for the patient. In cancer-related lymphedema, and especially in BCRL, a protocolized approach is useful because lymphatic awareness can be integrated into the cancer protocol. This gives the opportunity to start primary and secondary prevention programs on lymphedema from the outset. Much work has to be done to achieve this ambition.

Considerations in Manual Lymph Drainage

Only a few studies have been performed to study the additional effects of manual lymph drainage (MLD) over compression therapy in LE. Two controlled studies showed that compression therapy with or without additional MLD was equally effective for BCRL. Andersen et al.[8] performed a randomized controlled study in BCRL comparing MLD and compression ($n=20$) with a control group that was treated with only compression therapy ($n=20$). After 2 weeks, the control group actually had a greater percentage reduction in absolute edema (60%) compared with the MLD group (48%). Both groups experienced an equal reduction in the symptoms of heaviness and tightness, but the control group also had a reduction in reported discomfort. The reduction in absolute edema (66%) was maintained for 12 months' follow up (pooled data). Johansson et al.[9] studied the effect of short-stretch bandages with or without MLD in 38 female patients. Both groups showed significant improvement in volume reduction (−11% after 3 weeks) and fewer complaints.

A comparison of studies on MLD and compression therapy alone by Korpon et al.[10] found no difference in volume change.

In a systematic review, Kligman et al.[11] studied 10 randomized controlled trials of treatment for BCRL. In all of these studies, the authors could not go farther than stating that there was "some suggestion" that compression and MLD "may improve" LE. The effectiveness of the use of life-long compression garments was more obvious.

In daily practice, MLD is used in several therapeutic schemes, especially when it is combined with various forms of compression therapy, such as short-stretch multilayer bandaging applied after each MLD session.[12] Although MLD has been used widely for many decades and is assumed by many to be a panacea for the treatment of LE, there is currently no indisputable published evidence for its effectiveness or its mode of action in improving lymphatic drainage.

Controlled, comparative studies are currently not available for the effectiveness of each separate modality in the treatment of LE.

Moseley et al.[13] conducted an extensive review of the literature in 2006 for common non-operative treatment modalities for LE and concluded that despite the identified benefits, there was still a need for large-scale, clinical trials in this area. A combination of MLD with compression therapy improved the results. In most studies reviewed by Moseley et al. there was a mix of lymphedema types, mainly

BCRL, and specific outcome parameters were often not defined. Specific studies on primary lymphedema are not available.

In 2007, Hamner and Fleming[14] retrospectively studied 135 patients with BCRL who were receiving DLT. After 8 weeks, the volume reduction was about 18%. A surprisingly positive effect on pain was found: 76 patients experienced pain before treatment, and 56 were free of pain after treatment (76% reduction). It was concluded that LE continues to be a problem for patients with breast cancer. A program of lymphedema therapy can reduce the volume of edema and, in particular, reduce pain in this population. Badger et al.[15] compared the effects of treatment for 18 days with short stretch bandaging, followed by compression hosiery with those of compression hosiery alone for leg and arm lymphedema. They showed that initial compression therapy with subsequent use of hosiery was twice as effective as hosiery alone.

Measurement of the undergarment pressure was performed in some studies.[16,17] A major limitation of these studies is the discrepancy between the undergarment pressure claimed by the manufacturer and the actual interface pressure due to the large variety of types of garments and inter-individual variation in measuring garments. Vignes et al.[18] studied 682 patients treated for BCRL for four years in the maintenance phase. Treatment failure was associated with younger age and higher weight and body mass index. Treatment with diurnal garments and nocturnal bandaging decreased the risk of treatment failure significantly (hazard ratio, 0.53 [0.34–0.82], $p=0.004$), whereas the addition of MLD did not.

General Considerations for Compression

The pressure delivered by compression is different in the legs than in the arms. It is important to note that the hydrostatic pressure that must be overcome by external compression is much higher in the legs than in the arms. In a standing position, the venous pressure in the distal leg is equal to the weight of the blood column between the heart and the measuring point, which is about 80–100 mmHg. The high intravenous pressure in the upright body position always increases the lymphatic load by promoting increased fluid extravasation. High external pressure is necessary in order to counteract this extravasation. The venous pressure in the arm is much lower than that in the leg because of the lower weight of the blood column between the heart and the hand. Thus, less external compression will be needed to reduce extravasation into the tissue and to promote reabsorption of tissue fluid. The arm volume reduction from bandaging is probably due not only to a pressure-dependent shift in Starling's equilibrium, but also to stimulation of lymphatic drainage. Besides veno-dynamic issues, lympho-dynamic issues should also be considered. In healthy arms, the distance from the arm to the thoracic duct is short, and the intra-lymphatic pressure varies with the intra-thoracic pressure. Lymphatic drainage is stimulated with relatively low or even negative intra-lymphatic pressure. In BCRL, lymphatic drainage is deficient because of damage to the major lymph collectors and lymph nodes by surgery and/or radiation, leading to lymphatic congestion.[19]

Compression Therapy in the Arms

Although inelastic, multi-layer, multi-component compression bandages allow immediate reduction of volume in lymphedematous arms and is a mandatory part of treatment, studies to measure the interface pressure in arm LE has rarely been performed before. The deciding parameter of the interface pressure, which is the dosage of compression therapy, has been measured only in patients with chronic venous insufficiency[20] and there is a positive relation between pressure and volume reduction. In arm lymphedema, for example, the compression pressure required to obtain the highest volume reduction per unit of time is unknown.

Damstra and Partsch[21] showed that low sub-bandage pressures between 20 and 30 mmHg are effective and better tolerated than high-pressure bandages by the patient with arm lymphedema. In future, more research will be required to understand the therapeutic effect of types of compression therapy and materials in arm lymphedema.

Recently, published studies have shown the importance of compression therapy after circumferential suction-assisted lipectomy (the Brorson method)[22,23] in order to achieve a 100% volume reduction in end-stage arm lymphedema. The method consists of an operative intervention to remove the complete suprafascial component of the lymphedematous arm, which consists mainly of fat.[24] Postoperatively, compression therapy is provided by short stretch bandaging and garments, which should be worn lifelong, the same as in the conservative treatment of arm lymphedema. All garments are custom-fitted and flat knitted. Long-term results are highly favorable, with sustained complete volume reduction of the pre-operative volume excess, for up to 13 years of follow-up. In this procedure, manual lymph drainage is not necessary to maintain the result.

In lymphedema, intermittent pneumatic compression has been used for decades. Megens and Harris[25] reviewed the literature on physical therapy treatment of BCRL. Most studies were inappropriately designed and often lacked proper comparisons. They concluded that compression therapy should be performed with multi-chamber devices in combination with other therapeutic options, such as MLD and compression. Monotherapy with intermittent pneumatic compression was discouraged.

Bandaging and hosiery can provide compression. In general, hosiery is measured when the maintenance phase is reached. In this phase there is no further volume reduction despite proper LE treatment. The terms hosiery, garments, and sleeves are often used interchangeably and include gloves, gauntlets, Bermudas, and compression devices for toes. For LE, garments should always be custom-fitted and flat-knitted with a high static stiffness and should be measured routinely during long-term follow-up.[26]

References

1. Rockson SG, Miller LT, Senie R, brennan MJ, et al. American Cancer Society lymphedema workshop. Workgroup III: diagnosis and management of lymphedema. *Cancer.* 1998; 83(12 suppl American):2882-2885.

2. Damstra RJ, Kaandorp C. Multidisciplinary guidelines for early diagnosis and management. *J Lymphoedema*. 2006;1(1):37-65.

3. International Lymphoedema Framework. *Best Practice for the Management of Lymphedema. International Consensus*. London: MEP Ltd; 2006:1-60.

4. Shaw C, Mortimer PS, Judd PA. Randomized controlled trial comparing a low-fat diet with a weight-reduction diet in breast cancer-related lymphedema. *Cancer*. 2007;109(10): 1949-1956.

5. Meeske KA, Sullivan-Halley J, Ashley W, et al. Risk factors for arm lymphedema following breast cancer diagnosis in Black women and White women. *Breast Cancer Res Treat*. 2009;113(2):383-391.

6. Petrek JA, senie RT, peters M, Rosen PP. Lymphedema in a cohort of breast carcinoma survivors 20 years after diagnosis. *Cancer*. 2001;92(6):1368-1377.

7. Pain SJ, Purushotham AD, Barber RW, Ballinger JR, et al. Variation in lymphatic function may predispose to development of breast cancer-related lymphoedema. *Eur J Surg Oncol*. 2004;30(5):508-514.

8. Andersen L, Hojris I, Erlandsen M, Andersen J. Treatment of breast-cancer-related lymphedema with or without manual lymphatic drainage: a randomized study. *Acta Oncol*. 2000;39(3):399-405.

9. Johansson K, Albertsson M, Ingvar C, Ekdahl C. Effects of compression bandaging with or without manual lymph drainage treatment in patients with postoperative arm lymphedema. *Lymphology*. 1999;32(3):103-110; Comment in: Lymphology. 2000;33:69-70.

10. Korpon MI, Vacuriu G, Schneider B. Effects of compression therapy in patients after breast cancer surgery. Annual Congresses of the American College of Phlebology. San Diego, California, 2003; Online www.phlebology.org (Annual Meeting Abstracts).

11. Kligman L, Wong RKC, Johnston M, Laetsch NS. The treatment of lymphedema related to breast cancer: a systematic review and evidence summary. *Support Care Cancer*. 2004;12(6): 421-431.

12. Yamamoto R, Yamanoto T. Effectiveness of the treatment-phase of two-phase complex decongestive physiotherapy for the treatment of extremity lymphedema. *Int J Clin Oncol*. 2007;12(6): 463-468.

13. Moseley AL, Carrati CJ, Piller NB. A systematic review of common conservative therapies for arm lymphoedema secondary to breast cancer treatment. *Ann Oncol*. 2007;18(4):639-646.

14. Hamner JB, Fleming MD. Lymphedema therapy reduces the volume of edema and pain in patients with breast cancer. *Ann Surg Oncol*. 2007;14(6):1904-1908.

15. Badger CM, Peacock JL, Mortimer PS. A randomized, controlled, parallel-group clinical trial comparing multilayer bandaging followed by hosiery versus hosiery alone in the treatment of patients with lymphedema of the limb. *Cancer*. 2000;88(12):2832-2837.

16. Johansson K, Lie E, Ekdahl C, Lindfeldt J. A randomized study comparing manual lymph drainage with sequential pneumatic compression for treatment of postoperative arm lymphedema. *Lymphology*. 1998;31:56-64.

17. Swedborg I. Effects of treatment with an elastic sleeve and intermittent pneumatic compression in post-mastectomy patients with lymphoedema of the arm. *Scand J Rehabil Med*. 1984;16:35-41.

18. Vignes S, Porcher R, Arrault M, Dupuy A. Factors influencing breast cancer-related lymphedema volume after intensive decongestive physiotherapy. *Support Care Cancer*. 2010. doi: 10.1007/s00520-010-0906-x.

19. Modi S, Stanton AWB, Svensson WE, Peters A, Mortimer PS, Levick JR. Human lymphatic pumping measured in healthy and lymphedematous arms by lymphatic congestion lymphoscintigraphy. *J Physiol*. 2007;583(Pt 1):271-285.

20. Partsch H, Clark M, Mosti G, et al. Classification of compression bandages: practical aspects. *Dermatol Surg*. 2008;34(5):600-609.

21. Damstra RJ, Partsch H. Compression therapy in breast cancer related lymphedema. A randomized controlled, comparative study of relation between volume and interface pressure changes. *J Vasc Surg*. 2009;49:1256-1263.
22. Brorson H, Svensson H. Complete reduction of lymphoedema of the arm by liposuction after breast cancer. *Scand J Plast Reconstr Surg Hand Surg*. 1997;31:137-143.
23. Damstra RJ, Voesten HGJ, Klinkert P, Brorson H. Reduction surgery by Circumferential Suction-Assisted Lipectomy (Brorson method) in end stage breast cancer-related lymphedema: a prospective study. *Br J Surg*. 2009;96(8):859-864.
24. Brorson H, Ohlin K, Olsson G, Nilsson M. Adipose tissue dominates chronic arm lymphedema following breast cancer: an analysis using volume rendered CT images. *Lymphat Res Biol*. 2006;4:199-210.
25. Megens A, Harris SR. Physical therapist management of lymphedema following treatment for breast cancer: a critical review of its effectiveness. *Phys Ther*. 1998;78(12):1302-1311.
26. Lymphoedema Framework. *Template for Practice: Compression Hosiery in Lymphoedema*. London: MEP Ltd; 2006.

Chapter 36
Head and Neck Lymphedema

Anne-Marie Vaillant-Newman and Stanley G. Rockson

Introduction

Lymphedema is the complex, regional edematous state that ensues when lymph transport is insufficient to maintain tissue homeostasis;[1] it appears in settings where there is a relative failure of interstitial fluid clearance in the face of normal capillary filtration.[2] The predominant clinical presentation of lymphedema is characterized by the presence of regionalized edema; accordingly, it is not surprising that cases of isolated head and neck lymphedema will be encountered by the clinician.

As with other forms of this disease, lymphedema of the head and neck can be classified as either "primary" or "secondary," although hybrid forms will certainly be observed.[3,4] Primary lymphedema of the head and neck may be associated with limb lymphedema; however, when it occurs as a manifestation of the congenital, *praecox* or *tarda*, forms of lymphedema, the presence of head and neck lymphedema may suggest that the lymphatic insufficiency is quite widespread.[5]

Localized head and neck lymphedema may also occur as a consequence of recurrent episodes of skin infection or chronic inflammation. These pathological conditions alter the structure and function of the initial lymphatics and cause obstruction of lymphatic collectors. Head and neck lymphedema may also be an iatrogenic condition, occurring as a consequence of cancer therapeutics, including the sequelae of extensive surgical resection and radiotherapy. Additional contributing factors may include either infection or recurrent neoplastic involvement.[6]

Treatment of head and neck cancer typically invokes procedures such as modified radical neck dissection, total laryngectomy, neck radiotherapy, and chemotherapy. Singly and in aggregate, these interventions can create myriad complications.

A.-M. Vaillant-Newman (✉)
Division of Cardiovascular Medicine, Stanford University School of Medicine,
Falk Cardiovascular Research Center, Stanford, CA, USA

B.-B. Lee et al. (eds.), *Lymphedema*,
DOI 10.1007/978-0-85729-567-5_36, © Springer-Verlag London Limited 2011

Lymphedema of the head and neck is very common after radical neck dissection. Fortunately, most often the lymphedema is transient, improving as inflammation subsides and collateral lymphatic pathways open. However, lymphedema can also worsen, to the point of endangering the airway and blocking the pharynx.[6] It must be assessed and treated as early as possible to minimize functional, as well as emotional, issues.

In addition to regionalized lymphedema, dysphagia, mucositis, dermatitis, nutritional and metabolic changes, xerostomia, dysgeusia, speech impairment, hearing loss, vestibular disorders (when radiotherapy includes the temporal bone and the brain stem),[7] and shoulder dysfunction (when the spinal accessory nerve is injured) may occur.[6,8] Verbal communication, social interaction, and eating and breathing functions may be impaired.[7] All of these sequelae can have an impact on the approach to, and responsiveness of, the associated lymphedema.

Physical Treatment of Lymphedema of the Face and Neck

The physical treatment of lymphedema of the face and neck includes manual lymph drainage, multi-layered bandaging, stimulation of muscular activity, use of compression garment(s), education in precautions to observe to avoid exacerbation of symptoms and complications, and, if appropriate, education in self-treatment techniques (Table 36.1).

Manual Lymph Drainage (Leduc Method)

The superficial lymphatic collectors of the face chiefly carry lymph toward the para-auricular, sub-mandibular, and sub-mental lymph nodes. From these nodal sites, the lymph progresses to the supraclavicular lymph nodes, from which the treatment is initiated. However, in more complex cases, where involvement extends to the shoulder girdle, the treatment is initiated at the level of the axillary lymph nodes.

Table 36.1 Treatment of lymphedema of the face

The treatment of lymphedema of the face includes:
1. Manual lymph drainage
2. Multi-layered bandaging
3. Stimulation of muscular activity
4. Education in precautions to observe to avoid exacerbation of symptoms
5. Education in self-treatment
6. Assistance in improvement of quality of life of the patient and their family

Fig. 36.1 (**a, b**) Maneuver applied on the supra-clavicular lymph nodes

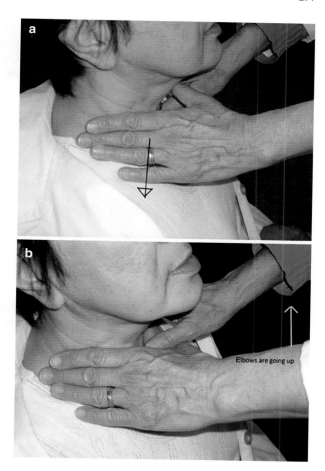

Description of the Maneuvers

- The maneuver performed on the lymph nodes consists of a slight mobilization of the skin overlying the nodes in question, in the direction of the major lymphatic drainage of the region under treatment, with manual application of a pressure equivalent to the weight of the hand. The flat hand is applied to the area, avoiding any rotation that would impart a shear force, which might generate a local inflammatory response. The maneuver is repeated ten times on each set of lymph nodes (Fig. 36.1).
- *The call-up maneuver* is applied either proximal to the lymphedematous area or, after completion of the reabsorption maneuver, in a distal-to-proximal direction on the lymphedematous, treated area. The radial or cubital aspect of the hand is brought into contact with the skin. The maneuver is intended, initially, to mobilize the skin in the direction of the main lymphatic flow, followed by the application of a gentle pressure by the full hand or several fingers, as dictated by the size

Fig. 36.2 (**a**, **b**) Call-up maneuver applied proximally toward the para-auricular lymph nodes

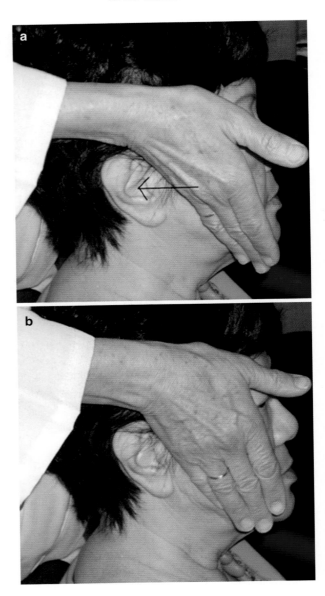

of the area involved. The maneuver will be repeated five times on each section of the treated site (Fig. 36.2).

- In the *reabsorption maneuver* the ulnar or radial aspect of the therapist's hand is brought into contact with the skin. A mobilization of the skin is performed in the direction of the lymphatic flow; thereafter, the full hand or several fingers, as dictated by the size of the treated area, applies a gentle pressure. This maneuver

Fig. 36.3 (a, b)
Reabsorption maneuver
applied proximally toward
the para-auricular lymph
nodes

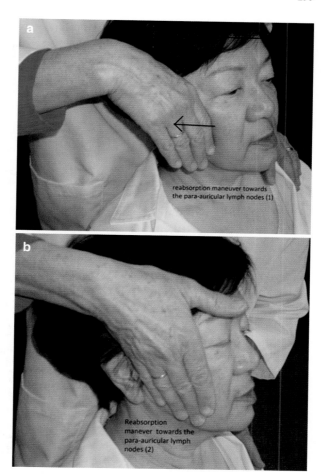

is performed proximal-to-distal on the lymphedematous area. It is repeated as many times as necessary, until a decrease in tension of the lymphedematous tissue is perceived (Fig. 36.3).

- Efficacy of the maneuvers described has been demonstrated through lympho-scintigraphic imaging.[9]

Protocol for Manual Treatment of Lymphedema of the Face and Neck

The protocol for the manual treatment of lymphedema requires the use of the maneuvers as described, with application in the following order:

1. Drainage of the *most proximal lymph nodes*. These receive the lymph flow derived from the area involved. In head and neck lymphedema, the proximal

lymph nodes are the supra-clavicular lymph nodes, or, if the lymphedema extends to the shoulder region, the axillary lymph nodes.

2. Drainage of the *intermediate lymph nodes* of the neck and face:
   (a) Sternocleidomastoid lymph nodes
   (b) Sub-mental lymph nodes
   (c) Sub-mandibular lymph nodes
   (d) Pre- and infra-auricular lymph nodes

3. These lymph node maneuvers are followed by the *maneuvers on the anastomotic or substitution pathways.* Several anastomotic pathways have been described (Olivier Leduc, unpublished observations). Two such pathways link the two sets of auricular lymph nodes, and are distributed above the upper lip and below the lower lip.

4. Once the maneuvers on the lymph nodes and along the anastomotic pathways have been completed, the *call-up maneuver* will be applied (if there is a lymphedema-free region between the most proximal lymph nodes and the lymphedematous zone). The call-up maneuver is applied initially to the lymphedema-free area and proximal to the lymphedematous site. This maneuver has been shown experimentally to enhance the efferent lymph flow from the lymphedematous area. Efficacy of the described maneuvers has been demonstrated through lymphoscintigraphic imaging.[9]

5. Next, the specific treatment of the lymphedematous area begins with application of the *reabsorption maneuver*, proximal-to-distal. The proximal end of the lymphedematous area is the aspect closest to the draining lymph nodes. The lymphedematous area will be divided into sections, each of which will be drained as previously described. The change in the consistency of tissues in the treated area is the factor that dictates when the maneuver can be considered complete, allowing the therapist to progress to the next, more distal section.

   The lymphedematous area will be drained toward the para-auricular lymph nodes as well as toward the sub-mandibular lymph nodes.

6. After all of the sections of the lymphedematous facial, neck or scalp area have been completely addressed with the *reabsorption technique*, the *call-up technique* is applied distal-to-proximal on each section.

7. At the end of the treatment, specific lymph node maneuvers, described above, will be applied successively to each set of lymph nodes from the most distal set to the most proximal set, concluding the treatment session.

Multi-Layered Bandaging Leduc Method

The multi-layered bandaging technique requires the application of a set of semi-rigid bandaging materials that provide a counter-pressure to the pressure generated by muscular contractions. The multi-layered bandaging technique includes the application of a stockinette (to protect the skin), foam, and low-stretch bandages applied to the area involved without exerting any tension.

Fig. 36.4 Multi-layered bandaging addressing lymphedema on the right hemi-face and neck

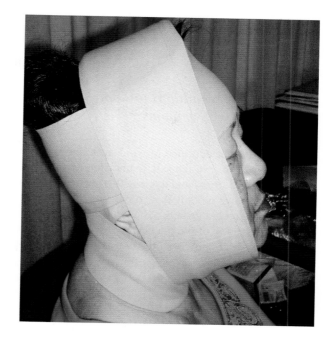

This bandage is effective when the subject is active and performs muscular contractions in the lymphedematous area.[10] In the context of head and neck lymphedema, it is assumed that the patient is not isolated and has some interactions with others, utilizes facial expressions and head movements, and performs speech. To address facial lymphedema, the multi-layered bandaging must be anchored in areas proximal and distal to the involved site. In between these two pieces a bridge applies pressure to the lymphedematous area (Fig. 36.4). The treatment is best performed in the home, to minimize stressful situations for the patient. Efficacy of the multi-layered bandaging on colloidal protein reabsorption during muscular activity has been demonstrated by lymphoscintigraphy.[10]

Stimulation of Muscular Activity

The patient should be educated in exercises of the facial musculature. These should be performed specifically while wearing the multi-layered bandaging. Asking the patient to repeat vowels in front of the mirror, 3–4 times a day, is an easily comprehended form of such exercise.

Compression Garment

To maintain the results gained by the manual lymph drainage and multi-layered bandaging a compression garment will be required. For mild cases of facial lymphedema, a ski mask can fulfill this function, but a medical garment for facial edema may be necessary. The garment is typically worn in the home.

Education in Precautions to Apply to Avoid Exacerbation of Symptoms

The patient must be educated to avoid sun exposure, as well as activities that expose the involved regions of the skin to abrasion, laceration or burn. The patient will be asked to practice strict hand hygiene to avoid self-contamination. Avoidance of skin scratching and eye rubbing is recommended.

Education in skin care is paramount, when one considers that infection is the major complication of lymphedema. Strict skin and hair hygiene is recommended, with, minimally, a daily evening shower. Regular use of a skin moisturizer is also strongly recommended.

Education in Self-Treatment

If the patient demonstrates a good understanding of the condition and is willing to participate in the lymphedema management, education in the approach to self-treatment is feasible. At times, a family member will volunteer to apply the manual technique. In the case of a child suffering from lymphedema, the parents will be educated. In these situations, the patient or parents will be educated in a simplified version of manual lymph drainage. Maneuvers are taught, to be applied by a family caregiver. The patient or family caregiver will be taught to initially apply the maneuver to the supraclavicular, sub-mental, sub-mandibular, and pre-auricular lymph nodes. The call-up and reabsorption maneuvers are not incorporated. Similarly, multi-layered bandaging is not incorporated into the self-treatment approach, which simply features skin mobilization combined with the application of very gentle pressure. The maneuver is undertaken by the patient or caregiver, progressing proximal-to-distal at the lymphedematous site. After the entire involved area has been treated, the maneuvers on the lymph nodes are repeated. The self-treatment should be closely monitored. The patient, or the parents of the patient, should be provided with a pictorial guide, including practical comments. If self-treatment education is feasible, it will be implemented early in the treatment intervention, to permit thorough training. Self-management techniques are not as effective as those applied by a physical or occupational therapist, but they do permit the patient, or family caregiver, to perceive changes in the consistency of tissues or in the skin temperature. The patient, or parents, should be made aware of the necessity to seek medical care if a change in tissue volume, tissue consistency, or skin temperature is detected. Erythema or pain in the area involved should also prompt medical consultation, as these symptoms may indicate the development of dermatolymphangioadenitis.

Multi-layered bandaging is purposefully not incorporated into the self-treatment approach, inasmuch as there is a risk that uneven pressure application and undesired pressure gradients will be created when the bandaging materials are applied by the patient or a family member.

In the Leduc method the notion of self-treatment is not considered to be appropriate. Initial and maintenance stages of the treatment are performed by the physical therapists.

An Example of Self-Treatment of Head and Neck Lymphedema

We will consider the case of a child affected by left-sided facial lymphedema. After initial instruction, the parents are photographed performing the technique.

These photographs are provided to the parents to guide their attempts at self-treatment.

In this case, the treatment begins with the *lymph node maneuver* on the supra-clavicular lymph node (Fig. 36.5), progressing to the nodes at the side of the neck, then to the sub-mental and sub-mandibular lymph nodes (Fig. 36.6), and, finally, the pre- and infra-auricular lymph nodes (Fig. 36.7).

Once the maneuver on the lymph nodes has been completed, *the maneuver on the anastomotic or substitution pathways* is performed. This maneuver consists of mobilization of the skin in the direction of the left, non-involved, pre-auricular, and infra-auricular lymph nodes. This mobilization is initially applied close to the left lymph nodes and progressively further from the non-involved auricular lymph nodes

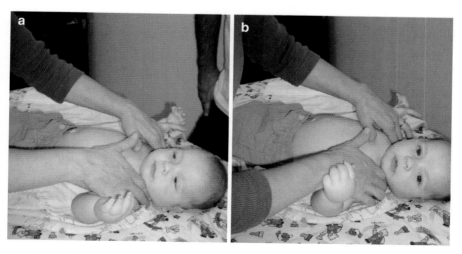

Fig. 36.5 (**a, b**) Maneuver of the supra-clavicular lymph nodes

Fig. 36.6 Maneuvers on the lymph nodes located along the jaw (sub-mandibular lymph nodes). Position your hand as illustrated on the picture. Apply gentle pressure and mobilize the skin (5-7 repetitions). Precautions: do not slide skin, do not rub skin, mobilize the skin gently, apply very gentle pressure, rhythm must be slow (example of documentation remitted to the parents to illustrate a specific maneuver)

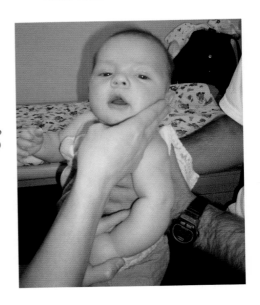

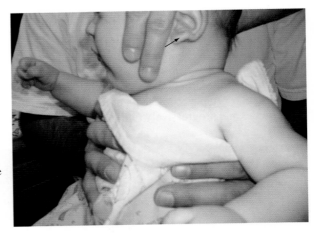

Fig. 36.7 Mobilization of the skin, combined with gentle pressure, toward the para-auricular lymph nodes, as indicated by the arrow

along a line running horizontally above the upper lip and simultaneously along a horizontal line running below the lower lip. When the fingers meet the involved area the maneuvers are interrupted.

The single maneuver described above is applied proximal-to-distal on the lymphedematous area, and repeated as many times as necessary to trigger a decrease in the tension of the lymphedematous tissues

The treatment will end with the lymph node maneuver, applied to the pre- and infra-auricular lymph nodes, the sub-mandibular and sub-mental lymph nodes, along the neck, and, finally, to the supra-clavicular lymph nodes. As mentioned above, the parents will be provided with a pictorial guide with practical comments (Fig. 36.6).

Rehabilitation to Address Functional Impairments

As mentioned initially, injury to the spinal accessory nerve may trigger denervation of the upper trapezius muscle and, sometimes, minor impairment of the sterno-cleidomastoid muscle. These nerve lesions generate shoulder drop and protracted, limited active range of motion, especially in shoulder flexion and, sometimes, in shoulder abduction, muscle strength impairment, and pain.[11] The medical literature amply documents the profound impact of shoulder dysfunction on quality-of-life in patients treated for head and neck cancer. Shah et al., in a study of short- and long-term quality of life after neck dissection, documented that shoulder dysfunction and neck tightness had the greatest negative impact.[12] Thus, post-surgical evaluation, with frequent, regular assessment of shoulder function should be implemented in these patients, in order to initiate immediate physical or occupational therapy when needed. During sessions of physical or occupational therapy, assessment of balance and strength should be implemented for early remediation or life style adaptations.

Quality of Life

As stated initially, treatment of head and neck cancers may trigger a variety of dysfunctional consequences beyond lymphedema. Patients receiving radiation-based therapy for locally advanced squamous carcinoma of the head and neck develop acute dysphagia consequent to pain, copious mucous production, xerostomia and tissue swelling. Early evaluation and treatment by speech and language pathologists permits the identification of patients with clinically significant aspiration; in these cases, a treatment plan that includes patient education and swallowing therapy can significantly enhance quality-of-life. Well-monitored dietary adaptations must be implemented to address swallowing and the risk of maladaptive feeding changes.[13]

Lymphedema of the face and neck generates emotional and social dysfunction which must be assessed and addressed in a timely fashion to maximally enhance the quality-of-life for patients and family.

References

1. Rockson SG. Diagnosis and management of lymphatic vascular disease. *J Am Coll Cardiol.* 2008;52(10):799-806.
2. Rockson S. Current concepts and future directions in the diagnosis and management of lymphatic vascular disease. *Vasc Med.* 2010;15(3):223-231.
3. Rockson SG. Secondary lymphedema: Is it a primary disease? *Lymphat Res Biol.* 2008;6(2): 63-64.
4. Rockson S. Lymphedema: evaluation and decision making. In: Cronenwett JL, Johnston KW, eds. *Rutherford's Vascular Surgery.* Philadelphia: Elsevier; 2010:1004-1016.
5. Mortimer PS. Managing lymphedema. *Clin Dermatol.* 1995;13(5):499-505.
6. Withey S, Pracy P, Vaz F, Rhys-Evans P. Sensory deprivation as a consequence of severe head and neck lymphoedema. *J Laryngol Otol.* 2001;115(1):62-64.
7. Fialka-Moser V, Crevenna R, Korpan M, Quittan M. Cancer rehabilitation: particularly with aspects on physical impairments. *J Rehabil Med.* 2003;35(4):153-162.
8. Murphy BA, Gilbert J, Cmelak A, Ridner SH. Symptom control issues and supportive care of patients with head and neck cancers. *Clin Adv Hematol Oncol.* 2007;5(10):807-822.
9. Leduc O, Bourgeois P, Leduc A. Manual lymphatic drainage scintigraphic demonstration of its efficacy on colloidal protein reabsorption. In: Partsch H, ed. *Progress in Lymphology.* Oxford: Elsevier; 1988:551-554.
10. Leduc O, Peters A, Bourgeiois P. Bandages: scintigraphic demonstration of its efficacy on colloidal protein reabsorption during muscle activity. *Lymphology.* 1990;12:421-423.
11. Cappiello J, Piazza C, Giudice M, De Maria G, Nicolai P. Shoulder disability after different selective neck dissections (levels II-IV versus levels II-V): a comparative study. *Laryngoscope.* 2005;115(2):259-263.
12. Shah S, Har-El G, Rosenfeld RM. Short-term and long-term quality of life after neck dissection. *Head Neck.* 2001;23(11):954-961.
13. Murphy BA, Gilbert J. Dysphagia in head and neck cancer patients treated with radiation: assessment, sequelae, and rehabilitation. *Semin Radiat Oncol.* 2009;19(1):35-42.

Chapter 37
Genital Lymphedema

Waldemar L. Olszewski

Introduction

The involvement of the external genitalia, leading to a marked increase in volume is an uncomfortable clinical situation, with impairment of movement, hygiene procedures, voiding in the standing position, and sexual intercourse.

Genital lymphedema develops as a consequence of:

(a) Stagnation of lymph flow in the skin and subcutaneous tissue of the scrotum, penis, labia, and hypogastrium after infection of external genitalia, inguinal lymphadenectomy in cancer of the penis, labia or perineal region, and radiotherapy of the inguinal and iliac areas as adjunctive cancer therapy (Fig. 37.1a, b).

(b) Chyloperitoneum with backflow of intestinal lymph to the peritoneal cavity, genitals, and lower limbs.

(c) Chyluria with oozing of lymph into the retroperitoneal space and backflow to the pelvis and genitalia.

Anatomy

Genital lymphedema usually affects the skin and subcutaneous tissue of the scrotum, penis, labia, and hypogastrium, but not the testes, uterus, or ovaries. The lymphatic drainage of genital skin is directed toward the inguinal nodes (Fig. 37.2).

W.L. Olszewski
Department of Surgical Research and Transplantology,
Medical Research Centre, Warsaw, Poland

B.-B. Lee et al. (eds.), *Lymphedema*,
DOI 10.1007/978-0-85729-567-5_37, © Springer-Verlag London Limited 2011

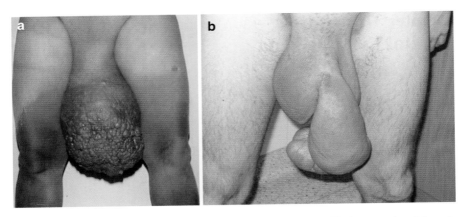

Fig. 37.1 (**a**) Lymphedematous scrotum hiding the penis. Papilloma-like hypertrophy of the epidermis and blisters containing stagnant lymph. Edema developed within 1 year and was followed by frequent septic attacks of dermato-lymphangio-adenitis. (**b**) Lymphedema of the penis and scrotum pulling down the hypogastrium skin. Swelling appeared after inflammation of the preputium

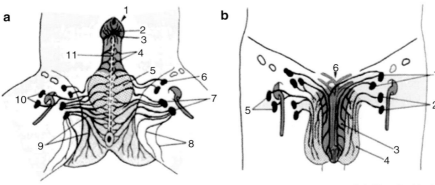

1 Glans penis
2 Lateral plexus of the frenulum (Oanezza's plexus)
3 Coronary trunk of the glans
4 Collectors of the skin of the penis
5 Scrotum
6 Superomedial superficial inguinal l.n.'s
7 Inferomedial superficial inguinal l.n.'s
8 Medial collectors of the thigh
9 Perineal collectors
10 Inferolateral inguinal l.n.'s
11 Raphe of the penis, scrotum, and perineum

1 Superomedial superficial inguinal l.n.'s
2 Inferomedial superficial inguinal l.n.'s
3 Skin of the penis
4 Scrotum
5 inferolateral inguinal l.n.'s
6 Superficial dorsal vein of the penis

Fig. 37.2 The anatomy of the lymphatic drainage of the perineum, scrotum, and penis. Note that the lymphatics drain the skin and subcutaneous tissue, but not the testes. The draining targets are the inguinal superficial nodes

Etiology

The etiology of genital lymphedema, except after surgery and irradiation, is usually postinflammatory and is caused by prior infection by microbes in the perineal and anal regions. The microbes entering the lymphatics are cocci in approximately 60% and bacilli in 40%. The most common are *Staphylococcus epidermidis* and *S. aureus*, *Enterococcus*, and *Micrococcus*. In the bacilli population *Pseudomonas*, *Acinetobacter*, *Proteus*, *Enterococcus*, *Enterobacter*, and *Corynebacteria* dominate.

Why only a few individuals develop infections is unclear; however, genetic predisposition is suspected.

The bacterial inflammatory process is followed by obliteration of afferent lymphatics and fibrosis of the inguinal lymph nodes. This is why, in some cases of genital lymphedema, lymphedema of the lower limbs also is seen.

Diagnosis

Diagnosis of genital lymphedema is based on:

(a) Physical examination revealing edema of the penis, scrotum or labia, disfigurement of these parts, erythema and increased temperature, and, not infrequently, oozing of lymph from epidermal blisters.
(b) Lymphoscintigraphy with intradermal injection of T99-Nanocoll.

Differential diagnosis between postinflammatory, chyloperitoneum, and chyluria with retroperitoneal backflow is based on:

(a) Histochemistry of oozing fluid: postinflammatory (presence of lymphocytes and dendritic cells with few granulocytes); chyloperitoneum (high concentration of lymphocytes and large macrophages).
(b) Chemistry of the fluid: presence of lipids determines intestinal origin of fluid (chyloperitoneum).
(c) Lymphoscintigraphy: postinflammatory (lack of absorption and flow of radioisotope from the skin of the swollen parts toward the inguinal area, chyloperitoneum (isotope accumulates in dilated lymphatics spreading toward the thigh, pelvis, and retroperitoneal space, chyluria (dilated genital lymphatic with isotope flow to the retroperitoneum and kidney pelvis).

Clinical Course

Genital lymphedema develops relatively quickly because of the ready accumulation of tissue fluid in loose subcutaneous tissue. The main complications are: (a) rapid increase in mass to several kilograms, (b) lymph oozing from epidermal blisters, and (c) recurrent attacks of acute inflammation followed by chronic inflammation.

Treatment

Conservative: (a) in each case administration of either long-term penicillin 1,200,000 IU, intramurally, every 3 weeks or amoxicillin + clavulanic acid 2 g for 3 days orally every 3 weeks, cleansing with antibacterial soap, (b) manual massage of the swollen parts toward the groin, (c) wearing a suspensory to support and compress the scrotum and penis.

Surgical

Postinflammatory: (a) removal of excess of skin and subcutaneous tissue after intraoperative elimination of the edema fluid from the penis, scrotum or labia toward the groin (Fig. 37.3)[1-8], (b) excision of fibrotic afferent lymphatics running toward the inguinal nodes, (c) in advanced cases, excision of the swollen skin and subcutis of the hypogastrium.

Chyloperitoneum: (a) laparotomy followed by (b) ligation and severing of retroperitoneal lymphatic bundles along the iliac veins (Fig. 37.4), (c) in advanced and recurrent cases, excision of half the length of the small bowel that produces stagnant lymph leaking into the peritoneal cavity, (d) postoperative injection of bleomycin or 3% aetoxisclerol into scrotal or labial blisters. In advanced edema of the genitals, plastic surgery is performed in the postinflammatory group.

Chyluria with genital edema: (a) retroperitoneal laparoscopic or open denudation of the kidney(s) and ligation of the dilated lymphatics running toward kidney pelvis (Fig. 37.4).

Technical hints: (a) scrotum: create a small anterior flap, leave as little skin as possible just to cover the denuded testes, remove afferent lymphatics with swollen tissues in the hypogastrium, use diathermy and avoid ligatures (foci of future abscesses),

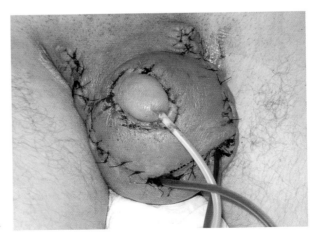

Fig. 37.3 Postoperative view of a reduced scrotum and exposure of the hidden penis. Small scrotal anterior flap. Circumcision of the penis. Elongation of the penis will require further plastic surgery

Fig. 37.4 Lymphoscintigram depicting iliac lymphatic bundles running along large pelvic veins. Lines crossing the bundles indicate where ligation and transection should take place. *Arrows* show sites of retroperitoneal lymphatics draining the kidneys and extravasated isotope in cases of chyluria

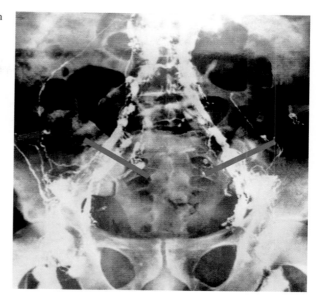

retain the urinary catheter until the wound has healed up, (b) penis: perform circumcision followed by longitudinal incision on the dorsum or lateral aspects and remove excess tissue, leave some more skin to allow future erection. Secondary plastic surgery of the penis is usually necessary. The application of a split-thickness skin graft involving the penile shaft promotes adequate skin coverage, with a penile girth compatible with sexual intercourse and little alteration in sensitivity. The zigzag suture of the graft on the ventral surface of the penis is aimed at avoiding scar contracture and subsequent ventral curvature of the penis. (c) Labia: remove as much tissue as possible, recurrence of edema is frequent.

Postoperative therapy: (a) antibiotics: long-term penicillin (bicillin) 1,200,000 IU, intramurally every seventh day for 1–2 months, followed by one injection every 3 weeks for 1 year or alternatively amoxicillin + clavulanic acid at a dosage of 1 g daily for 3 months and then 2 g for 3 days every 3 weeks, (b) manual massage of the remnant swollen tissues.

Postoperative complications: (a) slow recurrence of edema, (b) recurrence of local inflammatory episodes, (c) recurrence of lymph oozing, requiring injection of sclerosants, and (d) hidden penis requiring elongation.

References

1. Dandapat MC, Mohapatro SK, Patro SK. Elephantiasis of the penis and scrotum. A review of 350 cases. *Am J Surg*. 1985;149:686-690.
2. McDougal WS. Lymphedema of the external genitalia. *J Urol*. 2003;170:711-716.

3. Modolin M, Mitre AI, da Silva JC, et al. Surgical treatment of lymphedema of the penis and scrotum. *Clinics (Sao Paulo)*. 2006;61:289-294.
4. Halperin TJ, Slavin SA, Olumi AF, Borud LJ. Surgical management of scrotal lymphedema using local flaps. *Ann Plast Surg*. 2007;59:67-72.
5. Milanović R, Stanec S, Stanec Z, Zic R, Rudman F, Kopljar M. Lymphedema of the penis and scrotum: surgical treatment and reconstruction. *Acta Med Croat*. 2007;61:211-213.
6. Garaffa G, Christopher N, Ralph DJ. The management of genital lymphedema. *BJU Int*. 2008;102:480-484.
7. Zacharakis E, Dudderidge T, Zacharakis E, Ioannidis E. Surgical repair of idiopathic scrotal elephantiasis. *South Med J*. 2008;101:208-210.
8. Zugor V, Horch RE, Labanaris AP, Schreiber M, Schott GE. Penoscrotal elephantiasis: diagnostics and treatment options. *Urologe A*. 2008;47:472-476.

Chapter 38
Psychological Aspect: Compliance and Quality of Life

Cheryl L. Morgan

An estimated 99 million Americans live with chronic illness. The majority have not received effective treatment or optimal disease control.[1] Health services research indicates that it is the design of the care system, not the specialty of the physician or allied health professional, that is the primary determinant of the quality of chronic care.[2] Collaborative relationships with health care providers can help patients and families acquire effective medical, preventive, and health maintenance interventions.[3] Moreover, collaborative care between health care providers can help improve outcomes and adherence to self-care programs. Patient adjustment to requirements to maintain their health is improved when reinforced by each professional involved in his or her plan of care. They even develop adaptations to improve their own abilities to maintain the results achieved by treatment when accountability is emphasized by all members of their health care team.[4]

The term *compliance* has mostly been superseded by the term *adherence*, a similar concept, but one that has fewer negative connotations regarding the physician and patient relationship. Use of the term *compliance* has been strongly criticized because it was thought to convey a negative image of the relationship between patient and physician, in which the role of the physician was to issue the instructions and the patient's role was to follow the doctor's orders. Noncompliance, therefore, could be interpreted as patient incompetence with being unable to follow instructions or as deliberate, self-sabotaging behavior.[5]

The term *adherence* was introduced in an attempt to recognize a patient's right to choose, to participate actively in his or her plan of care, and to remove the concept of blame. It recognizes the need for patients, physicians, and allied health care professionals to work together to reach agreement and improve outcomes.[6] How we deal with this presents a major challenge for medicine, particularly in the management of chronic illnesses, such as lymphedema.

C.L. Morgan
Department of Rehabilitation Medicine,
Therapy Concepts Inc., Leawood, KS, USA

B.-B. Lee et al. (eds.), *Lymphedema*,
DOI 10.1007/978-0-85729-567-5_38, © Springer-Verlag London Limited 2011

The issue of one's quality of life for those living with chronic illness is important to consider when evaluating a patient's ability to manage lymphedema during treatment and thereafter. When possible, a comprehensive assessment would include not only a physical evaluation, but also would consider the psychological, emotional, and social concerns the patient may encounter.

Lymphedema patients are living an interrupted life replete with stages of emotional experiences and adaptive behavioral responses that correspond or collide with the individual's unique coping mechanisms. These emotional stages can range from feeling a violation of physical intactness to loss of autonomy. In some cases, lymphedema patients are dually threatened with death if they are suffering with cancer or other comorbidities complicating their recovery. Loss of activity, social isolation, and fear of stigmatization can threaten social identity and self worth.[7]

Adaptive behavioral responses can include resignation, disengagement or a refusal to help themselves. Some patients present with denial, avoidance, repressed anger or depression. These are largely unconscious responses that stop imagination or emotions from threatening a patient's sense of self. All represent defense mechanisms that can impair results of treatment if not addressed or are dismissed as noncompliance.[8]

Conscious coping mechanisms act as reality adjustors for the real world and are generally considered a more constructive overt behavior.[9] Stress research models have identified three fundamental types of conscious coping. *Information focused coping* is demonstrated by patients who seek instruments of emotional help. *Emotional focused coping* is observed in patients who vent emotions, denial, escape avoidance or acceptance of responsibility. Patients who utilize *problem-oriented coping* mechanisms will exercise active coping techniques, plan, and identify practical approaches to address stress.[10]

Consistent knowledge base and training of physicians and allied health professionals, paired with standardized information or resources, provide patients with confidence in the treatment approach and its demands. This is particularly important with protocols as demanding of time and resources as lymphedema management. Reliable direction helps prevents patients from pursuing unproven and often costly treatments. Obtaining incorrect or contradictory information promotes frustration and distrust and can lead to patients rejecting medical attention or non-adherence.[11]

Communication of expectations of therapeutic intervention involving family or caregivers in the selection of means of accountability fosters adherence with even strict protocols. Establishing reasonable outcomes and providing simple methods of measuring progress encourage patients and improve consistency with self care.[12] Instructions should be practical and individualized. Successful treatment is probable when a continuum of support and training is available to patients and active and sustained follow-up is available.[13]

Access to resources, treatment, literature, and supplies continues to encumber patients with lymphedema. Physician-directed care that is provided by experienced therapists, will enhance a patient's experience and provide superior results.[2] Support systems that provide additional resources are an important part of a successful program.[4] Without standardized educational requirements for health professionals or treatment protocols, lymphedema patients are often left on their own to learn about their condition and find treatment they can afford to pursue.

Improved communication between physicians and allied health professionals is increasing as awareness of the options for these patients increases. Once consensus on diagnosis, staging, and treatment of lymphedema can be reached, measureable outcomes can support the standardization of professional medical education, and improve reimbursement for treatment and supplies.[14]

Effective medical management of lymphedema is more likely to occur when collaborative care is consistently provided, and takes into consideration the patient's individual coping skills and variables that affect their quality of life and access to optimal treatment. Respecting each patient's autonomy, drawing out any concerns or ambivalence about pursuing treatment, and allowing the patient to develop and/or own the treatment plan greatly improve the odds of achieving positive clinical outcomes.[15] The growing population of chronically ill patients, such as patients with lymphedema, will require the development of successful systems and collaborative care.[16]

References

1. Rothman A, Wagner E, et al. Chronic illness management: What is the role of primary care? *Ann Intern Med.* 2003;138(3):256-261.
2. Casalino LP. Disease management and organization of physician practice. *JAMA.* 2005; 293(4):485-488.
3. Von Korff M, Gruman J, et al. Collaborative management of chronic illness. *Ann Intern Med.* 1997;127(12):1097-1102.
4. Cretin S, Shortell SM, Keeler EB. An evaluation of collaborative interventions to improve chronic illness care: framework and study design. *Eval Rev.* 2004;28(1):28-51.
5. Haynes RB, Sackett DL, Taylor DW. *Compliance in Healthcare.* Baltimore: Johns' Hopkins University Press; 1979.
6. World Health Organization. *Adherence to Long-Term Therapies: Evidence in Action.* Geneva: World Health Organization; 2003.
7. Redman BK. The ethics of self management for chronic illness. *Nurs Ethics.* 2005;12(4): 360-369.
8. Cramer P. *The Development of Defence Mechanisms: Theory, Research, and Assessment.* New York: Springer; 1991.
9. Faller H, Bülzebruck H, Drings P, Lang H. Coping, distress, and survival among patients with lung cancer. *Arch Gen Psychiatry.* 1999;56(8):756-762.
10. Lazarus RS, Folkman S. *Stress, Appraisal, and Coping.* New York: Springer; 1984.
11. Stille CJ, Jerant A, et al. Coordinating care across diseases, settings and clinicians. *Ann Intern Med.* 2005;142(8):700-708.
12. Zatzick D, Roy-Byrne P, et al. A randomized effectiveness trial of stepped collaborative care for acutely injured trauma survivors. *Arch Gen Psychiatry.* 2004;61(5):498-506.
13. Russell E, Wagner EH, Schaefer J, et al. Development and validation of patient assessment of chronic illness care (PACIC). *Med Care.* 2005;43(5):436-444.
14. Tretbar LL, Lee BB, Morgan CL, et al. *Lymphedema; Diagnosis and Treatment.* New York: Springer; 2007.
15. Butterworth S. Influencing patient adherence to treatment guidelines. *J Manag Care Pharm.* 2008;14(suppl S-b):S21-S25.
16. Wagner EH. Chronic disease care. *BMJ.* 2004;328(7433):177-178.

Part IX
Surgical Treatment:
Reconstructive Surgery

Chapter 39
General Overview – Historical Background

Waldemar L. Olszewski

Lymphovenous Microsurgical Shunts in Lower Limbs

Historically, limb lymphedema has been treated conservatively as far back as it has been found documented on ancient sculptures and scripts. Development of surgery in the nineteenth and twentieth centuries brought with it surgical methods for controlling lymphedema by improving tissue fluid and lymph drainage (e.g., through tissue bridging flaps, implantation of drains, etc.) and removal of excess of tissues in the advanced stages, such as elephantiasis. The results of lymph drainage by surgically created flow pathways turned out to be unsatisfactory and this is no longer practiced. In the 1960s modern microsurgery took its first steps based on the development of operating microscopes, microsurgical instruments, and refined sutures.

The idea came to my mind at that time to use microsurgical methods for the creation of artificial lymphovenous shunts that would mimic the natural communications between the two types of vessels. The physiological principles of the operation were based on the observations of natural anatomical lymphovenous communications in the retroperitoneal space in animals and in humans in cases of obstruction of the thoracic duct. In our project, the lymph node was cut transversely and lymph oozing started from the cortical sinuses. Bleeding from the node-supplying artery was stopped by coagulation. Then, the node was implanted end-to-side into an excised wall window of a neighboring vein (Fig. 39.1). The first operations were performed on dogs.[1,2] The mesenteric lymph node was transected and its distal part with afferent lymphatics was implanted into the inferior vena cava. Lymph flowed without resistance into the vein because blood pressure in the vena cava was slightly negative at inspiration (Fig. 39.1). These shunts created in dogs remained patent throughout life. The 12 months follow-up to the experiment was long enough to

W.L. Olszewski
Department of Surgical Research and Transplantology,
Medical Research Centre, Warsaw, Poland

B.-B. Lee et al. (eds.), *Lymphedema,*
DOI 10.1007/978-0-85729-567-5_39, © Springer-Verlag London Limited 2011

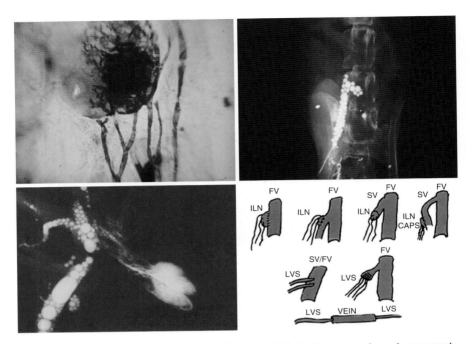

Fig. 39.1 Lymph node with afferent lymphatics (*upper left*). Cutting across the node exposes the lymphatic sinuses that implant into the vein and drain lymph into the blood circulation. Mesenteric lymph node in a dog was anastomosed with the inferior vena cava (*lower left*). Oily contrast medium was injected into the afferent mesenteric lymphatic and flowed to the vena cava (*large oil globules*). This can be better seen under higher magnification in the dog's vena cava and iliac veins (*upper right*). Various types of lympho-venous anastomoses have been developed by us since 1966. *ILN* inguinal lymph node, *FV* femoral vein, *SV* sapheous vein, *LVS* lymph vessel

convince us to perform the first human trials. In 1966, we carried out the first five operations of microsurgical lymphovenous shunts in humans, directing the stream of stagnant lymph of the lymphedematous lower limbs to the femoral vein.[1,3] The patients were women who had developed obstructive lymphedema of the lower limbs after the iliac dissection and radiotherapy of the pelvic region for cervical cancer. There was no postoperative venous thrombosis at the site of node insertion documented by phlebography. The decrease in limb volume was observed from the first postoperative day on. Surprisingly good results prompted us to perform our operation in patients with other types of lymphedema of the lower limbs such as postinflammatory, posttraumatic and the "idiopathic," known at that time as "the primary". The main questions at that time concerned the thrombosis at the site of anastomosis, lymph and venous blood pressure gradient and how many lymphatics were needed to drain the lymph into the vein to alleviate lymph stasis. Thrombosis of the femoral and great saphenous veins was not observed in our longest follow-ups. Lymph pressure in lymphatics was close to zero.[4,5] Blood pressure in the large limb veins was also close to zero when the patient was in a horizontal position.

It rose after the patient resumed an upright position, but was lowered by use of a muscular pump. Thus, the hydraulic conditions in the veins allowed lymph to flow into blood stream, at least in a supine position.

Over the course of time various modifications of the lymphovenous shunts have been introduced and tried by us and other authors (Fig. 39.1). Over the last 40 years, experience in microsurgical techniques, evaluation of early and late results, and correlation between the treatment by lymphovenous shunts and the clinical course of the disease have accumulated. It should be underlined that microsurgical shunting, alleviating tissue fluid and lymph outflow from the limb, is a palliative procedure. It only partially decompresses the overloaded lymphatic space and does not eliminate the etiological factor causing lymphedema, such as infections and scars. The transport capacity of the lymphatic vessel system remains partially insufficient because of the destruction of valves and impairment of the contractility of the lymph vessels.[5,6] Moreover, lymphedema is a condition characterized by an increase in extravascular fluid volume, proliferation of fibroblasts and keratinocytes, and the deposition of a large mass of extracellular matrix. The water content increases by 50% and the dry mass increases by 20%. The volume of the limb will never be the same as it was before lymphatic injury. All these factors should be taken into consideration during the evaluation of the results of microsurgical shunts. Moreover, the adjuvant therapy as manual and pneumatic massage and wearing of elastic garments further obscure objective evaluation of the result/response. Nevertheless, microsurgical anastomoses have established a definitive place among various therapeutic modalities for lymphedema, and with properly elaborated indications, they give excellent results.

The technique of microsurgical lympho-venous anastomoses for the treatment of lymphedema has undergone a steady evolution over the last 40 years and different modifications have been proposed.[7-23] A list of historical publications has been placed at the end of this chapter. The one man/one center experience, as in our case, has shown that even a small deviation from the elaborated technique results in closure of the anastomosis. Historically worked-out indications for the lympho-venous microsurgical shunt provide many hints on how the anastomoses should be performed and which factors affect the results.

Lympho-Venous Shunts (1966–2010)

Indications: Lower limb lymphedema at an early stage (I and II) of: post-surgical lymphedema (after cancer surgery and radiotherapy), post-inflammatory obstructive lymphedema (the most common, characterized by previous DLA attacks, often called cellulitis or erysipelas), hyperplastic lymphedema (inborn), or before debulking surgery, with at least one thigh lymphatic and a single inguinal or iliac lymph node on limb stress lymphoscintigraphy (performed during walking or pneumatic massage).
Contraindications: (a) recent attacks of dermato-lymphangio-adenitis (DLA), (b) skin ulcer.

Lack of indications: (a) stages III and IV with no lymphatics or nodes on lymphos-cintigraphy, (b) idiopathic lymphedema with soft skin, pitting edema, but no lymphatic structures on lymphoscintigraphy.

Pre- and Post-operative Pharmacological Treatment

(a) Long-term penicillin (bicillin) 1,200,000 IU intramurally 6 and 3 days before the operation and also postoperatively every 7th day for 1–2 months, followed by one injection every 3 weeks for 1 year or alternatively amoxicillin + clavulanic acid in a dosage of 2 g orally for 3 days before surgery followed by 1 g daily for 3 months and then 2 g for 3 days every 3 weeks (frequency depending on the number of previous DLA attacks).
(b) Postoperative LMWH (low molecular weight heparin) 80 mg subcutaneously daily for a period of 2 weeks.

Postoperative Physiotherapy

(a) Sequential pneumatic massage at a sleeve pressure of 120 mmHg, 1 h twice a day, for 10–30 days followed immediately by (b) putting on elastic stocking or pantyhose of II or III degree compression or elastic bandaging (40 mmHg) and (c) intensive walking.

Postoperative Evaluation Criteria

(a) Decrease in leg circumference
(b) Improved flexing in the ankle (to 80°) and knee joints (minimum 90°)
(c) Increase in the softness of the tissues (tonicity), measured with a deep tissue tonometer
(d) Subsidence of limb pain during long-lasting upright position
(e) Decreased frequency of DLA attacks

Objective Indirect Methods for the Evaluation of the Function of the Lympho-Venous Shunt

(a) Time of appearance of radioactivity over liver after Nanocoll toe web injection (less than 30 min in a horizontal position).
(b) Decreased tissue fluid pressure in leg subcutaneous tissue measured under standard conditions (test available in academic centers).

(c) Decreased volume of the interstitial space (postoperative intra-subcutaneous fluid volume infusion test; available in academic centers).

(d) Magnetic resonance measurement of tissue water content.

Note that evaluation should enclose both limbs. Temporary postoperative immobilization also brings about volume changes in a normal limb.

Direct Methods for Evaluation of Function of Lympho-Venous Shunt

Postoperative lymphoscintigraphic imaging of lymphatics (low level of sensitivity and specificity), also with venous occlusion above the shunt. In a few cases, radioactive tracer can be visualized in the draining vein (Fig. 39.2).

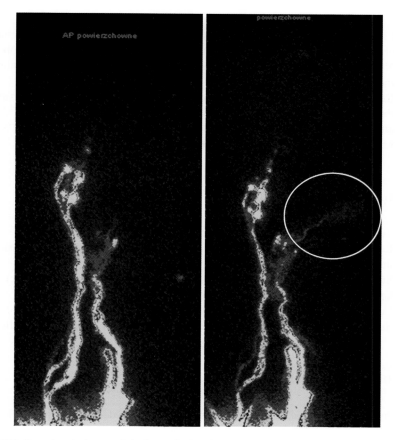

Fig. 39.2 Lymphoscintigram of the lower limbs of a patient with lymphedema of the left limb. The *circle* encompasses the site of the lymph vessel-to-vein anastomosis with radioisotope in the draining vein. Compare with the picture on the left before radioisotope injection

Factors Adversely Affecting the Patency
of Lymph-Venous Shunts

Local

(a) Infection of the operative wound
(b) Intraoperative damage to the afferent vessels
(c) Chronic inflammatory reaction at the site of anastomosis due to the nonabsorb-
    able sutures
(d) Formation of a parietal clot with subsequent organization (rare)
(e) A non-union of the lymphatic and venous endothelium

Distant

(a) Lack of lymph vessel contractility due to previous bacterial inflammatory
    changes (lymphangitis) and replacement of contractile elements by fibroblasts.
    Noncontracting vessels are not able to propel lymph along the lymphatics of
    the rest of the extremity.
(b) Lack of competent valves causing retrograde flow during muscular relaxation.
(c) Progression of inflammatory changes from distal lymphatics upward to the
    anastomosis (the "die-back phenomenon").
(d) Major fibrotic changes in the anastomosed lymph node.

Factors Affecting Evaluation of Clinical Results

(a) Lack of objective evaluation methods
(b) Recurrent dermatolymphangioadenitis attacks leading to sudden occlusion of
    the shunt
(c) Subjective judgment by the patient of limb movement freedom, decreased
    heaviness of leg, and softness of tissue
(d) Low patient compliance in using elastic support
(e) Supplementary multimodal therapy: massaging, elastic support, antibiotics

Results in General

Results should be evaluated separately in groups of lymphedema of various etiologies:

(a) The most satisfactory results have been obtained in the inborn hyperplastic
    lymphedema with large lymphatics not damaged by infection. The values reach

80–100% according to the clinical criteria of evaluation (see above). There is no increase in limb volume after operation if the operation was done at an early age.
(b) The results of lympho-venous shunts are also satisfactory in the group of patients after iliac and inguinal lymphadenectomy because of cancer and reach 80%. The afferent lymphatics have not been damaged by infection and their contractility is preserved.
(c) The results of the postinflammatory groups are low, not exceeding 30–40%, depending on the stage of lymphedema, and the frequency of recurrent attacks of DLA, and are evidently lower at the advanced stages. Skin and deep soft tissue infection damage the lymphatic wall and valves. Lymphatics become passive lymph conduits.
(d) In the group of post-traumatic lymphedema, prolonged healing and infection of injured tissues bring about major destructive changes in the lymphatics and regional lymph nodes. The indications for lympho-venous shunts are limited in this group.

References

1. Olszewski W. Experimental lympho-venous anastomoses. *Proceedings of the Congress, Polish Society of Surgeons.* Lodz; 1966, p. 62.
2. Nielubowicz J, Olszewski W. Experimental lymphovenous anastomosis. *Br J Surg.* 1968;55:449-451.
3. Nielubowicz J, Olszewski W. Surgical lympho-venous shunts in patients with secondary lymphedema. *Br J Surg.* 1968;55:440.
4. Politowski M, Bartkowski S, Dynowski J. Lympho-venous fistula for treatment of primary lymphedema of extremities. *Pol Med J.* 1970;9:438-444.
5. Olszewski WL. Surgical lympho-venous shunts for the treatment of lymphedema. In: Clodius L, ed. *Lymphedema.* Stuttgart: Thieme; 1977. p. 103.
6. Olszewski WL, Engeset A. Intrinsic contractility of prenodal lymph vessels and lymph flow in man. *Am J Physiol.* 1980;239:H775-H783.
7. Olszewski WL. *Lymph Stasis: Pathophysiology, Diagnosis and Treatment.* Boca Raton/Ann Arbor/Boston/Londyn/USA: CRC; 1991.
8. Olszewski WL. Contracility patterns of human leg lymphatic in various stages of obstructive lymphedema. *Ann NY Acad Sci.* 2008;1131:110-118.
9. Pokrovskij AV, Spiridonov AA, Thkor SN. Indications and technique of creating lympho-venous anastomosis in lymphedema of the extremities. *Klin Khir.* 1971;9:11-15.
10. Gilbert A, O'Brien BM, Vorrath JW, Sykes PJ. Lymphaticovenous anastomosis by microvascular technique. *Br J Plast Surg.* 1976;29:355-360.
11. O'Brien BM. Microlymphaticovenous surgery for obstructive lymphoedema. *ANZ J Surg.* 1977;47:284-291.
12. Petrovskii BV, Krylov VS, Stepanov GA, Milanov NO. Direct lymphovenous anastomosis making use of a microsurgical technic in secondary lymphedema of the extremities. *Klin Khir.* 1978;1:4-8. in Russian.
13. Kuzin MI, Anichkov MN, Zolotorevskii VIa, Savchenko TV, Zavarina IK. Direct lymphovenous anastomosis in disorders of lymph drainage in the extremities. *Khirurgiia (Mosk).* 1979;7:3-7. in Russian.
14. Krylov VS, Milanov NO, Abalmasov KG, Sandrikov VA, Sadovnikov VI. Role of lymphography in determining the indications for applying a direct lymphovenous anastomosis. *Khirurgiia (Mosk).* 1979;9:3-8. in Russian.

15. Gloviczki P, Kadar A, Soltesz L. Factors determining the patency of experimental anastomoses between lymphatic vessels and veins. *Morphol Igazságügyi Orv Sz*. 1980;20:250-255. in Hungarian.
16. Degni M. New microsurgical technique of lymphatico-venous anastomosis for the treatment of lymphedema. *Lymphology*. 1981;14:61.
17. Fox U, Montorsi M, Romagnoli G. Microsurgical treatment of lymphedemas of the limbs. *Int Surg*. 1981;66:53-56.
18. Jacobson JH 2nd. Microlymphaticovenous anastomosis for lymphedema. *J Microsurg*. 1982;3:255-257.
19. Huang GK, Hu RQ, Liu ZZ, Shen YL, Lan TD, Pan GP. Microlymphaticovenous anastomosis in the treatment of lower limb obstructive lymphedema: analysis of 91 cases. *Plast Reconstr Surg*. 1985;76:671-685.
20. Campisi C, Tosatti E, Casaccia M, et al. Microsurgery of the lymphatic vessels. *Minerva Chir*. 1986;41:469-481. in Italian.
21. Ipsen T, Pless J, Frederiksen PB. Experience with microlymphaticovenous anastomoses for congenital and acquired lymphedema. *Scand J Plast Reconstr Surg Hand Surg*. 1988;22:209-215.
22. Olszewski WL. The treatment of lymphedema of the extremities with microsurgical lympho-venous anastomoses. *Int Angiol*. 1988;7:312-321.
23. Campisi C. Use of autologous interposition vein graft in management of lymphedema: preliminary experimental and clinical observations. *Lymphology*. 1991;24:71-76.

Chapter 40
General Principles and Indications

Peter Gloviczki

Chronic lymphedema continues to be a challenge in both diagnosis and management. The diagnostic dilemma remains about how to best define detailed anatomy and lymphatic function, Whereas the problem with treatment remains our inability to cure chronic lymphedema. Still, both evaluation and treatment have greatly improved in recent years. Progress in genetics, imaging studies, physical therapy, and microsurgical techniques have sparked interest in chronic lymphedema, a disease long considered to be the stepchild of medicine. This textbook is testimony to the increasing interest in the investigation and treatment of lymphatic disorders.

The introduction of vascular microsurgery in the early 1960s by Jacobson established the possibility of surgical reconstruction of lymph vessels and lymph nodes.[1] The observations of Edwards and Kinmonth,[2] that, in lymphedema, spontaneous lymphovenous shunts in lymph nodes developed, and were likely to decompress the high pressure lymphatic system distal to an obstruction, led to early attempts to perform microsurgical lymphovenous anastomoses in patients with lymphedema. Lymph-vessel-to-vein[3-26] and lymph-node-to-vein anastomoses[27-30] were soon followed by lymphatic grafting to bypass the lymphatic obstructions.[31-36] In patients with lymphangiectasia, vein grafts with competent valves were used to drain the lymph and to prevent reflux of blood into the lymphatic system.[35,37,38] The free flap technique of lymph node transplantations was also developed.[39] Interest and enthusiasm for lymphatic microsurgery has waxed and waned during the last five decades, mostly because only a few centers around the world have had the expertise to perform these most difficult and challenging procedures (Fig. 40.1). In this section of the book we review the principles and indications, and briefly discuss the microsurgical techniques, results, and problems of the different types of lymphatic reconstructions.

P. Gloviczki
Division of Vascular and Endovascular Surgery, Gonda Vascular Center,
Mayo Clinic, Rochester, MN, USA

B.-B. Lee et al. (eds.), *Lymphedema*,
DOI 10.1007/978-0-85729-567-5_40, © Springer-Verlag London Limited 2011

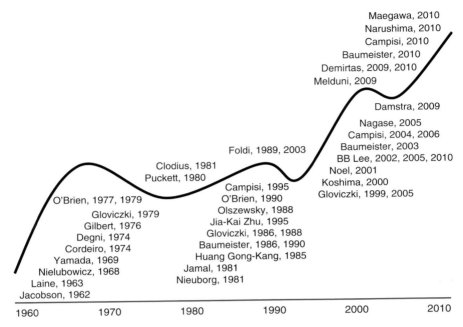

Maegawa, 2010
Narushima, 2010
Campisi, 2010
Baumeister, 2010
Demirtas, 2009, 2010
Melduni, 2009

Damstra, 2009
Nagase, 2005
Campisi, 2004, 2006
Baumeister, 2003
BB Lee, 2002, 2005, 2010
Noel, 2001
Koshima, 2000
Gloviczki, 1999, 2005

Foldi, 1989, 2003

Clodius, 1981
Puckett, 1980
Campisi, 1995
O'Brien, 1990
Olszewsky, 1988
Jia-Kai Zhu, 1995
Gloviczki, 1986, 1988
Baumeister, 1986, 1990
Huang Gong-Kang, 1985
Jamal, 1981
Nieuborg, 1981

O'Brien, 1977, 1979
Gloviczki, 1979
Gilbert, 1976
Degni, 1974
Cordeiro, 1974
Yamada, 1969
Nielubowicz, 1968
Laine, 1963
Jacobson, 1962

1960   1970   1980   1990   2000   2010

Fig. 40.1 Publications (first author, year) on microsurgical lymphatic reconstructions between 1962 and 2010 (By permission of Mayo Foundation for Medical Education and Reasearch)

Principles

In most patients chronic lymphedema is the result of acquired or congenital obstruction of the lymph vessels and the lymph–conducting elements of the lymph nodes. In some, valve incompetence of lymph vessels is the cause of poor lymph transport. The condition becomes clinically significant when the lymphatic collateral circulation is inadequate for draining lymph from the affected part of the body and lymph production exceeds the transport capacity of the lymphatic system. Other compensatory mechanisms, such as the tissue macrophage activity and drainage through spontaneous lymphovenous anastomosis, also are exhausted. The condition is aggravated by higher lymph production due to venous obstruction, venous valve incompetence, dependency of the limb, infection, or inflammation.

Surgical treatment of lymphedema includes excisional operations and lymphatic reconstructions.[40,41] Excisional surgery involves reduction of the volume of the limb by excision of the excess lymphatic tissue. This can be performed alone or with lymphatic reconstructions. Liposuction also has been used as an effective technique to decrease the excess volume of the affected limb.[42,43]

The goal of microsurgical lymphatic reconstructions is to restore or improve lymph transport in patients with chronic lymphedema. The ultimate goal is reduction of chronic swelling, decrease of the episodes of infection, and improvement of the quality of life of these patients.[44]

Indications

As discussed in ample detail in this book, multimodal complex decongestive physical therapy currently is recommended as first-line treatment for chronic lymphedema.[41,45] Successful therapy results in decreased volume, improved function, and improved quality of life. Considerations for surgery include no response to medical management after at least 6 months of therapy in surgically fit patients without recent episodes of cellulitis or lymphangitis and the availability of a center with an expert in lymphatic microvascular reconstructions. Severe pain is rare and it is a relative indication for surgery, whereas aesthetics alone is seldom an indication, although some patients are unwilling to undergo more conservative treatment, but are willing to proceed with experimental operations. The most suitable anatomy for lymphatic reconstructions is an acquired proximal (pelvic, axillary) lymphatic obstruction, with documented distal lymphatics on lymphoscintigraphy,[46,47] magnetic resonance lymphangiography,[48] or using the technique of indocyanine green injection and infrared scope imaging.[26]

Intrinsic contractility of the lymph vessels is one of the main factors responsible for normal lymphatic flow. Preserved contractility is ideal to assure good lymphatic flow against the higher pressure venous system. Activity and muscular contractions of the limb are also helpful and can generate intermittent pressures as high as 50 mmHg in the normal lymphatic system.[49] Unfortunately, compliance of the lymph vessels deteriorates in chronic lymphedema, and loss of contractility, especially when coupled with lymphatic obstructions or valvular incompetence, is an important reason why the response to lymphatic reconstructions in advanced stages of chronic lymphedema is so poor. Also, patients with lymphatic fibrosis, congenital hypoplasia, or even aplasia of the lymph vessels, as seen in those with primary lymphedema, are frequently poor candidates for lymphatic reconstructions.

Microsurgical Reconstructions

Three main techniques of lymphatic reconstructions have been developed. These include lymphovenous anastomosis, lymphatic grafting, and lymph node transplantations.

Lymphovenous Anastomosis

Lymphovenous anastomoses have been performed to drain lymph into the venous system in an area distal to the lymphatic obstruction.[3-30] Most patients have acquired or primary iliac lymphatic obstruction. Occasionally the operation is performed for congenital lymphangiectasia[37] or filariasis.[28,29] Two techniques have been introduced, lymph node-to-vein and lymph vessel-to-vein anastomoses (Fig. 40.2a, b).

Fig. 40.2 (a) End-to-end and
end-to-side lymph node-to-
vein anastomosis at the groin.
(b) End-to-end and end-to-
side microsurgical lymph
vessel-to-vein anastomosis.
(By permission of Mayo
Foundation for Medical
Education and Reasearch)

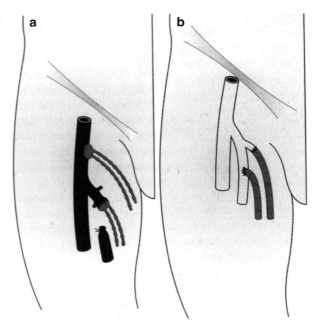

Lymph Node-to-Vein Anastomosis

Technique

Lymph node-to-vein anastomoses were first performed by Nielubowicz and
Olszewski in Poland in 1968.[27,50] During the operation transected inguinal lymph
nodes are anastomosed end-to-end or end-to-side to the saphenous or the femoral
veins (Fig. 40.2a).

Results

Clinical improvement after lymph-node-to-vein anastomoses has been reported in a
few uncontrolled studies,[27,30,50] but concerns about scarring over the cut surface of
the lymph nodes leading to failure prevented widespread application of this technique in most types of secondary lymphedema. In filariasis, however, lymphatics
are frequently enlarged even within the lymph nodes and lymph flow is high. Jamal
from India reported good results in 90% of patients with parasitic lymphatic infections.[28] Jamal also found that patients with congenital lymphangiectasia who underwent lymph node venous shunts constructed in the inguinal area, improved after the
procedure.[28,29]

Lymph Vessel-to-Vein Anastomosis

Microsurgical Technique

Earlier techniques of lymph vessel to vein anastomosis involved simple invagination of transected lymph vessels into large veins, like the saphenous, femoral, basilic, or brachial veins. This technique was popularized first in Brazil by Degni[51] and Cordeiro, and was used in a large number of patients by Campisi's group in Italy[16,18,52] (Fig. 40.3a, b). The same method of lymphatic reconstruction was also used in a recent prospective study by Damstra.[53] Variations of the invagination technique include pulling of the lymphatics into a vein graft and fixing with one or two sutures. Additional lymphatics distal to the obstruction can be pulled into the vein graft in an attempt to improve lymphatic drainage, and using the vein graft as a large lymphatic conduit to bypass the obstruction (Fig. 40.3b).

Most microsurgeons perform direct end-to-end or end-to-side lymphovenous anastomoses, using high power magnification and 8-10/0 microsutures (Fig. 40.2b).[3,7,12,54] The latest techniques of supermicroscopic surgery use very high power magnification. The introduction of intravascular stents and multiple configuration anastomosis, using both the proximal and distal ends of the transected lymph vessel (Figs. 40.4 and 40.5), enables better anastomosis of smaller (<1 mm) lymph vessels and likely contributes to improved patency rates and durable efficacy.[24-26,35,36,55] Reconstruction of larger lymph collectors and of the thoracic duct has also been reported.[23,56]

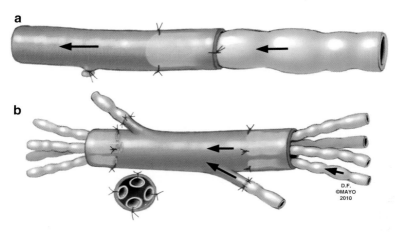

Fig. 40.3 Invagination techniques of Campisi. (**a**) Lymphovenous anastomosis, (**b**) lymphatic–venous–lymphatic anastomoses, performed using invagination of multiple lymphatics into an interposition vein graft. (By permission of Mayo Foundation for Medical Education and Reasearch)

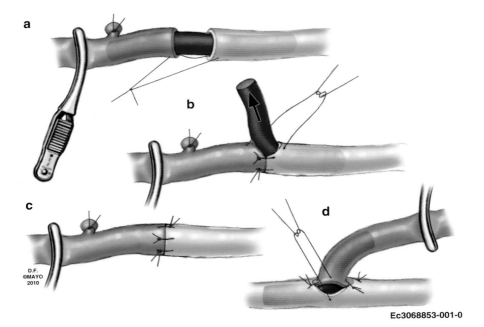

Fig. 40.4 Lymphovenous anastomoses performed with supermicroscopic technique, high-power magnification, and intravascular stents, according to Narushima. (**a, b, c**) Steps in performing end-to-end anastomosis with a stent. (**d**) End-to-side anastomosis. Stent is removed before completion of the anastomosis. (By permission of Mayo Foundation for Medical Education and Reasearch)

Results

Technically, lymphovenous anastomosis can be performed by experienced micro-surgeons, and in experiments anastomoses between normal femoral lymph vessels and a tributary of the femoral vein yielded a patency rate of 50% at 3–8 months after surgery.[7] The clinical effectiveness of this operation is more difficult to prove in humans, because almost all studies were uncontrolled and adjuvant compression therapy was used in most published series. In only five patients out of 14 on whom we operated in an earlier series maintained the initial improvement at an average of 46 months after surgery.[8] Patients with secondary lymphedema did better than those with primary lymphedema. In a group of 13 patients, 10 with primary and three with secondary lymphedema, Vignes et al.[57] failed to prove clinically significant long-term efficacy of the procedure. Damstra et al.,[53] in a similar, small cohort of 10 operated breast cancer patients with 11 procedures did not find a durable benefit of the invagination technique of lymphovenous anastomosis as described by Degni.

Experiences with large numbers of operated patients, however, suggest that clini-cal improvement can be achieved with lymphatic drainage procedures.[7-9,11-16] In O'Brien's series from Australia, 73% of the patients had subjective improvement

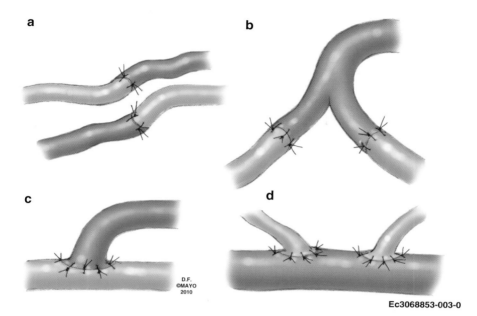

Ec3068853-003-0

Fig. 40.5 Techniques of Narushima for multiconfigurational lymphovenous anastomoses, with reconstruction of both the proximal and the distal ends of the transected lymph channels. (**a**) lymphovenous anastomosis with using both ends of the transected vessels. (**b**) anastomosis of two lymphatics with a bifurcated vein, end-to-end. (**c**) end-to-side vein – to-lymphatic anastomisis. (**d**) End-to-side anastomosis of two lymphatics into the same vein. (By permission of Mayo Foundation for Medical Education and Reasearch)

and 42% experienced long-term efficacy.[6] Campisi in Italy currently has the most experience with lymphatic microsurgery.[13-18,58,59] His team reported results in 665 patients with obstructive lymphedema using microsurgical lymphovenous anastomoses, with subjective improvement in 87% of the patients.[58,59] Four-hundred and forty-six patients were available for long-term follow-up: volume of the limb was reduced in 69%, conservative treatment was discontinued in a surprisingly high number of patients (85%). In 1,500 operated patients, using a variety of microsurgical reconstructions (Fig. 40.3), Campisi reported diminished volume of the operated limbs in 83% of the patients and decreased cellulitis in 87%.[60]

Significant recent progress in supermicroscopic surgical techniques has been documented in the past decade in publications by Koshima,[55] Demirtas,[24,25] and Narishima.[26] These authors have used high-power magnifications for direct lymphovenous anastomosis and lymphovenous implantations. Takeishi[61] suggested that lymphovenous anastomosis will prevent lymphedema in patients who undergo pelvic lymphadenectomy for cancer.

Narashima et al.[26] recently reported the use of temporary intravascular stents in 14 patients to ensure the patency of 39 multiconfiguration lymphaticovenous anastomoses capable of decompressing proximal, refluxing, and distal, antegrade lymphatic systems. These authors observed significant reduction in limb girth at a mean follow-up of 8.9 months, and found a greater decrease in the cross-sectional area with an increasing number of lymphaticovenous anastomoses per limb. Demirtas et al.[24,25] performed microlymphatic surgery in 80 lower extremities with primary and 21 with secondary lymphedema. Reduction of the edema occurred earlier in the secondary lymphedema group, but the mean change in the edema volume was comparable between the two groups. Although these results need confirmation by other investigators, this is the first promising study on using microsurgery with good results in patients with primary lymphedema.

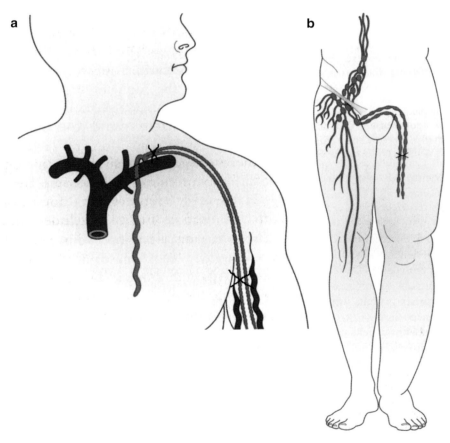

Fig. 40.6 Techniques of Baumeister: (**a**) Treatment of postmastectomy lymphedema with transplantation of two lymph channels from the lower to the upper extremity to by-pass the axillary lymphatic obstruction. (**b**) Cross-femoral lymph vessel transposition for unilateral lower extremity lymphedema. (By permission of Mayo Foundation for Medical Education and Reasearch)

Fig. 40.7 Lymphoscintigraphy 3 months after
cross-femoral lymphatic
transposition. Note
visualization of the left
inguinal nodes following
injection of isotope into the
right edematous foot. There
was no uptake prior to
operation. (By permission of
Mayo Foundation for
Medical Education and
Reasearch)

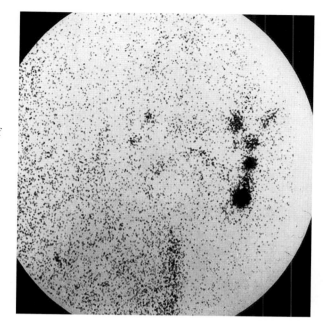

Lymphatic Grafting

Technique

Baumeister developed the technique of bypass with lymphatic grafts, harvested
from the unaffected lower limb. Two to three lymph vessels of the perisaphenous
superficial lymphatic bundle are harvested under magnification and used either as a
free graft for postmastectomy lymphedema to by-pass the axillary lymphatic
obstruction (Fig. 40.6a), or as a suprapubic cross-femoral transposition graft to treat
unilateral lower limb lymphedema in patients with iliac or iliofemoral lymphatic
obstruction (Fig. 40.6b).

Results

In a recent comprehensive review[34] of the subject, Baumeister, an experienced lymphatic microsurgeon, detailed the long-term results of these tedious operations. In
a group of 55 patients undergoing lymphatic grafting, improvement in limb volume
after a mean follow-up of 3 years was documented in 80% of the patients.[33] Patency
of transposed suprapubic lymph vessels can be documented with lymphoscintigraphy (Fig. 40.7). Using semiquantitative lymphoscintigraphy, significant improvement in lymphatic function could be demonstrated in 17 out of 20 patients at
8 years after the operation.[34,62] In a series of 127 patients suffering from arm edema,

a significant volume reduction was achieved with this technique, both at 8 days and at a mean of 2.6 years after surgery. In 81 patients with unilateral lower limb edema volume reduction after suprapubic transposition was significant, both early after surgery and at 1.7 years.[32]

Lymph Node Transplantation

Technique

Becker et al.[39,63] reported on the technique of lymph node transplantation, harvested from the groin as a free flap, to bridge the lymphatic obstruction in patients with postmastectomy lymphedema. The feeding artery and the draining vein of the flap are anastomosed to the appropriate vessels in the axillary fossa using a standard microsurgical technique.

Results

In 22 out of 24 patients the volume of the limb either decreased or returned to normal at 5 years or more after lymph node transplantation.[39,63] However, in only 5 out of 16 (31%), isotopic lymphoscintigraphy demonstrated activity of the transplanted nodes. Still, physiotherapy was discontinued in 15 patients (62.5%) and cure was demonstrated in 10 (41.6%).[39] The authors noted most improvement in patients with early stages of lymphedema. The use of this technique for lymphedema is appealing, but it needs independent confirmation by other microsurgical groups.

Problems with Microvascular Lymphatic Reconstructions

During the past few decades concerns and comments on the reasons for failures of lymphatic reconstructions have been voiced by Puckett,[64] Clodius,[65] and Foldi,[66,67] among others, and most recently by Damstra.[53] A thorough review of these publications by all experts who embark on the always challenging and sometimes unrewarding field of lymphatic microsurgery is strongly recommended.

One concern raised by critiques of lymphovenous anastomosis has been the lack of documented late patency. While lymphoscintigraphy is suitable to show patent lymphatic grafts[62,68] or transplanted lymph nodes,[39] this test can provide only indirect evidence of patency of lymphovenous anastomosis by showing improved lymph transport of the limb. Such improvement, however, can also be achieved by conservative measures. Observing contrast material during lymphangiography as it passes through the anastomosis is the only current way to document patency of lymphovenous shunts. Also, the droplets of the lipid-soluble contrast material are taken

Table 40.1 Guidelines of the American Venous Forum on surgical treatment of chronic lymphedema[40]

Number of guideline	Guideline	Grade of recommendation	Grade of evidence
6.4.1	All interventions for chronic lymphedema should be preceded by at least 6 months of non-operative compression treatment.	1	C
6.4.2	We suggest excisional operations or liposuction only to patients with late stage non-pitting lymphedema, who fail conservative measures	2	C
6.4.3	We suggest microsurgical lymphatic reconstructions in centers of excellence for selected patients with secondary lymphedema, if performed early in the course of the disease.	2	C

1 strong, *2* weak, *A* high quality, *B* moderate quality, *C* low or very low quality

away immediately by the venous blood stream; thus, the technique of cinelymphangiography is essential for documenting patency. In experiments, our group could demonstrate this,[6,7] but in patients, no firm data are available. In addition, assessment of the efficacy of microsurgical reconstructions is also hampered by the fact that the reported studies are uncontrolled, almost all are retrospective and, as pointed out by Damstra,[53] they lack a validated method of outcome evaluation. Damstra, disappointed by the negative results of his prospective study of 10 patients who underwent the Degni technique of lymphatic invagination, concluded that there was no convincing evidence of the success of lymphovenous anastomosis.[53] Another recent review of the literature[40] was somewhat more optimistic: it considered that evidence of the efficacy of surgery was there, but that it was of low or very low quality. Based on the available literature and consensus of experts, the American Venous Forum recently formulated recommendations for surgical treatment of lymphedema (Table 40.1).[40]

Finally, an observation on the clinical ineffectiveness of lymphovenous shunts in some patients deserves attention, as emphasized by Clodius, Piller, and Casley-Smith.[65] As these authors pointed out, some lymphatic microsurgeons consider the lymphatic system to be a canalicular system of drainage tubes and expect complete resolution of the edema by reestablishing lymph circulation using perfect microsurgical techniques. Unfortunately, in chronic lymphedema, inflammatory tissue changes occur that frequently will not reverse to even complete reconstruction of the lymph vessels or the lymph-conducting elements of the lymph nodes.

Conclusions

Conservative management with compression garments, decongestive lymphatic therapy, manual lymphatic drainage, bandaging, life-style modification, skin care, and treatment of infectious complications continues to be the mainstay of therapy for chronic lymphedema. Scientific evidence for the efficacy of lymphatic reconstructions to decrease limb swelling and improve the quality of life of patients with chronic lymphedema remains of very low quality. Most studies are uncontrolled and retrospective. Current recommendations for lymphatic microsurgery in patients with chronic lymphedema, non-responding to at least 6 months of intensive physical therapy, are weak. We suggest performing lymphatic reconstructions only in microsurgical centers of excellence in selected patients with obstructive, secondary lymphedema, early in the course of the disease.[40] Progress in the field of lymphatic microsurgery, however, has been noticeable and improvement in technique has been substantial. Interest in lymphatic microsurgery is increasing and supermicroscopic surgical techniques permit more reliable reconstructions of lymph vessels <1 mm in size. As non-invasive imaging techniques of the lymphatic system has also progressed, patient selection will likely be better and clinical improvement attributed solely to surgery can be documented in larger number of patients, in multiple centers. These are good reasons for being optimistic about treating chronic lymphedema effectively. However, until controlled prospective trials prove the clinical efficacy and durable function of lymphatic reconstructions, lymphatic microsurgery continues to remain an unfulfilled promise.

References

1. Jacobson JH 2nd. Founder's Lecture in plastic surgery. *Ann Plast Surg*. 2006;56(5):471-474.
2. Edwards JM, Kinmonth JB. Lymphovenous shunts in man. *Br Med J*. 1969;4(5683):579-581.
3. Gilbert A, O'Brien BM, Vorrath JW, Sykes PJ. Lymphaticovenous anastomosis by microvascular technique. *Br J Plast Surg*. 1976;29(4):355-360.
4. O'Brien BM. Microlymphaticovenous surgery for obstructive lymphoedema. *Aust NZ J Surg*. 1977;47(3):284-291.
5. O'Brien BM. The role of microsurgery in modern surgery. *Ann Plast Surg*. 1990;24(3):258-267.
6. Gloviczki P, Le Floch P, Hidden G. Lymphatico-venous experimental anastomosis (author's transl). *J Chir*. 1979;116(6-7):437-443.
7. Gloviczki P, Hollier LH, Nora FE, Kaye MP. The natural history of microsurgical lymphovenous anastomoses: an experimental study. *J Vasc Surg*. 1986;4(2):148-156.
8. Gloviczki P, Fisher J, Hollier LH, Pairolero PC, Schirger A, Wahner HW. Microsurgical lymphovenous anastomosis for treatment of lymphedema: a critical review. *J Vasc Surg*. 1988;7(5):647-652.
9. Laine JB, Howard JM. Experimental lymphatico-venous anastomosis. *Surg Forum*. 1963;14:111-112.
10. Degni M. New technique of lymphatic-venous anastomosis (buried type) for the treatment of lymphedema. *Vasa*. 1974;3(4):479-483.

11. Nieuborg L, Hoynck van Papendrecht A, Olthuis GA, van Dongen RJ. Treatment of secondary lymphedema with lymphatico-venous anastomosis. *Ned Tijdschr Geneeskd.* 1981;125(33):1330-1333.

12. Huang GK, Hu RQ, Liu ZZ, Shen YL, Lan TD, Pan GP. Microlymphaticovenous anastomosis in the treatment of lower limb obstructive lymphedema: analysis of 91 cases. *Plast Reconstr Surg.* 1985;76(5):671-685.

13. Campisi C. A rational approach to the management of lymphedema. *Lymphology.* 1991;24(2):48-53.

14. Campisi C. Lymphatic microsurgery: a potent weapon in the war on lymphedema. *Lymphology.* 1995;28(3):110-112.

15. Campisi C. Lymphoedema: modern diagnostic and therapeutic aspects. *Int Angiol.* 1999;18(1):14-24.

16. Campisi C, Boccardo F. Microsurgical techniques for lymphedema treatment: derivative lymphatic-venous microsurgery. *World J Surg.* 2004;28(6):609-613.

17. Campisi C, Davini D, Bellini C, et al. Lymphatic microsurgery for the treatment of lymphedema. *Microsurgery.* 2006;26(1):65-69.

18. Campisi C, Bellini C, Campisi C, Accogli S, Bonioli E, Boccardo F. Microsurgery for lymphedema: clinical research and long-term results. *Microsurgery.* 2010;30(4):256-260.

19. Koshima I, Yamamoto T, Narushima M, Mihara M, Iida T. Perforator flaps and supermicrosurgery. *Clin Plast Surg.* 2010;37(4):683-689. vii-iii.

20. Lee BB. Contemporary issues in management of chronic lymphedema: personal reflection on an experience with 1065 patients. *Lymphology.* 2005;38(1):28-31.

21. Lee BB, Kim DI, Whang JH, Lee KW. Contemporary management of chronic lymphedema—personal experiences. *Lymphology.* 2002;35:450-455.

22. Nagase T, Gonda K, Inoue K, et al. Treatment of lymphedema with lymphaticovenular anastomoses. *Int J Clin Oncol.* 2005;10(5):304-310.

23. Melduni RM, Oh JK, Bunch TJ, Sinak LJ, Gloviczki P. Reconstruction of occluded thoracic duct for treatment of chylopericardium: a novel surgical therapy. *J Vasc Surg.* 2008;48(6):1600-1602.

24. Demirtas Y, Ozturk N, Yapici O, Topalan M. Comparison of primary and secondary lower-extremity lymphedema treated with supermicrosurgical lymphaticovenous anastomosis and lymphaticovenous implantation. *J Reconstr Microsurg.* 2010;26(2):137-143.

25. Demirtas Y, Ozturk N, Yapici O, Topalan M. Supermicrosurgical lymphaticovenular anastomosis and lymphaticovenous implantation for treatment of unilateral lower extremity lymphedema. *Microsurgery.* 2009;29(8):609-618.

26. Narushima M, Mihara M, Yamamoto Y, Iida T, Koshima I, Mundinger GS. The intravascular stenting method for treatment of extremity lymphedema with multiconfiguration lymphaticovenous anastomoses. *Plast Reconstr Surg.* 2010;125(3):935-943.

27. Nielubowicz J, Olszewski W. Surgical lymphaticovenous shunts in patients with secondary lymphoedema. *Br J Surg.* 1968;55(6):440-442.

28. Jamal S. Lymphovenous anastomosis in filarial lymphedema. *Lymphology.* 1981;14(2):64-68.

29. Jamal S. Lymph nodo-venous shunt in the treatment of protein losing enteropathy and lymphedema of leg and scrotum. *Lymphology.* 2007;40(1):47-48.

30. Olszewski WL. The treatment of lymphedema of the extremities with microsurgical lympho-venous anastomoses. *Int Angiol.* 1988;7(4):312-321.

31. Baumeister RG, Seifert J. Microsurgical lymphvessel-transplantation for the treatment of lymphedema: experimental and first clinical experiences. *Lymphology.* 1981;14(2):90.

32. Baumeister RG, Frick A. The microsurgical lymph vessel transplantation. *Handchir Mikrochir Plast Chir.* 2003;35(4):202-209.

33. Baumeister RG, Siuda S. Treatment of lymphedemas by microsurgical lymphatic grafting: What is proved? *Plast Reconstr Surg.* 1990;85(1):64-74; discussion 5-6.

34. Baumeister R. Lymphedema: surgical treatment. In: Cronenwett JL, Johnston KW, eds. *Rutherford's Vascular Surgery.* 7th ed. Philadelphia: Saunders; 2010:1029-1043.

35. Maegawa J, Mikami T, Yamamoto Y, Hirotomi K, Kobayashi S. Lymphaticovenous shunt for the treatment of chylous reflux by subcutaneous vein grafts with valves between megalymphatics and the great saphenous vein: a case report. *Microsurgery*. 2010;30(7):553-556.
36. Maegawa J, Mikami T, Yamamoto Y, Satake T, Kobayashi S. Types of lymphoscintigraphy and indications for lymphaticovenous anastomosis. *Microsurgery*. 2010;30(6):437-442.
37. Noel AA, Gloviczki P, Bender CE, Whitley D, Stanson AW, Deschamps C. Treatment of symptomatic primary chylous disorders. *J Vasc Surg*. 2001;34(5):785-791.
38. Campisi C. Use of autologous interposition vein graft in management of lymphedema: preliminary experimental and clinical observations. *Lymphology*. 1991;24(2):71-76.
39. Becker C, Assouad J, Riquet M, Hidden G. Postmastectomy lymphedema: long-term results following microsurgical lymph node transplantation. *Ann Surg*. 2006;243(3):313-315.
40. Gloviczki P. Principles of surgical treatment of chronic lymphedema. In: Gloviczki P, ed. *Handbook of Venous Disorders: Guidelines of the American Venous Forum*. 3rd ed. London: Hodder Arnold; 2009:658-664.
41. Lee B, Andrade M, Bergan J, et al. Diagnosis and treatment of primary lymphedema. Consensus Document of the International Union of Phlebology (IUP)-2009. *Int Angiol*. 2010;29(5):454-470.
42. Brorson H, Svensson H. Liposuction combined with controlled compression therapy reduces arm lymphedema more effectively than controlled compression therapy alone. *Plast Reconstr Surg*. 1998;102(4):1058-1067; discussion 68.
43. Brorson H. From lymph to fat: complete reduction of lymphoedema. *Phlebology*. 2010;25(suppl 1):52-63.
44. Gloviczki P. Principles of surgical treatment of chronic lymphoedema. *Int Angiol*. 1999;18(1):42-46.
45. Gamble GL, Cheville A, Strick D. Lymphedema: medical and physical therapy. In: Gloviczki P, ed. *Handbook of Venous Disorders: Guidelines of the American Venous Forum*. 3rd ed. London: Hodder Arnold; 2009:649-657.
46. Gloviczki P, Calcagno D, Schirger A, et al. Noninvasive evaluation of the swollen extremity: experiences with 190 lymphoscintigraphic examinations. *J Vasc Surg*. 1989;9(5):683-689; discussion 90.
47. Cambria RA, Gloviczki P, Naessens JM, Wahner HW. Noninvasive evaluation of the lymphatic system with lymphoscintigraphy: a prospective, semiquantitative analysis in 386 extremities. *J Vasc Surg*. 1993;18(5):773-782.
48. Lohrmann C, Felmerer G, Foeldi E, Bartholoma JP, Langer M. MR lymphangiography for the assessment of the lymphatic system in patients undergoing microsurgical reconstructions of lymphatic vessels. *Microvasc Res*. 2008;76(1):42-45.
49. Olszewski WL. Physiology and microsurgery of lymphatic vessels in man. *Lymphology*. 1981;14(2):44-60.
50. Nielubowicz J, Olszewski W, Sokolowski J. Surgical lympho-venous shunts. *J Cardiovasc Surg*. 1968;9(3):262-267.
51. Degni M. New technique of lymphatic-venous anastomosis for the treatment of lymphedema. *J Cardiovasc Surg*. 1978;19(6):577-580.
52. Campisi C, Boccardo F. Role of microsurgery in the management of lymphoedema. *Int Angiol*. 1999;18(1):47-51.
53. Damstra RJ, Voesten HG, van Schelven WD, van der Lei B. Lymphatic venous anastomosis (LVA) for treatment of secondary arm lymphedema. A prospective study of 11 LVA procedures in 10 patients with breast cancer related lymphedema and a critical review of the literature. *Breast Cancer Res Treat*. 2009;113(2):199-206.
54. O'Brien BM, Shafiroff BB. Microlymphaticovenous and resectional surgery in obstructive lymphedema. *World J Surg*. 1979;3(1):3-15, 121-123.
55. Koshima I, Inagawa K, Urushibara K, Moriguchi T. Supermicrosurgical lymphaticovenular anastomosis for the treatment of lymphedema in the upper extremities. *J Reconstr Microsurg*. 2000;16(6):437-442.

56. Gloviczki P, Noel AA. Surgical treatment of chronic lymphedema and primary chylous disorders. In: Rutherford RB, ed. *Rutherford's Vascular Surgery*. 6th ed. Philadelphia: Elsevier; 2005:2428-2445.

57. Vignes S, Boursier V, Priollet P, Miserey G, Trevidic P. Quantitative evaluation and qualitative results of surgical lymphovenous anastomosis in lower limb lymphedema. *J Mal Vasc.* 2003;28(1):30-35.

58. Campisi C, Boccardo F, Zilli A, Maccio A, Napoli F. Long-term results after lymphatic-venous anastomoses for the treatment of obstructive lymphedema. *Microsurgery.* 2001;21(4): 135-139.

59. Campisi C, Boccardo F. Lymphedema and microsurgery. *Microsurgery.* 2002;22(2):74-80.

60. Campisi C, Eretta C, Pertile D, et al. Microsurgery for treatment of peripheral lymphedema: long-term outcome and future perspectives. *Microsurgery.* 2007;27(4):333-338.

61. Takeishi M, Kojima M, Mori K, Kurihara K, Sasaki H. Primary intrapelvic lymphaticovenular anastomosis following lymph node dissection. *Ann Plast Surg.* 2006;57(3):300-304.

62. Weiss M, Baumeister RG, Hahn K. Dynamic lymph flow imaging in patients with oedema of the lower limb for evaluation of the functional outcome after autologous lymph vessel transplantation: an 8-year follow-up study. *Eur J Nucl Med Mol Imaging.* 2003;30(2):202-206.

63. Becker C, Hidden G. Transfer of free lymphatic flaps. Microsurgery and anatomical study. *J Mal Vasc.* 1988;13(2):119-122.

64. Puckett CL, Jacobs GR, Hurvitz JS, Silver D. Evaluation of lymphovenous anastomoses in obstructive lymphedema. *Plast Reconstr Surg.* 1980;66(1):116-120.

65. Clodius L, Piller NB, Casley-Smith JR. The problems of lymphatic microsurgery for lymphedema. *Lymphology.* 1981;14(2):69-76.

66. Foldi E, Foldi M, Clodius L. The lymphedema chaos: a lancet. *Ann Plast Surg.* 1989;22(6): 505-515.

67. Foldi M, Foldi E, Kubik S. *Textbook of Lymphology for Physicians and Lymphedema Therapists*. Munchen: Urban & Fischer; 2003.

68. Weiss M, Baumeister RG, Hahn K. Planning and monitoring of autologous lymph vessel transplantation by means of nuclear medicine lymphoscintigraphy. *Handchir Mikrochir Plast Chir.* 2003;35(4):210-215.

Chapter 41
Lymphatic-Venous Derivative and Reconstructive Microsurgery

Corradino Campisi and Francesco Boccardo

General Considerations

Lymphedema that is refractory to nonoperative methods may be managed by surgical treatment. Indications include insufficient lymphedema reduction by well-performed medical and physical therapy (less than 50%), recurrent episodes of lymphangitis, intractable pain, worsening limb function, patient who are unsatisfied with the result obtained by nonoperative methods, and patients who are willing to proceed with surgical options.

The first microsurgical derivative operations were those using lymph node–venous shunts. These have been largely abandoned, except in endemic areas of lymphatic filariasis such as India, where thousands of these procedures have been performed. Lymphatic channels in lymph nodal–venous anastomoses are often widely dilated because of the high rate of anastomotic closures caused by the thrombogenic effect of lymph nodal pulp on the venous blood and the frequent re-endothelialization of the lymph node surface.[1] Because of the difficulties encountered with lymph nodal–venous shunts by surgeons worldwide, the next approach was to use lymphatic vessels directly anastomosed to veins.[2]

The technique consists of anastomosing lymphatic vessels to a collateral branch of the main vein with competent valvular function to secure the proper continence of the vein segment used for the anastomosis with no reflux. valvular competence warrants the mandated condition of lymph flow alone and not the blood within the venous segment, avoiding any risk of thrombosis of the anastomosis.[3]

C. Campisi (✉)
Department of Surgery, Section of Lymphology and Microsurgery,
University Hospital "San Martino", Genoa, Italy

B.-B. Lee et al. (eds.), *Lymphedema*,
DOI 10.1007/978-0-85729-567-5_41, © Springer-Verlag London Limited 2011

Fig. 41.1 Lymphatic–venous multiple anastomosis: several lymphatics are introduced inside a valved vein. The blue dye flowing into the vein demonstrates the patency of the vein. The well-functioning valve ensures the continence of the vein, avoiding blood reflux toward the lymphatics. This technical trick is important for the long-term patency of the anastomosis

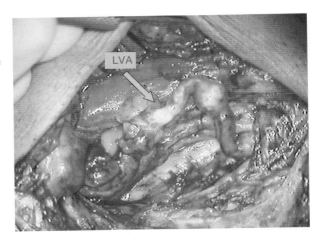

Clinical Experience and Surgical Techniques

The operations consisted of multiple microsurgical lymphovenous anastomoses. Healthy-appearing lymphatics found at the operation site are directly introduced together into the vein segment by a U-shaped stitch and then further secured to the vein's cut–end by means of additional stitches between the vein border and the peri-lymphatic adipose tissue. With the use of the Patent Blue dye, properly functioning lymphatics appear blue, and the passage of blue lymph into the vein branch verifies the patency of the lymphovenous anastomosis under the operating microscope when the anastomosis is completed (Fig. 41.1).

For patients with lower limb lymphedema, anastomoses are performed at the subinguinal region. Superficial lymphatic–lymph nodal structures are isolated, and all afferent lymphatics are used for the operation. Lymph nodes are subjected to histopathological examination. The usual finding in primary lower limb lymphede-mas is a varying grade of nodal fibrosclerosis and thickening of the nodal capsule, but with normal afferent lymphatic vessels.

For upper limb lymphedema, lymphovenous anastomoses are performed at the middle third of the volar surface of the arm, using both superficial and deep lym-phatic collectors, as demonstrated by the blue dye. Deep lymphatics are found among the humeral artery, vein, and the median nerve. The vein used for anastomo-ses is a patent branch of one of the humeral veins, and the technique most frequently performed is microsurgery (Fig. 41.2).

Primary lymphedemas largely include lymph node dysplasias (LAD II, accord-ing to Papendieck's classification[4]) consisting of hypoplastic lymph nodes with sinus histiocytosis and a thick and fibrous capsule with microlymphangioadenomy-omatosis. In these cases, lymph flow obstruction is apparent, as seen by alterations of the afferent lymphatics, which appear dilated and swollen with thickened walls and where smooth muscle cells are reduced in number and appear fragmented by associated fibrous elements.

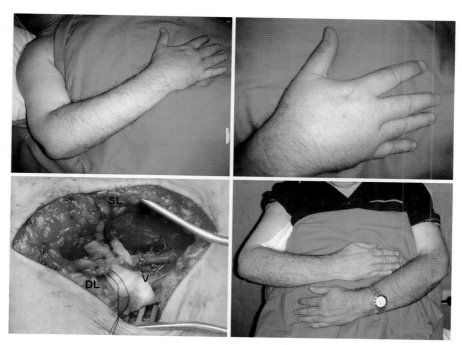

Fig. 41.2 Primary right upper limb lymphedema in a man treated with derivative lymphatic–venous anastomosis at the volar surface of the upper third of the arm. Superficial (SL) and deep (DL) lymphatics are prepared together with a vein (V) branch of one of the brachial veins with well-functioning valves. The result of the operation is immediate and the technique allowed stable results to be obtained at long-term follow-up

Secondary lymphedemas are largely due to lymphadenectomy and radiotherapy performed for oncological reasons (carcinoma of the breast, uterus, penis, bladder, prostate gland, and rectum and seminoma of the epididymis), as well as for complications of minor operations for varicose veins, crural and inguinal hernias, lipomas, tendinous cysts, or axillary and inguinal lymph node biopsies. Most of the lymphedemas treated by the microsurgery in our experience were at stages II (39%) and III (52%), whereas 3% of the patients were stage Ib and 6% were stages IV and V.

Lymphoscintigraphy, performed with 99mTc-labeled antimony sulfur colloid, is employed in the diagnostic work-up of patients with lymphedema and as a test for selecting patients for derivative microsurgical operations. Lymphoscintigraphy clearly determines whether or not edema was of lymphatic origin and also provides important data about the etiologic and pathophysiologic aspects of the lymphedema.

Echo Doppler is performed in all patients to identify any venous disorders possibly associated with lymphedema. In most patients, venous dysfunction is corrected at the same time as microlymphatico-venous anastomoses (i.e., valvuloplasty in the case of venous insufficiency) is performed. In other cases, the finding of

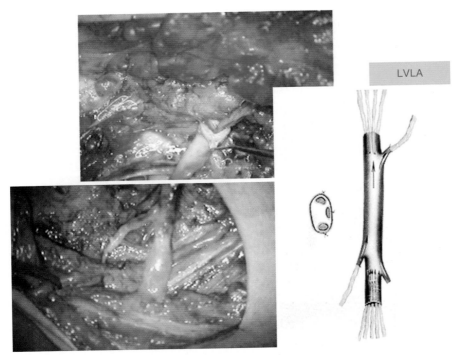

Fig. 41.3 Lymphatic–venous–lymphatic anastomoses used in those cases in which, owing to venous dysfunction, derivative technique are contraindicated. The technique consists in interposing a vein segment in between lymphatics above and below the obstacle to lymph flow[7]

venous dysfunction contraindicates derivative lympho-venous shunts, but at the same time facilitates referral of the patient for reconstructive microsurgical operations.

In those cases involving the lower limbs, where surgically uncorrectable venous disease exists, it is not advisable to use derivative lymphatic–venous techniques, and accordingly, reconstructive methods are used. The most commonly used technique is the interposition of an autologous vein graft between the lymphatics above and below the obstacle to lymph flow. Competent venous segments can be obtained from the same operative site or from the forearm (mostly the cephalic vein). The length of the graft is variable from 7 to 15 cm, and it is important to collect several lymphatics to connect to the distal cut end of the vein so as to ensure that the segment is filled with enough lymph and to avoid closure due to subsequent development of the fibrosis. The competent valves of the vein segments are essential for the correct direction of the lymphatic flow and to avoid gravitational backflow, or reflux. The technique of anastomosis is the microsurgery with introduction of the lymphatics inside the vein cut ends by a U-shaped stitch, which is then secured by additional peripheral stitches (Fig. 41.3).

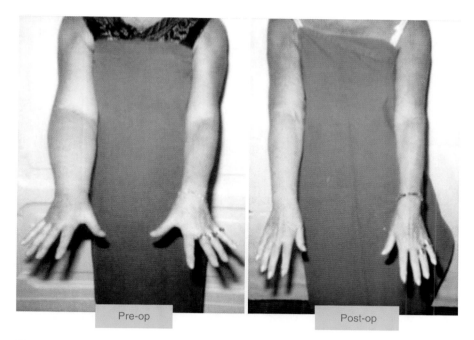

Fig. 41.4 Right upper limb lymphedema due to breast cancer treatment, managed by derivative lymphatic–venous microsurgical anastomoses at the arm (long-term follow-up)

Results and Final Considerations

Clinical outcome improves the earlier microsurgery is performed, owing to absent or minimal fibrosclerotic alterations of the lymphatic walls and surrounding tissues. Subjective improvement in our experience was noted in 87% of patients. Objectively, volume changes showed a significant improvement in 83%, with an average reduction of 67% of the excess volume. Of those patients followed up, 85% have been able to discontinue the use of conservative measures, with an average follow-up of more than 10 years and average reduction in excess volume of 69% (Figs. 41.4–41.8). There was an 87% reduction in the incidence of cellulitis after microsurgery.

Lymphoscintigraphy helped in verifying the patency of microanastomoses long term after operation by direct and indirect findings: reduction of dermal backflow together with the appearance of preferential lymphatic pathways not visible before microsurgery; disappearance of the tracer at the site of lymphatic–venous anastomoses because of direct tracer passage into the blood stream; and earlier liver uptake compared with pre-operative parameters (indirect patency test; Figs. 41.9 and 41.10).

Lymphatic microsurgery represents a means of bypassing the obstacle to lymph flow through lymphatic–venous drainage (lymphatic–venous anastomoses) or by

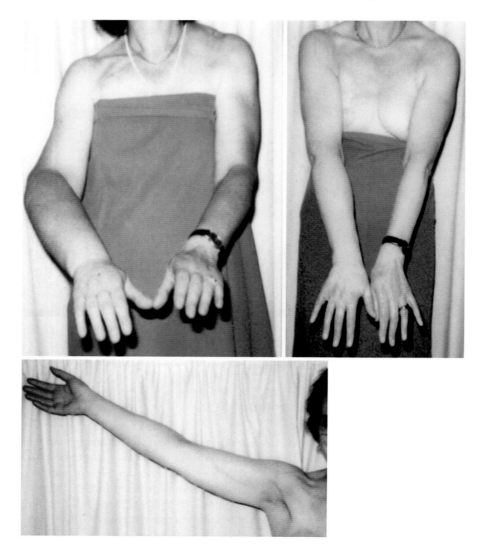

Fig. 41.5 Another case of secondary upper limb lymphedema. Of note is the good result at the hand and the favorable result from a cosmetic point of view

using venous grafts between lymphatic collectors below and above the obstruction (lymphatic–venous–lymphatic plasty). Combined physical therapy nonetheless represents the initial treatment of patients affected by peripheral lymphedema and it is best performed in specialized centers. The surgical timing follows completion of conservative treatment when further clinical improvement can no longer be achieved and/or recurrent lymphangitic attacks are not further reduced.[5] Microsurgical operations can then be performed and provide further improvement in the condition.[6,7]

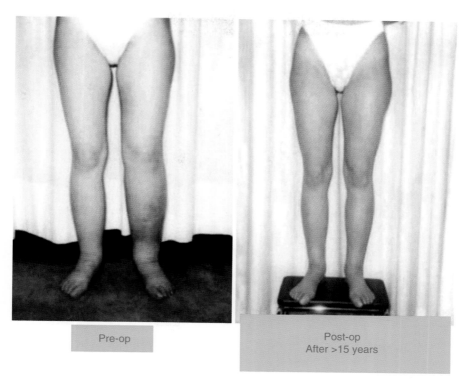

Pre-op

Post-op
After >15 years

Fig. 41.6 Bilateral lower limb primary lymphedema before and after 15 years from microsurgical derivative operation at the groin. The technique of lymphatic–venous anastomoses, if performed in the proper manner, represents a physiological, long-lasting repair of the lymphatic drainage of the extremity

The optimal indications for lymphatic microsurgery are represented by: early stages (Ib, II, early III); lymphoscintigraphy showing a low inguinal or axillary lymph nodal uptake and minimal or absent passage of the tracer beyond this proximal nodal area; excellent patient compliance; and a well-organized lymphedema center where the patient can be easily referred for additional care to a Center of Lymphatic Surgery to receive this specialized surgery.

At later stages (advanced III, IV, and V), with absent visualization of lymphatic channels and regional lymph nodes, it is necessary to reduce the stage of the lymphedema by non-operative methods before microsurgery. After the operation, it is particularly important for these patients to be kept under close follow-up with the regimen of complete lymphedema functional therapy – CLyFT[8]; such an approach is essential to improve the clinical outcome and maintain the short-term operative results for the long term (Fig. 41.11). In the case of poor patient compliance, the results may be unsatisfactory. Relative contraindications to lymphatic microsurgery are represented by cases of lymphatic–lymph nodal aplasia (extremely rare), diffuse metastatic disease, and advanced stage (V) not responsive to conservative therapy.

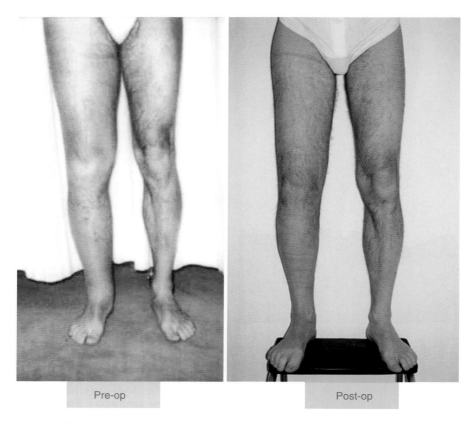

Fig. 41.7 Right lower limb lymphedema treated with derivative lymphatic–venous anastomoses at the inguino-crural region. These techniques allow the compression garments to be used irregularly thanks to the formation of preferential lymphatic pathways and to the positive lymphatic–venous pressure gradient

Traditional debulking operations are presently less frequently utilized to treat lymphedema except in cases of late-stage lymphedema to reduce skin folds after marked edema reduction obtained by conservative physical and microsurgical methods; in body regions relatively inaccessible to effective compression such as the genitalia; in advanced lymphatic filariasis at times combined with lymphatic–venous or nodal–venous anastomosis in the setting of widely dilated lymphatic channels; and in localized lipolymphedema associated with massive obesity and forced immobility.

In recent years, both primary and secondary peripheral lymphedemas have become better understood and more manageable problems, with increased awareness and early detection.[9-13] Nonetheless, apparent non-operative measures are aimed at minimizing morbidity without removing the cause of the underlying disturbance.[14,15] Microsurgical derivative and reconstructive operations can restore

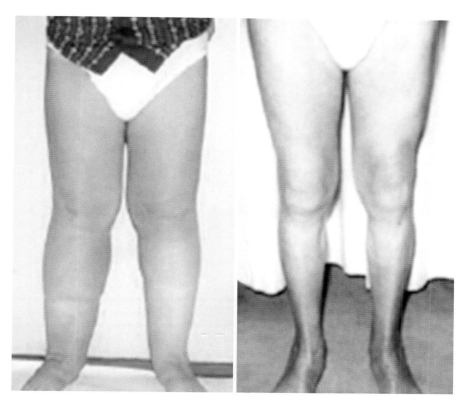

Fig. 41.8 Bilateral primary lower limb lymphedema with associated important venous dysfunction. In this case, reconstructive lymphatic–venous anastomoses was used bilaterally with a good long-term result. This technique can also be used in bilateral lymphedemas and does not determine any risk of secondary lymphedema at the harvesting site

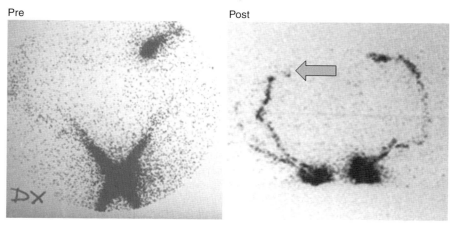

Fig. 41.9 Lymphoscintigraphic follow-up of an upper limb secondary lymphedema treated by derivative lymphatic microsurgery. Post-operatively, preferential lymphatic ways are evident and the tracer disappears at the site of anastomosis because of passage into the blood stream

Pre   Post

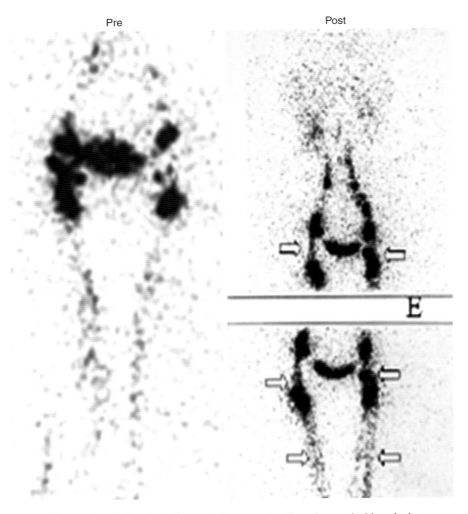

Fig. 41.10 Lymphoscintigraphy before and after reconstructive microsurgical lymphatic–venous technique performed in a bilateral lower limb lymphedema. Post-operatively, venous grafts are visualized in between lymphatic pathways below and above the inguinal region

lymphatic drainage, both in the short and long term, and the best results are obtained when these surgical procedures are combined with physical rehabilitative methods.

Finally, we recently proposed the use of lymphatic–venous anastomoses for primary prevention of arm lymphedema, performing anastomoses at the same time as axillary lymph nodal dissection for breast cancer treatment (the lymphatic microsurgical preventive healing approach – LyMPHA).[16] This technique was also used for preventing lower limb secondary lymphedema with vulvar carcinoma and melanoma of the trunk.

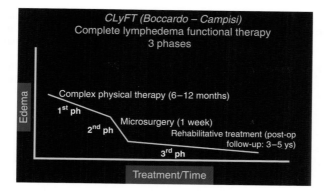

Fig. 41.11 Scheme of the complete lymphedema functional therapy (CLyFT) proposed for the combined non-operative and microsurgical treatment of lymphedema. This therapeutic association proved to supply the best and longest lasting results, combining the efficacy of non-operative methods with the results of microsurgical procedures and giving the patient the possibility of wearing compression garments irregularly at the beginning, and also to avoid the use of stockings and sleeves in the long run

References

1. Olszewski WL. The treatment of lymphedema of the extremities with microsurgical lymphovenous anastomoses. *Int Angiol*. 1988;7(4):312-321.
2. Campisi C, Boccardo F. Lymphedema and microsurgery (Invited Review). *Microsurgery*. 2002;22:74-80.
3. Campisi C, Boccardo F. Microsurgical techniques for lymphedema treatment: derivative lymphatic-venous microsurgery. *World J Surg*. 2004;28(6):609-613.
4. Papendieck CM. The big angiodysplastic syndromes in pediatrics with the participation of the lymphatic system. *Lymphology*. 1998;31(suppl):390-392.
5. Dellachà A, Boccardo F, Zilli A, Napoli F, Fulcheri E, Campisi C. Unexpected histopathological findings in peripheral lymphedema. *Lymphology*. 2000;33:62-64.
6. Campisi C, Eretta C, Pertile D, et al. Microsurgery for treatment of peripheral lymphedema: long-term outcome and future perspectives. *Microsurgery*. 2007;27(4):333-338.
7. Campisi C, Boccardo F, Tacchella M. Reconstructive microsurgery of lymph vessels: the personal method of lymphatic-venous-lymphatic (LVL) interpositioned grafted shunt. *Microsurgery*. 1995;16(3):161-166.
8. Campisi C, Boccardo F. Terapia Funzionale Completa del Linfedema (CLyFT: Complete Lymphedema Functional Therapy): efficace strategia terapeutica in 3 fasi. *Linfologia*. 2008;1:20-23.
9. Bellini C, Boccardo F, Taddei G, et al. Diagnostic protocol for lymphoscintigraphy in newborns. *Lymphology*. 2005;38(1):9-15.
10. Bourgeois P, Leduc O, Leduc A. Imaging techniques in the management and prevention of posttherapeutic upper limb edemas. *Cancer*. 1998;83(12 suppl American):2805-2813.
11. Mariani G, Campisi C, Taddei G, Boccardo F. The current role of lymphoscintigraphy in the diagnostic evaluation of patients with peripheral lymphedema. *Lymphology*. 1998;31(S):316.
12. Pecking AP, Gougeon-Bertrand FJ, Floiras JL. Lymphoscintigraphy. Overview of its use in the lymphatic system. *Lymphology*. 1998;31(S):343.
13. Witte C, McNeill G, Witte M. Whole-body lymphangioscintigraphy: making the invisible easily visible. In: Mitsumas N, Uchino S, Yabuki S, eds. *Progress in Lymphology XII*. Amsterdam/London/Tokyo: Elsevier; 1989:123.

14. Campisi C. Use of autologous interposition vein graft in management of lymphedema: preliminary experimental and clinical observations. *Lymphology.* 1991;24(2):71-76.
15. Campisi C. Rational approach in the management of lymphedema. *Lymphology.* 1991;24: 48-53.
16. Boccardo F, Casabona F, De Cian F, et al. Lymphedema microsurgical preventive healing approach: a new technique for primary prevention of arm lymphedema after mastectomy. *Ann Surg Oncol.* 2009;16(3):703-708.

Chapter 42
Lymphatic-Lymphatic Reconstructive Microsurgery

Ruediger G.H. Baumeister

Introduction

A direct approach to the lymphatic vessels was considered unthinkable for a long time. However, on the basis of high-power operating microscopes and increasing ability to anastomose small arteries and veins, the lymphatic vessels also became possibly suturable vessels.

Lympholymphatic anastomoses and microsurgically performed lymphovenous anastomoses using grafts were described by Cordeiro et al.[1]

In extensive experimental studies the use of lymphatic grafts for reconstruction purposes within the lymphatic vascular system and their patency could be demonstrated as well.[2]

Subsequently, lymphatic grafting was introduced into the treatment protocol for the patients with localized lymphatic interruptions, and was performed for the first time in June 1980 in Munich.[3]

Correlation With the Pathophysiology of Lymphedemas

The origin of the development of lymphedemas can be described as an imbalance between the lymphatic load and the lymphatic transport capacity.[4,5] In western countries, most jeopardized lymph transport capacity is due to surgical and/or radiation injuries. Therefore, the obstruction of the lymphatic system is limited to a localized area, mostly at the root of an extremity, e.g., in the axilla or the groin.

R.G.H. Baumeister
Professor of Surgery, the Ludwig Maximilians University, Munich, Germany
Consultant of Lymphology,
Chirurgische Klinik Muenchen Bogenhausen
Drozzaweg 6, D 81375 Muenchen, Bavaria, Germany
e-mail: baumeister@lymphtransplant.com

B.-B. Lee et al. (eds.), *Lymphedema*,
DOI 10.1007/978-0-85729-567-5_42, © Springer-Verlag London Limited 2011

For such limited interruption of the lymphatic vessels, a bypass has been considered as an option that could lead to full recovery of the reduced transport capacity because the bypass surgery has been well accepted as a viable treatment in other vascular systems with obstruction.

However, especially in advanced lymphedemas, secondary tissue damages/changes have a serious impact on the outcome of the therapy. Therefore, preferably at an early stage, after maximum conservative treatment, a reconstruction should be offered to the patient as an optional treatment to provide further improvement of the condition. Because edemas also can subside spontaneously within approximately 6 months, this time period should be used for this kind of treatment.

If the early interventional option was missed and the lymphedema accompanied heavy tissue change with fat and connective tissue deposits, an improvement in the transport capacity by reconstruction of the lymphatic interruption should be attempted first. Thereafter, further treatment to restore the original volume and shape of the extremity may be added with various invasive methods/resection including the suctioning out of the surplus tissue when indicated.

However, a great concern regarding suction is the potential risk of lymphatic tissue damage, and, therefore, it should be performed with great care to spare the lymphatics as much as possible.[6] In addition, lymphedematous tissue is quite different from normal fatty tissue, which can be sucked out in aesthetic indications. Therefore, this procedure should be named properly, with consideration of the underlying lymphatic problem, and should not be called just liposuction[7] but rather "lipo-lymphosuction" at best.

In this way, the surgical procedure follows the pathophysiology. The reconstruction of the interrupted lymphatic system is attempted first, and thereafter the sequelae of the primary cause are dealt with, the deposit of fat and connective tissue when indicated.

Experimental Basis

Reconstruction of lymphatics is based on extensive experimental investigations.[2,3]

Anastomosing procedures were tested in the rat model at the abdominal thoracic duct.

Lymphatic vessels are relatively resistant against longitudinal traction, but most fragile under oblique tension. Therefore, the "tension-free anastomosing technique" was developed. The ends of the lymphatic vessel remain in place to maintain a tension-free condition. First, the corner stitch opposite the surgeon is performed. Then, for the back wall stitches, the vessel is minimally lifted as necessary to handle the needle. The second corner stitch and the front wall are made subsequently without moving the vessel. In small lymphatic vessels, only three stitches can be applied in the same manner (Figs. 42.1–42.3).

Absorbable suture material seemed to be of advantage. Histological studies showed within several weeks almost no foreign body reactions using this material,

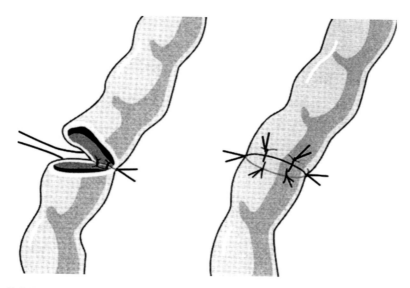

Fig. 42.1 Lympho-lymphatic end-to-end anastomoses under tension-free anastomosing technique without turning the vessel

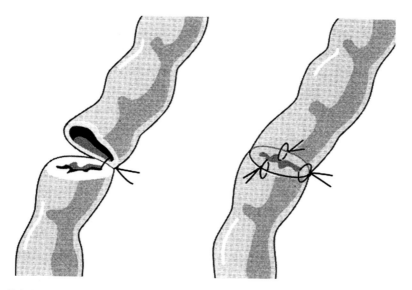

Fig. 42.2 Lympho-lymphatic end-to-end anastomoses between the graft with a thin wall and the lymph vessel with long-standing lymphedema with heavy fibrosis using three stitches

whereas non-absorbable suture material remained long after the intervention with a remarkable foreign body reaction close to the small lymphatic vessels. Therefore, we prefer absorbable suture material for the anastomoses, even though it is available only in a larger size compared with non-absorbable material.

Fig. 42.3 Lympho-lymphatic
end-to-side anastomoses

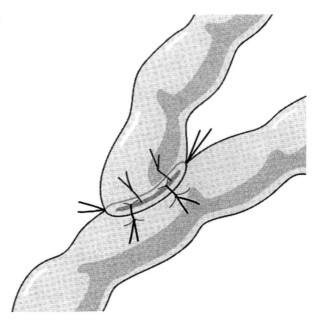

   The patency of the lympho-lymphatic anastomoses has been proved by surgical
reinterventions, direct lymphographies, patent-blue injections, and electron
microscopy.

   The rate of patency reached 100% checked by histological examinations, which
indirectly reflects that the lymphatic collectors are able to help to maintain patency
following microsurgery. The findings of the Danese et al., who only approximated
lymphatic vessels and found spontaneous communication, also support this
impression.[8]

   The patency and effect of lymphatic transplants were checked in the rat as
well as in the dog model using surgical reinterventions, direct lymphography,
dye injections, isotopic tracers, volume estimations, and intralymphatic pressure
measurements. Thereby, high patency rates and high functional benefits could
be demonstrated. After removal of the lymphatic transplant, as a control study,
the opposite effect was seen. The volume of the affected extremity immediately
increased again.

   By measuring the intralymphatic pressure, we investigated the effect of low
molecular dextran as well. We documented an increase in the pressure and assumed
it to be an effect of flushing through the newly created anastomoses. Therefore, we
also administer this or similar drugs to the patients for several days after the intervention to keep increased lymph flow through the anastomoses.

   Also, we compared different materials like autogenic veins, allogeneic lymphatics, small PTFE grafts, together with autogenous lymphatic grafts. This showed the
clear superiority of autologous lymphatic grafts. This was confirmed in a study of
the canine model by Yuwono.[9]

Indications for Lymphatic Reconstruction Using Lymphatic Grafts

Secondary lymphedemas due to a locally interrupted lymphatic system are the main indication for lymphatic grafting.[10,11]

Arm edemas after axillary node dissection are a predominant form of chronic lymphedema in the countries outside the tropical region and are those mostly treated in our series.

Leg edema after the interventions in the inguinal or pelvic region is also common in developed countries generally as unilateral lymphedema. This iatrogenic condition can also be treated by transposing the lymphatic vessels from the healthy to the affected side. One leg has to serve as the harvesting side.

In primary lymphedemas, a selected group with unilateral atresias of the inguinal and/or pelvic region can be treated by lymphatic grafting as well.

In cases with a history of malignancies, the patient must be tested to be tumor-free.

Since the burden of surgery is comparable to that of venous interventions in the subcutaneous tissue, there is almost no known general restriction for this type of surgery.

Each patient should report adequate conservative treatment before the surgery of at least 6 months' duration. During that time period, spontaneous regression of the edema is also reported.

Therefore, before the reconstructive surgery is performed, the patient has to get a complete set of lymphatic decongestion therapy, including manual lymphatic drainage, elastic stockings, and compression bandage therapy for at least half a year.

Operative Technique

The grafts are harvested from the medial aspect of the thigh (Fig. 42.4). As many as 16 lymphatic vessels can be found within the ventromedial bundle. About one to three vessels are used as grafts, but should be harvested with caution avoiding the narrowing portions of the lymphatic system at the groin and at the knee region.

The lymph nodes at the knee region as well as the groin are not touched or removed to spare the lymphatic system as much as possible.

The number of lymphatic collectors, used for grafting, is sufficient for reconstructive purposes, since anatomical studies also showed that only one preserved lymphatic collector of the long lateral bundle of the upper arm is able to prevent a patient after axillary node dissection from developing arm edema.[12]

To facilitate the preparation, about 15 min before the incision, Patent blue® is injected subdermally into the first to second web space. The joints are moved to improve the transport of the dye.

The incision is started medial to the palpable vessels beneath the inguinal ligament. The incision is extended distally step-by-step following the direction of the stained vessels.

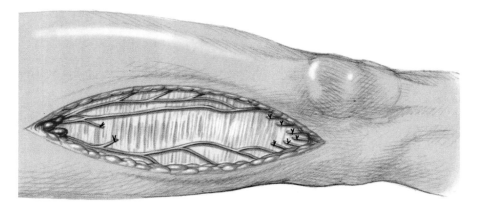

Fig. 42.4 Harvesting lymphatic vessels from the patient's thigh

Also, the ramifications of the main lymphatic collectors can be saved to use for anastomosing purposes. Therefore, more lympho-lymphatic anastomoses can be performed at the affected extremity as the equivalent of the number of the harvested main collectors. For safety reasons, it is necessary that stained lymphatic vessels also remain untouched.

Depending on the length of the thigh, the grafts can be harvested up to a length of about 30 cm. The grafts are secured at the proximal end with 6–0 sutures and transected proximally and distally. Distally on the transected side, the proximal ends of incoming lymphatic vessels are ligated to avoid lymphatic leakages.

In arm edemas (Fig. 42.5), an oblique incision is performed at the inner aspect of the upper arm. Under the microscope, the tissue is searched for lymphatic vessels. Since the transport of dye is disturbed in lymphedema, no staining is performed.

At the neck, an oblique incision is made at the dorsal rim of the sternocleidomastoid muscle. Prior to this step, a dye injection is performed cranial to the ear to enhance the chance of dyeing the lymphatic vessels at the neck. Behind the muscle up to the lateral border of the internal jugular vein, thin-walled lymphatic vessels can be found. Often, it is easier to prepare several lymph nodes.

In between the incisions at the upper arm and the neck, a tunnel is created by blunt dissection, and a silicon tube is temporarily inserted, and with its help, the grafts are pulled through. Finally, the tube is removed, and the grafts lie in the subcutaneous tissue without friction.

The anastomoses are performed under the "tension-free" anastomosing technique in an end-to-end or end-to-side fashion with 10–0 absorbable suture material. In the neck region lympho-lymphonodular anastomoses can also be performed.

In unilateral lymphedema of the lower extremities (Fig. 42.6), the grafts remain attached to the inguinal lymph nodes on the harvesting side. Ascending lymphatics are dissected via an incision below the inguinal ligament on the affected side. The grafts are placed in a technique similar to that in arm edemas. After microsurgical lympho-lymphatic anastomosing, the lymph flows via the grafts to the healthy side.

Fig. 42.5 Bridging a
lymphatic gap at the axilla
with autogenous lymphatic
vessels by lympho-lymphatic
anastomoses at the upper arm
and the neck

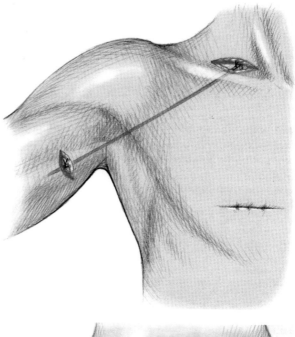

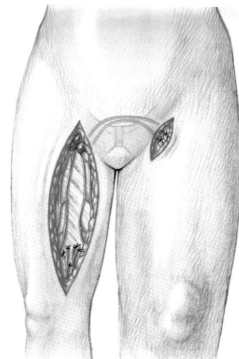

Fig. 42.6 Lymphatic grafting in unilateral
lymphedema of lower extremities; the
grafts remain attached to the inguinal
lymph nodes

In penile and scrotal edemas with at least one edema-free leg, short lymphatic collectors, remaining attached to the inguinal lymph nodes can be anastomosed with draining lymphatic vessels at the route of the penis and the scrotum.

Post-operative Procedures

The limbs are elevated, and bed rest is recommended for 3 days. For about 5 days, antibiotics are given, and infusions of low molecular dextran or HAES are administered. Elastic bandaging is applied, and elastic stockings should be worn for 6 months. In addition, a prophylaxis against erysipelas is recommended for the same time period. Thereafter, we try to discontinue the additional therapy.

Results

In patients, follow-up studies included volume measurement of the affected extremity as well as of the harvesting area, lymphoscintigraphic studies, quality of life interrogations; more invasive procedures like indirect lymphographies using water soluble contrast medium and MRI lymphographies using gadolinium are undertaken among selected patients.[11,13]

As complications, one patient developed a lymph cyst at the groin that was treated with puncture drainage. One patient developed a swelling of the lower leg due to the venous thrombosis and two patients showed postoperative erysipelas in the first series of our patients prior to the routine post-operative administration of antibiotics.

Starting in June 1980 and continuing until January 2009, a total of 329 patients were treated: 187 suffered from arm edemas, 132 from leg edemas, and 10 from scrotal and penile lymphedema.

In arm edemas as well as in leg edemas, more than 60% of the patients showed a reduction in volume difference to the healthy side of more than 50% after a mean follow-up period of more than 2 years.

In 100 arm edemas after a follow-up of more than 1 year a significant reduction in volume from $3,234 \pm 78$ cm^3 to $2,597 \pm 66$ cm^3 compared with a volume of the healthy contralateral arm of $2,181 \pm 46$ ($p < 0.001$) was demonstrated.

Follow-up in arm edemas up to at least 10 years also showed a significant reduction after this long period of time (mean volumes: $2,918 \pm 141$–$2,243 \pm 147$ cm^3 compared with $1,890 \pm 88$ cm^3 in the healthy arm).

The patency of the graft was confirmed in an indirect way via lymphoscintigraphy.[13] In arm edemas, the route of the grafts was able to track down along the visible tracts of the tracer activity, whereas no such activity has been found prior to the transplantation. In edemas of the lower extremities, the radioactive tracer activity was able to be tracked toward the contralateral groin where the transposed cross-over grafts remained attached to the nodes following the injection of radiotracer only to the affected limb.

The proof of long-term patency was also possible after more than 10 years with indirect lymphography in the upper and lower extremities, and more than 7 years with MRI lymphoscintigraphies in the lower extremities.

Lymphoscintigraphy also enabled us to calculate the overall function of the lymphatic system of an extremity.[14,15]

The lymphatic transport index was also feasible to estimate the function of the graft.[13] Hereby, the investigators of the department of nuclear medicine summarized the findings as a score between 0 and 45:0 for the best and 45 for the worst outflow. The difference between normal and pathological status is calculated based on the transport index of 10.

A follow-up study within 7 years showed a score of 10 in the group with a clearly visible activity of the transplants, which means it reached the value of a normal lymphatic outflow. Since the decrease in limb volume runs parallel to the improvement shown on lymphoscintigraphy, it suggests a potential chance for a cure and freedom from further additional treatment.[15]

In long-standing lymphedemas with excess accumulation of adipose and fibrous tissue, additional removal of surplus tissue with lymphatic sparing suction might be added to get closer to the condition/shape of the healthy extremity without continuous treatment.

References

1. Cordeiro AK, Bracat FF, Al Assal F. Transplantation of lymphatic ducts, preliminary and experimental report. In: Abstract VII Congress of Lymphology Florence; 1979.
2. Baumeister RGH, Seifert J, Wiebecke B. Transplantation of lymph vessels on rats as well as a first therapeutic application on the experimental lymphedema of the dog. *Eur Surg Res.* 1980;12(suppl 2):7.
3. Baumeister RGH, Seifert J, Wiebecke B, Hahn D. Experimental basis and first application of clinical lymphvessel transplantation of secondary lymphedema. *World J Surg.* 1981;5:401-407.
4. Földi M. Physiologie des Lymphgefäßsystems. *Angiologica.* 1971;8:212.
5. Földi M, Földi E. Physiology and pathophysiology of the lymphatic system. In: Földi M, Földi E, eds. *Földi's Textbook of Lymphology.* 2nd ed. Munich: Mosby/Elsevier; 2006.
6. Frick A, Hoffmann JN, Baumeister RGH, Putz R. Liposuction technique and lymphatic lesions in lower legs – anatomic study to reduce risks. *Plast Reconstr. Surg.* 1999;103:1868-1873
7. Brorson H, Svensson H. Complete reduction of lymphedema of the arm by liposuction after breast cancer. *Scand J Plast Reconstr Surg Hand Surg.* 1997;31:137-143.
8. Danese C, Bower R, Howard J. Experimental anastomosis of lymphatics. *Arch Surg.* 1962;84:24.
9. Yuwono HS, Klopper PJ. Comparison of lymphatic and venous interpositional autografts in experimental microsurgery of the canine lymphatics. *Plast Reconstr Surg.* 1990;86:752-757.
10. Baumeister RG, Siuda S. Treatment of lymphedemas by microsurgical lymphatic grafting: what is proved? *Plast Reconstr Surg.* 1990;85:64-74.
11. Baumeister RGH, Frick A. Die mikrochirurgische Lymphgefäßtransplantation. *Handchir Mikrochir Plast Chir.* 2003;35:202-209.
12. Kubik S. Zur klinischen Anatomie des Lymphsystems. *Verh Anat Ges.* 1975;69:109-116.

13. Kleinhans E, Baumeister RGH, Hahn D, Siuda S, Buell U, Moser E. Evaluation of transport kinetics in lymphoscintigraphy: follow-up study in patients with transplanted lymphatic vessels. *Eur J Nucl Med*. 1985;10:349-352.
14. Notohamiprodjo M, Baumeister RG, Jakobs TF, et al. MR-lymphangiography at 3.0 T— a feasibility study. *Eur Radiol*. 2009;19(11):2771-2778. Epub Jun 6, 2009.
15. Weiss M, Baumeister RGH, Hahn D. Post-therapeutic lymphedema: scintigraphy before and after autologous lymph vessel transplantation 8 years of long term follow-up. *Clin Nucl Med*. 2002;27(11):788-792.

Chapter 43
Lymph Node-Venous Microvascular Reconstructive Surgery: Filariasis Lymphedema

Gurusamy Manokaran

Lymphatic filariasis is one of the most chronic, incapacitating diseases; once it was believed that there was no treatment. Ancient sculptures and scriptures depict lymphatic filariasis of the lower limb and still can be seen in many temples in India. According to Manusrithi's 300 BC written in Hindu mythology it was mentioned, and some native treatments also have been mentioned. It was considered to be caused by Karma (result of sins from a previous life), but through science and technology we have been able to identify the organism and its transmission to human beings from the mosquito. Initially, a lot of medical and surgical treatments were done unsuccessfully and this disease was classified as "neglected tropical disease." Because exicisional surgery has not given good results, during the era of microvascular reconstructive surgery in 1963 Niclubowicz, Olszewski developed this nodovenal anastomosis in artificial lymphedema produced in dogs; subsequently this procedure was tried in various parts of world in human beings with lymphedema. This procedure is a surgery of choice for treatment of early lymphedema in some centers and in cases of elephantiasis before performing cyto-reductive/debulking procedures. This nodovenal anastomosis is more of a physiological procedure[1-10] and is very useful when there is a deformity or disease of the afferent lymphatics to connect to the efferent lymphatics (e.g., lymphatic filariasis, posttraumatic lymphedema, postinflammatory lymphedema). This is not useful in disease for which there is no lymphatics or lymph node (e.g., after mastectomy, after irradiation, and congenital lymphedemas).

Thus, in developed countries, where lymphedema is mainly due to mastectomy, irradiation, and congenital etiology, this procedure is not very popular, although it has been introduced in Europe.

G. Manokaran
Department of Plastic and Reconstructive Surgery and Lymphologist,
Apollo Hospitals, 21, Greams Road, Chennai, India

B.-B. Lee et al. (eds.), *Lymphedema*,
DOI 10.1007/978-0-85729-567-5_43, © Springer-Verlag London Limited 2011

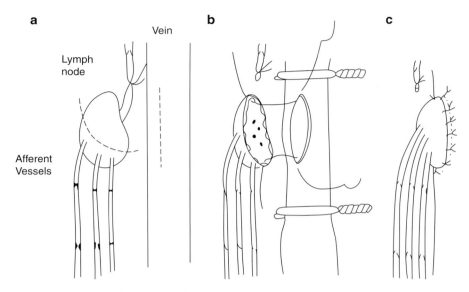

Fig. 43.1 Diagrammatic representation of a nodovenous by-pass (micro-vascular anastomosis) (**a**) vein and node showing (dotted lines) the area to be shaved (**b**) anastomosis of node-vein end to side (**c**) completion of anastomosis

NodoVenal Shunt

Indications

1. Patients with competent saphenofemoral junction.
2. Patients without inguinal abscess or sepsis.
3. All grades of lymphedema.
4. There should be a healthy and functioning lymph node (lymphoscintigraphy or ultrasound finding).

Surgical Techniques

There are two methods of anastomosis: end to end or end to side (Fig. 43.1).

End-to-End Anastomosis

Nodovenal shunting for lower limb lymphedema is carried out with the patient in a supine position under general or regional anesthesia. A vertical incision of 3 cms is made, in the upper part of the thigh just medial to the femoral pulsations, and the long saphenous vein or a good caliber vein is exposed. Ligate the distal end with chromic catgut and the upper end is cut open like a fish mouth. There should not be any retrograde flow in the proximal segment, proving that there is no sapheno-femoral incompetence. Identify a vertical group of inguinal lymph nodes, these nodes must be reasonably big (at least 1 cm in diameter) and pink in color. No dissection is performed around the lymph node so that both afferent and efferent lymphatics are preserved. Shave the upper capsule of the lymph nodes and you can see the lymph ooze from the cut surface. Avoid using diathermy; if it is urgently needed use bipolar diathermy, so that it causes less damage to the surroundings. Anastomose the proximally cut long saphenous vein to the cut surface of the capsule of the node using 6-0 or 7-0 nylon continuous suture. Then the wound is closed in layers after perfect hemostasis. No drain is required.

End-to-Side Anastomosis

A nodovenal shunt can be placed end-to-side also. In this method a vertical stab incision of 0.5–1 cm is made, depending upon the vein caliber, with an 11-sized blade. The stab incision is made after applying vascular clamps proximally and distally and the cut surface of the node is anastomosed with the vertical stab incision into the vein using 8-0 nylon, interrupted sutures. Clamps are released and observed for filling of the vein. Continuous irrigation of the anastomosis site with heparinized saline should be performed because clot formation is common with this technique. When there is no healthy or reasonable sized lymph node in the inguinal region, multiple lymphatic channels can be buried into the continuous vein at three or four places. The open end of the lymphatics are left in the venous lumen to float (use an 18-gauge needle to stab); lymphatic vessels are anchored with 8–0 nylon as a single suture. This technique is known as lymphatic venous anastomosis.

Contraindications

1. No visible lymph node in lymphoscintigraphy or in ultrasound
2. Associated varicose veins or sapheno-femoral incompetence
3. No reduction of circumferential measurements of the leg at any given point, even after 6 days of MLD (manual lymph drainage)
4. Acute ADL (adeno-dermo-lymphangitis)
5. Elderly patients
6. Associated medical diseases

Complications

1. Seroma
2. Lymphorrohea
3. Lymphocele
4. Wound dehiscence

Free Omental Transfer[11,12]

This procedure is carried out in lymphatic filariasis, post-traumatic, and postsurgical lymphedemas. In lymphatic filariasis with lower limb lymphedemas, through a vertical, upper thigh mid-line incision, the GSV, superficial circumflex iliac artery, and the inguinal lymph nodes or lymphatics are exposed and prepared for microvascular anastomosis. The abdomen is opened with a lower transverse incision and the omentum is dissected with its artery, vein, and lymphatics, which can be anastomosed with the respective artery, vein, and lymphatics. A small window during the closure of the thigh incision is left open for assessment of the viability of the omentum, which can be closed secondarily. The abdomen is closed in layers after perfect hemostasis.

The tunneling of the omentum into the inguinal region (omentoplasty), was initially popular with Russian surgeons in the management of various types of lymphedemas, but was subsequently abandoned, because of the increased incidence of lymphangitis of the leg, leading to peritonitis as the omentum was kept in continuity. Surgery for lymphedema should not cause mortality, although a certain amount of morbidity is acceptable.

References

1. Campisi C, Boccardo F. Microsurgical techniques for lymphedema treatment: derivative lymphatic-venous microsurgery. *World J Surg*. 2004;28(6):609-613.
2. Clodius L, Piller NB, Casley-Smith JR. The problems of lymphatic microsurgery for lymphedema. *Lymphology*. 1981;14(2):69-76.
3. Olszewski WL. The treatment of lymphedema of the extremities with microsurgical lymphovenous anastomoses. *Int Angiol*. 1988;7(4):312-321.
4. Gloviczki P. Microsurgical lymphovenous anastomosis for treatment of lymphedema: a critical review. *J Vasc Surg*. 1988;7(5):647-652.
5. Gloviczki P. The natural history of microsurgical lymphovenous anastomoses: an experimental study. *J Vasc Surg*. 1986;4(2):148-156.
6. Zolotorevskii VIa. Late results of lymphovenous anastomoses in lymphedema of the lower extremities. *Khirurgiia (Mosk)*. 1990;5:96-101.
7. O'Brien BM. Long-term results after microlymphaticovenous anastomoses for the treatment of obstructive lymphedema. *Plast Reconstr Surg*. 1990;85(4):562-572.
8. Yamamoto Y. Microsurgical lymphaticovenous implantation for the treatment of chronic lymphedema. *Plast Reconstr Surg*. 1998;101(1):157-161.
9. Manokaran G. Management of genital manifestations of lymphatic filariasis. *Indian J Urol*. 2005;21(1):39-43.
10. Huang GK. Results of microsurgical lymphovenous anastomoses in lymphedema—report of 110 cases. *Langenbecks Arch Chir*. 1989;374(4):194-199.
11. Binoy C, GovardhanaRao Y, Ananthakrishnan N, Kate V, Yuvaraj J, Pani SP. Omentoplasty in the management of filarial lymphoedema. *Trans R Soc Trop Med Hyg*. 1998;92(3):317-319.
12. Goldsmith HS, de los Santos R, Beattie EJ. Relief of chronic lymphedema by omental transposition. *Ann Surg*. 1967;166:572.

Chapter 44
Lymph Nodes Transfer Microvascular Reconstructive Surgery

Corinne Becker, Gael Piquilloud, and Byung-Boong Lee

Introduction

Manual lymphatic drainage – based complex decongestive therapy has become the mainstay of chronic lymphedema management for many decades, as reviewed extensively in Chaps. 9 and 10.

Complex decongestive therapy (CDT) is now the treatment of choice regardless of the severity/clinical stage. Unfortunately, however, CDT-based management is only able to delay the progress during the treatment period; to maintain long-term control, continuous patient commitment with a lifetime pledge is mandatory.

Therefore, surgical treatment, either for curative/reconstructive or palliative/excisional purposes, has been pursued as an alternative method of controlling chronic lymphedema for decades. Indeed, reconstructive surgery in particular is theoretically optimal for restoring normal function.

Reconstructive surgery, regardless of its method, is aimed at relieving lymphatic hypertension to improve lymphatic function at best, although there is a theoretical chance of a cure when performed under ideal conditions, as reviewed in Chap. 11.

Free lymph node transplantation surgery (FLTS)[1-5] is an "indirect approach" to lymphatic reconstruction, which is relatively new compared with the "direct approach" with various lymphovenous anastomotic surgeries that were reviewed in sections of Chap. 11.

The concept of lymph node transplantation seems to be a logic approach for the reconstruction of a damaged lymph transport system after radical mastectomy/axillary lymph node dissection in particular.[1-5]

Based on extensive experimental studies,[6-8] including anatomical studies,[9] 1,000 patients with different types of lymphedema, both primary and secondary,[10,11] were treated and had excellent outcomes.[1-5]

C. Becker (✉)
Department of Academy of Surgery, Hopital Universitaire
Europeen Georges Pompidou, Paris, France and
Department of Plastic Surgery, Jouvenet Hospital, Paris, France

B.-B. Lee et al. (eds.), *Lymphedema*,
DOI 10.1007/978-0-85729-567-5_44, © Springer-Verlag London Limited 2011

Secondary Lymphedema

In developed countries, the etiology of chronic lymphedema is mostly secondary to the lymphadenectomy as a part of cancer management. Such surgical excision of the lymph nodes often is combined with postoperative radiation therapy to the lymphadenectomy site, which will result in further damage to the remaining lymph nodes and lymph-transporting system and will further jeopardize normal function. Hence, this approach to restore the lost function by replacement with normal lymph nodes is naturally a more logical approach.

The free fatty flap containing lymph nodes for lymph node transplantation provides various benefits:

- Abundant interconnections in the nodes with the venous circulation
- The germinal cells in the nodes as a critical part of the immune system
- Abundant cytokines within the fatty tissue around the nodes, promoting lymph angiogenesis

Furthermore, the dissection of postsurgical/postradiation fibrosis in the axillary or inguinal region and subsequent free fatty flap interposition improve the venous flow as well.

Lymphedema of the Arm: Upper Extremity

Indication for Node Grafting

Manual lymphatic drainage-based CDT is the mainstay of treatment to control edema. However, when the lymphedema becomes resistant to this conventional therapy, such a condition may become an indication for lymph node grafting as an additional procedure.

Preoperative evaluation warrants thorough clinical description and physical examination, and radionuclide lymphoscintigraphy, which would provide a road map for the subsequent surgery; it is mandatory to know whether there are any drainage pathways. If drainage is absent, the indication for free node transfer is established.[12,13]

Operative Technique

The same incision as for the previous adenectomy is generally sufficient to prepare the lymph node graft recipient site, but occasionally the old incision needs to be extended for appropriate preparation when severe fibrosis is involved.

The axillary region is then carefully dissected to identify the thoracic-dorsal branch, which is located distal to the branch the dorsalis muscle, is selected and prepared for the micro-anastomosis. The local thoracic nerves are neurolyzed in case neuromas develop following previous surgery and cause pain.

To harvest the nodes for grafting from the inguinal region, an incision is made above the inguinal ligament from the iliac crest to the pubic region.

The fat under the fascia cribriformis is elevated from the muscular layer in the direction of the point of emergence of the circumflex iliac vessels. This flap generally contains four to five nodes and includes neither the deep nodes nor the nodes under the inguinal ligament. The size of the flap is comparable to the size of a palm of a hand.

The flap is then imported to the graft recipient site/axillary region, where the micro-anastomosis is performed under a microscope (with 10–0 nylon). The flap is then placed along the axillary vein before closure of the wound.

The manual lymphatic drainage should be started immediately after the operation; during the postoperative 3-month period, it has to be given daily in advanced cases or every other day in mild cases to prevent lymph stasis along the graft site.

Results

The long-term results after 5 years among "less advanced" lymphedema patients, have shown complete relief of the lymphedema in 40% of the cases with a normal lymphoscintigraphy (Fig. 44.1a). In 20%, the clinical results are better than on the images of the radioisotopes. However, the overall results show 98% with improvement, and 2% with no change (Fig. 44.1b).

In the 2% with no clinical improvement following surgery, the operation did not worsen the pre-existing lymphedema.

The incidence of erysipelas also decreased drastically to 2% without any prophylactic antibiotics from 68% of all the patients presenting chronic infections.

The postoperative lymphoscintigraphy at 1 year has shown the uptake of technetium in the transplanted nodes, or the new pathways, or both (Fig. 44.2).

Longstanding lymphedema of more than 20 years shows substantial improvement, although the results are proportional to the quality of the dermis (thickness, fibrosis destruction, etc.). Even after 30 years, we can observe significant improvement, in terms of volume, quality of the skin, and infections (Fig. 44.1b).[14]

Plexopathy

An additional benefit of the free fatty flap is it can improve radiotherapy-induced pain and progressive palsy by new vascularization of the nerves. Some young patients can recover in 2 years while older patients can experience stabilization of the palsy. Occasionally, when the lymphedema disappears, tendon transfers can reinforce some movements if some of the muscles are strong enough.

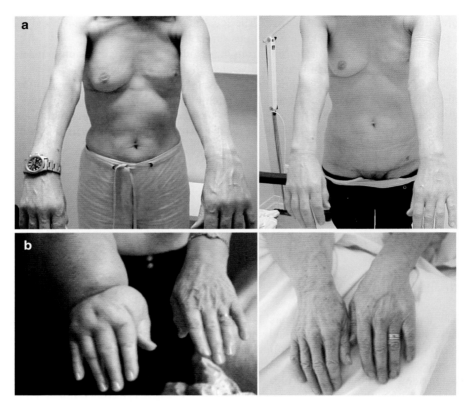

Fig. 44.1 (**a**) Moderate lymphedema involving the upper limb: preoperatively (*left*) and postoperatively 2 years (*right*). (**b**) Preoperative finding of advanced lymphedema along the right upper limb (*left*) and postoperative (4 years) finding (*right*) following lymph node transplantation, showing complete relief

The pain in the thoracic and breast region, induced by the surgery, disappears immediately after the neurolysis of those branches.[15,16]

Breast Reconstruction Combined with Lymphedema Treatment

The deep inferior epigastric perforator (DIEP) flap or even transverse rectus abdominis muscle (TRAM) flap can be elevated with some external inguinal nodes.[17]

The nodes are inserted into the previous adenectomy site, and the abdominal skin is folded to rebuild the breast. The anastomosis of the vessels of the flap (deep epigastric or superficial epigastric vessels) is performed in the axillary region, to the thoracodorsal vessels, or on the internal mammary vessels. The fibrosis in the axillary region must be dissected before implanting nodes, and if needed, epineurolysis of the brachial plexus can be added, before insertion of the nodes (Fig. 44.3).

The results are exactly identical to those obtained with only the inguinal flap.

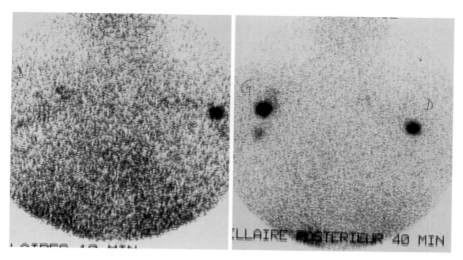

Fig. 44.2 Lymphoscintigraphic findings before (*left*) and after (*right*) lymph node transplantation to the right axilla

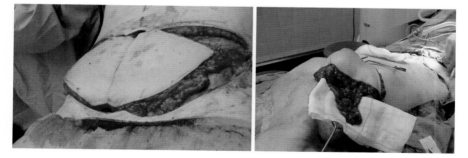

Fig. 44.3 Deep inferior epigastric perforator (DIEP) flap elevated together with internal mammary vessels (*left*), with nodes ready to implant to the adenectomy site (*right*)

Lymphedema of the Leg: Lower Extremity

The lymphadenectomy and radiotherapy in the inguinal and iliac region can induce either unilateral or bilateral leg lymphedema.

- Pelvic surgery combined with radiotherapy: extended hysterectomies, extended prostatectomy for cancer management
- Lymph node resections in the inguinal region for melanoma
- Radiotherapy and adenectomy to inguinal lymph nodes for Hodgkin's disease

The release of the fibrotic tissues followed by transplanting lymph nodes also seems a logic approach to improving the lymphedema if the cases are unilateral, so that use of the contralateral iliac drainage can be expected.

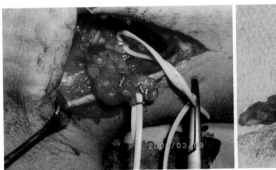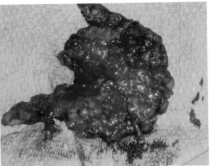

Fig. 44.4 Thoracic flap based on branches of the thoracodorsal vessels

Operative Technique

The inguinal region is opened. The scars are evaluated and all the fibrotic tissues are released. The inguinal ligament region is explored. Recipient vessels – mainly the circumflex iliac or superior epigastric vessels – are isolated for microanastomosis.[18,19]

The donor flap is obtained either from the thoracic region (90%), or the cervical region.

The thoracic flap is isolated along the thoracodorsal vessels, giving a vascularization to an average of four to five nodes, just under the branch for the dorsalis muscle. This flap does not include the nodes around the axillary vein and thus does not interfere with the drainage of the arm (Fig. 44.4).

The cervical flap depends on the branch of transverse cervical artery, and is elevated just under the sternocleidomastoid muscle (Fig. 44.5).

The flap is then elevated with the vessels and isolated to make microscopic anastomosis to the receiving/recipient vessels.

Results

The results are similar to those of the arm, but, because the pathways are longer, it takes more time to show clinical improvement. On average, the perimeter of the leg decreases 1–2 cm/month, but lymphedema with recent onset or with no radiotherapy involved is relieved more quickly.

The bandages and manual drainage are important as postoperative care, especially during the first 3 months following the surgery (Fig. 44.6). Compression stockings are also useful later to maintain the outcome when sitting or standing for a long time.

Moderately advanced lymphedema can have substantial benefit if the skin was not destroyed, and the infection rates decreases to 2% among patients with previous chronic infections.

Fig. 44.5 Cervical flap based on the transverse cervical artery

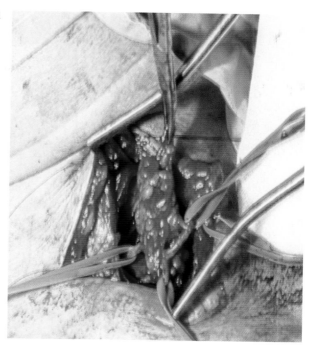

Primary Lymphedema

The principle and concept of lymph node transplantation among primary lymphedema as a clinical manifestation of (congenital) lymphatic malformation[20-23] are the same as those for secondary lymphedema. However, primary lymphedema involving the lymphatic vessels (e.g., aplasia, hypoplasia, and hyperplasia) is well known for being difficult to manage because of variations in lymphatics and lymph nodes; surgery outcomes are generally known to be variable and the procedures are generally not as effective as those seen in patients with secondary lymphedema. Depending upon the extent and severity of the defect involving lymphatic system-collecting and transporting vessels and nodes, though, the new lymph node grafting could be the optimal solution with a chance of permanent cure.

At the same time, the fatty tissue around the grafting nodes is known to contain various cytokines that induce the regeneration of lymphatic vessels. The addition of lymph nodes would help not only the lymphatic drainage of the limb, but also the overall function of the immune system.

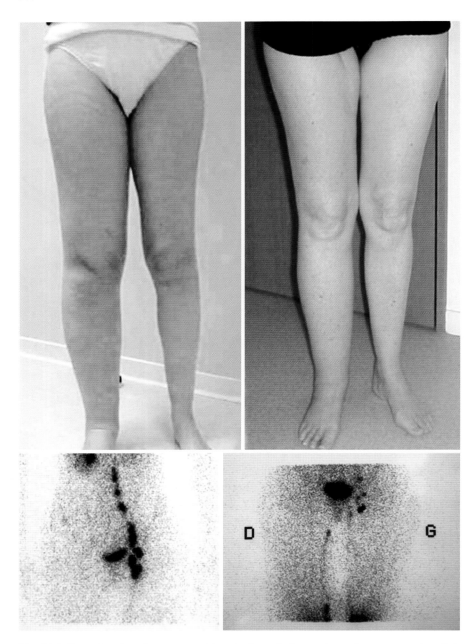

Fig. 44.6 Secondary (post-hysterectomy) lymphedema: *Left two photos* show preoperative clinical and lymphoscintigraphic findings. *Right two photos* show clinical and lymphoscintigraphic findings following the lymph node transplant in the inguinal region (1-year result)

Indications

When lymphedema appears at birth, or in the first years of life, physiotherapy is very important, but compressive bandages are often difficult for a growing child, and subsequently the skin can become thickened very early. Therefore, if the donor flap is technically feasible, and there is no additional illness, free node transplant must be carried out as soon as possible.[24,25]

If the lymphedema occurs in puberty and is resistant to conventional physiotherapy the free flap of node transplantation should be considered as soon as possible to avoid recurrent infections. If the edema involves the lower part of the leg, the flap will be placed at the knee. Combination with resection is sometimes indicated.

Operative Technique

The recipient site of the node transplantation should be chosen based on the type of lymphedema and the lymphangioscintigraphy findings.

If the whole leg is swollen, the inguinal level will be preferred to the knee level as the first site of implantation of the nodes. If the lymphedema is limited below the knee, the free flap will be inserted into the popliteal region of the knee level. For the free flap to the inguinal region, the circumflex iliac vessels are preferred for the anastomosis. However, if the flap is inserted at the knee level, the venous anastomosis is performed to one of the branches of greater saphenous vein. The donor free flap can be best harvested with the thoracic flap based on branches of the thoracodorsalis vessels, but the cervical flap is still another option when use of the thoracic flap is not feasible.

Results

For the moderately advanced lymphedema limited to below the knee level that appeared at puberty, full recovery to restore normal lymphatic function can be expected in 40%.

All other cases are improved to various degrees and the majority experience less pain and less infection. Quality of life is also improved substantially within 2 years following the surgery in the majority (Fig. 44.7).

All the patients showed a reduction in the diameter of the treated limb at 2 years postoperative follow-up assessment: 7.5 at the ankle level and 10 cm at a 10-cm higher level.

Postoperative lymphoscintigraphy showed well functioning transplanted lymph nodes with new lymph drainage pathways[26] (Fig. 44.6). The inguinal nodes, not visible before the operation, became visible in some cases as well (Fig. 44.2).

When the lymphedema is improved following node transplantation, it also brings about a substantial change in lipedema; the biopsies show normal fat.

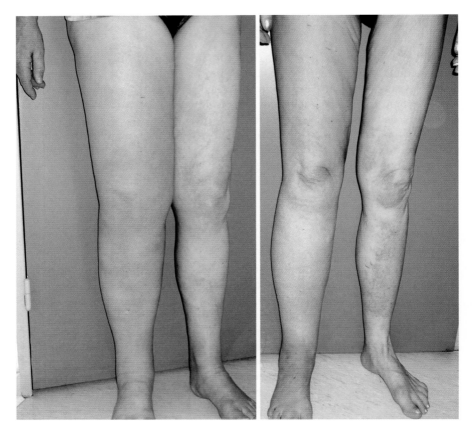

Fig. 44.7 Primary lymphedema since the age of 20 years. Pre-operative (*left*) and post-operative (1 year; *right*) clinical findings following lymph node transplantation

Conclusion

This new approach with free lymph node grafting can provide substantial benefit to either primary or secondary lymphedema. For the surgeon who is well-trained in microscopic anastomosis, the failure rate does not exceed 2% of the cases. If the lymphedema has not advanced to too fibrotic a condition, complete, or near complete, relief can be expected. This flap can be included in the DIEP or TRAM to combine lymphedema treatment with reconstruction of the breast. Complications of plexopathy can also be improved by neurolysis through this free flap surgery.

References

1. Bestian JM, Becker C, Cognet J. La transplantation ganglionnaire, traitement chirurgical des lymphoedemes. *Phlébologie*. 2007; 60(1):17-22.

2. Lee BB. Current issue in management of chronic lymphedema: personal reflection on an experience with 1065 patients commentary. *Lymphology*. 2005;38:28-31.
3. Lee BB. Surgical management of lymphedema. In: Tredbar LL, Morgan CL, Lee BB, Simonian SJ, Blondeau B, eds. *Lymphedema-Diagnosis and Treatment*. London: Springer; 2008:55-63: chap 6.
4. Becker C, Hidden G, Godart S, Maurage H, Pecking A. Free lymphatic transplantation. *Eur J Lymphology Relat Probl*. 1991;6/2:75-80.
5. Becker C, Hidden G, Maurage H, Leduc O, Cognet JM. Free lymphatic transplantation. Vth International Congress of Hand Surgery; 1992; Paris:244.
6. Becker C. Anatomie du système lymphatique du membre supérieur et conséquences thérapeutiques. *Cahier d'enseignement de la société française de la chirurgie de la main*. Elsevier; 2001;13:27-33.
7. Becker C, Hidden G. Transfer of free lymphatic flaps. Microsurgery and anatomical study. *J Mal Vasc*. 1988;13:119-122.
8. Becker C, Hidden G, Pecking A. Transplantation of lymphnodes: an alternative method for treatment of lymphoedema. *Prog Lymphology*. 1990;XI:487-493.
9. Becker C, Gilbert A. Free vascularized lymphatic node transplantation for lymphoedema. In: Tubiana R, Gilbert A, eds. *Bone and Skin Disorders*. UK: M. Dunitz; 2002:541-547.
10. Becker C. Transplantation of lymphnodes; an alternative method for treatment of lymphoedema. *Linfologia*. 1996;8:54.
11. Becker C. Treatment of lymphoedema. Questions of reconstruction of microsurgery (Russia). 2008;2(25):5-10.
12. Brun B, Becker C. Pluridisciplinary staff evaluation for treatment of lymphoedema. *Eur J Lymphology*. 2008;19(54):19-21.
13. Becker C. Traitements des lymphoedemes du membre supérieur après adénectomie et raiothérapie. *Lett Sénologue*. 2009;44:18-21.
14. Becker C, Assouad J, Riquet M, Hidden G. Postmastectomy lymphedema: long-term results following microsurgical lymph node transplantation. *Ann Surg*. 2006;243:313-315.
15. Becker C, Pham DN, Assouad J, Badia A, Foucault C, Riquet M. Postmastectomy neuropathic pain: results of microsurgical lymph nodes transplantation. *Breast*. 2008;17:472-476.
16. Assouad J, Becker C, Riquet M. Treatment of lymphoedema combined with reconstruction of the breast. *Eur J Lymphology*. 2001;9:34.
17. Assouad J, Becker C, Hidden G, Riquet M. The cutaneo-lymph node flap of the superficial circumflex artery. *Surg Radiol Anat*. 2002;24:87-90.
18. Becker C, Becker C, Godart S, Maurage H, Pecking A. *Transferts Lymphatiques Libres*. Paris: Masson; 1995.
19. Becker C. Les transferts lymphatiques. *Ann Chir Plast Esthét*. 2000.
20. Lee BB, Kim DI, Whang JH, Lee KW. Contemporary issues in management of chronic lymphedema: personal reflection on an experience with 1065 patients. *Lymphology*. 2005 Mar;38(1):28-31.
21. Lee BB. Classification and staging of lymphedema. In: Tredbar LL, Morgan CL, Lee BB, Simonian SJ, Blondeau B, eds. *Lymphedema—Diagnosis and Treatment*. London: Springer; 2008:21-30: chap 3.
22. Lee BB, Villavicencio JL. Primary lymphedema and lymphatic malformation: Are they the two sides of the same coin? *Eur J Vasc Endovasc Surg*. 2010;39:646-653.
23. Lee BB, Andrade M, Bergan J, et al. Diagnosis and treatment of primary lymphedema: consensus document of the International Union of Phlebology (IUP)-2009. *Int Angiol*. 2010;29(5):454-470, v.
24. Becker C. The treatment of lymphoedema with free nodes transplantations. *Int Angiol*. 2000;19:114.
25. Becker C. La chirurgie du lymphoedeme, effet des greffes ganglionnaires. *e-Mém Acad Natl Chir*. 2008;7(1):55-64.
26. Bourgeois P, Munk D, Becker C. A three phase lymphoscintigraphic investigation protocol for evaluation of lower limb oedema. *Eur J Lymphology Relat Probl*. 1997;6(21):10-21.

Chapter 45
Current Dilemmas and Controversy

Byung-Boong Lee, James Laredo, and Richard F. Neville

The ideal treatment for the lymphedematous limb should restore both function and a normal cosmetic appearance regardless of its etiology. Unfortunately, it is impossible to achieve these goals with the currently available treatment modalities.[1]

Manual lymphatic drainage (MLD) – based complex decongestive therapy (CDT)[2-4] has long been accepted as the mainstay of treatment in the contemporary management of chronic lymphedema. Its clinical validity and its legitimacy is reviewed in two additional Sections VII and VIII – total 13 chapters altogether – supporting its role as the de facto leader in contemporary lymphedema management.

Because of the ease of availability and accessibility, in addition to having no risk to add "harm" to an already deranged lymphatic system, its value has been overestimated as the sole treatment modality for long-term management. Unfortunately, one crucial aspect of CDT has been neglected: "CDT is neither a panacea nor a curative method." It is only effective in slowing progression at best and never restores the lost function. This remains its Achilles heel. When CDT is discontinued, the lymphedematous condition deteriorates at a faster rate, requiring a lifetime commitment that, again, only slows progression.[5,6]

Such reliance on CDT-based therapy was partly due to the old concept that chronic lymphedema is a simple "static" condition characterized by soft tissue swelling of the affected limb/region after the blockage of the lymph-transporting/collecting system. This is the major flaw: chronic lymphedema is *not* a static condition, but is actually a steadily progressing condition independent of the efficacy of CDT.[7,8]

Chronic lymphedema is now accepted to be a "continuously changing" condition of degenerative and inflammatory processes involving the skin, lymphatics, and lymph nodes. This condition is characterized by recurrent episodes of dermato lymphoadenitis, resulting in diffuse, irreversible tissue fibrosis. What began as a

B.-B. Lee (✉)
Department of Surgery, Division of Vascular Surgery,
George Washington University School of Medicine, Washington, DC, USA

B.-B. Lee et al. (eds.), *Lymphedema*,
DOI 10.1007/978-0-85729-567-5_45, © Springer-Verlag London Limited 2011

simple phenomenon of accumulation of lymph fluid eventually becomes a disabling and distressing limb condition affecting the entire surrounding soft tissue beyond the lymphatic system.[5,7,8]

With a better understanding of the disease process, contemporary treatment of lymphedema has evolved into an approach that is focused on strategies aimed at preserving and improving quality of life for better social, functional, and psychological adaptation.[9]

The role of reconstructive lymphatic surgery has also changed in that its new, different role is to provide improvement of patient quality of life as a whole.[1,9] Various surgical treatments for curative and reconstructive purposes have been introduced throughout the last century as additional methods to control chronic lymphedema.[10-13] Detailed information regarding these surgical treatments is reviewed in other chapters.

Indeed, reconstructive surgery has been known to be the optimal treatment to restore normal lymphatic function with a chance of a "cure" of the chronic lymphedema. This treatment remains controversial mainly because of poor reproducibility and a wide variety of mixed outcomes, and these are most likely due to variation in the selection of patients and variability in the indications for treatment by different surgical teams in different countries.[14]

Among the various criteria required for successful outcome, optimal timing of the surgical procedure is the most critical. Optimal timing of surgery is important because the reconstructive surgery is only successful when performed at the "earlier" stage of chronic lymphedema, before residual lymphatic vessels are damaged by prolonged lymphatic hypertension. Injured lymphatic vessels (not yet destroyed) can be effectively rejuvenated and restored to normal function by continuous MLD-based CDT postoperatively.

Reconstructive surgery is most effective when performed in the earlier stage of lymphedema, when residual lymphatic vessels remain functionally intact with the ability to relieve lymphatic obstruction and lymph stasis after successful lymphatic reconstruction.

In contemporary practice, the majority of ideal lymphatic surgery candidates are never offered reconstructive surgery and are instead, treated with CDT decompression. When reconstructive lymphatic surgery is considered, it is often after the window of opportunity has already passed and the patient is left with an unsalvageable condition with damaged and paralyzed lymphatic vessels.

Furthermore, reconstructive lymphatic surgery requires a continuing commitment by a dedicated and experienced microsurgical team skilled at lymphovenous and lympho-lymphatic anastomosis, in order to achieve successful long-term results. Such a commitment requires significant resources that are often far beyond what is available at the majority of many capable medical centers.

Therefore, reconstructive surgery has many practical limitations and due to its time constraints, has been extremely limited to a few select patients. Although there is no doubt that it is more theoretically sound and ideal than CDT, with a definite chance of a "cure," it is still far from being a practical treatment in the day-to-day management of chronic lymphedema. Reconstructive surgery may serve as the sole treatment option in the ideal situation or as a supplemental therapy to boost CDT-based physical therapy among its poor responders.[15,16]

In reality, many medical centers only offer reconstructive surgery to patients who are poor to non-responders to conventional CDT-based treatment. CDT-based treatment is often effective in the majority of chronic lymphedema patients. The Institutional Review Board, therefore, encourages delaying surgical therapy until CDT-based therapy has been completely exhausted with no further improvement. Reconstructive surgery is often recommended by a multidisciplinary care team only after properly documenting that the patient has failed extensive CDT, and is then determined to have "treatment failure" and in addition, has experienced steady progression of the disease for preferably 2 years.

Patients in whom CDT-based therapy fails and are then considered a candidate for additional reconstructive surgical therapy, typically fall under the later parts of clinical stage II or III, based on our own experience. This stage of lymphedema is generally too advanced and is long after the ideal time period for reconstructive surgery to be curative.

Therefore, reconstructive surgery is now limited to a supplemental role in the management of lymphedema in the non- to poor-responding group of CDT patients. It is now an adjunctive treatment in the management of lymphedema along with CDT-based treatment. Both treatment modalities have mutually complementary effects. Reconstructive surgical therapy requires maintenance CDT. Therefore, the success of reconstructive surgical therapy is dependent on patient compliance with postoperative CDT.[1,16]

Patient compliance with life-long maintenance CDT is the single most important factor that directly influences the long-term results of reconstructive surgical therapy. A comprehensive treatment plan incorporating both treatment modalities as part of a multidisciplinary approach to the treatment of lymphedema, will produce the most effective results.[17]

The various modes of surgical therapy have recently been found to be more effective when combined with CDT, which is in line with the new concept of a multidisciplinary approach to the treatment of lymphedema.[18]

Clinical Experiences (Personal)

Among 1,065 lymphedema patients (131 male and 934 female; 259 primary and 806 secondary; age range 2 months to 82 years), a total of 32 patients were selected for lymphovenous anastomotic surgery (LVAS; $n = 19$ patients), and free lymph node transplant surgery (FLTS; $n = 13$ patients), during a 10 year period (January 1995 to December 2004).[5,16]

All 32 patients were selected due to failure of CDT alone to relieve intractable symptoms with various indications. Various non-invasive tests including lymphoscintigraphy were performed to determine clinical and laboratory staging in all surgical candidates.

The inclusion criteria and indications for reconstructive surgery were:

- Failure to respond to therapy at clinical stage I or II
- Progression of the disease to an advanced stage (e.g., stage I to stage II or stage II to III) in the setting of CDT-based treatment
- Chylo-reflux combined extremity lymphedema
- High recurrence of local and systemic infection
- Poor tolerance to CDT-based conservative treatment

We NEVER initiated surgery as the primary mode of therapy. We selected the various reconstructive surgical therapies as supplemental treatment.

For lymphovenous anastomotic surgery (LVAS), candidates were offered surgery when CDT-based treatment failed or when it was not sufficient to prevent the rapid progression of the disease: clinical stage I to II, or early stage II to late stage II.

All patients selected met all the inclusion criteria for this additional treatment, particularly among the "secondary" lymphedema patients. Nineteen patients (mean age 49 years; female = 18, male = 1; primary = 4, secondary = 15) underwent a minimum of 3–4 anastomoses between healthy, well-functioning collecting lymph vessels and competent branches of the saphenous vein.

At 6 months, 16 out of 19 LVAS patients with good compliance to maintain postoperative MLD/compression therapy had clinically satisfactory improvement, while the other non-compliant 3 failed. At 24 months, 8 out of 16 were compliant and 8 were not. The non-compliant patients showed progressive deterioration, while the compliant patients maintained their improvement.

At 48 months, 2 out of the 8 compliant patients dropped out. Three of the remaining 6 maintained satisfactory clinical and lymphoscintigraphic improvement.

For free lymph node transplant surgery (FLTS), candidates were selected based on the same indications as for LVAS, but preferably for "primary" lymphedema with progress from clinical stage II to III. Thirteen patients (mean age 34 years, female = 10, male = 3; primary = 6, secondary = 7) at clinical stage II or III underwent FLTS using a microsurgical free grafting technique when LVAS could not be performed.

At 12 months, 10 of the 13 FLTS patients with good compliance to MLD showed clinical improvement with a successful graft, but the remaining 2 with poor compliance with the MLD failed.

At 24 months, 8 patients were compliant and 5 were not. Compliant patients maintained clinical improvement while the remaining non-compliant patients showed progressive deterioration.

Conclusion

Reconstructive surgery is a viable option in the management of chronic lymphedema. Postoperative CDT and/or compression therapy is required as supplemental therapy in the group of poor responders to CDT. It is more crucial when instituted at a less ideal/later stage of lymphedema.

Long-term maintenance of satisfactory clinical improvement following the surgical therapy to this less ideal group in particular is totally dependent on the patient's "compliance" in maintaining postoperative CDT/compression therapy.

References

1. Lee BB. Chronic lymphedema, no more step child to modern medicine! *Eur J Lymphology.* 2004;14(42):6-12.
2. Leduc O, Bourgeois P, Leduc A. Manual of lymphatic drainage: scintigraphic demonstration of its efficacy on colloidal protein reabsorption. In: Partsch H, ed. *Progress in Lymphology IX.* Amsterdam: Elsevier/Excerpta Medica; 1988.
3. Hwang JH, Kwon JY, Lee KW, et al. Changes in lymphatic function after complex physical therapy for lymphedema. *Lymphology.* 1999;32:15-21.
4. Foldi E, Foldi M, Weissletter H. Conservative treatment of lymphedema of the limbs. *Angiology.* 1985;36:171-180.
5. Lee BB, Kim DI, Whang JH, Lee KW. Contemporary management of chronic lymphedema – personal experiences. *Lymphology.* 2002;35(suppl):450-455.
6. Hwang JH, Lee KW, Chang DY, et al. Complex physical therapy for lymphedema. *J Kor Acad Rehabil Med.* 1998;22:224-229.
7. Olszewski WL. Episodic dermatolymphangioadenitis (DLA) in patients with lymphedema of the lower extremities before and after administration of benzathine penicillin: a preliminary study. *Lymphology.* 1996;29:126-131.
8. Choi JY, Hwang JH, Park JM, et al. Risk assessment of dermatolymphangioadenitis by lymphoscintigraphy in patients with lower extremity lymphedema. *Korean J Nucl Med.* 1999; 33(2):143-151.
9. Lee BB, Bergan JJ. New clinical and laboratory staging systems to improve management of chronic lymphedema. *Lymphology.* 2005;38(3):122-129.
10. Baumeister RGH, Siuda S. Treatment of lymphedemas by microsurgical lymphatic grafting: What is proved? *Plast Reconstr Surg.* 1990;85:64-74.
11. Becker C, Hidden G, Godart S et al. Free lymphatic transplant. *Eur J Lymphol.* 1991;6:75-80.
12. Krylov VS, Milanov NO, Abalmasov KG, Sandrikov VA, Sadovnikov VI. Reconstructive microsurgery in treatment of lymphoedema in extremities. *Int Angiol.* 1985;4(2):171-175.
13. Campisi C, Boccardo F, Zilli A, Maccio A, Napoli F. Long-term results after lymphatic-venous anastomoses for the treatment of obstructive lymphedema. *Microsurgery.* 2001;21(4): 135-139.
14. Gloviczki P. Review. Principles of surgical treatment of chronic lymphoedema. *Int Angiol.* 1999;18(1):42-46.
15. Gloviczki P, Fisher J, Hollier LH, Pairolero PC, Schirger A, Wahner HW. Microsurgical lymphovenous anastomosis for treatment of lymphedema: a critical review. *J Vasc Surg.* 1988; 7(5):647-652.
16. Lee BB. Current issue in management of chronic lymphedema: personal reflection on an experience with 1065 patients. *Lymphology.* 2005;38:28.
17. Lee BB. Surgical management of lymphedema. In: Tredbar LL, Morgan CL, Lee BB, Simonian SJ, Blondeau B, eds. *Lymphedema—Diagnosis and Treatment.* London: Springer; 2008:55-63, chap 6.
18. Lee BB, Kim YW, Kim DI, Hwang JH, Laredo J, Neville R. Supplemental surgical treatment to end stage (stage IV –V) of chronic lymphedema. *Int Angiol.* 2008;27(5):389-395.

Chapter 46
Prospects for Lymphatic Reconstructive Surgery

Victor S. Krylov

To get a better prospect of reconstructive microlymphatic surgery we need further improvement of the diagnosis and use of the appropriate classification. The most useful practical classification allows us to divide all lymphatic disorders into primary and secondary.

Primary lymphatic insufficiency, which is of hereditary origin, cannot be successfully cured with reconstructive microsurgery. The creation of the new lymphatic vessels in congenital cases is a matter for the future. Genetic research in this field will hopefully yield valuable information for future practical use.[1]

Secondary lymphatic insufficiency assumes that before the damage or disease occurred, the patient had a normal lymphatic system. In many cases the damage can be corrected with the help of modern reconstructive microsurgery.

We also have to keep in mind that contemporary conservative treatment, when properly indicated and carried out, such as well-organized and systematized manual lymphatic drainage,[2] must be tried first, before the patient is offered any reconstructive surgery. Today, only 20–25% of patients with secondary lymphedema can benefit from modern reconstructive microsurgery of the lymphatic system. The remaining 75–80% of the patients are candidates for conservative palliation, which, if carried out thoroughly enough and with the cooperation of the patient, can offer a quite tolerable quality of life.[3,4]

The lack of a system in manual lymphatic drainage considerably discredits the conservative treatment, which is sometimes the only hope for the patient.

Lymphatico-venous anastomosis – the microsurgical operation of the direct junction of the lymphatic vessel to the adjacent systemic vein – has been in practice since the late 1970s[5] and now can offer up to 83–87%[6] of properly selected patients stable benefit through reduction, or full elimination, of the edema or cessation of the erysipelas (cellulitis).

V.S. Krylov
Vascular Research Laboratory, Department of Surgery, University of Tennessee,
Graduate School of Medicine, Knoxville, TN, USA

B.-B. Lee et al. (eds.), *Lymphedema*,
DOI 10.1007/978-0-85729-567-5_46, © Springer-Verlag London Limited 2011

Sometimes the situation during surgery does not allow the creation of the direct anastomosis between the lymphatic vessel and the systemic vein. In these case such maneuvers like interposition of the auto-vein graft is a very important innovation, which will to improve results considerably. The auto-vein interposition technique provides a connection between the afferent lymphatic vessels, bringing the lymph from the extremity with the outflow tract – either the adjacent vein or the efferent lymphatic vessels, or the lymph node.[7] Using this technique today can improve remote results by offering subjective improvement in 87% of the patients and objective improvement in 83%. Reduction of 67% of the excess volume in the extremity was achieved with this technique. In 87% of the patients there were no new episodes of erysipelas. This perspective of technical innovation, interposition of the vein between two lymphatic vessels, or connection of the lymph vessel with the vein, makes it possible to overcome technical difficulties in many cases. Both microsurgical techniques are prospective and progress is only limited by organizational difficulties.

Microsurgery is one of the highly specialized parts of today's surgery and we cannot expect the required facilities to be available everywhere. Because microsurgical technique requires the surgeon to maintain an appropriate level of training – so-called technical optimum – it is not currently used as widely as it deserves. Future development and refinement of this technique can be accomplished in the centers where these operations are performed often. This can significantly improve the results, even at the present level of the diagnostic and surgical technique.

The most common reason for secondary lymphedema is the treatment of breast cancer. One promising technique to prevent secondary lymphedema after treatment for breast cancer has been suggested. This suggested technique consists of not blocking the lymph outflow after axillary dissection and performing prophylactic creation of the lymphovenous anastomosis using the afferent lymphatic vessels in the axillary area during the primary cancer operation.[8]

This direction in reconstructive microlymphatic surgery is very significant, considering the number of patients suffering with breast cancer.

The situation after treatment of breast cancer is characterized not only by the lesion of the lymphatic vessels and lymph nodes, but often by the involvement of the venous system. This may be characterized by stenosis and/or occlusion of the axillary vein with corresponding venous hypertension and also by involvement of the brachial plexus (radiation plexitis). Sometimes there is also radiation dermatitis in a region of the clavicle. The lesion is called "postmastectomy syndrome"[9] and correction of the lymphatic insufficiency in such a case is indicated only after correction of the venous hypertension.

In some cases, intervention on the brachial plexus (microsurgical endoneurolysis)[10] and excision of damaged skin and radiation ulcers with subsequent free flap transfer could also be indicated. In this area, the composite free flap is often the best solution. For instance, after the brachial plexus neurolysis combined with the excision of the skin (radiation dermatitis), the nerve trunks can be successfully covered with the greater omentum free flap, and the flap itself is covered with the split skin graft (Fig. 46.1).

One important question remains unsolved in the literature – how stable are the remote results of the lymphatico-venous reconstruction? To get the stable and

Fig. 46.1 Lymphogram with contrast media showing the transport of the lymph through the free flap with the lymph node (original picture)

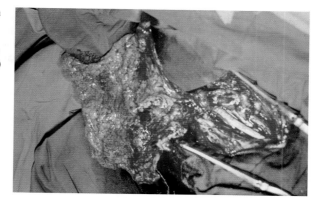

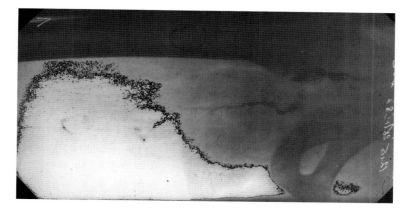

Fig. 46.2 Greater omentum free flap is vascularized in the axillary area to cover the trunks of the brachial plexus after microsurgical endoneurolysis (personal observation)

long-lasting function of the LVA there must be a pressure gradient between the lymphatic vessel and the adjacent vein. When there is successful functioning of the anastomosis, the pressure gradient is decreased and theoretically we must assume that when the gradient falls to zero the flux of the lymph from the lymph vessel into the vein will stop.

There is also another possible outcome, which is the reverse flow of the blood from the vein into the lymph vessel followed by thrombosis of the anastomosis.

Research must be continued in order to study the remote results of the lympho-venous reconstructive microsurgery.

Microsurgical reconstructive operations on the lymph nodes, a very prospective direction in the reconstructive lymphatic microsurgery, has its own history. The first attempts to transfer the lymphatic nodes were made in the hope of helping patients with primary lymphedema of the lower extremity and the lymph nodes were taken as part of the free flap of the greater omentum (Fig. 46.2).[5]

Later, a free transplantation of the lymph node was successfully reported by a few authors.[11] The transplantation of the lymphatic nodes is best accomplished by forming the flap of the tissue with the incorporation of one or several lymphatic nodes. The greater omentum can be considered the most reliable and safe. The laparotomy in this case can be minimal with a very low postoperative complication rate.

In conclusion, as conservative treatment of lymphedema offers only temporary palliation, there is no alternative to the radical approach, namely, reconstructive microsurgical intervention, which already helps more than 80% of the patients with secondary lymphedema with good remote results. Preventive microsurgical operations can significantly improve the remote results.

References

1. Bellini C, Witte MH, Campisi C, Bonioli E, Boccardo F. Congenital lymphatic dysplasias: genetics review and resources for the lymphologist. *Lymphology*. 2009;42(1):36-41.
2. Foldi M. *Foldi's "Textbook of Lymphology"*. 2nd ed. Munchen: Elsevier; 2006.
3. Boccardo FM, Ansaldi F, Bellini C, et al. Prospective evaluation of a prevention protocol for lymphedema following surgery for breast cancer. *Lymphology*. 2009;42(1):1-9.
4. Campisi C, Davini D, Bellini C, et al. Is there a role for microsurgery in the prevention of arm lymphedema secondary to breast cancer treatment? *Microsurgery*. 2006;26(1):70-72.
5. Abalmasov KG. *Microsurgery and plastic surgery* (point of view). In: Microsurgery in Russia ed. Krylov VS. Geotar Moscow, 2005;189-263.
6. Campisi C, Eretta C, Pertile D, et al. Microsurgery for treatment of peripheral lymphedema: long-term outcome and future perspectives. *Microsurgery*. 2007;27(4):333-338.
7. Campisi C, Davini D, Bellini C, et al. Lymphatic microsurgery for the treatment of lymphedema. *Microsurgery*. 2006;26(1):65-69.
8. Boccardo F, Casabona F, De Cian F, et al. Lymphedema microsurgical preventive healing approach: a new technique for primary prevention of arm lymphedema after mastectomy. *Ann Surg Oncol*. 2009;16(3):703-708.
9. Milanov NO. *Postmastectomy Syndrome and Its Surgical Correction* [doctoral dissertation]. Moscow; 1984. In: Microsurgery in Russia CD disc. Moscow Geotar, 2005.
10. Becker C, Pham DN, Assouad J, Badia A, Foucault C, Riquet M. Postmastectomy neuropathic pain: results of microsurgical lymph nodes transplantation. *Breast*. 2008;17(5):472-476.
11. Becker C, Assouad J, Riquet M, Hidden G. Postmastectomy lymphedema: long-term results following microsurgical lymph node transplantation. *Ann Surg*. 2006;243(3):313-315.

Part X
Surgical Treatment: Excisional/Cytoreductive Surgery

Chapter 47
Historical Background – General Overview

Waldemar L. Olszewski

Introduction

Over the last 200 years, not to mention in more ancient times, the Charles procedure, the buried dermal flap, and the staged subcutaneous excision beneath flaps
were the main surgical options for advanced stages of lymphedema of the lower
limbs.[1-11] Classic operations such as total denuding of the limb down to the fascia
and covering with epidermal grafts turned out to be unsatisfactory because of acute
infections of the remaining foot skin, epidermal ulcerations, and plasma leakage
from the uncovered surfaces. So far, the subcutaneous excision beneath skin flaps
has offered the most reliable and consistently beneficial means of surgically
decreasing the size of a limb and controlling recurrences of infective episodes, as
shown in Fig. 47.1.

The Morphological Changes in Advanced Lymphedema

Morphological changes include (a) hyperkeratosis and fibrosis of the skin,
(b) fibrosis of the subcutaneous tissue, (c) lack of lymphatic channels with formation of numerous tissue fluid lakes (Fig. 47.2), (d) fibrosis of inguinal lymph nodes,
(e) growth of fat tissue, (f) tissue fluid subepidermal blisters with leakage,
(g) superficial skin ulcers, and (h) doubling or tripling limb weight with subsequent
destruction of the hip and knee joints.

W.L. Olszewski
Department of Surgical Research and Transplantology,
Medical Research Centre, Warsaw, Poland

B.-B. Lee et al. (eds.), *Lymphedema*,
DOI 10.1007/978-0-85729-567-5_47, © Springer-Verlag London Limited 2011

Fig. 47.1 The stage IV obstructive lymphedema of the lower limb with overgrowth of fat and fibrous tissue. It developed over a 2-year period after foot skin abrasion. Although a infrequent case in the western hemisphere, it is quite common in other parts of the world and creates a challenge for surgeons

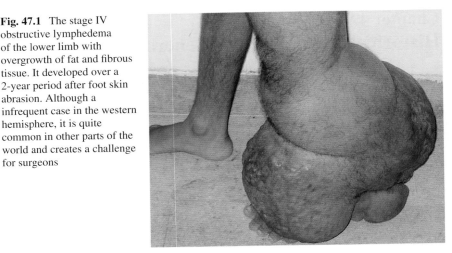

Fig. 47.2 Specimen of skin and subcutaneous tissue of 10 cm in thickness containing fibrous and fat tissue and thousands of fluid-filled blisters, some large (*arrows*). Patent Blue injected subdermally spreads around in the tissue and does not visualize lymphatics. This is proof that the lymphatics are obliterated and that the tissue-containing stagnant fluid and microbes should be removed

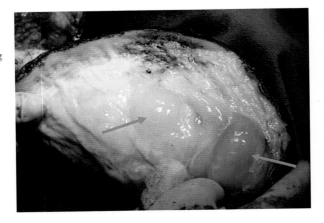

Indications for Debulking

The changes qualifying for debulking procedures, as they have evolved over the years, are (a) overall changes, as described in the section "The Morphological Changes in Advanced Lymphedema"; (b) recurrent local skin infections in the toe web, foot, and lower calf; (c) recurrent septic attacks of dermatolymphangioadenitis (DLA) of increasing frequency (>3 per year).

Bacteriology of Skin and Deep Tissues

Advanced stages of lymphedema are characterized by colonization of toe web and skin crevices by fungi and environmental bacteria. Deep tissues and tissue fluid contain a number of bacterial species. They include *S. epidermidis*, *S. aureus*,

Bacilli, Pseudomonas, Enterobacter, Enterococcus, and *Acinetobacter.*[12] Colonization of tissue requires proper antibacterial preparation before planned surgery. Frequent attacks of DLA are the consequence of colonization and limited capillary filtration of immune proteins and the cessation of immune cell extravasation. Infection of the lymphedematous tissues is an inherent factor of the disease and requires proper preoperative preparations.

Surgical Technique

Preparatory procedures: (a) Antibiotics: patients usually remain on long-term penicillin administration at a dosage of 1,200,000 IU every 3 weeks. Additionally, they should be given oral amoxicillin+clavulanic acid at a dosage of 1 g for 30 days before surgery or alternatively 1 g of ciprofloxacin as well as 0.5 g daily of oral metronidazole. This low dosage of antibiotics controls deep bacterial flora and lowers the postoperative wound infection rate. (b) Two-week limb manual massage and elevation in bed.

According to our years-long experience, surgery is divided into three stages (Fig. 47.3). (a) Lymph node–vein shunt (if lymph is oozing from the cut node) or

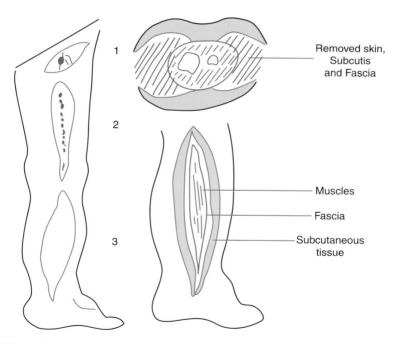

Fig. 47.3 Excisional operation in the advanced stages of lymphedema is divided into three stages. Stage 1: lymphovenous shunt or, if there is no lymph flow from the cut node, removal of fibrotic nodes and afferent lymphatics. Stage 2: excision of the obliterated lymphatics on the anterior aspect of the thigh. Stage 3: subdermal excision of the subcutaneous tissue and fascia of the calf. This procedure is routinely consecutively done on the medial, lateral, and posterior aspects of the calf. Operation stages can be combined depending on the individual situation

removal of the fibrotic inguinal lymph nodes and optionally vessels down to the knee level. (b) 3–4 weeks later, depending on the advancement of the lymphedema, surgical excision of fibrotic lymphatics down to the knee level together with a large mass of the neighboring fibrous infected tissues beneath the skin. (c) 3 months later the excision under the skin of the subcutaneous tissue with the fascia on the lateral side of the calf. (d) 3 months later the excision under the skin on the posterior side of the calf. Continuous intradermal non-absorbable suture retained for 30–40 days prevents dehiscence or later expansion of the scar. Overall, the entire procedure relies on three longitudinal excisions under the skin at the anteromedial, posterior, and lateral aspects of the calf. Note that the muscular fascia in advanced lymphedema could be 1–2 cm thick and should be removed. Skin flaps cover the denuded muscle and the wound heals up quickly. Large mass on the dorsum of the foot can also be removed subdermally. (e) Subcutaneous suction drainage, as long as there is free subdermal tissue fluid. (f) Bed-confined limb elevation. (g) Continuation of 1 g of amoxicillin+clavulanic acid or 1 g of ciprofloxacin for another month, followed later by long-lasting penicillin. (h) Elastic support (pressure grade III) after wound healing.

New elements in debulking surgery introduced by us: (a) long-term systemic antibiotic preparation (1–3 months, depending on the frequency rate of DLA episodes), (b) inguinal lymphovenous shunt or removal of fibrotic nodes and obliterated afferent lymphatics, (c) resection of redundant skin and subcutaneous tissue (with fibrotic lymphatics) beneath the skin leaving pedunculated flaps, (d) excision of fibrotic calf muscular fascia, (e) postoperative long-term low-dose antibiotics.

Postoperative complications: They include: (a) partial wound dehiscence usually at the lower end of the wound (rare), (b) wound inflammation (rare after antibiotic preparation), (c) occasionally tissue fluid leakage.

References

1. Charles RH. Elephantiasis scroti. In: Latham A, English TC, eds. *A System of Treatment*, vol. 3. London: Churchill; 1912.
2. Dellon AL, Hoopes JE. The Charles procedure for primary lymphedema. *Plast Reconstr Surg.* 1977;60:589.
3. Mavili ME, Naldoken S, Safak T. Modified Charles operation for primary fibrosclerotic lymphedema. *Lymphology.* 1994;14:20.
4. Kim DI, Huh S, Lee SJ, Lee BB. Excision of subcutaneous tissue and deep muscle fascia for advanced lymphedema. *Lymphology.* 1998;31:190-194.
5. Kondoleon E. Ultimate results of Kondoleon operation for elephantiasis. *Arch Fr Belg Chir.* 1924;27:104.
6. Sistrunk WE. Experiences with the Kondoleon operation for elephantiasis. *JAMA.* 1918;71:800.
7. Savage RC. The surgical management of lymphedema. *Surg Gynecol Obstet.* 1985;160:283-290.
8. Kobayashi MR, Miller TA. Lymphedema. *Clin Plast Surg.* 1987;14:303-313.
9. Miller TA, Wyatt LE, Rudkin GH. Staged skin and subcutaneous excision for lymphedema: a favorable report of long-term results. *Plast Reconstr Surg.* 1998;102:1486-1498.

10. van der Walt JC, Perks TJ, Zeeman BJ, Bruce-Chwatt AJ, Graewe FR. Modified Charles procedure using negative pressure dressings for primary lymphedema: a functional assessment. *Ann Plast Surg*. 2009;62:669-675.
11. Campbell W, Harkin DW. Surgical debulking in a case of chronic lymphoedema. *Ir J Med Sci*. 2009;178:227-229.
12. Olszewski WL, Jamal S, Manokaran G, et al. Bacteriologic studies of skin, tissue fluid, lymph, and lymph nodes in patients with filarial lymphedema. *Am J Trop Med Hyg*. 1997;57:7-15.

Chapter 48
General Principles

Gurusamy Manokaran

The debulking surgical procedure in lymphatic filariasis – lymphedema – is carried out in grade IV lymphedemas with nodules, warty growths, and ulcers. The basic principles in lymphedema surgery are (a) augment the lymphatic drainage using a physiological procedure, and (b) reduce the lymphatic load by debulking the lymphedematous, lymph-producing surface. In this chapter, we will be talking about our strategy for lymphedema surgery, followed by a review of the existing forms of debulking surgery.[1-16]

Our strategy for debulking is always done after establishing a lymphatic drainage procedure, namely complete decongestive therapy (CDT) for 1 week, followed by a permanent drainage surgical procedure, such as nodovenal shunt, lymphovenal shunt, free omental transfer, or *supramicrovascular surgery* of transplanting a myocutaneous flap with arterial, venous, and lymphaticolymphatic anastomosis. Once permanent lymphatic drainage is established, the huge grade IV lymphedema with or without skin changes shrinks, leaving only the subcutaneous fat, fibrous tissue, and the soft tissues like muscle and fascia. We wait for 10–14 days and then debulk the excess skin, fat, and subcutaneous tissue up to the level of the deep fascia under tourniquet control. This debulking surgery may have to be done periodically at a minimum interval of 6 weeks to 3 months, depending upon the entire size of the limb, until near normal shape and size are achieved. We try to use the same skin to resurface without using a split-thickness skin graft (STSG). The same remaining skin with subcutaneous tissues containing the subdermal lymphatics drains the reshaped limb and maintains the contour for a long time with a pressure garment, leg elevation, elimination of the focus of sepsis, and prevention of secondary infection by periodic, cyclic antibiotics like penicillin, doxycycline, and quinolones (ciprofloxacin, ofloxacin, etc.), depending upon the sensitivity pattern of the drug and patient.

G. Manokaran
Department of Plastic and Reconstructive Surgery and Lymphologist,
Apollo Hospitals, 21, Greams Road, Chennai, India

B.-B. Lee et al. (eds.), *Lymphedema,*
DOI 10.1007/978-0-85729-567-5_48, © Springer-Verlag London Limited 2011

The entire outcome of debulking surgery depends upon the methodical preoperative preparation and postoperative follow-up with the above-mentioned recommendations. If the patient does not follow the postoperative instructions meticulously, secondary infection can occur. Secondary infection leading to lymphangitis and cellulitis is the main cause of recurrence and progress of lymphedemas. This above-mentioned technique has been followed by us for the last 25 years, and we have been able to achieve very good results and maintain the shape and size of the limb in our long-term follow-ups. If any patient comes to us with recurrence or progress of the lymphedema, we repeat a lymphoscintigram and find out the status of the lymphatics, lymph nodes, and drainage. Most were found to have had repeated attacks of lymphangitis due to their negligence and experienced recurrence. We motivate these people again to meticulously follow the conservative, nonsurgical methods like manual lymphatic drainage and CDT, by which most of the patients get better and get back the original shape and size of the limb, and we maintain it with a pressure garment or bandaging techniques. Very few patients (approximately 5–6%) need a revision surgical procedure, like redoing a nodovenal or lymphaticovenous shunt.

This debulking procedure is always done under tourniquet control to avoid blood loss, hematoma, and infection. The tourniquet can be used safely for 2 h in the lower limb and 1 h in the upper limb. Once the excision is made, the tourniquet is released and perfect hemostasis secured before retaining the suction drain and closing the wound in layers. The incision is always made as a reverse hockey stick on the medial side of the limb. The edges of the skin surface are examined for viability after the excess skin has been trimmed. We always try to go through the same scar for any subsequent reduction surgeries so that patient does not have multiple unsightly scars on the limbs. The excision always stops short of the deep fascia. We never open the deep fascia because it allows the muscle to bulge into the subcutaneous plane and makes wound closure difficult, causing a lot of pain during the postoperative period and even blocking the drains.

The other debulking procedures that has been practiced for a long time is Charles excisional surgery, wherein the lymphedematous tissue (skin, subcutaneous tissue up to the fascia) is excised circumferentially and then STSG is done to cover the raw area. As there is no subdermal plexus for drainage and the STSG is stuck to the fascia, it produces much worse edema distal to the excision, usually in the foot. Because of the unaesthetic outcome and a *bottle neck deformity*, this procedure has almost been abandoned these days. The Kondolean excision is also technically similar to the Charles procedure; therefore, this technique has also almost been abandoned due to the cobble stone appearance of the operated leg (unaesthetic appearance).

Thomson's procedure was claimed to be a physiological procedure as the de-epithelialized dermal flap is buried under the opposite skin flap and sutured in two layers. The disadvantage of this procedure is that if the dermal flap sutured as a deeper layer becomes necrosed, then the skin closure will not heal. Thus, we have to re-open the flaps and salvage the necrosed skin flap and then provide skin cover. This causes morbidity to the affected limb and it takes a longer time for the leg wound to get settled.

The older techniques of debulking surgeries such as the Thomson, Kondolean and Charles procedures have been abandoned because of poor outcome. Many patients are scared to undergo surgery after seeing this unsightly results. In many of the centers where debulking surgery is performed for lymphedema, it is always carried out as a secondary procedure, following lymphatic drainage. These days simple elliptical excisions of multiple stages, following a microvascular lymphatic drainage procedure, and maintained by conservative multimodality therapies like periodic antibiotics to prevent secondary infections, regular foot hygiene, CDT, and pressure garments provide the most acceptable long-term results.

References

1. Miller TA. Charles procedure for lymphoedema: a warning. *Am J Surg.* 1980;139(2):290-292.
2. Dumanian GA, Futrell JW. Radical excision and delayed reconstruction of a lymphoedematous leg with a 15 year follow-up. *Lymphology.* 1996;29(1):20-24.
3. Revis Don R Jr. Lymphedema: treatment. http://www.lymphedemapeople.com.
4. Silkie. Complications of the Thompson's procedure. www.Lymphoedemapeople.com/wiki
5. Kondoleon E. Die Operative Behandlung der elephantiastichen Oedeme. *Zentralbl Chir.* 1912;39:1022.
6. Servelle M. Surgical treatment of lymphedema: a report on 652 cases. *Surgery.* 1987;101:484.
7. Sawhney CP. Evaluation of Thompson's buried dermal flap operation for lymphoedema of the limbs: a clinical and radioisotopic study. *Br J Plast Surg.* 1974;27:278-283.
8. Lee BB, Kim DI, Whang JH, Lee KW. Contemporary management of chronic lymphedema – personal experiences. *Lymphology.* 2002;35(Suppl):450-455.
9. Huh SH, Kim DI, Hwang JH, Lee BB. Excisional surgery in chronic advanced lymphedema. *Surg Today.* 2003;34:434-435.
10. Lee BB. Surgical management of lymphedema. In: Tredbar, Morgan, Lee, Simonian, Blondeau, eds. *Lymphedema—Diagnosis and Treatment.* London: Springer; 2008:55-63, chap 6.
11. Lee BB, Kim YW, Kim DI, Hwang JH, Laredo J, Neville R. Supplemental surgical treatment to end stage (stage IV –V) of chronic lymphedema. *Int Angiol.* 2008;27(5):389-395.
12. Auchincloss H. New operation for elephantiasis. *Puert Rico J Publ Health Trop Med.* 1930;6:149.
13. Dellon Al, Hoopes JE. The Charles procedure for primary lymphedema. *Plast Reconstr Surg.* 1977;60:589.
14. Homans J. The treatment of elephantiasis of the legs. *N Engl J Med.* 1936;215:1099.
15. Kim DI, Huh S, Lee SJ, Hwang JH, Kim YI, Lee BB. Excision of subcutaneous tissue and deep muscle fascia for advanced lymphedema. *Lymphology.* 1998;31:190-194.
16. Sistrunk WE. Further experiences with the Kondoleon operation for elephantiasis. *JAMA.* 1918;71:800.

Chapter 49
Contemporary Indications and Controversies

Byung-Boong Lee, James Laredo, and Richard F. Neville

Chronic lymphedema was once considered to be a relatively benign condition of limb swelling associated with minimal morbidity. However, this old concept has been proven to be totally erroneous; the condition is steadily progressive and affects not only the lymphatic system itself, but also the entire surrounding soft tissue, resulting in a unique condition of clinically significant dermato lipofibrosclerosis.[1,2]

Once chronic lymphedema progresses to its end stage (stages IV–V, equivalent to International Society of Lymphology (ISL) stage III),[3,4] the effectiveness and efficacy of complex decongestive therapy (CDT)[5,6] is curtailed substantially. The fibrosis of the soft tissue reduces the efficacy of CDT and the massively swollen limb becomes increasingly difficult to wrap properly with compression bandaging. The extremity is often grotesquely disfigured with a severely deformed contour (Fig. 49.1).

Chronic lymphedema becomes a disabling and distressing condition that is unresponsive to CDT. This results in frequent bacterial and fungal infections in a limb with a chronic inflammatory condition affecting the skin and soft tissue.[7,8]

Once the local/regional sepsis begins, the risk of systemic sepsis is increased and may become a potentially life-threatening condition. The chronic inflammation associated with lymphedema also predisposes patients to an immunodeficiency and wasting condition resulting in malignancies such as Kaposi sarcoma and lymphangiosarcoma.

The associated morbidity and potentially serious complications of chronic lymphedema have significant physical, psychological, social, and financial burdens that have an impact on patients' lives, resulting in poor quality of life in the advanced stage.[4] Hence, a new treatment regimen was desperately needed in an effort to prevent such a disastrous outcome.

B.-B. Lee (✉)
Department of Surgery, Division of Vascular Surgery,
George Washington University School of Medicine,
Washington, DC, USA

B.-B. Lee et al. (eds.), *Lymphedema*,
DOI 10.1007/978-0-85729-567-5_49, © Springer-Verlag London Limited 2011

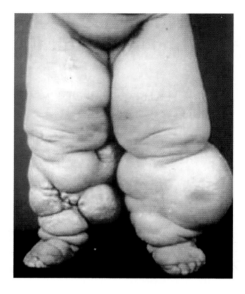

Fig. 49.1 Clinical appearance of the bilateral lower limbs with chronic lymphedema at its end stage (clinical stage III to IV) before the excisional surgery. The resection of grotesquely disfigured fibro-edematous tissue was mandated to improve complex decongestive therapy (CDT)-based management

As part of a new approach to the treatment of chronic lymphedema, various excisional surgeries were revisited during the last decade to reassess their potential role as a new treatment.[7-9] Careful review determined that the poor outcomes associated with excisional surgery throughout the last century was mostly due to a cavalier approach by surgeons, a lack of appropriate knowledge about lymphedema and lymphatic function, and improper indications.

Excisional surgery,[10-13] once condemned by many surgeons because of severe postoperative morbidity, now has been resurrected with limited use among patients with end-stage chronic lymphedema with strictly controlled indications. However, many remain skeptical and biased against excisional surgery based on previous experiences of it as a sole independent therapy.

Excisional surgery plays an auxiliary role in supplementing failing CDT. The reduction and excision of fibrosclerotic, overgrown soft tissue improves the efficacy of subsequent CDT and compression bandaging. In addition, there is no more risk of injury to the remaining salvageable lymphatic vessels by the excision procedure at this advanced stage.[9] For example, excisional surgery may be performed in a patient with intractable end-stage lymphedema associated with recurrent local and systemic sepsis that is refractory to maximum CDT combined with compression therapy. The outcome of excisional surgery is dependent on the appropriate postoperative CDT and patient compliance.[7-9]

Clinical Experience

A total of 1,065 patients (131 men and 934 women; 259 primary lymphedemas and 806 secondary lymphedemas; age range, 2 months to 82 years) were assessed between January 1995 to December 2004 with various noninvasive tests, including lymphoscintigraphy, to determine proper clinical and laboratory staging.[14]

Twenty-two patients (mean age, 46 years; three men, 19 women; five primary lymphedemas and 17 secondary lymphedemas) at stage IV or advanced stage III underwent excisional surgery on 33 limbs (11 unilateral; 22 bilateral) as supplemental therapy; indications were for palliation, to reinforce failing CDT, to improve the local condition to facilitate proper CDT and/or compression therapy, and to reduce the incidence of sepsis.

Indications for excisional surgery as an additional/supplemental therapy[9,14]:

- Failure to implement proper care with the CDT at clinical stage III or IV (end stage)
- Progression of the disease to end stage, despite maximal treatment for a minimum of 2 years and declared a "treatment failure" by a multidisciplinary care team
- Increased frequency and/or severity of local and/or systemic sepsis
- Treatment failure and subsequent progression of the disease despite maximal therapy for 2 years and properly declared per recommendation by IRB to become a candidate for excisional surgery

Evaluation confirmed end-stage chronic lymphedema (stage IV or late stage III) with increased difficulty in providing effective CDT and increased frequency and severity of local and/or systemic sepsis (3–4 episodes per year) despite prophylactic antibiotic administration.

A modification of Auchincloss-Homan's operation[15,16] was used to excise a generous amount of grotesquely disfigured tissue with advanced dermato-lipo-fibro-sclerotic change, including the whole skin layer, subcutaneous tissue, and muscle fascia in order to re-establish the normal limb contour and to allow proper postoperative compression therapy (Fig. 49.2).

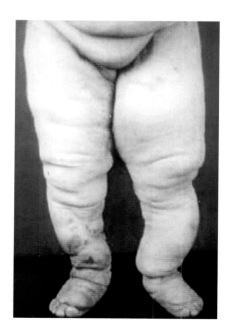

Fig. 49.2 Clinical appearance of the bilateral lower limbs with fully restored normal contour following excisional surgery. The efficacy of CDT was markedly improved postoperatively

Postoperative MLD and compression therapy were performed in all patients. Pre- and postoperative evaluation were based on clinical improvement (patient satisfaction index), four-level limb circumference measurements, infrared optical limb volume determination, and lymphoscintigraphy.[7-9]

Follow-up assessment was made every 6 months for a mean of 4 years. An additional clinical evaluation was performed during each episode of local and/or systemic sepsis.

At 12 months, 28 out of the 33 limbs in 22 patients with good compliance in maintaining postoperative compression therapy reported satisfactory improvement.

At 24 months, 18 out of 28 limbs with good compliance were able to maintain successful results while 10 with poor compliance failed.

At 48 months, 8 limbs in 6 patients were compliant and maintained satisfactory improvement. Among the remaining 25 limbs, 9 were lost to follow-up and 16 noncompliant patients experienced further deterioration.

Our own experience has shown that excisional surgery is a very effective method of establishing optimal conditions for CDT. Patients report satisfactory improvement initially, but most do not experience long-term improvement without postoperative CDT and/or compression therapy.

Satisfactory clinical improvement following surgery showed that patient compliance with postoperative CDT was once again confirmed as the single most important factor that determined long-term outcome. Compliant patients maintained successful results, whereas noncompliant patients experienced further deterioration.

Compliance of the patient and the commitment to life-long CDT are crucial in order to achieve satisfactory long-term results among our candidates. Full integration with CDT-based therapy as a part of a multidisciplinary team approach following surgical therapy is the only means of achieving the most effective control of chronic lymphedema.

Excisional surgery plays a new supplemental role in the non- to poorly- responding CDT group of chronic lymphedema patients. As adjunctive therapy in most situations, together with CDT it plays a critical role in the management of chronic lymphedema. Surgery and CDT have mutually complementary effects.

At the present time, CDT-oriented treatment is still first-line therapy, although it is not curative. It effectively prevents disease progression and produces a satisfactory outcome in the majority of chronic lymphedema patients who are compliant and maintain self-motivated home treatment following hospital-initiated care. Patient compliance with maintenance CDT is the most important factor in the treatment of chronic lymphedema. Prevention and treatment of systemic and/or local infection (e.g., cellulitis, erysipelas) is the next most important factor in the successful management of chronic lymphedema with this combined approach, with excisional surgery reserved for end-stage disease.[17]

Based on the same principle, percutaneous liposuction was introduced as a less radical surgical approach to avoid the complications and morbidity associated with the traditional excisional technique.[18,19]

Instead of resecting all soft tissue with fibrosclerotic overgrowth using a conventional open surgical method, liposuction aims to remove excessive adipose tissue alone in order to obliterate the epifascial compartment by "circumferential" suction-assisted lipectomy. This technique, however, requires more vigorous compression therapy following the procedure to maintain the reduced limb volume.

Initial results of liposuction to remove excessive adipose tissue in the early stage of lymphedema have been reported, with excellent long-term results, despite lingering doubt regarding the risk of damage to the remaining lymphatic system.

This new approach remains to be proven. Its efficacy, long-term results, durability, and safety remain to be determined. The effect of liposuction and the risk of collateral damage to the viable lymph vessels are still unclear.

Conclusion

Excisional surgery is a viable option as supplemental therapy in the treatment of intractable lymphedema at its end stage by improving the postoperative CDT in order to break the vicious cycle of deteriorating CDT and increasing sepsis. Long-term maintenance of satisfactory clinical improvement following excisional surgery is totally dependent on patient compliance with maintenance postoperative CDT/compression therapy.

References

1. Olszewski WL. Episodic dermatolymphangioadenitis (DLA) in patients with lymphedema of the lower extremities before and after administration of benzathine penicillin: a preliminary study. *Lymphology*. 1996;29:126-131.
2. Lee BB. Chronic lymphedema, no more stepchild to modern medicine! *Eur J Lymphology*. 2004;14(42):6-12.
3. Lee BB. Classification and staging of lymphedema. In: Tredbar LL, Morgan CL, Lee BB, Simonian SJ, Blondeau B, eds. *Lymphedema—Diagnosis and Treatment*. London: Springer; 2008: 21-30, chap 3.
4. Lee BB, Bergan JJ. New clinical and laboratory staging systems to improve management of chronic lymphedema. *Lymphology*. 2005;38(3):122-129.
5. Casley-Smith JR, Mason MR, Morgan RG, et al. Complex physical therapy for the lymphedematous leg. *Int J Angiol*. 1995;4:134-142.
6. Hwang JH, Kwon JY, Lee KW, et al. Changes in lymphatic function after complex physical therapy for lymphedema. *Lymphology*. 1999;32:15-21.
7. Lee BB, Kim DI, Whang JH, Lee KW. Contemporary management of chronic lymphedema – personal experiences. *Lymphology*. 2002;35(Suppl):450-455.
8. Lee BB. Current issue in management of chronic lymphedema: personal reflection on an experience with 1065 patients. *Lymphology*. 2005;38:28.
9. Lee BB, Kim YW, Kim DI, Hwang JH, Laredo J, Neville R. Supplemental surgical treatment to end stage (stage IV –V) of chronic lymphedema. *Int Angiol*. 2008;27(5):389-395.
10. Homans J. The treatment of elephantiasis of the legs. *N Engl J Med*. 1936;215:1099.
11. Sistrunk WE. Further experiences with the Kondoleon operation for elephantiasis. *JAMA*. 1918;71:800.
12. Kinmonth JB, Patrick J II, Chilvers AS. Comments on operations for lower limb lymphedema. *Lymphology*. 1975;8:56-61.

13. Dellon Al, Hoopes JE. The Charles procedure for primary lymphedema. *Plast Reconstr Surg.* 1977;60:589.
14. Lee BB. Surgical management of lymphedema. In: Tredbar LL, Morgan CL, Lee BB, Simonian SJ, Blondeau B, eds, *Lymphedema-Diagnosis and Treatment.* London: Springer; 2008: 55-63, chap 6.
15. Auchincloss H. New operation for elephantiasis. *Puerto Rico J Publ Health Trop Med.* 1930;6:149.
16. Huh SH, Kim DI, Hwang JH, Lee BB. Excisional surgery in chronic advanced lymphedema. *Surg Today.* 2003;34:434-435.
17. Lee BB, Andrade M, Bergan J, et al. Diagnosis and treatment of primary lymphedema. Consensus document of the International Union of Phlebology (IUP)-2009. *Int Angiol.* 2010;29(5):454-470.
18. Brorson H, Svensson H. Liposuction combined with controlled compression therapy reduces arm lymphedema more effectively than controlled compression therapy alone. *Plast Reconstr Surg.* 1998;102(4):1058-1067; discussion 1068.
19. Brorson H, Svensson H, Norrgren K, Thorsson O. Liposuction reduces arm lymphedema without significantly altering the already impaired lymph transport. *Lymphology.* 1998;31(4):156-172.

Chapter 50
Surgical Treatment of Postmastectomy Lymphedema – Liposuction

Håkan Brorson

Excess Subcutaneous Adiposity and Chronic Lymphedema

There are various possible explanations for adipose tissue hypertrophy in lymphedema. There is a physiological imbalance of blood flow and lymphatic drainage, resulting in the impaired clearance of lipids and their uptake by macrophages.[1,2] There is increasing support, however, for the view that the fat cell is an endocrine organ and a cytokine-activated cell,[3,4] and chronic inflammation plays a role here.[5,6]

For more information about relationship between slow lymph flow and adiposity, as well as that between structural changes in the lymphatic system and adiposity, see Harvey et al.[7] and Schneider et al.[8]

Other indications for adipose tissue hypertrophy include:

- The findings of increased adipose tissue in intestinal segments in patients with inflammatory bowel disease (Crohn's disease), known as "fat wrapping," have clearly shown that inflammation plays an important role.[5,9,10]
- Consecutive analyses of the content of the aspirate removed under bloodless conditions using a tourniquet showed a high content of adipose tissue (mean 90%).[11]
- In Graves' ophthalmopathy with exophthalmos, adipocyte-related immediate early genes are overexpressed and cysteine-rich, angiogenic inducer 61 may play a role in both orbital inflammation and adipogenesis.[12]

H. Brorson
Department of Clinical Sciences in Malmö, Lund University,
Plastic and Reconstructive Surgery, Skåne University Hospital,
SE-205 02 Malmö, Sweden
e-mail: hakan.brorson@med.lu.se

B.-B. Lee et al. (eds.), *Lymphedema*,
DOI 10.1007/978-0-85729-567-5_50, © Springer-Verlag London Limited 2011

- Tonometry can distinguish if a lymphedematous arm is harder or softer than the normal one. Patients with a harder arm compared with the healthy one have excess adipose tissue.[13]
- Volume-rendered computed tomography and dual X-ray absorptiometry have shown adipose tissue excess of 81% and 73%, respectively, in the swollen arm.[14-16]

The common misunderstanding among clinicians is that the swelling of a lymphedematous extremity is purely due to the accumulation of lymph fluid, which can be removed by use of noninvasive conservative regimens, such as complete decongestive therapy and controlled compression therapy (CCT). These therapies work well when the excess swelling consists of accumulated lymph, but do not work when the excess volume is dominated by adipose tissue.[17] The same may apply to microsurgical procedures using lymphovenous shunts and lymph vessel transplantation,[18-20] which do not remove adipose tissue.

The Outcome of Liposuction

Today, chronic nonpitting arm lymphedema of up to 4 L in excess can be effectively removed by use of liposuction without any further reduction in lymph transport.[21] Complete reduction is mostly achieved in between 1 and 3 months. Long-term results have not shown any recurrence of the arm swelling (Fig. 50.1a, b).[17,22-24] Promising results also can be achieved for leg lymphedema (Fig. 50.2a, b), for which complete reduction is usually reached at around 6 months.[25,26]

How to Perform Liposuction for Lymphedema

Surgical Technique

Made-to-measure compression garments (two sleeves and two gloves) are measured and ordered 2 weeks before surgery, using the healthy arm and hand as a template.

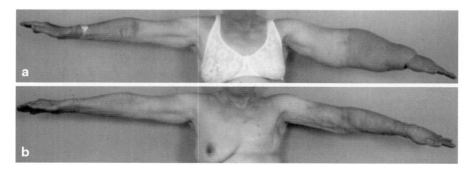

Fig. 50.1 (**a**) A 74-year-old woman with non-pitting arm lymphedema lasting for 15 years. Preoperative excess volume was 3,090 mL. (**b**) Postoperative result

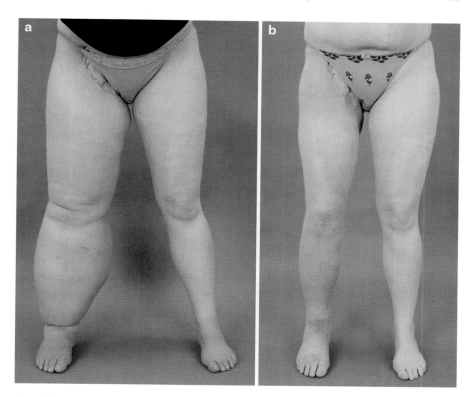

Fig. 50.2 (**a**) Secondary lymphedema: preoperative excess volume 7,070 mL. (**b**) Postoperative result after 6 months where excess volume is −445 mL i.e., the treated leg is somewhat smaller than the normal one

Nowadays we use power-assisted liposuction because the vibrating cannula facilitates the liposuction, especially in the leg, which is more demanding to treat.

Initially the "dry technique" was used.[27] Later, to minimize blood loss, a tourniquet was utilized in combination with tumescence, which involves infiltration of 1–2 L of saline containing low-dose adrenaline and lignocaine.[28,29]

Through approximately 15–20, 3-mm-long incisions, liposuction is performed using 15- and 25-cm-long cannulas with diameters of 3 and 4 mm (Fig. 50.3). When the arm distal to the tourniquet has been treated, a sterilized made-to-measure compression sleeve is applied (Jobst® Elvarex BSN medical, compression class 2) to the arm to stem bleeding and reduce postoperative edema. A sterilized, standard interim glove (Cicatrex interim, Thuasne®, France), in which the tips of the fingers have been cut to facilitate gripping, is put on the hand. The tourniquet is removed and the most proximal part of the upper arm is treated using the tumescent technique.[28,29] Finally, the proximal part of the compression sleeve is pulled up to compress the proximal part of the upper arm. The incisions are left open to drain through the sleeve. The arm is lightly wrapped with a large absorbent compress covering the whole arm (60×60 cm, Cover-Dri, www.attends.co.uk). The arm is kept at heart level on a large pillow. The compress is changed when needed.

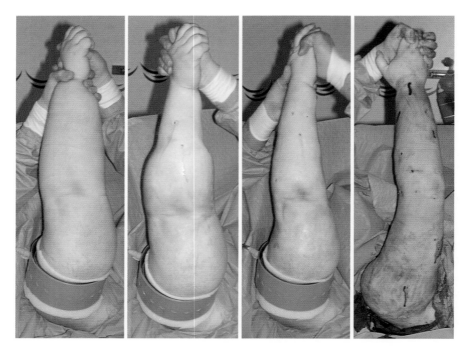

Fig. 50.3 Liposuction of arm lymphedema. The procedure takes about 2 h. From preoperative to postoperative state (*left to right*). Note the tourniquet, which has been removed at the right, and the concomitant reactive hyperemia

The following day, a standard gauntlet (a glove without fingers but with a thumb) (Jobst® Elvarex BSN medical, compression class 2) is put over the interim glove after the thumb of the gauntlet has been cut off to ease the pressure on the thumb. Operating time is, on average, 2 h.

Postoperative Care

Garments are removed 2 days postoperatively so that the patient can take a shower. Then, the other set of garments is put on and the used set is washed and dried. The patient repeats this after another 2 days before discharge. The standard glove and gauntlet is usually changed to the made-to-measure glove at the end of the hospital stay.

The patient alternates between the 3 sets of garments (2 sleeves and 2 gloves) during the 2 weeks postoperatively, changing them daily or every other day so that a clean set is always put on after showering and lubricating the arm. After the 2-week control, the garments are changed every day after being washed. Washing "activates" the garment by increasing the compression due to shrinkage.

Controlled Compression Therapy

A prerequisite to maintaining the effect of liposuction and, for that matter, conservative treatment, is the continuous use of a compression garment.[17,22] After initiating compression therapy, the custom-made garment is taken in at each visit using a sewing machine to compensate for reduced elasticity and reduced arm volume. This is most important during the first 3 months when the most notable changes in volume occur, but even later it is important to adapt the garment to compensate for wear and tear. This can often be managed by the patient him or herself. At the 1- and 3-month visits the arm is measured for new custom-made garments. This procedure is repeated at 6, 9, and 12 months. If complete reduction has been achieved at 6 months, the 9-month control may be omitted. If this is the case, garments are prescribed for the next 6 months, which normally means double the amount that would be needed for 3 months. When the excess volume has decreased as much as possible – usually the treated arm becomes somewhat smaller than the normal arm – and a steady state is achieved, new garments can be prescribed using the latest measurements. In this way, the garments are renewed 3 or 4 times during the first year. Two sets of sleeve and glove garments are always at the patient's disposal: one is worn while the other is washed. Thus, a garment is worn permanently, and treatment is interrupted only briefly when showering and, possibly, for formal social occasions.

The life span of 2 garments worn alternately is usually 4–6 months. Complete reduction is usually achieved after 3–6 months, often earlier. After the first year, the patient is seen again after 6 months (1.5 years after surgery) and then at 2 years after surgery. Then the patient is seen once a year only, when new garments are prescribed for the coming year, usually 4 garments and 4 gloves (or 4 gauntlets). For active patients, 6–8 garments and the same amount of gauntlets/gloves a year are needed. Patients without preoperative swelling of the hand can usually stop using the glove/gauntlet after 6–12 months postoperatively.

For legs, the author's team often uses up to 2 or 3 compression garments on top of each other, depending on what is needed to prevent pitting. A typical example is Elvarex® compression class 3 (or 3 Forte), Jobst Bellavar® compression class 2 (or Elvarex® compression class 2), and Elvarex® compression class 2 (BSN Medical); the latter being a below-the-knee garment. Thus, such a patient needs 2 sets of 2–3 garments. One set is worn while the other is washed. Depending on the age and activity of the patient, 2 such sets can last for 2–4 months. That means that they must be prescribed 3–6 times during the first year. After complete reduction has been achieved, the patient is seen once a year when all new garments are prescribed for the coming year.

Volume Measurements

Volumes of both extremities are always measured at each visit using water plethysmography, and the difference in volumes is designated as the excess volume.[17,22]

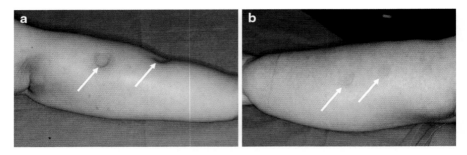

Fig. 50.4 (**a**) Marked lymphedema of the arm after breast cancer treatment, showing pitting several centimeters in depth (grade I edema). The arm swelling is dominated by the presence of fluid, i.e., the accumulation of lymph. (**b**) Pronounced arm lymphedema after breast cancer treatment (grade II edema). There is no pitting in spite of hard pressure by the thumb for 1 min. A slight reddening is seen at the two spots where pressure has been exerted. The "edema" is completely dominated by adipose tissue. The term "edema" is unsuitable at this stage since the swelling is dominated by hypertrophied adipose tissue and not by lymph. At this stage, the aspirate contains either no, or a minimal amount, of lymph

When to Use Liposuction to Treat Lymphedema

A surgical approach, removing the hypertrophied adipose tissue, seems logical when conservative treatment has not achieved satisfactory reduction of the excess volume and the patient has subjective discomfort of a heavy arm or leg.

Liposuction should never be performed in a patient with a pitting edema, as it is dominated by accumulated lymph, which can be removed by conservative treatment.

The first and most important goal is to transform a pitting edema into a non-pitting one by conservative regimens like complete decongestive theraphy or CCT. "Pitting" means that a depression is formed after pressure on the edematous tissue by the fingertip, resulting in lymph being squeezed into the surroundings (Fig. 50.4a). To standardize the pitting test, one presses as hard as possible with the thumb on the region to be investigated for 1 min, the amount of depression being estimated in millimeters. A swelling, which is dominated by hypertrophied adipose tissue, shows little or no pitting (Fig. 50.4b).[23]

Around 4–5 mm of pitting in an arm lymphedema, and 6–8 mm in a leg lymphedema can be accepted. The reason for not performing liposuction for a pitting edema is that liposuction is a method to remove fat, not fluid, even if theoretically it could remove all the accumulated fluid in a pitting lymphedema without excess adipose tissue formation.

Liposuction improves patients' quality of life[17,30] and reduces the incidence of erysipelas.[31]

Summary

There need be no tension between those who favor conservative treatment and proponents of liposuction. Accumulated lymph should be removed using the well-documented conservative regimens until minimal or no pitting is seen. If there is still significant excess volume, it can be removed by the use of liposuction. Continuous wearing of a compression garment prevents recurrence. To date, the author has trained and approved several teams from several countries. A recent publication from the Dutch team shows the same favorable outcome as from our clinic.[32]

Key Points

- Excess volume without pitting means that adipose tissue is responsible for the swelling.
- Adipose tissue can be removed with liposuction. Conservative treatment and microsurgical reconstructions cannot do this.
- As in conservative treatment, the lifelong use (24 h a day) of compression garments is mandatory for maintaining the effect of treatment.

References

1. Vague J, Fenasse R. Comparative anatomy of adipose tissue. In: Renold AE, Cahill GF, eds. *American Handbook of Physiology, Section 5*. Washington DC: American Physiology Society; 1965:25-36.
2. Ryan TJ. Lymphatics and adipose tissue. *Clin Dermatol*. 1995;13:493-498.
3. Mattacks CA, Sadler D, Pond CM. The control of lipolysis in perinodal and other adipocytes by lymph node and adipose tissue derived dendritic cells in rats. *Adipocytes*. 2005;1:43-56.
4. Pond CM. Adipose tissue and the immune system. *Prostaglandins Leukot Essent Fatty Acids*. 2005;73:17-30.
5. Borley NR, Mortensen NJ, Jewell DP, Warren BF. The relationship between inflammatory and serosal connective tissue changes in ileal Crohn's disease: evidence for a possible causative link. *J Pathol*. 2000;190:196-202.
6. Sadler D, Mattacks CA, Pond CM. Changes in adipocytes and dendritic cells in lymph node containing adipose depots during and after many weeks of mild inflammation. *J Anat*. 2005;207:769-781.
7. Harvey NL, Srinivasan RS, Dillard ME, et al. Lymphatic vascular defects promoted by Prox1 haploinsufficiency cause adult-onset obesity. *Nat Genet*. 2005;37:1072-1081.
8. Schneider M, Conway EM, Carmeliet P. Lymph makes you fat. *Nat Genet*. 2005;37:1023-1024.
9. Jones B, Fishman EK, Hamilton SR, et al. Submucosal accumulation of fat in inflammatory bowel disease: CT/pathologic correlation. *J Comput Assist Tomogr*. 1986;10:759-763.
10. Sheehan AL, Warren BF, Gear MW, Shepherd NA. Fat-wrapping in Crohn's disease: pathological basis and relevance to surgical practice. *Br J Surg*. 1992;79:955-958.

11. Brorson H, Åberg M, Svensson H. Chronic lymphedema and adipocyte proliferation: clinical therapeutic implications. *Lymphology*. 2004;37(Suppl):153-155.
12. Lantz M, Vondrichova T, Parikh H, et al. Overexpression of immediate early genes in active Graves' ophthalmopathy. *J Clin Endocrinol Metab*. 2005;90:4784-4791.
13. Bagheri S, Ohlin K, Olsson G, Brorson H. Tissue tonometry before and after liposuction of arm lymphedema following breast cancer. *Lymphat Res Biol*. 2005;3:66-80.
14. Brorson H, Ohlin K, Olsson G, Nilsson M. Adipose tissue dominates chronic arm lymphedema following breast cancer: an analysis using volume rendered CT images. *Lymphat Res Biol*. 2006;4:199-210.
15. Brorson H. Adipose tissue in lymphedema: the ignorance of adipose tissue in lymphedema. *Lymphology*. 2004;37:135-137.
16. Brorson H, Ohlin K, Olsson G, Karlsson MK. Breast cancer-related chronic arm lymphedema is associated with excess adipose and muscle tissue. *Lymphat Res Biol*. 2009;7:3-10.
17. Brorson H, Svensson H. Liposuction combined with controlled compression therapy reduces arm lymphedema more effectively than controlled compression therapy alone. *Plast Reconstr Surg*. 1998;102:1058-1067. discussion 1068.
18. Baumeister RG, Siuda S. Treatment of lymphedemas by microsurgical lymphatic grafting: what is proved? *Plast Reconstr Surg*. 1990;85:64-74. discussion 75-76.
19. Baumeister RG, Frick A. The microsurgical lymph vessel transplantation. *Handchir Mikrochir Plast Chir*. 2003;35:202-209.
20. Campisi C, Davini D, Bellini C, et al. Lymphatic microsurgery for the treatment of lymphedema. *Microsurgery*. 2006;26:65-69.
21. Brorson H, Svensson H, Norrgren K, Thorsson O. Liposuction reduces arm lymphedema without significantly altering the already impaired lymph transport. *Lymphology*. 1998;31: 156-172.
22. Brorson H, Svensson H. Complete reduction of lymphoedema of the arm by liposuction after breast cancer. *Scand J Plast Reconstr Surg Hand Surg*. 1997;31:137-143.
23. Brorson H. Liposuction in arm lymphedema treatment. *Scand J Surg*. 2003;92:287-295.
24. Brorson H, Ohlin K, Olsson G, Svensson B. Liposuction of postmastectomy arm lymphedema completely removes excess volume: a thirteen year study (Quad erat demonstrandum). *Eur J Lymphol*. 2007;17:9.
25. Brorson H, Freccero C, Ohlin K, Svensson B. Liposuction normalizes elephantiasis of the leg. A prospective study with a 6 years follow up. *Eur J Lymphol*. 2009;20:29.
26. Brorson H, Ohlin K, Svensson B, Svensson H. Controlled compression therapy and liposuction treatment for lower extremity lymphedema. *Lymphology*. 2008;41:52-63.
27. Clayton DN, Clayton JN, Lindley TS, Clayton JL. Large volume lipoplasty. *Clin Plast Surg*. 1989;16:305-312.
28. Klein JA. The tumescent technique for liposuction surgery. *Am J Cosm Surg*. 1987;4: 263-267.
29. Wojnikow S, Malm J, Brorson H. Use of a tourniquet with and without adrenaline reduces blood loss during liposuction for lymphoedema of the arm. *Scand J Plast Reconstr Surg Hand Surg*. 2007;41:243-249.
30. Brorson H, Ohlin K, Olsson G, Långström G, Wiklund I, Svensson H. Quality of life following liposuction and conservative treatment of arm lymphedema. *Lymphology*. 2006;39:8-25.
31. Brorson H, Svensson H. Skin blood flow of the lymphedematous arm before and after liposuction. *Lymphology*. 1997;30:165-172.
32. Damstra RJ, Voesten HG, Klinkert P, Brorson H. Circumferential suction-assisted lipectomy for lymphedema after surgery for breast cancer. *Br J Surg*. 2009;96:859-864.

Part XI
Lymphedema and Congenital Vascular Malformation

Chapter 51
Primary Lymphedema as a Truncular Lymphatic Malformation

Byung-Boong Lee, James Laredo, and Richard F. Neville

Definition

Primary lymphedema has been treated successfully for many decades and is one of the two main types of chronic lymphedema; the other is secondary lymphedema.[1,2] Primary and secondary lymphedema are two different diseases with different etiologies, clinical behavior, response to treatment, and prognosis. Throughout the last decade, substantial progress has been made in the understanding of the true nature of primary lymphedema as a type of congenital vascular malformation (CVM)[3,4] affecting the lymphatic system.

Primary lymphedema has been classified as a "congenital" disorder because the majority of patients present with a congenital defect of the lymph-transporting system. This lymphatic congenital defect is often a hypoplastic, hyperplastic, or aplastic lesion of the lymph vessels and/or lymph nodes.[5,6]

Indeed, the majority of "primary" lymphedema patients present with the clinical manifestations of a "truncular" type of lymphatic malformation (LM) that arises during the later stages of lymphangiogenesis.[7,8]

Nevertheless, not all primary lymphedema patients have anatomically evident truncular defects in the lymphatic system. For example, "hereditary familial lymphedema," known as Milroy's disease,[9] does not have a gross macrostructural defect of the lymphatic vessels. Initial and collecting lymphatics are present, but there is impairment of absorption at the level of the initial lymphatics reflecting a functional defect. "Lymphedema–distichiasis syndrome"[10] lacks only intraluminal valves of the lymphatic collectors, resulting in lymph reflux. These conditions are further discussed in detail in Section II – Embryology, Anatomy, and Histology.

B.-B. Lee (✉)
Department of Surgery, Division of Vascular Surgery,
George Washington University School of Medicine, Washington, DC, USA

B.-B. Lee et al. (eds.), *Lymphedema*,
DOI 10.1007/978-0-85729-567-5_51, © Springer-Verlag London Limited 2011

There is also some controversy about the current classification of primary lymphedemas based on the time of onset of clinical manifestations: congenital, praecox, and tarda to constitute one spectrum of the disease where an arbitrary end point of age 35 is used to separate tarda from praecox. However, there are some conditions classified as tarda that can hardly fit as a primary disorder (see Chap. 3).[11]

By the same token, some congenital lymphedemas by classification are not true congenital defects but postnatal obliterations of lymph collectors/lymph nodes that simply mimic the congenital/prenatal condition. In a true sense, these are not malformations of the lymphatic system, but nonetheless they are classified as congenital lymphedema since they are found at birth.[12,13]

Nevertheless, primary lymphedema should be considered as an LM until proven otherwise, not only for its clinical management, but also from the point of view of its prognosis.

Classification

LM is one of the two most common forms of CVM,[14,15] the other being venous malformations. LM exists either as an independent lesion, or as a combined lesion with other CVMs: venous malformations,[16,17] arteriovenous malformations (AVMs),[18,19] and capillary malformations.[20] Such a combined condition is classified separately in the Hamburg Classification[21] as a hemolymphatic malformation (HLM).[22,23]

LM is further classified into two subgroups based on the embryological stage when developmental arrest occurred. "Extratruncular" lesions develop at an earlier stage of embryogenesis and "truncular" lesions originate at a later stage. The truncular LM is better known as primary lymphedema, whereas extratruncular lesions are known as cystic/cavernous lymphangiomas.[5,24]

These two different types of LMs resulting from different embryological stages are often mistakenly identified as two different disease entities without relationship. However, extratruncular LM lesions and truncular LM lesions are inseparable and often coexist, affecting each other in a profound manner.

Extratruncular Lymphatic Malformation Lesions

Extratruncular lesions are the result of premature embryonic tissue that fails to involute and remains in the condition of earlier stages of embryonic life (e.g., the reticular stage). The extratruncular lesion represents the pretruncal embryonic tissue remnant before the lymphatic trunks are formed.[25,26]

Therefore, extratruncular lesions maintain the unique embryonic characteristics of the mesenchymal cells that respond/grow when provoked or stimulated by various conditions such as trauma, menarche, pregnancy, surgery, or hormonal changes. They will never disappear and will remain throughout adult life and, because of their origin, and will continue to grow.

Clinically, extratruncular lesions present as diffuse infiltrating conditions that exert mechanical pressure on surrounding tissues and organs, including nerves and muscles (e.g., cystic hygroma). Such lesions usually form a closed system independent of normal lymph-conducting pathways without direct communications, although they could coexist with lymphedema-causing truncular lesions.

Truncular Lymphatic Malformation Lesions

In contrast, truncular lesions are the result of developmental arrest occurring at later stages of fetal development during the formation of the lymphatic trunks, vessels, and nodes long after the reticular stages of vascular development have ceased. These are termed *posttruncal fetal lesions* (cf. pretruncal extratruncular lesions).[25,26]

Truncular lesions, therefore, no longer have the evolutional power to grow or recur. They have lost the embryonic characteristics of mesenchymal cells and bear no risk of recurrence, but they have a significant lymphodynamic impact on the lymph transport system involved.

Truncular lesions occur in various clinical conditions as the result of an incomplete development of the axial or truncal lymphatic vessels. Depending on the severity or extent of the abnormality occurring during the last maturation period of the lymphatic system, various conditions may result, such as aplasia, hypoplasia, or hyperplasia of lymphatic vessels and/or lymph nodes. These may clinically manifest as obstruction or dilatation. When the endoluminal valves are absent or defective, lymphatic reflux becomes the most important clinical manifestation.

Clinical Evaluation

Detailed information about the clinical evaluation of primary lymphedema as a chronic lymphedema together with secondary lymphedema is presented in Section IV – Clinical Diagnosis, Section V – Laboratory/Imaging Diagnosis, and Section VI – Infection.

Once the differential diagnosis has excluded secondary lymphedema, further evaluation of primary lymphedema as a truncular LM is required in addition to staging of the condition as a chronic lymphedema.[27,28]

Clinical evaluation should begin with a basic evaluation of the CVM as a whole, followed by a more focused, separate investigation into the possible coexistence of an extratruncular LM. Further evaluation of the potential risk of other occurring CVM lesions should be considered when the overall results of the investigation are suggestive (e.g., Klippel–Trenaunay syndrome).[22,23]

Based on the initial assessment with history and physical examination, an appropriate combination of non- to minimally invasive tests can be performed.[29-32] Usually, a few basic tests (e.g., lymphoscintigraphy [LSG]) will provide all the information necessary to ensure an adequate diagnosis and lead to a correct multidisciplinary treatment strategy. However, a few additional tests can be added to provide more specific and detailed information.[33,34]

Radionuclide (LSG)[35,36] is the most essential test and remains the gold standard for evaluation of lymphatic function. Periodic LSG findings provide adequate laboratory staging, which is essential to supplement clinical staging necessary for proper clinical management.

Together with LSG, Duplex ultrasound[31] for evaluation of venous function/status is indicated in every case of primary lymphedema. Accurate assessment of venous function is essential to rule out accompanying abnormal venous conditions that often act as predisposing factors for deterioration of the LM condition (e.g., aplasia/hypoplasia of the ilio-femoral-venous system).

Invasive tests are necessary in certain situations and provide more information for an accurate differential diagnosis among the CVMs. These tests should be considered to help guide subsequent therapy.[11]

Direct puncture percutaneous lymphangiography to verify the status of an extratruncular LM can be generally deferred until needed to refine the diagnosis or to provide information if surgical or other invasive therapeutic measures are considered.[11]

Conventional oil contrast lymphangiography is useful in selecting patients with chylous dysplasia and gravitational reflux disorders to better define the extent of the pathological alterations and sites of lymphatic and chylous leakage.[11]

Lymphedema in children can be a part of the syndrome if there are other concomitant phenotypic abnormalities. Detailed information about the genetic testing and related evaluation is presented in Chaps. 3 and 59.

Clinical Management

Primary lymphedema management is essentially the same as that for secondary lymphedema when it is due to an independent truncular LM. Detailed information has been presented in Section VII through Section X.

However, when both truncular LM (primary lymphedema) and extratruncular LM (lymphangioma) lesions occur together, treatment should be focused on the extratruncular LM lesion. The extratruncular lesion often accelerates the deterioration of the truncular lesion by increasing the lymphatic burden to an already jeopardized lymphatic system.

When the two different LM lesions coexist with other CVMs, the treatment should be focused on the other malformation such as the venous malformation or AVM if they are clinically significant "major" lesions. Further detailed information on combined CVM conditions is presented in Chap. 52.

Conservative (Physical) Therapy

Detailed discussion is presented in Section VII – Physical and Medical Management, and Section VIII – Practical issue on Physical Therapy.

The management of truncular LM aims to control the clinical manifestation as primary lymphedema. Complex decongestive therapy (CDT) is still the most effective form of therapy for truncular LM lesions, whether alone or combined with extratruncular LM lesions.

Surgical Therapy: Reconstructive Surgery

Although ample discussion on the role of reconstructive surgery in chronic lymphedema is presented in Section IX – Surgical treatment – Reconstructive Surgery, there is one critical and unique issue where primary lymphedema is caused by truncular LM.[37] Truncular LMs have an extremely variable number and type of lymph vessels and lymph nodes, as exemplified by the various forms of dysplasias such as lymphangiodysplasia, lymphadenodysplasia, and lymphangioadenodysplasia.[38]

Candidates for reconstructive surgery are, therefore, rare among primary lymphedemas because of the variable anatomy involved with the truncular defect, although some colleagues reported different findings.[39] Surgery outcomes are also variable, but generally not as successful as those of secondary lymphedema patients who have surgically correctable lesions along the major lymphatics/collectors.[8,33]

Hence, the role of reconstructive surgery is further limited in patients with primary lymphedema, even as an adjunctive therapy to CDT at best with a specific indication.

Surgical Therapy: Ablative/Excisional Surgery

As discussed in Section X – Surgical treatment – Excisional/Cytoreductive Surgery thoroughly for the role of excisional surgery in chronic lymphedema when the condition reaches the later/end stage (stages III and IV), most of the normal tissues have become fibrosclerotic and all the remaining lymph vessels are severely damaged, leading to an unsalvageable condition. Therefore, the etiology/cause does not matter from a treatment/excision point of view at this stage.[11,40]

Excisional surgery becomes a treatment of last resort in such a condition once the CDT-based therapy fails to arrest lymphedema progression toward the end stages with evidence of steady deterioration despite maximum treatment.

Liposuction: Circumferential Suction-Assisted Lipectomy

As presented in Section X – Surgical treatment – Excisional/Cytoreductive Surgery, this procedure has been used for treatment of secondary lymphedema following mastectomy. The procedure utilized liposuction to remove excessive, overgrown adipose tissue. However, this less-invasive approach is only effective when performed in the early stage of secondary lymphedema. It is not effective in advanced cases of lymphedema where tissue fibrosis predominates. Circumferential suction-assisted lipectomy requires intensive compression therapy post-procedure and its results are short-lived when compression therapy is discontinued. Its role in the treatment of primary lymphedema is still unknown and its efficacy remains to be proven.

Prospect: Primary Lymphedema as Lymphatic Malformation

This critical part was also presented in Section XIV: Chap. 59.

Conclusion

The primary lymphedema represents a clinical manifestation of the truncular type of lymphatic malformation (LM) arising during the later stages of lymphangiogenesis. A clear understanding of its contemporary classification as a vascular malformation is necessary, because embryological staging information of the LM is critical for proper management of the primary lymphedema as one of the CVMs.

References

1. Lee BB, Villavicencio JL. Primary lymphedema and lymphatic malformation: Are they the two sides of the same coin? *Eur J Vasc Endovasc Surg.* 2010;39:646-653.
2. Lee BB. Lymphedema-angiodysplasia syndrome: a prodigal form of lymphatic malformation (LM). *Phlebolymphology.* 2005;47:324-332.
3. Lee BB, Kim YW, Seo JM, et al. Current concepts in lymphatic malformation (LM). *Vasc Endovascular Surg.* 2005;39(1):67-81.
4. Lee BB. Lymphatic malformation. In: Tredbar LL, Morgan CL, Lee BB, Simonian SJ, Blondeau B, eds. *Lymphedema—Diagnosis and Treatment.* London: Springer; 2008: 31-42, chap 4.
5. Lee BB, Laredo J, Lee TS, Huh S, Neville R. Terminology and classification of congenital vascular malformations. *Phlebology.* 2007;22(6):249-252.
6. Lee BB, Laredo J, Seo JM, Neville R. Treatment of lymphatic malformations. In: Mattassi R, Loose DA, Vaghi M, eds. *Hemangiomas and Vascular Malformations.* Milan: Springer; 2009:231-250. chap. 29.
7. Lee BB. Critical issues on the management of congenital vascular malformation. *Ann Vasc Surg.* 2004;18(3):380-392.
8. Lee BB, Kim DI, Whang JH, Lee KW. Contemporary management of chronic lymphedema – personal experiences. *Lymphology.* 2002;35(Suppl):450-455.
9. Eliachar E, Servelle M, Tassy R, Gamerman H. Hereditary lymphedema (Milroy's disease). *Ann Pediatr (Paris).* 1970;17(11):750-753.
10. Erickson RP. Lymphedema-distichiasis and FOXC2 gene mutations. *Lymphology.* 2001; 34(1):1.

11. Lee BB, Andrade M, Bergan J, et al. Diagnosis and treatment of primary lymphedema: consensus document of the International Union of Phlebology (IUP)-2009. *Int Angiol.* 2010;29(5): 454-470.
12. Witte MH, Jones K, Wilting J, et al. Structure function relationships in the lymphatic system and implications for cancer biology. *Cancer Metastasis Rev.* 2006;25(2):159-184.
13. Rockson SG. Diagnosis and management of lymphatic vascular disease. *J Am Coll Cardiol.* 2008;52:799-806.
14. Lee BB, Laredo J, Lee SJ, Huh SH, Joe JH, Neville R. Congenital vascular malformations: general diagnostic principles. *Phlebology.* 2007;22(6):253-257.
15. Lee BB. Statues of new approaches to the treatment of congenital vascular malformations (CVMs) – single center experiences – (editorial review). *Eur J Vasc Endovasc Surg.* 2005; 30(2):184-197.
16. Lee BB, Kim DI, Huh S, et al. New experiences with absolute ethanol sclerotherapy in the management of a complex form of congenital venous malformation. *J Vasc Surg.* 2001;33:764-772.
17. Lee BB, Do YS, Byun HS, Choo IW, Kim DI, Huh SH. Advanced management of venous malformation with ethanol sclerotherapy: mid-term results. *J Vasc Surg.* 2003;37(3):533-538.
18. Lee BB, Do YS, Yakes W, et al. Management of arterial-venous shunting malformations (AVM) by surgery and embolosclerotherapy. A multidisciplinary approach. *J Vasc Surg.* 2004;39(3):590-600.
19. Lee BB, Laredo J, Deaton DH, Neville RF. Arteriovenous malformations: evaluation and treatment. In: Gloviczki P, ed. *Handbook of Venous Disorders: Guidelines of the American Venous Forum.* 3rd ed. London: A Hodder Arnold Ltd; 2009.
20. Berwald C, Salazard B, Bardot J, Casanova D, Magalon G. Port wine stains or capillary malformations: surgical treatment. *Ann Chir Plast Esthét.* 2006;51(4–5):369-372. Epub 2006 Sep 26.
21. St B. Classification of congenital vascular defects. *Int Angiol.* 1990;9:141-146.
22. Gloveczki P, Driscoll DJ. Klippel-Trenaunay syndrome: current management. *Phlebology.* 2007;22(6):291-298.
23. Villavicencio JL. Congenital vascular malformations – Predominantly venous? The syndrome of Klippel-Trenaunay. *Scope Phlebology Lymphology.* 2000;71(1):116-125.
24. Lee BB. Classification and staging of lymphedema. In: Tredbar LL, Morgan CL, Lee BB, Simonian SJ, Blondeau B, eds. *Lymphedema—Diagnosis and Treatment.* London: Springer; 2008; 21-30, chap. 3.
25. Bastide G, Lefebvre D. Anatomy and organogenesis and vascular malformations. In: Belov ST, Weber J, eds. *Vascular Malformations.* Reinbek: Einhorn-Presse; 1989:20-22.
26. Leu HJ. Pathoanatomy of congenital vascular malformations. In: Belov S, Loose DA, Weber J, eds. *Vascular Malformations*, vol. 16. Reinbek: Einhorn-Presse; 1989:37-46.
27. International Society of Lymphology. The diagnosis and treatment of peripheral lymphedema. 2009 Consensus document of the International Society of Lymphology. *Lymphology.* 2009;42:51-60.
28. Lee BB, Bergan JJ. New clinical and laboratory staging systems to improve management of chronic lymphedema. *Lymphology.* 2005;38(3):122-129.
29. Lee BB, Mattassi R, Kim BT, Kim DI, Ahn JM, Choi JY. Contemporary diagnosis and management of venous and AV shunting malformation by whole body blood pool scintigraphy (WBBPS). *Int Angiol.* 2004;23(4):355-367.
30. Lee BB, Mattassi R, Kim BT, Park JM. Advanced management of arteriovenous shunting malformation with transarterial lung perfusion scintigraphy (TLPS) for follow up assessment. *Int Angiol.* 2005;24(2):173-184.
31. Lee BB, Mattassi R, Choe YH, et al. Critical role of Duplex ultrasonography for the advanced management of a venous malformation (VM). *Phlebology.* 2005;20:28-37.
32. Lee BB, Choe YH, Ahn JM, et al. The new role of MRI (Magnetic Resonance Imaging) in the contemporary diagnosis of venous malformation: Can it replace angiography? *J Am Coll Surg.* 2004;198(4):549-558.

33. Lee BB. Current issue in management of chronic lymphedema: personal reflection on an experience with 1065 patients. *Lymphology*. 2005;38:28.
34. Lee BB, Villavicencio L. General considerations. Congenital vascular malformations. Arteriovenous anomalies (Sect 9). In: Cronenwett JL, Johnston KW, eds. *Rutherford's Vascular Surgery*. 7th ed. Philadelphia: Saunders Elsevier; 2010: 1046-1064, chap. 68.
35. Olszewski WL. Lymphoscintigraphy helps to differentiate edema of various etiologies (inflammatory, obstructive, posttraumatic, venous). *Lymphology*. 2002;35(Suppl):233-235.
36. Choi JY, Hwang JH, Park JM, Kim DI, Lee BB, Kim BT. Risk assessment of dermatolymphangioadenitis by lymphoscintigraphy in patients with lower extremity lymphedema. *Korean J Nucl Med*. 1999;33(2):143-151.
37. Lee BB. Surgical management of lymphedema. In: Tredbar LL, Morgan CL, Lee BB, Simonian SJ, Blondeau B, eds. *Lymphedema—Diagnosis and Treatment*. London: Springer; 2008: 55-63, chap. 6.
38. Papendieck CM. Lymphangiomatosis and dermoepidermal disturbances of lymphangioadenodysplasias. *Lymphology*. 2002;35(Suppl):478.
39. Campisi C, Da Rin E, Bellini C, Bonioli E, Boccardo F. Pediatric lymphedema and correlated syndromes: role of microsurgery. *Microsurgery*. 2008;28(2):138-142.
40. Lee BB, Kim YW, Kim DI, Hwang JH, Laredo J, Neville R. Supplemental surgical treatment to end stage (stage IV –V) of chronic lymphedema. *Int Angiol*. 2008;27(5):389-395.

Chapter 52
Primary Lymphedema and Klippel-Trénaunay Syndrome

Byung-Boong Lee, James Laredo, Richard F. Neville, and Raul Mattassi

The majority of primary lymphedemas[1,2] are due to a congenital, independent lesion of the lymphatic system resulting in dysfunction. Primary lymphedema due to a truncular lymphatic malformation (LM) has been thoroughly reviewed in Chap. 51.

Primary lymphedema less commonly presents as a component of multiple congenital vascular malformations (CVMs) producing a clinical condition. One such condition was named after Maurice Klippel and Paul Trenaunay, based on their description in 1900 of a complex CVM. Klippel–Trenaunay syndrome (KTS) became a synonym for a complicated condition due to CVMs for more than a century.[3,4]

This old eponym originally described a clinical triad: port wine stain, soft tissue, and bone hypertrophy of the lower limb, and atypical, mostly lateral varicosities. These various soft tissue, bone, and vein lesions are due to the underlying vascular malformations involved. This original description failed to specify the type of vascular malformations involved (Fig. 52.1).

The vascular malformation components of KTS are venous malformation (VM),[5,6] LM,[7,8] and capillary malformation (CM).[9] When an arteriovenous malformation (AVM)[10,11] is further involved, it is known as Parkes–Weber Syndrome (PWS; Fig. 52.2).

Such eponyms like KTS or PWS failed to meet the requirements for advanced management of various CVMs based on a new contemporary concept. These eponyms have been replaced with new terminology based on the Hamburg Classification (Table 52.1).[12,13]

The VM component of the KTS is classified as a hemolymphatic malformation (HLM) and represents a combined condition of VM, LM, and CM, resulting in the various presentations seen in patients with KTS.[14,15]

B.-B. Lee (✉)
Department of Surgery, Division of Vascular Surgery,
George Washington University School of Medicine, Washington, DC, USA

B.-B. Lee et al. (eds.), *Lymphedema*,
DOI 10.1007/978-0-85729-567-5_52, © Springer-Verlag London Limited 2011

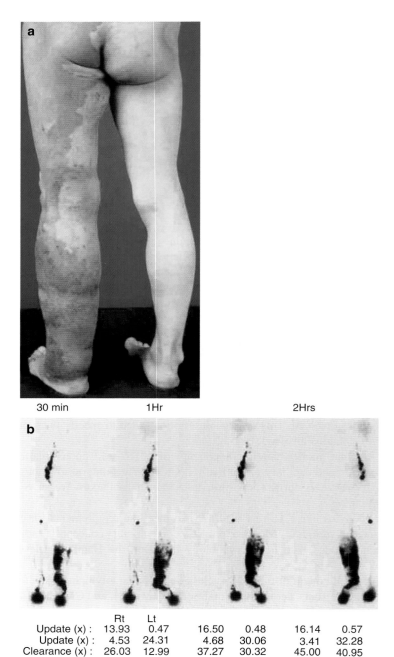

		Rt	Lt				
Update (x) :		13.93	0.47	16.50	0.48	16.14	0.57
Update (x) :		4.53	24.31	4.68	30.06	3.41	32.28
Clearance (x) :		26.03	12.99	37.27	30.32	45.00	40.95

Fig. 52.1 Klippel–Trenaunay syndrome (KTS). (**a**) Clinical appearance of KTS involving the left lower extremity. Various non-invasive tests confirmed all four different vascular malformation components: truncular LM (primary lymphedema) by radionuclide lymphoscintigraphy (**b**) and MR-T2 weighted image (**d**), extratruncular LM by direct puncture lymphangiography (**g**), extratruncular VM by whole-body blood pool scintigraphy (**c**), and truncular VM (marginal vein) by Duplex ultrasound (**e**) and MR venography (**f**)

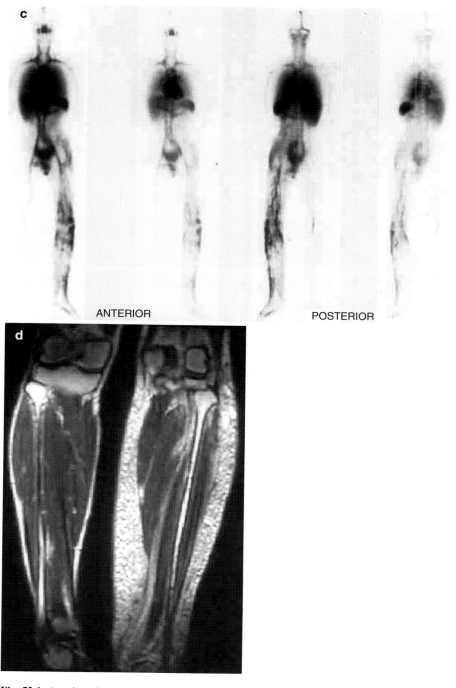

Fig. 52.1 (continued)

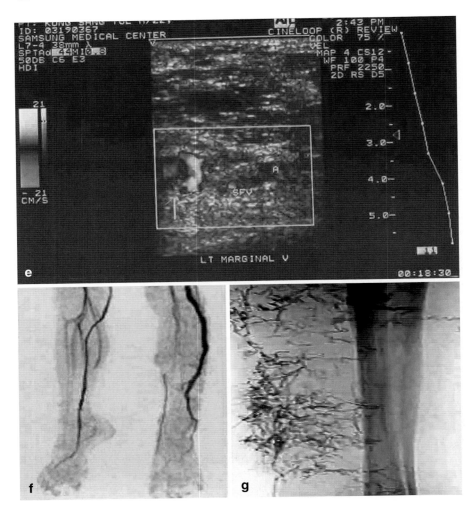

Fig. 52.1 (continued)

Looking at primary lymphedema from a VM point of view, it is natural to have a mixed condition with other CVMs because they are a group of various birth defects after developmental arrest along any of peripheral vascular systems during the various stages of embryogenesis. It can therefore, affect more than one vascular system: the capillary, arterial, venous, and/or lymphatic systems, producing a mixture of various defects with different characteristics. These defects may occur as either an extratruncular or truncular type of lesion.[16,17]

The clinical significance of the two different embryological subtypes – extratruncular and truncular – was thoroughly reviewed in Chap. 51. Its critical importance in the clinical management of CVMs cannot be overemphasized.

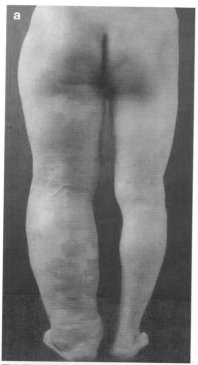

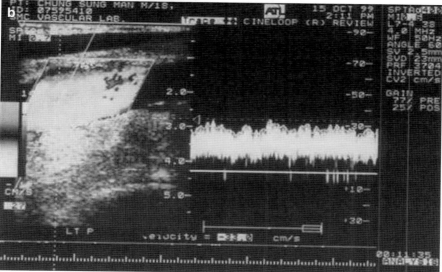

Fig. 52.2 Parkes–Weber Syndrome (PWS). (**a**) Clinical condition of the PWS involving the left lower extremity. In addition to the VM, LM, and CM components like KTS, the AVM lesion was confirmed as an additional vascular malformation component. Duplex ultrasound (**b**) displays high flow condition along the femoropopliteal vein by AV shunting lesion along the knee area; the lesion was subsequently confirmed as a micro-shunting AVM with the arteriography (shunting percentage to 69% by transarterial lung perfusion to make scintigraphy (**c**)

Fig. 52.2 (continued)

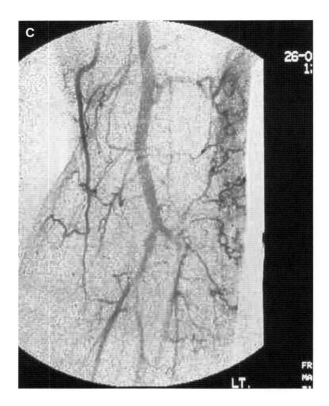

Whenever lymphedema is caused by a truncular LM, the likelihood that another type of LM (extratruncular LM), as well as a VM and CM, is also present increases, producing the VM component of KTS.

Hence, clinical investigation and management of primary lymphedema as a part of the KTS is required. This unique, complicated condition often involves two different embryological subtypes of LM as well as VM, making a total of four different VMs.

There is significant variability in clinical presentation, ranging from a simple condition of one LM and one VM subtypes to a complicated condition with all four lesions: extratruncular LM and truncular LM, and extratruncular VM and truncular VM, in addition to the CM.

Capillary malformation,[9] also known as a port wine stain, has a unique distinction that whenever it is present, another CVM is always present. Depending on its location (e.g., the face), it may be present with a serious intracranial lesion (e.g., Sturge–Weber syndrome[18]). In addition, CMs are well known to be associated with more frequent wound complications after surgical treatment of other coexisting CVMs (e.g., keloid formation).

The CM lesion itself has limited clinical significance in general and often presents as a cosmetic problem alone, where its management is relatively straight

Table 52.1 Hamburg classification of congenital vascular malformation (CVM), modified

Main classification based on its predominant vascular component:
• Predominantly arterial defects
• Predominantly venous defects
• Predominantly AV (arteriovenous) shunting defects
• Predominantly lymphatic defects
• Predominantly capillary malformation
• Combined vascular defects
Subclassification based on the embryological stage of the defect:
• Extratruncular forms – developmental arrest at the earlier stages of embryonal life:
– Diffuse, infiltrating
– Limited, localized
• Truncular forms – developmental arrest at the later stages of embryonal life:
– Obstruction
◦ Hypoplasia; aplasia; hyperplasia
◦ Stenosis; membrane; congenital spur
– Dilatation
◦ Localized (aneurysm)
◦ Diffuse (ectasia)

Both extratruncular and truncular forms may exist together in the same vascular malformation, and may be combined with other various malformations (e.g., capillary, arterial, AV shunting, venous, hemolymphatic, and/or lymphatic). Based on the consensus on the CVM classification through the international workshop in Hamburg, Germany, 1988, which was upheld by the subsequently founded ISSVA (International Society for Vascular Anomaly).

forward with the laser-based therapy, and therefore, this chapter will be limited to the combined VM and LM.

The other two vascular components of KTS, VM and LM, typically present as a clinically complicated condition due to the interwinding of the four different components and subtypes: extratruncular VM, truncular VM, extratruncular LM, and truncular LM, presenting in various combinations and locations with differing severity and extent. Fortunately, the majority of KTS patients do not all have four different subtypes of LM and VM. More frequently encountered is a single type of VM presenting with a single type of LM.

With regard to the VM component of KTS, the extratruncular VM is relatively rare. In contrast, the truncular VM is more common (e.g., marginal or lateral embryonic vein). The marginal vein has direct and indirect effects on an already dysfunctional lymphatic system caused by LM lesion(s). The marginal vein does not have any venous valves resulting in venous reflux and chronic venous insufficiency. Furthermore, these KTS patients often have a poorly developed, uncompensated deep venous system.[19,20]

Similar to the VM component of KTS, the LM component is often a truncular LM as a cause of primary lymphedema. The extratruncular LM, better known as a "cavernous or cystic lymphangioma", is occasionally found in KTS patients, presenting either alone or combined with a truncular LM (primary lymphedema), and makes the clinical management more complicated.

Table 52.2 Laboratory diagnosis – primary pathological features of KTS

I. Non- to less-invasive study – basic (standard)
  • T1- and T2-weighted MR image study
  • Duplex ultrasound
  • Whole-body blood pool scintigraphy (WBBPS)
  • Radionuclide lymphoscintigraphy
II. Non- to less-invasive study – optional
  • Transarterial lung perfusion scintigraphy (TLPS)
  • MR venography and/or arteriography
  • Ultrasound and/or MR lymphangiography
  • CT
III. Selective invasive study
  • Ascending and/or segmental venography
  • Standard and/or selective arteriography
  • Percutaneous direct puncture phlebography
  • Percutaneous direct puncture lymphangiography

The diagnosis of KTS, therefore, should begin with the clinical evaluation of its primary etiology and determination of the different vascular malformation components that are present.[21,22]

Proper assessment and evaluation of the direct and indirect secondary effects of the primary pathological condition (HLM) on the various organ systems should include:

• Gastrointestinal system (e.g., GI bleeding, chylo-ascites, malabsorption syndrome)
• Cardiopulmonary system (e.g., pleural effusion, chylothorax)
• Musculoskeletal system (e.g., long bone length discrepancy, scoliosis, pelvic tilt)
• Genito-urinary system (e.g., lymph leak: chyluria, chylorrhagia).

Hence, the diagnostic tests for KTS are aimed at characterizing all four vascular malformation components (Table 52.2). Diagnostic testing of the truncular LM is limited to radionuclide lymphoscintigraphy, which was discussed in Sect. V and Chap. 51.

For management of primary lymphedema in KTS, precise assessment of the extent and severity of each VM and LM lesion should follow proper identification of each CVM component of the KTS. Following identification and assessment of each CVM component of KTS, treatment priority should be determined by the relative clinical significance of the VM and LM lesions.

The VM lesion is usually the more clinically significant lesion in KTS patients, except in cases of lymph leakage and sepsis due to a LM lesion. VM lesions have more serious hemodynamic effects directly on the venous system and indirectly on the lymphatic system.[16,23] Treatment of the VM lesion usually proceeds first, followed by treatment of the LM lesion.

An aggressive approach to the marginal vein utilizing a one-stage resection in a KTS patient will lead to an acute increase in deep venous flow following excision of the marginal vein. A KTS patient with a normal deep venous system can easily accommodate the acute increase in deep venous flow. In contrast, a KTS patient with hypoplasia of the deep venous system has limited capacity and cannot accommodate the acute increase in deep venous flow. As a consequence, resection of the marginal vein in the presence of a hypoplastic deep venous system often results in acute venous hypertension and secondary lymphatic hypertension.

When an extratruncular VM lesion occurs with a truncular VM lesion, the extratruncular lesion (often an infiltrating lesion) should be treated first in order to reduce its hemodynamic effects on the deep venous system, before treating the truncular VM. In addition, follow-up after treatment is required to monitor for lesion recurrence. Extratruncular VM lesions are derived from embryonic tissue from an early stage of embryogenesis, and exhibit mesenchymal cell characteristics, including the ability to proliferate when stimulated.[24,25]

Primary lymphedema due to a truncular LM in KTS is generally resistant to complex decongestive therapy (CDT) alone, compared with primary lymphedema in patients without KTS. Treatment of the VM lesion in KTS patients is especially important and almost always required in addition to CDT for management of lymphedema.[26,27]

The extratruncular LM is easily affected by the treatment of VM as mentioned above. Treatment of the extratruncular LM often exacerbates overall lymphatic dysfunction with an increased burden to the lymph transport system.

If an extratruncular LM is present with an extratruncular VM, both lesions should be treated together. In the unique situation where all four different subtypes of LM and VM are present in the KTS patient, extreme precaution should be exercised in order to minimize this unwanted imbalance between the venodynamics and lymphodynamics. Appropriate preparation to prevent or minimize anticipated complications and morbidity should be undertaken prior to initiating therapy.

References

1. Lee BB, Villavicencio JL. Primary lymphedema and lymphatic malformation: Are they the two sides of the same coin? *Eur J Vasc Endovasc Surg.* 2010;39:646-653.
2. Lee BB, Andrade M, Bergan J, et al. Diagnosis and treatment of primary lymphedema: consensus document of the International Union of Phlebology (IUP)-2009. *Int Angiol.* 2010;29(5):454-470.
3. Klippel M, Trenaunay J. Du noevus variqueux et osteohypertrophique. *Arch Gén Méd.* 1900;3: 641-672.
4. Servelle M. Klippel and Trenaunay's syndrome. *Ann Surg.* 1985;201:365-373.
5. Lee BB, Do YS, Byun HS, Choo IW, Kim DI, Huh SH. Advanced management of venous malformation (VM) with ethanol sclerotherapy: mid-term results. *J Vasc Surg.* 2003;37(3):533-538.
6. Lee BB, Bergan J, Gloviczki P, et al. Diagnosis and treatment of venous malformations – consensus document of the International Union of Phlebology (IUP)-2009. *Int Angiol.* 2009;28(6):434-451.
7. Lee BB, Kim YW, Seo JM, et al. Current concepts in lymphatic malformation (LM). *Vasc Endovasc Surg.* 2005;39(1):67-81.
8. Lee BB, Laredo J, Seo JM, Neville R. Hemangiomas and vascular malformations. In: Mattassi R, Loose DA, Vaghi M, eds. *Treatment of Lymphatic Malformations.* Milan: Springer; 2009: 231-250, chap. 29.

9. Berwald C, Salazard B, Bardot J, Casanova D, Magalon G. Port wine stains or capillary malformations: surgical treatment. *Ann Chir Plast Esthét.* 2006;51(4–5):369-372. Epub 2006 Sep 26.
10. Lee BB, Villavicencio L. General considerations. Congenital vascular malformations. Arteriovenous anomalies (Sect 9). In: Cronenwett JL, Johnston KW, eds. *Rutherford's Vascular Surgery.* 7th ed. Philadelphia: Saunders Elsevier; 2010: 1046-1064, chap. 68.
11. Lee BB, Laredo J, Neville R. Arterio-venous malformation: How much do we know? *Phlebology.* 2009;24:193-200.
12. Lee BB, Laredo J, Lee TS, Huh S, Neville R. Terminology and classification of congenital vascular malformations. *Phlebology.* 2007;22(6):249-252.
13. St B. Classification of congenital vascular defects. *Int Angiol.* 1990;9:141-146.
14. Gloviczki P, Driscoll DJ. Klippel–Trenaunay syndrome: current management. *Phlebology.* 2007;22:291-298.
15. Jacob AG, Driscoll DJ, Shaughnessy WJ, Stanson AW, Clay RP, Gloviczki P. Klippel-Trenaunay syndrome: spectrum and management. *Mayo Clin Proc.* 1998;73(1):28-36.
16. Lee BB. Critical issues on the management of congenital vascular malformation. *Ann Vasc Surg.* 2004;18(3):380-392.
17. Lee BB. Lymphedema-angiodysplasia syndrome: a prodigal form of lymphatic malformation (LM). *Phlebolymphology.* 2005;47:324-332.
18. Moore GJ, Slovis TL, Chugani HT. Proton magnetic resonance spectroscopy in children with Sturge-Weber syndrome. *J Child Neurol.* 1998;13(7):332-335.
19. Kim YW, Lee BB, Cho JH, Do YS, Kim DI, Kim ES. Haemodynamic and clinical assessment of lateral marginal vein excision in patients with a predominantly venous malformation of the lower extremity. *Eur J Vasc Endovasc Surg.* 2007;33(1):122-127.
20. Mattassi R, Vaghi M. Vascular bone syndrome-angi-osteodystrophy: current concept. *Phlebology.* 2007;22:287-290.
21. Lee BB. Lymphatic malformation. In: Tredbar LL, Morgan CL, Lee BB, Simonian SJ, Blondeau B, eds. *Lymphedema—Diagnosis and Treatment.* London: Springer; 2008:31-42, chap. 4.
22. Lee BB, Laredo J, Lee SJ, Huh SH, Joe JH, Neville R. Congenital vascular malformations: general diagnostic principles. *Phlebology.* 2007;22(6):253-257.
23. Lee BB, Bergan JJ. Advanced management of congenital vascular malformations: a multidisciplinary approach. *Cardiovasc Surg.* 2002;10(6):523-533.
24. Lee BB, Laredo J, Kim YW, Neville R. Congenital vascular malformations: general treatment principles. *Phlebology.* 2007;22(6):258-263.
25. Lee BB. Changing concept on vascular malformation: no longer enigma. *Ann Vasc Dis.* 2008;1(1):11-19.
26. Lee BB, Kim DI, Whang JH, Lee KW. Contemporary management of chronic lymphedema – personal experiences. *Lymphology.* 2002;35(Suppl):450-455.
27. Lee BB. Current issue in management of chronic lymphedema: personal reflection on an experience with 1065 patients. *Lymphology.* 2005;38:28.

Chapter 53
Special Issues in Pediatric Primary Lymphedema

Cristobal Miguel Papendieck

Definition and Classification

Primary lymphedema in the pediatric group has a special position among the congenital vascular malformation (CVM), because the majority represent a clinical manifestation of the "truncular" type of lymphatic malformation (LM; Figs. 53.1 and 53.2).

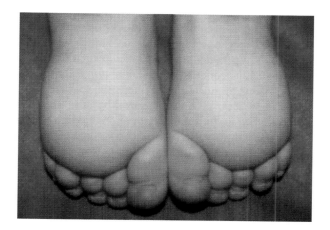

Fig. 53.1 Bilateral primary lymphedema

C.M. Papendieck
Angiopediatria, Buenos Aires, Argentina

B.-B. Lee et al. (eds.), *Lymphedema*,
DOI 10.1007/978-0-85729-567-5_53, © Springer-Verlag London Limited 2011

Fig. 53.2 Unilateral primary lymphedema with lymphangiomatosis

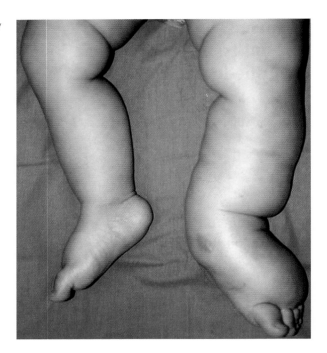

Therefore, proper understanding of the mechanism of the formation of the lymphatic system is essential; the right interpretation of the primary/congenital lymphedema is warranted, because this condition is one of the results of the cellular work led by the endothel of the initial lymphatics.

The lymph originates in the interstitial space following the intercellular and transcellular process; it is characterized by at least +0.9 g% of proteins that can be incorporated into the flow only through the cannalicular system of the lymphatics.[1]

A defect in this system would result in interstitial stagnation of the fluids, and would manifest clinically as an edema, the condition known as lymphedema.[2] At the beginning, lymphedema is soft, dry, and without abnormalities in temperature and color.

The increase in the volume along the compromised body segment initially accompanies the increase in density and interstitial pressure, which is usually painless, if not inflammatory. However, its worst expression is the consequence of the intracellular accumulation/edema resulting in the condition hydrops.[3]

There is no pathognomic sign for primary lymphedema per se, but there are two findings/signs that are well accepted as clinical signs of the primary lymphedema among the pediatric group. However, the Stemmer sign[4] is always positive, whereas pitting edema is not always positive in the Fovea or Godet test (Figs. 53.3 and 53.4).

Fig. 53.3 Primary lymphedema
with Stemmer sign

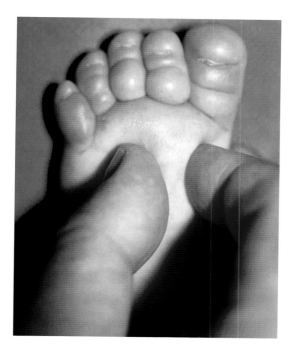

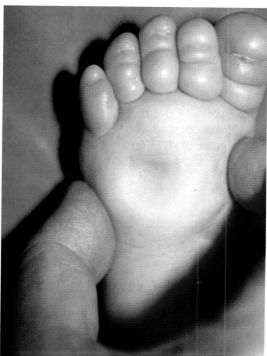

Fig. 53.4 Primary lymphedema with
a positive pitting test (Fovea)

However, both signs are nonspecific and present in other edematous conditions. The Stemmer sign is also constant in segmentary corporeal hypertrophies, lipedemas, and lipodysplasias, and the pitting edema reflects an acute clinical appearance of a primary lymphedema or an inflammatory process.

The first segment of the lymphatic system is the initial lymphatics, which is lined with "endothelial" cells[5] without a basal membrane. Its functional failure generates "interstitial" dysfunction to cause canalicular lymphatic hypertension.

From the post interstitial level (initial lymphatics) to the left thoracic duct draining site, blockage of the lymphatic transit may occur. This may be functional or organic, with or without involvement of secondary components of the lymphatic system, such as the lymph nodes or the lymphatic trunks (lymph node or truncular angiodysplasias).

On the basis of this new concept/interpretation, primary lymphedema can be further classified into three groups:

1. Primary lymphedema due to the interstitial lymphatic endothelial dysplasia and dysfunction
2. Primary lymphedema due to lymphangiodysplasia and dysfunction
3. Primary lymphedema due to lymphadeno- or nodal dysplasia and dysfunction

It will result in various conditions of the defective lymphatic system from the initial lymphatics to the lymphatic vessel and/or lymph nodes resulting in lymphangio dysplasias (LAD I) and lymphadenodysplasias (LAD II).[6-9]

LAD I: hypoplasia, hyperplasia/ectasia, lymphangiomatosis, lymphangioleiomyomatosis, dysvalvulosis, avalvulosis, lymphangio-neurosis cause organic or functional neurovegetative disturbance of the lymph vessels, and lymphangioma

LAD II: hypoplasia, global, central, and peripheral fibrosis, lymphangiomatosis, nodal angiomatosis, hemangiomatosis, follicular or medullary hyperplasia

LAAD: LAD I+LAD II, combined lymph system dysplasias

Primary lymphedema (1°L) due to interstitial dysfunction or hypoplasia of the initial lymphatics, or both are now named as three different syndromes[10] with proper identification of specific gene mutations as the cause.

1. Milroy (Nonne–Milroy) disease: lymph capillary hypoplasia by defective VEGFR-3[11]
2. Lymphedema–distichiasis syndrome: FOXC2[12]
3. The lymphedema–hypotrichosis–telangiectasia syndrome: SOX18[13]

There are 41 syndromes with peripheral primary lymphedema, added to 85 syndromes with primary generalized lymphedema[14]:

1. Noonan syndrome[15]
2. Turner syndrome[16]
3. Yellow nail syndrome[17]
4. Nevo syndrome[18]
5. Aplasia cutis + 1°L (Bronspiegel syndrome)[19]

6. Cholestasis + 1°L (Aagenaes syndrome)[20]
7. Progressive encephalopathy with edema, hypsarrhythmia, and optic atrophy (PEHO) Syndrome[21]
8. Cerebral arteriovenous malformation + 1°L (Avasthey syndrome)[22]
9. Cleft palate + 1°L (Figueroa syndrome)[23]
10. Hypoparathyroidism + 1°L (Dahlberg syndrome)[24]
11. Distichiasis + 1°L syndrome[25]
12. Microcephaly + 1°L[26]

These 12 syndromes are most frequently mentioned among many others.[27] Such syndromes are often detected among the newborns and month-old pediatric patients, with primary lymphedema combined with various conditions: uni- or bilateral Wilm's tumor, unilateral suprarenal cysts, superficial and deep venous malformations, the Klippel–Trenaunay–Servelle syndrome,[28] Klippel–Trenaunay–Weber and F.P. Weber syndromes with micro and macro AV shunts, neurofibromatosis I and II, and combined angiodysplastic syndromes.

Rarely, such a condition becomes more complicated with "the phantom bone disease": Gorham–Stout[29] syndrome, Haferkamp syndrome,[30] the Proteus syndrome (tri-dermal and tri-systemic vascular dysplasia),[31] lipodysplasias, lipoblastomatosis,[32] exudative enteropathies, and chylus reflux syndromes.

The classification of primary lymphedema into three groups of congenital, praecox, and tarda types[33] is based on the age at first clinical manifestation, but they all have similar dysplastic and or functional causes. Instead, primary lymphedema can be graded based on its expression in grades (0–3)[34]; frequently grade 0 or 1 is not recognized or is transitory among pediatric patients.

Diagnosis

Diagnostic evaluation of primary lymphedema in the pediatric group follows the general principle, which is reviewed in detail in Sections IV and V. It would be based on various imaging tests, including radioisotope lymphoscintigraphy to confirm its clinical diagnosis and/or intersticial Lymphography with MRI.

Although the genetic information would support the diagnosis, a certain condition of dysplasia and or dysfunction would need a biopsy of a nodal or lymph vessel to establish a anatomopathological pattern.

Secondary lymphedema among the pediatric group is also fully reviewed through Section IV - Clinical Diagnosis, and Section V - Laboratory/Imaging Diagnosis together with primary lymphedema.

Depending on their cause, they can be presented as a localized, regional or systemic condition by a functional or mechanical blockage at one or multiple levels.

Various factors are known to provoke a normal lymph system resulting in damage and consequent dysfunction (e.g., parasites, trauma, chronic infection, venous disorder, podoconiosis etc.).[35-39]

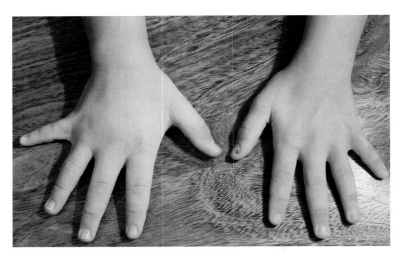

Fig. 53.5 Congenital asymmetric 1° Lymphedema on the right hand in a Turner syndrome with HGH treatment

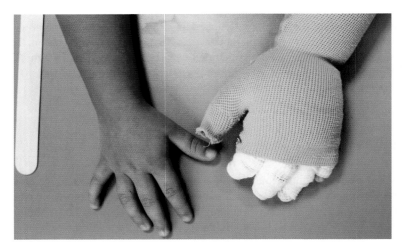

Fig. 53.6 Congenital syndromatic asymmetric 1° Lymphedema on upper limbs after and during physical treatment

Management

Detailed review of various issues for the management of primary lymphedema in the pediatric group is included in Chaps. 8–12. However, the treatment regimen with manual lymph drainage (MLD)-based complex decongestive physical therapy (CDP) are all indicated for pediatric lymphedema, and the LF(Lymphedema Framework)[40] and ISL[41] consensus documents remain a useful guideline (Figs. 53.5–53.7).

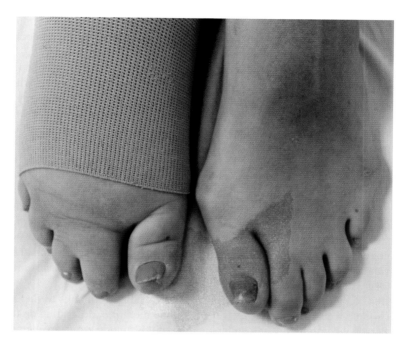

Fig. 53.7 Congenital bilateral asymmetric 1° Lymphedema in a young girl on the feet with elastic support, with bilateral syndactilia (II-III)

According to the Latin American Consensus,[42] phlebotropic agents are beneficial when primary lymphedema is associated with venous anomalies. In all primary lymphedemas, a lymph node micro-biopsy is essential as well as a thorough phlebographic study, lymphochromy, and Doppler ultrasound to explore the possibility of a lymphovenous anastomosis.

Various surgical options are possible, but are not easy in pediatric patients.[43-45] We, therefore, prefer the contralateral Palma techinique[46] for the lower extremity so as not to worsen the edema in the compromised side.

General Considerations

There are more than 250 million lymphedema patients throughout the world according to the WHO data and a third are of the pediatric age group.

The impact of this lifelong pathological condition on this pediatric group is much greater than that on the adult patient group; the psychological, physical, and also social impacts are much harder, not only for the affected child, but also for the whole family in various respects.

However, the condition is manageable, with a remarkable response to multidisciplinary treatment, including specific conditions such as head, face and neck lymphedema, genital lymphedema, lymph leakage, etc.

The big difference from the adult patients with mostly secondary lymphedema is that this condition among the children is a pathological condition for life; when the child grows, it grows with this condition as well. Therefore, all therapy regimens must be adjusted constantly, although new measurements incur much higher costs (e.g., babies with bandages and elastic supports). Also, the increased risk of cancer development cannot be ignored through this lifetime chronic illness.

Lack of social knowledge/interest in this disease often gives the wrong belief/prejudice that it is a contagious if not hereditary condition, which should be eradicated to provide reasonable quality of life to the children through full integration into school. This condition must be recognized as a part of mandatory social welfare.

Whenever possible, the children should be treated through a separate center and not mix with the adult patients. The suffering of the adult patients often gives severe psychological trauma to adolescent patients who are at a critical moment in their life and psychologically most sensitive. Proper recognition of all these issues makes it easier to assist pediatric patients in specialized centers.[47]

Results of the treatments in this group are well achieved, thanks to the confluence of simple well-planned steps in diagnosis and therapies, depending on the etiology. Personal commitment and understanding of this unique group are elementary for the proper management of this pediatric lymphedema.

References

1. Foldi M, Foldi E. *Foldi's Textbook of Lymphology*. 2nd ed. Munich: Elsevier; 2006.
2. Olszewski W. *Lymph Stasis: Pathophysiology, Diagnosis and Treatment*. Florida: CRC Press Inc; 2001:348-377.
3. *Dorlands Medical Dictionary*. Philadelphia: W.B. Saunders; 1957.
4. Stemmer R. *The Angiologycal Dictionary*. Bonn: Kagerer Kommunikation; 1997.
5. Zoltzer H. Initial lymphatics, morphology and functions of the endothelial cells. *Lymphology*. 2003;36(1):7-25.
6. Papendieck CM, Barbosa ML, Pozo P. Angiodysplasias em Pediatria. In: Thomaz JB, Belczack CEQ, eds. *Tratado de Flebologia e Linfologia*. Rio de Janeiro: Livraría e Editora Rubio Ltda; 2006:767-785. chap. 65.
7. Barbosa ML, Papendieck CM. Linfangioadenodisplasias en pediatria. *Patologia Vascular*. 2000;6(4):323-327.
8. Papendieck CM. Lymphatic dysplasias in pediatrics. *Int Angiol*. 1999;18(1):5-9.
9. Papendieck CM, Barbosa L, Pozo P. Síndromes Angiodisplasicos en Pediatria. In: Simkin R, ed. *Tratado de Patología Venosa y Linfatica*. Buenos Aires: Medrano Ediciones; 2008. chap. 41.
10. International Consensus. *Best Practice for the Management of Lymphedema. MEP*. London: Thames Valley University; 2006:6-7.
11. Online Mendelenian Inheritance on Man 153100.
12. Online Mendelenian Inheritance on Man 153400.
13. Online Mendelenian Inheritance on Man 607823.

14. Hennekam RC. Syndromic lymphatic maldevelopment. 2000. *4 International Conference National Lymphedema Network*. Florida, USA. Abstract 11-12.
15. Allanson JE. Noonan syndrome. *J Med Genet*. 1987;24:9-13.
16. Turner H. A syndrome of infantilism. Congenital webbed neck and cubitus valgus. *Endocrinology*. 1938;23:566.
17. Witte MH, Dellinger M, Bernas M, Jones KA, Witte CH. In: Foldi M, Foldi E, ed. Molecular lymphology and genetics of lymphedema-angiodysplasia syndromes. *Foldis Textbook of Lymphology*. Mosby; 2006:497-523, chap. 16.
18. Dumik M. Nevo syndrome. *Am J Med Genet*. 1998;76:67-70.
19. Bronspiegel N. Aplasia cutis-lymphedema. *Am J Dis Child*. 1985;139:509-513.
20. Aagenaes O. Cholestasis-lymphedema syndrome. *Scand J Gastroenterol*. 1998;33:335-341.
21. Somer M. Diagnostic criteria and genetics of the PEHO syndrome. *J Med Genet*. 1993;30:932-936.
22. Avasthey P. Lymphedema-cerebral AV malformations. *Br Heart J*. 1968;30:769-775.
23. Figueroa A. Lymphedema-cleft palate syndrome. *Cleft Palate*. 1983;20:153-157.
24. Dahlberg P. Lymphedema-hypoparathyroidism. *Am J Med Genet*. 1983;16:88-104.
25. Temple K. Distichiasis lymphedema syndrome. *Clin Dysmorphol*. 1994;3:139-142.
26. Crowe C. Lymphedema-microencephaly syndrome. *Am J Med Genet*. 1986;24:131-135.
27. Papendieck CM. Linfedema primario, cuando y porque? *Linfologia*. 2009;42(14):13-18.
28. Papendieck CM, Barbosa L, Pozo P, Braun D. Klippel trenaunay servelle syndrome in pediatrics. *Lymphat Res Biol*. 2003;1(1):81-85.
29. Gorham LW, Stout AP. massive osteolysis. *Bone Joint Surg*. 1955;37A:985-1004.
30. Mulliken JB, Young AE. *Vascular Birthmarks. Haemangioma and Malformations*. Philadelphia: WB Saunders; 1988.
31. Wiedemann HR. The Proteus syndrome. *Eur J Pediatr*. 1983;140:5.
32. Bertana S, Parigi GP, Giuntoli M, et al. Lipoblastoma and lipoblastomatosis. In children. *Minerva Pediatr*. 1999;51:159-166.
33. Foldi M, Foldi E, Kubik S. *Lehrbuch der Lymphologie*. 6th ed. Munich: Elsevier; 2005.
34. International Consensus. *Best Practice for the managements of Lymphoedeme*. London: MEP; 2006:6-7.
35. Jamal S. Lymphatic filariasis and the ISL consensus document. *Lymphology*. 2005;38(4):193-196.
36. Papendieck CM. Malformaciones venosas en pediatria. *RACCV*. 2004;2(1):46-55.
37. Price EW. *Podoconiosis. Non-filarial Elephantiasis*. Oxford: Oxford Medical Publication; 1990:1-35.
38. Papendieck CM. Linfedema en pediatria. Classification y etiopatogenia. *Rev Hosp Niños B Aires*. 2003;45(201):14-22.
39. Hamade A. *The Puffy Hand Syndrome*. Hinterzrten, Germany: GEL XXXII; 2006.
40. MEP. Lymphoedema Framework Best practice for the management of Lymphoedema. International Consensus MEP Ltd 2006: 2. Thames Valley Univ., London, p. 206.
41. ISL Consensus Document. The diagnosis and treatment of peripheral lymphedema. *Lymphology*. 2009;43(2):51-60.
42. Consenso Latinoamericano para el tratamiento del Linfedema. Servier Argentina.Dir. Ciucci JL. Doc. I.II.III. 2003–2009.
43. Campisi C, Boccardo F, Zilli A, Maccio A. Long term results alter lymphatic venous anastomosis for the treatment of obstructive lymphedema. *Microsurgery*. 2001;21:1135-1139.
44. Becker C, Hidden G, Pecking A. Transplantation of lymphnodes: an alternative method for treatment of lymphedema. *Prog Lymphology*. 1990;6:487-493.
45. Baumeister R, Frick A. Autogenous lymph vessel transplantation. *Eur J Lymphology*. 1995;5:17-18.
46. Palma E. Das postphlebitische syndrome-operative Therapie. *Documenta Angiologorum*. 1983;XV.
47. Todd J. *The Big Book of Lymphoedema*. The Leeds Teaching Hospitals UK NHS Trust, Charitable Foundation, 2009.

Part XII
Management of Chylous Reflux

Chapter 54
Medical Management

Francine Blei

Chylorrhea ("Chyle leak") occurs when chyle (see Table 54.1), a milky, triglyceride-rich liquid, extravasates, most commonly into the peritoneal cavity (chylous ascites) or pleural space (chyloperitoneum). Chyle leakage can also result in chyluria (chyle in the urine), chyloptysis (chyle in the sputum), chylopericardium, or cutaneous chyle leakage.

Chyle is a creamy white fluid formed in intestinal lacteals during digestion. It is normally transported through the lymphatics, entering the venous circulation via the thoracic duct. Chyle is rich in triglycerides, protein, and white blood cells, especially T lymphocytes. Accordingly, patients with chylorrhea have low serum levels of protein, lymphocytes, and fat-soluble vitamins, and develop a metabolic acidosis due to electrolyte imbalances. Immune dysfunction can arise through loss of immunoglobulins and lymphocytes[1] (Table 54.2).

Obstruction or direct trauma to the lymphatics may lead to leakage of chyle into the pleural or peritoneal cavity. Chyle leaks can occur in the prenatal, pediatric, and adult populations, with age-related etiological correlation. In adults, chyle leaks are more commonly related to malignancy. Symptoms of chyle leak can be acute or insidious, ranging from nonspecific discomfort to respiratory distress and abdominal distension. During normal digestion, chylomicrons are absorbed by the small intestines, then traverse the omental lymphatics to the cisterna chyli, anterior to the lumbar vertebrae. The cisterna chyli connects to the lumbar, thoracic, and hepatic lymphatics, ultimately forming the thoracic duct, which deposits lymph (all but that from the right chest, arm, neck, and head) into the venous system. When normal lymphatic vessels are obstructed (e.g., hypoplasia, extrinsic compression, fibrosis), or damaged (e.g., trauma), chylous leaks (also called chylous effusions) can occur.

Chylothorax can result from trauma (after cardiac, pulmonary, esophageal, or head and neck surgery; thoracic duct trauma; cardiopulmonary resuscitation; central

F. Blei
Vascular Birthmark Institute,
Roosevelt Hospital, New York, NY, USA

B.-B. Lee et al. (eds.), *Lymphedema*,
DOI 10.1007/978-0-85729-567-5_54, © Springer-Verlag London Limited 2011

Table 54.1 Properties of chyle

High protein (albumin)
High triglyceride level (>110 mg/dL)
White blood cells – especially T cells

Table 54.2 Consequences of chyle leak

Hypoproteinemia (e.g., loss of albumin)
Lymphopenia
Hypocalcemia
Hyponatremia
Metabolic acidosis
Deficiencies of fat-soluble vitamins (A, D, E, K)
Immunocompromise/susceptibility to infection (loss of immunoglobulins, T lymphocytes)

venous catheter placement; or diaphragmatic hernia repair), malignancy, congenital defects, or infections (e.g., tuberculosis). Trauma-related chyle leaks can be due to blunt damage to the thoracic duct or to incomplete ligation of the lymphatic vessels. Chylothorax may also result from lymphatic malformations, lymphangiectasia, lymphangioleiomyomatosis, lymphatic obstruction (e.g., due to congenital anomalies or hypoplasia, or as a consequence of malignancy).[2-5] Chylothorax has a high morbidity, often presenting as a pleural effusion, and diagnosis can be made by analysis of fluid from pleurocentesis. Chylothorax may be associated with chyloptysis or chyle-containing sputum.[6]

Lymphoscintigraphy or lymphangiography may be useful to define anatomy.[7,8] Shackcloth recommends administration of ingested cream to patients prior to esophageal surgery, because this intervention helps to identify the thoracic duct and surrounding lymphatic channels, decreasing the chance of trauma and post-operative chylothorax.[9]

Chylothorax can be identified (and treated) prenatally.[10] Caserio, reported 29 cases of congenital chylothorax, 94% diagnosed in utero, 66.7% of which had fetal hydrops, with an overall survival rate of 56% at 3 years of age.[11] Ergaz reported 11 neonates with congenital chylothorax, nine of whom were diagnosed prenatally, five of whom underwent intrauterine pleurocentesis.[12] Most of the patients (8) had chromosomal abnormalities.

Chylous ascites, due to disruption of the abdominal lymphatics, can manifest as abdominal distention or dyspnea. In adults, this is most commonly due to malignant obstruction. Other etiologies include lymphangiectasia, cirrhosis, trauma, and lymphangioleiomyomatosis.[13] Trauma-induced chylous ascites may be due to secondary portal hypertension, which can disrupt the integrity of the lymphatics. Retroperitoneal lymph node dissection, abdominal aortic aneurysm, and renal surgeries are most commonly associated with chylous ascites (Table 54.3).[14]

Treatment of chylorrhea often begins with dietary modification: enteral nutrition with either a no fat or a low-fat diet and medium chain triglycerides (MCT)

Table 54.3 Etiologies of chyle leakage

Chylous pleural effusion	Chylous ascites
Cardiac surgery	Abdominal, spinal, renal surgery
Trauma to thoracic duct or lacteals	Trauma to lacteals
Radiation	Radiation
Malignancy	Malignancy
Indwelling intravenous port placement	Cirrhosis, chronic liver disease
Lymphangiectasia	Lymphangiectasia
Lymphangioleiomyomatosis	Lymphangioleiomyomatosis
Lymphatic malformation	Lymphatic malformation
Congenital anomalies of thoracic duct or lymphatics	
Infection (e.g., tuberculosis)	

oil. MCTs are directly absorbed into the portal system, bypassing the lymphatics. Total parenteral nutrition with bowel rest may also ameliorate chyle leaks. If nutritional measures are inadequate, medical or surgical interventions may be effective.

Medical Therapies for Chylorrhea

Octreotide (Sandostatin, Novartis Pharmaceuticals) is a long-acting somatostatin analog that inhibits many hormones (including growth hormone, glucagon, and insulin), diminishes secretions from the intestine and pancreas, and decreases intestinal motility. This drug is approved by the Food and Drug Administration for the treatment of acromegaly and carcinoid syndrome; however, there are many published reports documenting efficacy in managing primary or secondary chylothorax and chylous ascites,[5,14-25] including in newborns.[26] Octreotide may indirectly decrease chyle secretion via binding to lymphatic somatostatin receptors and reducing bile acid secretion into the intestine. It has also been effective in traumatic thoracic duct trauma-related chyle leak.[27]

There are several reports of successful antenatal (in utero) treatment with intrapleural OK-432 (Picibanil) for fetal chylothorax.[28-30] Matsukum showed successful results with postnatal treatment with OK-432 for unrelenting octreotide-resistant congenital chylothorax in newborns.[31]

Intravenous etilefrine hydrochloride was shown to decrease chyle leaks in eight out of ten patients. The authors conclude: "by inducing contraction of the smooth muscle fibres present in the wall of the main thoracic chyle ducts, etilefrine can be considered as a useful adjunct in the management of post-operative chyle leak."[32] One report demonstrates that sirolimus (Rapamycin, Wyeth Pharmaceuticals) ameliorated after lung transplant chylothorax in a patient with lymphangioleiomyomatosis.[33] There is one report of Factor XIII infusion for recalcitrant chylothorax after lung transplantation in a patient with underlying lymphangioleiomyomatosis.[34]

Percutaneous embolization may be effective[35-37] for recurrent chylothorax after neck surgery, with percutaneous thoracic duct embolization as primary treatment.

What is evident is that there is no consensus for the management of chylorrhea, nor have there been any randomized case control studies.[22,38]

Non-surgical treatments for chylorrhea
Octreotide
OK432
Etiliefrine
Sirolimus
Factor XIII
Sclerotherapy
Radiation

References

1. Spain D, McCLure S. Chylothorax and chyous ascites. In: Gottschlich M, Fuhrman M, Hammond K, eds. *The Science and Practice of Nutrition Support: A Case-Based Core Curriculum*. Dubuque: Kendall/Hunt Publishing; 2000:479-489.
2. McGrath EE, Blades Z, Anderson PB. Chylothorax: aetiology, diagnosis and therapeutic options. *Respir Med*. 2010;104(1):1-8.
3. Teichgraber UK, Nibbe L, Gebauer B, Wagner HJ. Inadvertent puncture of the thoracic duct during attempted central venous catheter placement. *Cardiovasc Intervent Radiol*. 2003;26(6):569-571.
4. Fishman SJ, Burrows PE, Upton J, Hendren WH. Life-threatening anomalies of the thoracic duct: anatomic delineation dictates management. *J Pediatr Surg*. 2001;36(8):1269-1272.
5. Soto-Martinez M, Massie J. Chylothorax: diagnosis and management in children. *Paediatr Respir Rev*. 2009;10(4):199-207.
6. Lim KG, Rosenow EC 3rd, Staats B, Couture C, Morgenthaler TI. Chyloptysis in adults: presentation, recognition, and differential diagnosis. *Chest*. 2004;125(1):336-340.
7. Le Pimpec-Arthes F, Badia A, Febvre M, Legman P, Riquet M. Chylous reflux into localized pulmonary lymphangiectasis. *Ann Thorac Surg*. 2002;74(2):575-578.
8. Sashida Y, Nishizeki O, Higaonna K, Arashiro K. Blunt thoracic duct injury in the neck diagnosed by lymphoscintigraphy. *J Plast Reconstr Aesthet Surg*. 2008;61(9):1114-1115.
9. Shackcloth MJ, Poullis M, Lu J, Page RD. Preventing of chylothorax after oesophagectomy by routine pre-operative administration of oral cream. *Eur J Cardiothorac Surg*. 2001;20(5):1035-1036.
10. Dendale J, Comet P, Amram D, Lesbros D. Prenatal diagnosis of chylothorax. *Arch Pediatr*. 1999;6(8):867-871.
11. Caserio S, Gallego C, Martin P, Moral M, Pallas C, Galindo A. Congenital chylothorax: from foetal life to adolescence. *Acta Paediatr*. 2010;99(10):1571-1577.
12. Ergaz Z, Bar-Oz B, Yatsiv I, Arad I. Congenital chylothorax: clinical course and prognostic significance. *Pediatr Pulmonol*. 2009;44(8):806-811.
13. Gaba RC, Owens CA, Bui JT, Carrillo TC, Knuttinen MG. Chylous ascites: a rare complication of thoracic duct embolization for chylothorax. *Cardiovasc Intervent Radiol*. 2010;34(suppl 2):245-249.
14. Ferrandiere M, Hazouard E, Guicheteau V, et al. Chylous ascites following radical nephrectomy: efficiency of octreotide as treatment of a ruptured thoracic duct. *Intensive Care Med*. 2000;26(4):484-485.

15. Ulibarri JI, Sanz Y, Fuentes C, Mancha A, Aramendia M, Sanchez S. Reduction of lymphor-rhagia from ruptured thoracic duct by somatostatin. *Lancet.* 1990;336(8709):258.
16. Bliss CM, Schroy IP. Primary intestinal lymphangiectasia. *Curr Treat Options Gastroenterol.* 2004;7(1):3-6.
17. Maayan-Metzger A, Sack J, Mazkereth R, Vardi A, Kuint J. Somatostatin treatment of congenital chylothorax may induce transient hypothyroidism in newborns. *Acta Paediatr.* 2005;94(6):785-789.
18. Chan SY, Lau W, Wong WH, Cheng LC, Chau AK, Cheung YF. Chylothorax in children after congenital heart surgery. *Ann Thorac Surg.* 2006;82(5):1650-1656.
19. Siu SL, Lam DS. Spontaneous neonatal chylothorax treated with octreotide. *J Paediatr Child Health.* 2006;42(1–2):65-67.
20. Barili F, Polvani G, Topkara VK, et al. Administration of octreotide for management of postoperative high-flow chylothorax. *Ann Vasc Surg.* 2007;21(1):90-92.
21. Mincher L, Evans J, Jenner MW, Varney VA. The successful treatment of chylous effusions in malignant disease with octreotide. *Clin Oncol (R Coll Radiol).* 2005;17(2):118-121.
22. Panthongviriyakul C, Bines JE. Post-operative chylothorax in children: an evidence-based management algorithm. *J Paediatr Child Health.* 2008;44(12):716-721.
23. Pratap U, Slavik Z, Ofoe VD, Onuzo O, Franklin RC. Octreotide to treat postoperative chylothorax after cardiac operations in children. *Ann Thorac Surg.* 2001;72(5):1740-1742.
24. Valentine CN, Barresi R, Prinz RA. Somatostatin analog treatment of a cervical thoracic duct fistula. *Head Neck.* 2002;24(8):810-813.
25. Markham KM, Glover JL, Welsh RJ, Lucas RJ, Bendick PJ. Octreotide in the treatment of thoracic duct injuries. *Am Surg.* 2000;66(12):1165-1167.
26. Bulbul A, Unsur EK. Octreotide as a treatment of congenital chylothorax. *Pediatr Pulmonol.* 2010;45(6):628. author reply 9–30.
27. Rosing DK, Smith BR, Konyalian V, Putnam B. Penetrating traumatic thoracic duct injury treated successfully with octreotide therapy. *J Trauma.* 2009;67(1):E20-E21.
28. Takahashi M, Kurokawa Y, Toyama H, Hasegawa R, Hashimoto Y. The successful management of thoracoscopic thoracic duct ligation in a compromised infant with targeted lobar deflation. *Anesth Analg.* 2001;93(1):96-97.
29. Chen M, Chen CP, Shih JC, et al. Antenatal treatment of chylothorax and cystic hygroma with OK-432 in nonimmune hydrops fetalis. *Fetal Diagn Ther.* 2005;20(4):309-315.
30. Nygaard U, Sundberg K, Nielsen HS, Hertel S, Jorgensen C. New treatment of early fetal chylothorax. *Obstet Gynecol.* 2007;109(5):1088-1092.
31. Matsukuma E, Aoki Y, Sakai M, et al. Treatment with OK-432 for persistent congenital chylothorax in newborn infants resistant to octreotide. *J Pediatr Surg.* 2009;44(3):e37-e39.
32. Guillem P, Papachristos I, Peillon C, Triboulet JP. Etilefrine use in the management of postoperative chyle leaks in thoracic surgery. *Interact Cardiovasc Thorac Surg.* 2004;3(1):156-160.
33. Ohara T, Oto T, Miyoshi K, et al. Sirolimus ameliorated post lung transplant chylothorax in lymphangioleiomyomatosis. *Ann Thorac Surg.* 2008;86(6):e7-e8.
34. Shigemura N, Kawamura T, Minami M, et al. Successful factor XIII administration for persistent chylothorax after lung transplantation for lymphangioleiomyomatosis. *Ann Thorac Surg.* 2009;88(3):1003-1006.
35. Repko BM, Scorza LB, Mahraj RP. Recurrent chylothorax after neck surgery: percutaneous thoracic duct embolization as primary treatment. *Otolaryngol Head Neck Surg.* 2009;141(3):426-427.
36. Patel N, Lewandowski RJ, Bove M, Nemcek AA Jr, Salem R. Thoracic duct embolization: a new treatment for massive leak after neck dissection. *Laryngoscope.* 2008;118(4):680-683.
37. Itkin M, Kucharczuk JC, Kwak A, Trerotola SO, Kaiser LR. Nonoperative thoracic duct embolization for traumatic thoracic duct leak: experience in 109 patients. *J Thorac Cardiovasc Surg.* 2010;139(3):584-589. discussion 9–90.
38. Smoke A, Delegge MH. Chyle leaks: Consensus on management? *Nutr Clin Pract.* 2008; 23(5):529-532.

Chapter 55
Surgical Management

Richard G. Azizkhan and Jesse A. Taylor

Introduction

This chapter focuses on surgical interventions for treating chyle reflux. As with many areas of vascular medicine, multidisciplinary management is the norm, with surgeons, medical specialists, and interventional radiologists all playing important roles. An understanding of chyle transportation from the bowel lacteals to the thoracic duct and venous system is important in planning treatment. When flow is disrupted, the anatomic location of a blockage or rupture in this ductal system may translate into chylous ascites, chylothorax, chylous cyst, chylopericardium, chyloptysis, chyluria, and skin lesions with chylorrhea. The goal of therapy is to restore balance to the lymphatic system through decreased lymph production, facilitation of physiological lymphatic pathways, or removal of regions of lymphatic dysplasia.

Drainage Procedures

Removal of pooled chylous fluid is another adjunct to surgical treatment. For example, compression garments and mechanical massage have shown good results in limiting and/or controlling lymphedema, cellulitis, and lymphangitis in extremities.[1] When disrupted flow results in a chylothorax or chylous ascites, thoracentesis and paracentesis may be used to relieve symptoms of respiratory failure and improve hemodynamics. Wheeler et al.[2] have described thoracentesis as a means of treating life-threatening neonatal tension chylothorax. To obtain continuous drainage, tube thoracostomy has been shown to be effective. In a study of 29 patients, Marts et al.[3]

R.G. Azizkhan (✉)
Department of Surgery and Pediatrics,
Cincinnati Children's Hospital Medical Center,
Cincinnati, OH, USA

B.-B. Lee et al. (eds.), *Lymphedema*,
DOI 10.1007/978-0-85729-567-5_55, © Springer-Verlag London Limited 2011

were able to combine medium chain triglyceride (MCT) therapy with chest tube placement for a cure rate of 79% of adult patients presenting with a traumatic or iatrogenic chylothorax. Though there is no consensus as to when drainage procedures should be abandoned in favor of surgery, most authors recommend surgery for persistent disease after two attempts at drainage.[1-3]

The literature does not support drainage procedures as primary treatment for cutaneous chyle reflux, especially in the setting of lymphangiomyomatosis.[4,5] Converting an internally draining system into an externally draining system may worsen chyle losses and hasten malnutrition.

Image-Guided Approaches

Dilated lymphatic channels and resultant chylorrhea are often the most symptomatic manifestation of chyle reflux. The cutaneous manifestation presents as milia-like lesions often in the external genitalia, thigh, or trunk.[6,7] To address megalymphatics, dilated channels, and "lakes," luminal obliteration has become increasingly utilized. Toxic agents may be directly injected into the lumen of such vessels, causing obliterative lymphangitis. Commonly employed agents include tetracycline, doxycycline, alcohol, OK-432, and bleomycin.[8,9] Alternatively, vessels may be obliterated by placing intraluminal coils. Two teams have advocated percutaneous lymphangiography-guided cannulation and embolization as primary treatment for chylous leak of the thoracic duct after head and neck surgery.[10,11] Superficial lesions with lower degrees of lymphatic dilation have been successfully managed with the use of radiation therapy and lasers such as the carbon dioxide, yttrium aluminum garnet, and potassium titanyl phosphate laser. Carati et al.[12] summarized their experience in a double-blinded randomized control trial with a low-level 904-nm laser in which one third of postmastectomy lymphedema patients demonstrated decreased limb volume and limb hardness.

Open Surgical Approaches

Treatment of Cutaneous Chylorrhea and Chylorrhagia

Removing a region of lymphatic dysplasia is often the most expedient route to symptomatic relief. This principle is true in almost all regions of the body, including the skin, bowel, thorax, and abdomen.[13] Ruptured lymphatics are identified after the patient ingests a fatty meal and the leaking lymphatic ducts are ligated, oversewn, clipped, or excised with diathermy. Cutaneous lesions in the groin area have a high rate of recurrence, and multimodal therapy with excision and laser or sclerotherapy works well (Fig. 55.1).[14] Percutaneous drainage tubes are often employed in the

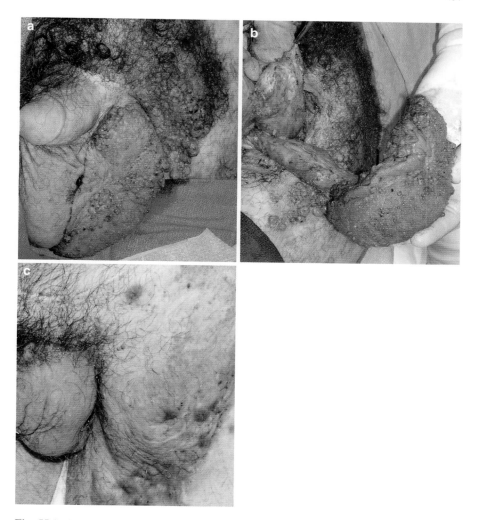

Fig. 55.1 An 18-year-old male patient with a complex capillary venolymphatic malformation involving the groin, pelvis and left leg. Patient was draining more than 300 mL/day of lymphatic fluid from the lymphatic vesicles in the pubic region and experienced numerous episodes of life-threatening sepsis. (**a**) Photograph just prior to hemiscrotal resection. (**b**) Intraoperative photograph demonstrating a massive lymphatic varix to the resected hemiscrotum. (**c**) 6 months following a second operative resection of residual suprapubic involvement and following CO_2 laser treatment of residual vesicles

postoperative phase to decrease the incidence of seroma formation. As previously stated, such drains transform an internally draining system into an externally draining system, and the amount of drainage must be monitored closely to avoid complications associated with high volume chyle loss.

A second surgical option is to reconstruct damaged lymphatics in an attempt to restore "physiological" lymphatic flow. The goal of physiological surgical intervention is to bypass disrupted or malformed lymphatics and to restore physiological balance to the lymphatic system. Prior to undergoing physiological intervention, Kim et al.[13] recommend that patients first undergo a trial of complex physical therapy (CPT) that includes manual lymph drainage, compression bandages, stockings or serial compression devices. Used primarily for its high rate of symptom amelioration, CPT also delays progression of chyle reflux to chronic interstitial edema, which is not amenable to reconstruction.[15] However, Campisi[16] believes that compression does not affect the microcirculation and attributes high nonresponse rates of 30–40% to this failure. Consequently, microsurgical techniques have been developed to create super-microsurgical anastomoses between lymphatics and venules.

The most common surgical approaches are through lymphaticovenous anastomoses and lymphatico-veno-lymphatic anastomoses. Both can be performed end-to-end or end-to-side, and both have been reported at vessel diameters of as little as 0.3 mm.[17] In a report of 39 cases, Narushima[18] found a positive correlation between the number of anastomoses to symptomatic improvement and decreased limb diameter. In another study, Kobayashi[15] described a technique in which he telescoped, or invaginated, multiple small lymphatic channels into a single venule. Like Narushima, he documented both symptomatic and functional improvement in his cohort. The downside to microsurgical techniques is their technical difficulty and variable long-term patency rates.[18]

Treatment of Chylothorax

With the development of a chylothorax, chest tube drainage is often implemented first to alleviate respiratory dysfunction. MCT diet, thoracentesis, and percutaneous obliteration follow as definitive therapy and/or helpful adjuncts. Videoscopic-assisted thoracoscopy (VATS) is a safe and effective technique to evaluate the entire thorax and allow for intervention based on the amount and location of output of the chylous leak.[19] When output is less than 500 mL/day, pleural abrasion and pleurodesis with talc or other agents has been shown to be effective.[20] Fibrin glue can be used during the VATS procedure to help manage chylous leakage when no focal drainage point can be determined.[21] With diffuse drainage, partial pleurectomy has also been demonstrated to resolve symptoms.[22]

For high output chylous drainage or drainage exceeding 1 L/day, ligation of the thoracic duct can be achieved with VATS or thoracotomy. The technique may involve the injection of methylene blue dye or consumption of a high fat content material, such as a butter/cream mixture, and observation for focal output. If diffuse drainage is seen, en masse tissue ligation can be undertaken as the thoracic duct generally follows posterior to the esophagus, and anteromedial to the azygos vein in the lower chest.[23] Studies have shown a 90% resolution of the leak and earlier chest tube removal when the thoracic duct is ligated in both pediatric and adult populations.[24,25] Alternatively, cannulation of the cysterna chyli with coil embolization of the thoracic duct may be performed. Partial or full response has been shown to be around 95% when either the cysterna chyli or thoracic duct can be identified and accessed.[19]

Congenital chylothorax secondary to lymphatic aplasia, hypoplasia, fibrosis, and superior vena caval obstruction remains a clinical challenge. Serial thoracentesis was the classic treatment, but increased risk of infection, patient discomfort and the psychological effects of repeated trauma in children led to the development of new shunting procedures. The first clinical pleuroperitoneal shunts were reported in 1983 with a low-pressure ventriculoperitoneal shunt catheter system in five ventilator-dependent babies.[26] Resolution of pulmonary failure and chylothorax was evident in four of the five patients. The Denver pleuroperitoneal shunt, which requires the patient to manually pump the fluid with a subcutaneous pump, has also been used for difficult cases of chylothorax.[27] Side effects to these shunts include skin erosion, infection, and, most commonly, occlusion. In 1999, Wolff et al.[28] described a modification of the pleuroperitoneal shunt with externalization of the pumping chamber that increased efficacy and comfort in utilizing this approach.

Retrograde chyle flow resulting from thoracic duct obstruction may be managed by a thoracic duct to azygos vein anastomosis. The procedure involves the lower thoracic duct (usually around 2–3 mm) and an end-to-end anastomosis with 8-0 or 10-0 non-absorbable suture.[29]

Treatment of Chylous Ascites

As with other disorders of chyle reflux, multimodal treatment is the rule with chylous ascites. Percutaneous procedures, aimed at embolizing retroperitoneal lymphatics with needle disruption, are a first-line therapy in conjunction with an MCT diet. Cope et al.[30] have shown a response in up to 42 (73.8%) of the study patients with percutaneous techniques. Patients with symptomatic chylous ascites can be initially managed through serial paracentesis. However, if the drainage persists, a peritoneal–venous shunt can be utilized. The "LeVeen Shunt," developed in 1974 to combat cirrhotic ascites, consists of a one-way pressure valve that shunts fluid from the peritoneal cavity to the internal or external jugular vein.[31] However, complications in a nutritionally sub-optimal patient include high rates of wound infection, peritonitis, asymptomatic coagulopathy, disseminated intravascular coagulation (DIC), subclavian vein thrombosis, and electrolyte disturbances.[32]

Adjuncts to Surgical Management of Recalcitrant Chyle Reflux

Octreotide, a somatostatin analog, has been shown in multiple studies to slow chylothorax output and hasten chylous fistula closure.[31] The mechanism of action is thought to be a result of mild vasoconstriction of splanchnic vessels and the reduction in gastrointestinal secretions. The treatment can be delivered intravenously or subcutaneously. Side effects of this therapy include hypothyroidism, necrotizing enterocolitis, renal impairment, hyperglycemia, cramps, loose stools, and liver dysfunction.[32–35]

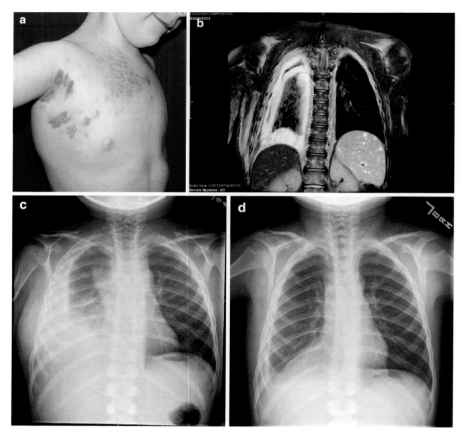

Fig. 55.2 A 7-year-old male with a diffuse microcystic lymphatic malformation involving the entire right hemithorax including the chest wall, right pleura, and mediastinum. This was associated with persistent chylothorax and respiratory distress. Failure to create pleural symphysis using doxycycline through thoracostomy tubes and subsequent failure of surgical decortication led 3 months later to using rapamycin as a salvage therapy. (**a**) Patient showing chest wall involvement. (**b**) MRI showing an extensive and transmural right chest wall and mediastinal lesion. (**c**) Chest radiograph prior to any intervention. (**d**) Chest radiograph 3 months after initiating oral rapamycin

Unpublished cases have shown promising results through the use of rapamycin in the inhibition of lymphangiomatosis. Rapamycin is a lipophylic macrolide antibiotic that inhibits mTOR, a serine/threonine kinase involved in VEGF-A expression and angiogenesis.[32] Primarily investigated for its role in preventing tumor cell metastasis within the lymphatic system, rapamycin has been used to treat life-threatening lymphatic malformations at our institution (Fig. 55.2).

Summary

Treatment of chyle reflux, like most areas of vascular medicine, is in rapid evolution. Multidisciplinary management is the norm, with surgeons, medical specialists, and interventional radiologists all playing important roles.

References

1. Campisi C, Eretta C, Pertile D, Da Rin E, Campisi C, et al. Microsurgery for treatment of peripheral lymphedema: long-term outcome and future perspective. *Microsurgery*. 2007; 27(4):333-338.
2. Wheeler AD, Tobias JD. Tension chylothorax in two pediatric patients. *Paediatr Anaesth*. 2007;17(5):488-491.
3. Marts BC, Naunheim KS, Fiore AC, Pennington DG. Conservative versus surgical management of chylothorax. *Am J Surg*. 1992;164:532-534.
4. Lim ST, Ngan H, Wong KK, Ong GB. Leakage of lymph through scrotal skin. *J Urol*. 1981;125(6):889-890.
5. Sales F, Trepo E, Brondello S, Lemaitre P, Bourgeois P. *Eur J Surg Oncol*. 2007;33(8): 1042-1043.
6. Kinmonth JB, Taylor GW. Chylous reflux. *Br Med J*. 1964;I:529-532.
7. Johnson WT. Cutaneous chylous reflux: the weeping scrotum. *Arch Dermatol*. 1979;115: 164-166.
8. Alomari AI, Karian VE, Lord DJ, Padua HM, Burrows PE. Percutaneous sclerotherapy for lymphatic malformations: a retrospective analysis of patient-evaluated improvement. *J Vasc Interv Radiol*. 2006;17:1639-1648.
9. Dasgupta R, Adams AD, Elluru R, Wentzel MS, Azizkhan RG. Noninterventional treatment of selected head and neck lymphatic malformations. *J Pediatr Surg*. 2008;43(5):869-873.
10. Scorza LB, Goldstein BJ, Mahraj RP. Modern management of chylous leak following head and neck surgery: a discussion of percutaneous lymphangiography-guided cannulation and embolization of thoracic duct. *Otolaryngol Clin North Am*. 2008;41(6):1231-1240.
11. Repko BM, Scorza LB, Mahraj RP. Recurrent chylothorax after neck surgery: percutaneous thoracic duct emobolization as primary treatment. *Otolaryngol Head Neck Surg*. 2009;141(3): 426-427.
12. Carati CJ, Anderson SN, Gannon BJ, Piller NB. Treatment of postmastectomy lymphedema with low-level laser therapy: a double blind, placebo-controlled trial. *Cancer*. 2003;98(6):1114-1122. Erratum in: Cancer. 2003 Dec 15; 98(12):2742.
13. Kim NR, Lee SK, Suh YL. Primary intestinal lymphangiectasia treated by segmental resections of small bowel. *J Pediatr Surg*. 2009;44(10):e13-e17.
14. Connolly M, Archer CB. Chylous reflux presenting with minimal milia-like lesions on the thigh. *J Am Acad Dermatol*. 2006;55(6):1108-1109.
15. LeVeen HH, Wapnick S, Diaz C, Grosber S, Kinney M. Ascites: its correction by peritoneovenous shunting. *Curr Probl Surg*. 1979;16:1-61.
16. Campisi C, Boccardo F, Zilli A, Maccio A, Gariglio A, et al. Peripheral lymphedema; new advances in microsurgical treatment and long-term outcome. *Microsurgery*. 2003;23:522-555.
17. Koshima I, Inagawa K, Urushibara K, Moriguchi T. Super-microsurgical lymphaticovenular anastomosis for treatment of lymphedema in the upper extremities. *J Reconstr Microsurg*. 2000;16:437-442.
18. Narushima M, Mihara M, Yamamoto Y, Lida T, Koshima I, et al. The intravascular stenting method for treatment of extremity lymphedema with multiconfiguration lymphaticovenous anastomoses. *Plast Reconstr Surg*. 2010;125(3):935-943.

19. Maldonado F, Cartin-Ceba R, Hawkins FJ, Ryu JH. Medical and surgical management of chylothorax and associated outcomes. *Am J Med Sci*. 2010;339(4):314-318.
20. Paul S, Altorki NK, Port JL, Stiles BM, Lee PC. Surgical management of chylothorax. *Thorac Cardiovasc Surg*. 2009;57(4):226-228.
21. Nguyen D. Successful management of postoperative chylothorax with fibrin glue in a premature neonate. *Can J Surg*. 1994;37(2):158-160. Review.
22. Barret DS. Pleurectomy for chylothorax associated with intestinal lymphangiectasia. *Thorax*. 1987;42:557-558.
23. Robinson CL. The management of chylothorax. *Ann Thorac Surg*. 1985;39:90-95.
24. Nath DS, Savla J, Khemani RG, Nussbaum DP, Greene CL, et al. Thoracic duct ligation for persistent chylothorax after pediatric cardiothoracic surgery. *Ann Thorac Surg*. 2009;88(1):246-251. discussion 251-252.
25. Cerfolio RJ, Allen MS, Deschamps C, Trastek VF, Pairolero PC. Postoperative chylothorax. *J Thorac Cardiovasc Surg*. 1996;112:1361-1366.
26. Azizkhan RG, Canfield J, Alford BA, Rodgers BM. Pleuroperitoneal shunts in the management of neonatal chylothorax. *J Pediatr Surg*. 1983;18(6):842-850.
27. Podevin G, Levard G, Larroquet M, Gruner M. Pleuroperitoneal shunt in the management chylothorax caused by thoracic lymphatic dysplasia. *J Pediatr Surg*. 1999;34:1420-1422.
28. Wolff AB, Silen ML, Kokoska ER, Rodgers BM. Treatment of refractory chylothorax with externalized pleuroperitoneal shunts in children. *Ann Thorac Surg*. 1999;68:1053-1057.
29. Barili F, Polvani G, Topkara VK. Administration of octreotide for management of postoperative high-flow chylothorax. *Ann Vasc Surg*. 2007;21(1):90-92.
30. Rasiah SV, Oei J, Lui K. Octreotide in the treatment of congential chylothorax. *J Paediatr Child Health*. 2004;40:585-588.
31. Roehr CC, Jung A, Proquitte H, Blankenstein O, Hammer H, et al. Somatostatin or octreotide as treatment options for chylothorax in young children: a systematic review. *Intensive Care Med*. 2006;32:650-657.
32. Kobayashi T, Kishimoto T, Kamata S, Otsuka M, Miyazaki M, et al. Rapamycin, a specific inhibitor of the mammalian target of rapamycin, suppresses lymphangiogenesis and lymphatic metastasis. *Cancer Sci*. 2007;98(5):726-733.
33. Noel AA, Gloviczki P, Bender CE, Whitley D, Stanson AW, et al. Treatment of symptomatic primary chylous disorders. *J Vasc Surg*. 2001;34(5):785-791.
34. Cope C, Kaiser LR. Management of unremitting chylothorax by percutaneous embolisation and blockage of retroperitoneal lymphatic vessels in 42 patients. *J Vasc Interv Radiol*. 2002;13:1139-1148.
35. Leveen HH, Christoudias G, Ip M, Luft R, Falk G, Grosberg S. Peritoneo-venous shunting for ascites. *Ann Surg*. 1974;180(4):580-591.

Part XIII
Filariasis Lymphedema

Chapter 56
Epidemiology

LeAnne M. Fox

Lymphatic filariasis is caused by infection with three species of parasite: *Wuchereria bancrofti, Brugia malayi,* and *Brugia timori*. Currently, there are an estimated 1.3 billion people living in endemic areas in 81 countries and 120 million people are infected. More than 90% of these infections are caused by *W. bancrofti* for which humans are the only natural host.

Lymphatic filariasis is endemic in Africa, Asia, the Indian subcontinent, the western Pacific Islands, focal areas of Latin America, and the Caribbean, particularly Haiti and the Dominican Republic (see Table 56.1).[1] Of these, the greatest numbers of infected persons live in sub-Saharan Africa, south Asia, and the western Pacific. Both China and the Republic of Korea were considered endemic until recently, but declared elimination of lymphatic filariasis as a public health problem in 2007 and 2008 respectively.[2] Infection with *B. malayi* is limited to Asia (India, Malaysia, and formerly China) and several Pacific island groups (Indonesia and the Philippines), and there are fewer than 10–20 million persons in these areas who are infected with *B. malayi*. Unlike *W. bancrofti, B. malayi* has feline and primate reservoirs. *B. timori* is only found on the Timor island of Indonesia.

The distribution of lymphatic filariasis is highly focal within an endemic area. This is due to the different feeding behaviors of the mosquito vectors that are capable of transmitting lymphatic filariasis as well as to the local ecological factors that favor the breeding of mosquito vectors. For example, *W. bancrofti* is transmitted in much of rural Africa by *Anopheles* species,[3] whereas in many urban areas of the world, including India and in the western hemisphere, *W. bancrofti* is transmitted by *Culex* mosquitoes.[4] Other vectors include *Aedes* species and *Mansonia*.[5] Lymphatic filariasis is less commonly transmitted than other vector-borne parasitic infections and therefore less commonly infects travelers with short-term exposure in endemic

L.M. Fox
Division of Parasitic Diseases and Malaria, Center for Global Health,
Centers for Disease Control and Prevention, Atlanta, GA, USA

Table 56.1 Characteristics of filarial parasites of humans

Most common tissue location

Species	Adult	Microfilaria	Geographic distribution	Estimated no. infected	Vector	Periodicity
Wuchereria bancrofti	Lymphatics	Blood	Tropics worldwide	115 million	Mosquitoes	Nocturnal or subperiodic
Brugia malayi	Lymphatics	Blood	Southeast Asia	13 million	Mosquitoes	Nocturnal or subperiodic
Brugia timori	Lymphatics	Blood	Indonesia	Thousands	Mosquitoes	Nocturnal

areas.[6] The microfilariae of *W. bancrofti* and *B. malayi* have a nocturnal periodicity whereby large numbers of the organisms are present in the peripheral circulation between 9 p.m., and 2 a.m., which coincides with the time when most mosquito vectors take their blood meal.[7] In contrast, there is no clear-cut periodic cycle for *Aedes*-transmitted microfilariae in the South Pacific.

At the time of feeding, infective L3 larvae escape from the proboscis of the mosquito, penetrate the skin, and home to lymph nodes and lymphatic vessels. It then takes between 6 and 12 months for the L3 larvae to become sexually mature adult female worms (L5 stage) capable of producing first-stage L1 larvae called microfilariae that circulate in the blood. The adult worms can live in the lymphatic vessels and produce microfilaria for 5–10 years. Microfilariae are taken up in the blood meal of mosquitoes and develop into infective L3 larvae in the thorax of the mosquito over a period of 7–21 days and are then ready to infect another host.

Infection with lymphatic filariasis is most often clinically unapparent, although it has been demonstrated that even asymptomatic infected individuals have underlying lymphatic damage in the form of lymphatic dilatation and dysfunction.[8,9] Initial infection, detected as the presence of circulating filarial antigen, commonly occurs between the ages of 2 and 4 years in highly endemic areas.[10,11] In these areas of intense transmission, the prevalence of microfilaremia in the population increases rapidly between the ages of 5 and 10 years and continues to increase until the third and fourth decades of life.

A recently discovered biological feature of several human filarial parasites, including *W. bancrofti* and *Brugia* species, relates to the fact that these nematodes possess the bacterial endosymbiont *Wolbachia*.[12] *Wolbachia* are rickettsia-like endosymbiotic bacteria that are involved in the normal development, viability, and fertility of the adult worm.[13] They have been investigated as potentially important chemotherapeutic targets as well as disease-causing organisms for lymphatic filariasis.[14-16]

The chronic clinical manifestations of lymphatic filariasis, including lymphedema, elephantiasis, and hydrocele, occur infrequently in persons younger than 10 years of age and generally increase in frequency with age.[11] It is estimated that of the 120 million persons infected worldwide, approximately one third, or 40 million, have some form of clinically overt disease: 25 million with hydrocele and 15 million with lymphedema or elephantiasis.[1] In addition to the chronic clinical manifestations of lymphatic filariasis, patients may also exhibit acute manifestations, particularly acute filarial lymphangitis (AFL) and acute dermatolymphangioadenitis (ADLA). AFL involves acute inflammation of a lymphatic vessel that progresses distally along the vessel and is thought to be caused by the death of the adult worm.[17] ADLA is a separate and clinically distinct syndrome that is caused by bacterial infection of the small collecting lymphatic vessels in areas of lymphatic dysfunction.[17,18] Unlike filarial lymphangitis, this syndrome develops in a reticular rather than a linear pattern and is more commonly associated with severe pain, fever, and chills. Factors postulated to be involved in the progression of filarial lymphedema to elephantiasis include: repeated attacks of acute dermatolymphangioadenitis,[19] the intensity of filarial transmission within a population,[20] and the presence of *Wolbachia*.[21] Lymphedema management involves leg hygiene, early treatment of bacterial and fungal infections, elevation, and exercises.[22] Clinical and histopathological studies suggest that lymphedema management can both decrease the number of ADLA episodes and halt or, in some cases, partially reverse disease progression.[23,24] The chronic clinical manifestations of lymphatic filariasis lead to adverse psychological and economic consequences, making lymphatic filariasis one of the leading causes of disability[25] and an impediment to economic and social development.[26]

Recognition that lymphatic filariasis can be eradicated using currently available chemotherapies has led to the 1997 World Health Assembly (WHA) resolution to eliminate lymphatic filariasis as a public health problem (WHA 50.29, 13 May 1997).[27] After this resolution in 2000, the Global Programme for the Elimination of Lymphatic Filariasis (GPELF) was launched with the dual goals of (1) interrupting transmission by annual mass drug administration (MDA) of diethylcarbamazine or ivermectin plus albendazole to the entire population in endemic areas and (2) alleviating the suffering of people affected by chronic disease through morbidity management. (http://www.filariasis.org/progress/elimination_strategy.html). Drug donations of ivermectin by Merck and Co. and albendazole by GlaxoSmithKline have been critical to making the global elimination program a reality. Since the inception of the GPELF, there has been a steady increase in the number of countries implementing MDA from 12 in 2000 to 52 out of 81 lymphatic filariasis endemic countries in 2009.[2] In the first 8 years of the global elimination program, more than 1.9 billion treatments were provided via yearly MDA to a minimum of 570 million individuals, thus protecting more than 16 million people from filarial infection or progression of clinical disease and averting 32 million disability adjusted life years.[28] In addition, it has been estimated that during the first 8 years of the GPELF, US $21.8 billion of direct economic benefits has been gained, making global elimination of lymphatic filariasis one of the "best buys" in public health.[29]

References

1. Michael E, Bundy DAP, Grenfell BT. Re-assessing the global prevalence and distribution of lymphatic filariasis. *Parasitology*. 1996;112:409-428.

2. World Health Organization. Global Programme to Eliminate Lymphatic Filariasis (GPELF) Progress Report 2000–2009 and Strategic Plan 2010–2020. 2010; 6–8.
3. Merelo-Lobo AR, McCall PJ, Perez MA, et al. Identification of the vectors of lymphatic filariasis in the Lower Shire Valley, southern Malawi. *Trans R Soc Trop Med Hyg.* 2003;97(3):299-301.
4. Ramaiah KD, Das PK. Seasonality of adult *Culex quinquefasciatus* and transmission of bancroftian filariasis in Pondicherry, south India. *Acta Trop.* 1992;50(4):275-283.
5. Chang MS. Operational issues in the control of the vectors of Brugia. *Ann Trop Med Parasitol.* 2002;96(2):S71-S76.
6. Lipner EM, Law MA, Barnett E, et al. Filariasis in travelers presenting to the GeoSentinel Surveillance Network. *PloS Negl Trop Dis.* 2007;1(3):e88.
7. O'Conner FW. Filarial periodicity with observations and on the mechanisms of migration of the microfilariae and from parent worm to the blood stream. *PR Public Health Trop Med.* 1931;6:263.
8. Shenoy RK, Suma TK, Kumaraswami V, et al. Lymphoscintigraphic evidence of lymph vessel dilation in the limbs of children with *Brugia malayi* infection. *J Commun Dis.* 2008;40(2):91-100.
9. Fox LM, Furness BW, Haser JK, et al. Ultrasonographic examination of Haitian children with lymphatic filariasis: a longitudinal assessment in the context of antifilarial drug treatment. *Am J Trop Med Hyg.* 2005;72:642-648.
10. Lammie PJ, Reiss MD, Dimock KA, et al. Longitudinal analysis of the development of filarial infection and antifilarial immunity in a cohort of Haitian children. *Am J Trop Med Hyg.* 1998;59:217-221.
11. Witt C, Ottesen EA. Lymphatic filariasis: an infection of childhood. *Bull World Health Org.* 2001;6:582-606.
12. Taylor MJ, Hoerauf A. *Wolbachia* bacteria of filarial nematodes. *Parasitol Today.* 1999;15: 437-442.
13. Hise AG, Gillette-Ferguson I, Pearlman E. The role of endosymbiotic *Wolbachia* bacteria in filarial disease. *Cell Microbiol.* 2004;6:97-104.
14. Hoerauf A, Mand S, Fischer K, et al. Doxycycline as a novel strategy against bancroftian filariasis-depletion of *Wolbachia* endosymbionts from *Wuchereria bancrofti* and stop of microfilaria production. *Med Microbiol Immunol.* 2003;192:211-216.
15. Cross HF, Haarbrink M, Egerton G, et al. Severe reactions to filarial chemotherapy and release of *Wolbachia* endosymbionts into blood. *Lancet.* 2001;358:1873-1875.
16. Debrah AY, Mand S, Marfo-Debrekyei Y, et al. Macrofilaricidal effect of 4 weeks of treatment with doxycycline on *Wuchereria bancrofti*. *Trop Med Int Health.* 2007;12(12):1433-1441.
17. Dreyer G, Medeiros Z, Netto MJ, et al. Acute attacks in the extremities of persons living in an area endemic for bancroftian filariasis: differentiation of two syndromes. *Trans R Soc Trop Med Hyg.* 1999;93:413-417.
18. Olszewski WL, Jamal S, Manokaran G, et al. Bacteriologic studies of blood, tissue fluid, lymph, and lymph nodes in patients with acute dermatolymphangioadenitis (DLA) in course of 'filarial' lymphedema. *Acta Trop.* 1999;73:217-224.
19. Dreyer G, Noroes J, Figueredo-Silva J, et al. Pathogenesis of lymphatic disease in bancroftian filariasis: a clinical perspective. *Parasitol Today.* 2000;16:544-548.
20. Kazura JW, Bockarie M, Alexander N, et al. Transmission intensity and its relationship to infection and disease due to *Wuchereria bancrofti* in Papua New Guinea. *J Infect Dis.* 1997;176:242-246.
21. Debrah AY, Mand S, Specht S, et al. Doxycycline reduces plasma VEGF-C/sVEGFR-3 and improves pathology in lymphatic filariasis. *PLoS Pathog.* 2006;2(9):e92.
22. Dreyer G, Addiss DG, Dreyer P, et al. *Basic Lymphoedema Management: Treatment and Prevention of Problems Associated with Lymphatic Filariasis.* Hollis: Hollis Publishing Co.; 2002.
23. Addiss DG, Louis-Charles J, Roberts J, et al. Feasibility and effectiveness of basic lymphedema management in Leogane, Haiti, an area endemic for bancroftian filariasis. *PloS Negl Trop Dis.* 2010;4(4):e688.

24. Kerketta AS, Babu BV, Rath K, et al. A randomized clinical trial to compare the efficacy of three treatment regimens along with footcare in the morbidity management of filarial lymphoedema. *Trop Med Int Health.* 2005;10:698-705.
25. WHO. Informal consultation on preventing disability from lymphatic filariasis, WHO, Geneva, August 2006. *Wkly Epidemiol Rep.* 2006;81:373-383.
26. Evans DB, Gelband H, Vlassoff C. Social and economic factors and the control of lymphatic filariasis: a review. *Acta Trop.* 1993;53:1-26.
27. Ottesen EA. The global programme to eliminate lymphatic filariasis. *Trop Med Int Health.* 2000;5:591-594.
28. Ottesen EA, Hooper PJ, Bradley M, et al. The global programme to eliminate lymphatic filariasis: health impact after 8 years. *PloS Negl Trop Dis.* 2008;2(10):e317.
29. Chu BK, Hooper PJ, Bradley MH, et al. The economic benefits resulting from the first 8 years of the Global Programme to Eliminate Lymphatic Filariasis (2000–2007). *PloS Negl Trop Dis.* 2010;4(6):e708.

Chapter 57
Etiology and Pathophysiology

Waldemar L. Olszewski

Lymphatic filariasis is caused by *Wuchereria bancrofti*, *Brugia malayi*, and *Brugia timori*.[1,2] The adult worms live in the lymphatic vessels and are responsible for the primary lesions causing lymph stasis. Lymph stasis predisposes to bacterial infections and host inflammatory response. Adult worms die after some time, but bacterial colonization of tissues continues. The pathological changes in tissues develop further, leading to an increase in limb volume, hyperkeratosis, and fibrosis.

Morphology

The adult *W. bancrofti* are 4–10 cm long, whereas *B. malayi* are shorter (3–5 cm long). The males are smaller than the females. The life-span ranges from 7 to 15 years. The female worm discharges eggs (microfilaria) into the lymphatics that circulate in the blood. The microfilaria vary in length from 200–300 µm. Humans are the only known definitive hosts for *W. bancrofti*, but *B. malayi* is also seen in animals.

Life Cycle

The *W. bancrofti* microfilariae are ingested by mosquitoes as Culex or Anopheles and *B. malayi* by Mansonia and Anopheles. The adult worms do not multiply in the host, nor do the larvae multiply in the mosquitoes. The microfilariae are ingested by mosquitoes. In the mosquitoes the microfilaria mature to become the infective form. Depending on the temperature and humidity of the environment, this process takes 10–14 days. The infective L3 larvae are 1.4–2.0 mm long. They migrate to the

W.L. Olszewski
Department of Surgical Research and Transplantology,
Medical Research Centre, Warsaw, Poland

B.-B. Lee et al. (eds.), *Lymphedema*,
DOI 10.1007/978-0-85729-567-5_57, © Springer-Verlag London Limited 2011

Fig. 57.1 Lymphoscintigram of a filaria-infected patient with lymphedema of both lower limbs. The toeweb-injected Nanocoll T99 spreads in the dilated calf lymphatics (left leg). It flows along the superficial lymphatics to the inguinal lymph nodes and along the deep vessels, through multiple enlarged popliteal nodes in both limbs. In normal conditions only 1–2 small nodes are seen in this region

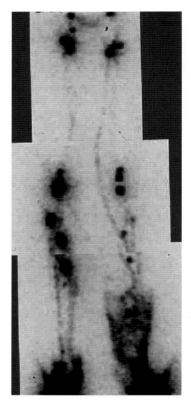

proboscis to be deposited at the bite wound by the mosquito. The larvae enter the skin at puncture sites and reach the lymphatics to grow, mature, and mate. Microfilariae appear in circulation 6–12 months after entry of the larvae. They remain viable for 2–3 months, after which they die and are removed by host macrophages.

Pathology

Gross Pathology

Filarial lymphedema is most commonly seen in the lower limbs (Fig. 57.1). It may also affect the upper limbs, breast, scrotum, and urinary tract. It is a chronic, progressive condition leading to major tissue changes.

The volume of the limb steadily increases, accumulating tissue fluid in the subcutaneous tissue. Skin growth and deposition of collagen further increase limb mass. Hyperkeratosis develops, first on the toes, and then on the dorsum of the foot. Papillomatosis is observed in the late stages. Epidermal vesicles filled with lymph break and ooze fluid. Maceration of the epidermis develops in the interdigital spaces.

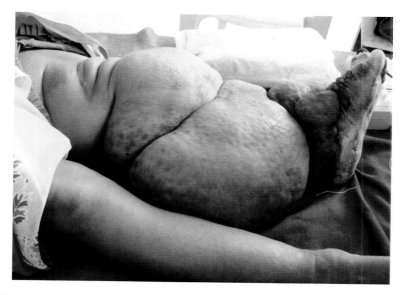

Fig. 57.2 Gigantic lymphedema of the left lower limb of a woman from the filaria-endemic area. Hyperkeratotic warty foot skin, hypertrophy of the calf skin, and subcutaneous tissue in the swollen part. Duration of lymphedema, 3 years

Breaks in the sole skin change into chronic crevices colonized by bacteria and fungi. The mechanisms of the uncontrolled growth of the epidermis remain unclear. Microbial etiology is likely because long-term administration of antibiotics mitigates this process.

The movements in ankle joints become limited due to hardening of the skin and formation of a hanging calf tissue fold. Gradually, the volume of the calf increases and the skin becomes thicker and harder, limiting at the later stages the knee joint movements. The inguinal lymph nodes first become enlarged and then decrease in size and harden.

The changes in the limb superficial lymphatic system can be seen on lymphoscintigrams (Fig. 57.2). At the initial stages, there is dilatation of the lymphatic collectors and enlargement of the lymph nodes. Later, the lymphatics are obliterated. Recurrent attacks of dermato-lymphangio-adenitis (DLA) accelerate this process. The lymph nodes shrink, and become impermeable for the radioisotope. Collateral lymphatics bypassing nodes can be seen.

Ultrasound shows dilated lymphatic trunks in the calf and thigh. In some cases the "dancing microfilariae" can be seen.

A filaria-infected scrotum enlarges, in some cases to a size limiting walking ability. As a rule, there is leakage of stagnant lymph from multiple epidermal vesicles.

Dysfunction of the lymphatics of the spermatic cord and the para-aortic lymph nodes leads to accumulation of fluid to the tunica vaginalis testis and hydrocele.

Rupture of dilated mesenteric lymphatics and cisterna chyli results in formation of chyloperitoneum and transudation of milky lymph to the scrotum and thighs. Leakage of lymph from the thigh skin occurs frequently.

Rupture of the overloaded retroperitoneal lymphatics to the kidney pelvis leads to loss of lymph with chyluria.

All tissues and organs affected by lymph stasis are sites for development of lymphangitis. It is observed in the lower and upper limbs, scrotum, spermatic cord, testes, inguinal and axillary lymph nodes, intestine, and urinary tract.

Changes Attributed to Filariae

The adult worms living in the lymphatic collectors are considered to be responsible for the changes in these vessels. The severity of the pathological condition depends on the number of adult worms and the host immune response. Not all infected individuals reveal microfilaremia and lymphatic lesions. The largest group of affected individuals are asymptomatic, despite the presence of microfilariae in the blood.

Live adult worms cause dilatation of the lymphatics. This can be seen using ultrasound. There is evidence of chronic inflammation of tissues and the draining lymph nodes.[3] On histology, hyperkeratosis is characterized by an increase in the number of keratinocyte layers (8–10) and desquamation. In the dermis mononuclear infiltrates around blood capillaries and at the epidermal–dermal junctions are seen. There is dilatation and increase in the number of lymphatic capillaries of the subepidermal plexus. Lymph nodes are hard and enlarged. The microscopical pictures show dense cellularity in the subcapsular cortex, enlarged follicles with B cells and paracortical regions with T cells. Multiple large macrophage-like cells are seen disseminated in all areas, but most densely in the medullary portion of the node.

Changes Ascribed to Bacterial Infections

Skin abrasion, moisture, and barefoot walking predispose to bacterial penetration of the filarial lymphedematous limb. The common ports of entry are the interdigital spaces, but any other foot skin damage may also facilitate bacterial colonization. Dilatation of collecting lymphatic trunks is responsible for the later dysfunction and subsequent lymph stasis. Stasis predisposes to secondary bacterial infection and tissue colonization. Lack of elimination of microbes brings about host immune response diagnosed as DLA.[4] Acute attacks of DLA are followed by chronic DLA characterized by hyperkeratosis, fibrosis of the skin, and increase in limb volume. The mixed bacterial flora of the patient's own skin is presumably responsible for this condition.[4] The tissue fluid, lymph and lymph node specimens obtained from lower limbs show the presence of bacterial isolates in 70% of cases. The dominant strains are coagulase-negative staphylococci and bacilli. Bacterial infections in lymph stasis are easily controlled by antibiotics. Long-term administration of, for example, benzathine penicillin at a dose of 1,200,000 IU every 21 days has decreased the recurrence rate of DLA attacks by 80%, without a change in sensitivity to antibiotics.[5,6] The reported presence of endosymbiotic bacteria of the genus *Wolbachia* in the adult filarial worms may be an additional indication for antibiotic treatment.[7]

Immunology

Filaria evoke the host immune response.[8,9] Although the adult worm remains in the lymphatics for long periods this response is rather weak. Most studies have been devoted to the humoral reaction, among others, production of IgG4 and its effects on IgE[10,11] and synthesis of interleukins 4, 5, and 17 by T lymphocytes. The cellular reaction involves T suppressor cells[12] and T regulatory cells (Treg).[13]

References

1. Ottesen EA. The Wellcome Trust lecture: infection and disease in lymphatic filariasis: an immunological perspective. *Parasitology*. 1992;104:S71-S79.
2. Report of the Scientific Working Group on Filariasis, 2005 TDR/SWG/057: Addiss DG, Brady MA. Morbidity management in the global programme to eliminate lymphatic filariasis: a review of the scientific literature. *Filaria J.* 2007; 6:2
3. Olszewski WL, Jamal S, Manokaran G, et al. Bacteriological studies of blood, tissue fluid, lymph and lymph nodes in patients with acute dermatolymphangioadenitis (DLA) in course of "filarial" lymphedema. *Acta Trop.* 1999;73:217-224.
4. Olszewski WL, Jamal S, Manokaran G, et al. Bacteriologic studies of skin, tissue fluid, lymph, and lymph nodes in patients with filarial lymphedema. *Am J Trop Med Hyg.* 1997;57:7-15.
5. Olszewski WL. Episodic dermatolymphangioadenitis (DLA) in patients with lymphedema of the lower extremities before and after administration of benzathine penicillin: a preliminary study. *Lymphology.* 1996;29:126-131.
6. Olszewski WL, Jamal S, Manokaran G, et al. The effectiveness of long-acting penicillin (penidur) in preventing recurrencies of dermatolymphangiodenitis (DLA) and controlling skin, deep tissues, and lymph bacterial flora in patients with "filarial" lymphademia. *Lymphology.* 2005;38:66-80.
7. Taylor MJ, Makunde WH, McGarry HF, et al. Macrofilaricidal activity after doxycycline treatment of *Wuchereria bancrofti*: a double-blind, randomized placebo-controlled trial. *Lancet.* 2005;365:2116-2121.
8. Allen JE, Maizels RM. Immunology of human helminth infection. *Int Arch Allergy Immunol.* 1996;109:3-10.
9. Jackson JA, Friberg IM, Little S, Bradley JE. Review series on helminthes, immune modulation and the hygiene hypothesis: immunity against helminthes and immunological phenomena in modern human population: Coevolutionary legacies? *Immunology.* 2008;126:18-27.
10. Ottesen EA, Skvaril F, Tripathy SP, et al. Prominence of IgG4 in the IgG antibody response to human filariasis. *J Immunol.* 1985;134:2707-2712.
11. Kurniawan A, Yazdanbakhsh M, van Ree R, et al. Differential expression of IgE and IgG4 specific antibody responses in asymptomatic and chronic human filariasis. *J Immunol.* 1993;150:3941-3950.
12. Piessens WF, Ratiwayanto S, Tuti S, et al. Antigen-specific suppressor cells and suppressor factors in human filariasis with *Brugia malayi*. *N Engl J Med.* 1980;302:833-837.
13. Taylor MD, LeGoff L, Harris A, et al. Removal of regulatory T cell activity reverses hyporesponsiveness and leads to filarial parasite clearance in vivo. *J Immunol.* 2005;174:4924-4933.

Chapter 58
Clinical Overview-Diagnosis and Management

Gurusamy Manokaran

There are about 120 million people at risk for and 70 million people have established lymphatic filariasis, of which 40 million are suffering from lymphedema; thus, it is very important for medical, paramedic and health planners to understand this disease and to provide morbidity control including surgery for these unfortunate patients. The World Health Organization is working toward elimination of lymphatic filariasis by 2020.[1-17]

Lymphatic filariasis is a chronic debilitating parasitic disease caused by *Wuchereria bancrofti*, *Brugia malayi*, and *Brugia timori*. This is transmitted by the culex mosquito to humans. Prevention and elimination of this disease is vital, but it will take a long time because the third-world countries are struggling to cope up with the basic needs of drinking water, food, and shelter (Figs. 58.1 and 58.2).

We have presented the most common manifestation of lymphatic filariasis, namely, lymphedema and its present management strategies.

Manifestations

Lymphatic filariasis can manifest as (a) hydrocele, (b) lymphedema of both upper and lower limbs, (c) chylothorax, (d) chyluria, (e) chylascitis, (f) genital manifestations (filarial scrotum, Ramp horn penis genital vesicles, and edema), and (g) *atypical lymphatic filariasis* in the form of fleeting joint pains and lymphangitis (string sign). It can affect the breast, gluteal region, abdomen, and suprapubic region in the form of isolated lesions. The lower limb is the commonest manifestation, and women are more frequently affected than men (Figs. 58.3 and 58.4).[18-23]

G. Manokaran
Department of Plastic and Reconstructive Surgery and Lymphologist,
Apollo Hospitals, 21, Greams Road, Chennai, India

B.-B. Lee et al. (eds.), *Lymphedema*,
DOI 10.1007/978-0-85729-567-5_58, © Springer-Verlag London Limited 2011

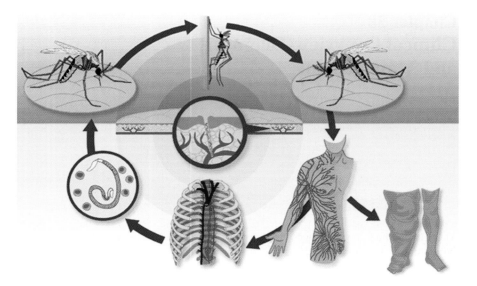

Fig. 58.1 Life cycle of *Wucheraria bancrofti*

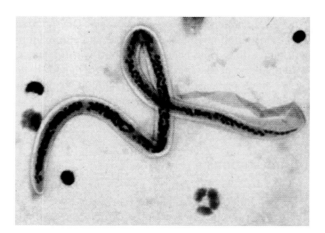

Fig. 58.2 *Wucheraria bancrofti*

The chemotherapeutic management[24] of these problems are either diethyl car-bamazine [DEC]) alone or in the following combinations – DEC + albendazole, DEC + ivermectin, along with periodic antibiotics like penicillin, doxycyline, and sulfonamides. Doxycycline is very useful in symbiotic bacterial infections called *Wolbachia*,[25-29] (Figs. 58.5 and 58.6) which reside inside the parasite and cause resistance to antifilarial drugs. The entire topic of lymphatic filariasis is beyond the scope of this chapter, which will be restricted to the management of filarial lymphedema.

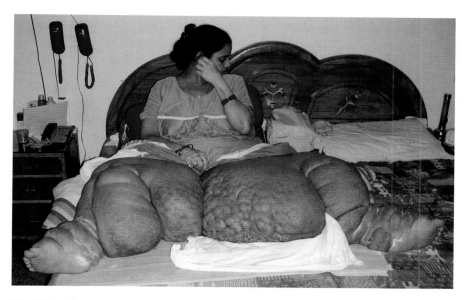

Fig. 58.3 A female patient with bilateral lymphedema due to lymphatic filariasis (elephantiasis)

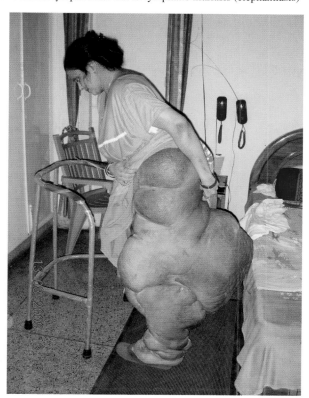

Fig. 58.4 The same patient –
lateral view

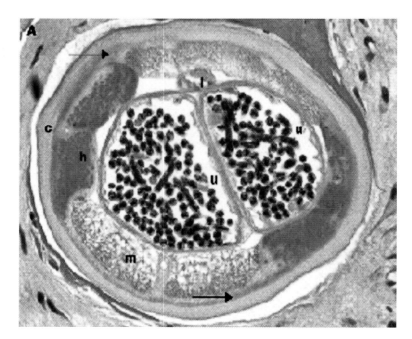

Fig. 58.5 Symbiotic infection with *Wolbachia*

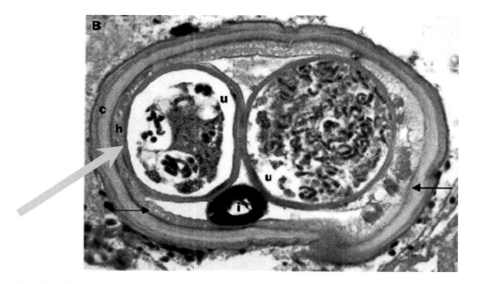

Fig. 58.6 Wolbachia eliminated after chemotherapy

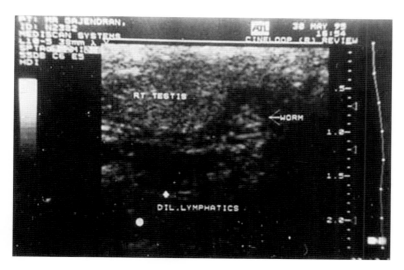

Fig. 58.7   Ultrasound showing the worm in the scrotum

Diagnosis

When diagnosing a case of filarial lymphedema, history is very important because it provides an indication regarding the cause of lymphedema. Careful clinical examination involving color of the skin, the texture of the skin, and skin changes are very important in staging the disease. Circumferential measurements at fixed points of both upper and lower limbs are documented. Height and weight of the patient also are recorded.

The Immuno Chromatographic Test (ICT)[30,31] card test gives a bedside test for lymphatic filariasis, which is highly sensitive for *W. bancrofti* 90–95%.

Ultrasound[32-35] in lymphatic filariasis is used in endemic areas as a screening test that can sometimes can show *dancing adult worms* in the scrotum in men and in the breast in women. Patients positive for adult worms on ultrasound may not have had any clinical signs and symptoms; thus removing the adult worms surgically from these patients will prevent the occurrence of lymphatic filariasis (Fig. 58.7).

Lymphoscintigraphy[20,36-39] is the single most useful investigation in establishing diagnosis grading and etiology. This investigation can tell us about the outcome of this treatment both after chemotherapy and postsurgical results (Fig. 58.8).

Magnetic resonance imaging[40] will be useful when there are associated problems.

For practical purposes we divide filarial lymphedema into four clinical grades:

Grade 1: edema appears and disappears spontaneously, pitting in nature, uniform in size.

Grade 2: edema persisting, pitting, and uniform.

Grade 3: edema persisting, non-pitting, and uniform.

Grade 4: giant lymphedema with complications like ulcers, warty growth, and loss of limb shape (elephantiasis).

Fig. 58.8 Lymphoscintigraphy of lower limb grade III lymphedema. Showing multiple, dilated, lymphatic channels with dermal back flow

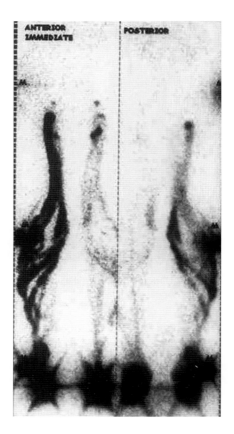

Management

Basic Management

For all four grades of lymphedema the recommendations below should be followed.

Grades 1 and 2 of lymphatic filariasis lymphedema are the only forms of lymphedema that are reversible after this protocol of treatment, which has been demonstrated by lymphoscintigraphy before and after treatment (Fig. 58.9).

Recommendations for Grades I and II

– Foot care
– Avoiding injury and injections to the affected limb
– Elimination of the focus of sepsis caries teeth, intertrigo – fungal infection
– Complete decongestive therapy with bandaging followed by
– Pressure garments

Fig. 58.9 Dr. G. Manokaran's protocol of management

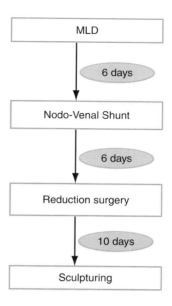

- Elevation of the affected part
- Cyclical chemotherapy (antibiotic and antifilarial) to prevent secondary infections

Secondary infections from injury or focus of sepsis like intertrigo and caries in teeth are responsible for the progress of lymphedema and not lymphatic filariasis. Avoid injection, blood sampling and tight garments in the affected limb. Thus, prevention of secondary infection in the initial stages of lymphatic filariasis can completely reverse the damage done by the parasite (Dr. G. M's observation).

Management of Grades III and IV

Apart from the basic recommendations listed earlier, surgical correction has to be undertaken. Our policy is to combine physiological surgery like a nodo venous shunt or a lympho venal shunt immediately followed by a reduction or debulking procedure without skin grafting. In our experience of 25 years, we have evolved the technique where the functional and aesthetic aspect of the limb is preserved. Although microvascular surgery like free lymphatic channel transfer, lymph node transfer, omental transfer and supra-microvascular surgery like lymphatico-lymphatic anastomosis is useful in congenital and postsurgical lymphedemas, this did not play much of a role in filarial lymphedemas.

Nodovenal Shunt

In Chap. 43 all the detailed information on about lymph nodovenous anastomosis, including the crucial technical aspect, was thoroughly reviewed.

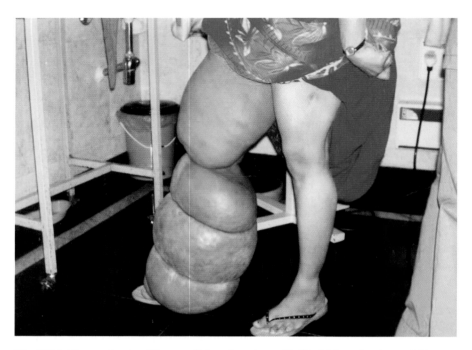

Fig. 58.10 Picture showing 27 years old female patient with Filarial Lymphoedema of 20 years duration

Reduction Surgery (Dr. G. M's Technique)

Under tourniquet control we usually use incision only on the medical side of the limb. We use an elliptical incision for excising the redundant skin and subcutaneous tissue followed by a nodovenal shunt; we do not go below the fascial level. We try to use the same skin as far as possible, unless there is an ulcer or warty growth, which will be either included in the ellipse or a tangential excision is made (sculpturing). In the case shown in the photograph we have used multiple circular incisions up to the subdermal level and retained the subcutaneous fat of reasonable thickness; no undermining of the skin was made, which gives a functional and cosmetically acceptable outcome. As far as the thigh is concerned we make a vertical medial incision and reduce the size of the thigh (Figs. 58.10–58.13) (Dr. G. M's technique).

Although this is the most useful protocol, that gives the best acceptable results in lymphedema due to lymphatic filariasis, we have to modify our technique or time duration depending upon individual patients. All patients are advised to follow foot hygiene, eliminate the focus of the sepsis, avoid injury to the affected limb, and retain the shape of the limb with the help of pressure garments postoperatively.

Stage III and IV lymphedema cannot be cured, it can only be controlled.

The older debulking procedures like the Charles, Kondolean, and Thomson procedures are no longer performed because the long-term results are not good and

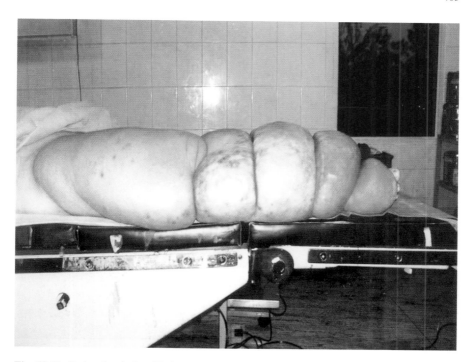

Fig. 58.11 Patient just before Nodo-venal shunt

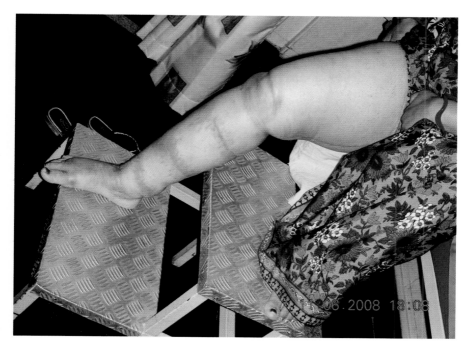

Fig. 58.12 Patient after the author's technique of reduction

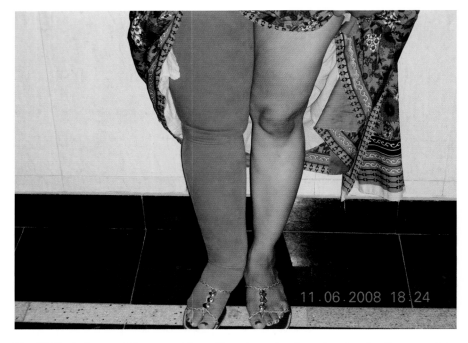

Fig. 58.13 At 3 years follow-up, with stockings (note that the patient is using footwear of the same size on both the feet)

they produce a bottleneck deformity and cobble stone appearance; this is due to the excision of the skin and subcutaneous tissue up to the fascia, which eliminates all the lymphatics in the subdermal layers.

Further detailed discussion was provided in Chap. 48: "Principle of Debulking Procedures".

Complications

    Lymphorrhea
    Lymphocele
    Wound dehiscence and flap necrosis
    Hemorrhage

These are the possible complications in this kind of surgery. Although there were a few morbidities, there was no mortality resulting from these surgical procedures. A good preoperative assessment and preparation avoid all unwanted complications postoperatively.

References

1. Molyneux DH, Zagaria N. Lymphatic filariasis elimination: progress in global programme development. *Ann Trop Med Parasitol.* 2002;96:S15-S40.
2. Ottesen EA, Duke BOL, Karam M, Behbehani K. Strategies and tools for the elimination of lymphatic filariasis. *Bull World Health Organ.* 1997;75:491-503.
3. Ottesen EA. Lymphatic filariasis: treatment, control and elimination. *Adv Parasitol.* 2006;61:395-441.
4. World Health Organization. Global programme to eliminate lymphatic filariasis: progress report for 2004. *Wkly Epidemiol Rec.* 2005;80:202-212.
5. World Health Organization. Global programme to eliminate lymphatic filariasis: progress report on mass drug administrations in 2005. *Wkly Epidemiol Rec.* 2006;22:221-232.
6. World Health Organization. Global programme to eliminate lymphatic filariasis: progress report on mass drug administration in 2006. *Wkly Epidemiol Rec.* 2007;82:361-380.
7. World Health Organization. Global programme to eliminate lymphatic filariasis: progress report on mass drug administration in 2007. *Wkly Epidemiol Rec.* 2008;83:333-348.
8. World Health Organization (2002) Annual Report on Lymphatic Filariasis 2001. Geneva. http://whqlibdoc.who.int/hq/2002/WHO_CDS_CPE_CEE_2002.28.pdf.
9. World Health Organization (2003) Annual Report on Lymphatic Filariasis 2002. Geneva. http://whqlibdoc.who.int/hq/2003/WHO_CDS_CPE_CEE_2003.38.pdf.
10. World Health Organization (2004) Annual Report on Lymphatic Filariasis 2003. Geneva. http://whqlibdoc.who.int/hq/2005/WHO_CDS_CPE_CEE_2005.52.pdf.
11. Dreyer G, Ottesen EA, Galdino E, Andrade L, Rocha A, et al. Renal abnormalities in microfilaremic patients with Bancroftian filariasis. *Am J Trop Med Hyg.* 1992;46:745-751.
12. Dreyer G, Figueredo-Silva J, Carvalho K, Amaral F, Ottesen EA. Lymphatic filariasis in children: adenopathy and its evolution in two young girls. *Am J Trop Med Hyg.* 2001;65: 204-207.
13. Schlemper BR, Steindel M, Grisard EC, Carvalho-Pinto CJ, Bernardini OJ, et al. Elimination of bancroftian filariasis *(Wuchereria bancrofti)* in Santa Catarina state, Brazil. *Trop Med Int Health.* 2000;5:848-854.
14. Bockarie MJ, Ibam E, Alexander NDE, Hyun P, Dimber Z, et al. Towards eliminating lymphatic filariasis in Papua New Guinea: impact of annual single-dose mass treatment on transmission of *Wuchereria bancrofti* in East Sepik Province. *PNG Med J.* 2000;43:172-182.
15. Grady CA, de Rochars MB, Direny AN, Orelus JN, Wendt J, et al. Endpoints for lymphatic filariasis programs. *Emerg Infect Dis J.* 2007;13:608-610.
16. Chhotray GP, Ranjit MR, Mohapatra M. Occurrence of asymptomatic microscopic haematuria in a filarial endemic area of Orissa, India. *J Commun Dis.* 2000;32:85-93.
17. Dreyer G, Addiss D, Dreyer P, Noroes J. *Basic Lymphedema Management: Treatment and Prevention of Problems Associated with Lymphatic Filariasis.* Hollis: Hollis Publishing Company; 2002.
18. Ottesen EA. Infection and disease in lymphatic filariasis: an immunological perspective. *Parasitology.* 1992;104:S71-S79.
19. Dreyer G, Ottesen EA, Galdino E, et al. Renal abnormalities in microfilaremic patients with bancroftian filariasis. *Am J Trop Med Hyg.* 1992;46:745-751.
20. Freedman DO, de Almeida Filho PJ, Besh S, et al. Lymphoscintigraphic analysis of lymphatic abnormalities in symptomatic and asymptomatic human filariasis. *J Infect Dis.* 1994;170: 927-933.
21. Noroes J, Addis D, Amaral F, et al. Occurrence of living adult Wuchereria bancrofti in the scrotal area of men with microfilaremia. *Trans R Soc Trop Med Hyg.* 1996;90:55-56.
22. Pani SP, Yuvaraj J, Vanamail D, et al. Episodic adenolymphangitis and lymphoedema in patients with bancroftian filariasis. *Trans R Soc Trop Med Hyg.* 1992;89:72-74.
23. Ottesen EA, Nutman TB. Tropical pulmonary eosinophilia. *Annu Rev Med.* 1992;43: 417-424.

24. Molyneux DH, Bradley M, Hoerauf A, Kyelem D, Taylor MJ. Mass drug treatment for lymphatic filariasis and onchocerciasis. *Trends Parasitol.* 2003;19(11):516-522.
25. Bosshardt SC et al. Prophylactic activity of tetracycline against *Brugia pahangi* infection in jirds (*Meriones unguiculatus*). *J Parasitol.* 1993;79:775-777.
26. McCall JW et al. *Wolbachia* and the antifilarial properties of tetracycline. An untold story. *Ital J Zool.* 1999;66:7-10.
27. Bandi C et al. Effects of tetracycline on the filarial worms *Brugia pahangi* and *Dirofilaria immitis* and their bacterial endosymbionts *Wolbachia*. *Int J Parasitol.* 1999;29:357-364.
28. Hoerauf A. et al. Targeting of *Wolbachia* in *Litomosoides sigmodontis*: comparison of tetracycline with chloramphenicol, macrolides and ciprofloxacin. *Trop Med Int Hlth* (in press)
29. Townson S et al. The activity of rifampicin, oxytetracycline and chloramphenicol against *Onchocerca lienalis* and *O. gutturosa*. *Trans R Soc Trop Med Hyg.* 1999;93:123-124.
30. Schuetz A, Addiss DG, Eberhard ML, Lammie PJ. Evaluation of the whole blood filariasis ICT test for short-term monitoring after antifilarial treatment. *Am J Trop Med Hyg.* 2000;62(4):502-503.
31. Weil GJ, Lammie PJ, Weiss N. The ICT Filariasis Test: a rapid-format antigen test for diagnosis of bancroftian filariasis. *Parasitol Today.* 1997;13(10):401-404.
32. Amaral F, Dreyer G, Figueredo-Silva J, et al. Live adult worms detected by ultrasonography in human Bancroftian filariasis. *Am J Trop Med Hyg.* 1994;50:753-757.
33. Dreyer G, Santos A, Noroes J, Amaral F, Addiss D. Ultrasonographic detection of living adult *Wuchereria bancrofti* using a 3.5-MHz transducer. *Am J Trop Med Hyg.* 1998;59:399-403.
34. Homeida MA, Mackenzie CD, Williams JF, Ghalib HW. The detection of onchocercal nodules by ultrasound technique. *Trans R Soc Trop Med Hyg.* 1986;80:570-571.
35. Leichsenring M, Troger J, Nelle M, Buttner DW, Darge K, Doehring-Schwerdtfeger E. Ultrasonographical investigations of onchocerciasis in Liberia. *Am J Trop Med Hyg.* 1990;43:380-385.
36. Shelley S, Manokaran G, Indirani M, Gokhale S, Anirudhan N. Lymphoscintigraphy as a diagnostic tool in patients with lymphedema of filarial origin—an Indian study. *Lymphology.* 2006;39(2):69-75.
37. Szuba A, Shin WS, Strauss HW, Rockson S. The third circulation: radionuclide lymphoscintigraphy in the evaluation of lymphedema. *J Nucl Med.* 2003;44:43-57.
38. Sherman A, Ter-Pogossian M. Lymph node concentration of radioactive colloidal gold following interstitial injection. *Cancer.* 1953;6:1238-1240.
39. Nawaz K, Hamad MM, Sedek S, Awdeh M, Eklof B, Abdel-Dayem HM. Dynamic lymph flow imaging in lymphedema: normal and abnormal patterns. *Clin Nucl Med.* 1986;11:653-658.
40. Werner GT, Scheck R, Kaiserling E. Magnetic resonance imaging of peripheral lymphedema. *Lymphology.* 1998;31:34-36.

Part XIV
Genetic Prospects for Lymphedema Management

Chapter 59
Genetic Prospects for Lymphedema Management

Stanley G. Rockson

Angiogenic revascularization of the lymphatics is an emerging research area that is likely to be important to the future therapeutics of lymphedema and other pathological conditions of the lymphatic vasculature.[1,2] The potential to modulate the growth of lymphatic vessels also represents an important aspect of the biological response to the problem of tumor metastasis. Promising pro-lymphangiogenic gene therapy and exogenous molecular treatment methods are under current, active investigation.

The growth of lymphatic vessels is regulated by a large number of growth factors (Fig. 59.1),[3] a developmental process called *lymphangiogenesis*. This topic is discussed in greater detail in Chap. 2. Among the identified lymphangiogenic factors, the vascular endothelial growth factor (VEGF) family occupies a central position.[4,5] Of these, VEGF-C is the chief lymphangiogenic factor, with a less well-defined role for the other VEGFR-3 ligand, VEGF-D[6,7]; VEGF-A stimulates lymphangiogenesis in an indirect manner.[8]

Beyond the VEGFs, several additional growth factors have been identified to play a potential role in the process of lymphangiogenesis. Fibroblast growth factor-2, hepatocyte growth factor, platelet-derived growth factor-B, and insulin-like growth factor-1 (IGF-1) and -2 (IGF-2) can induce experimental lymphangiogenesis.[9]

The angiopoietins also play a potential role as growth regulators of lymphatic vessels. The Ang1 receptor, Tie2, is expressed both in lymphatic endothelial cells and in intact lymphatic vessels.[10,11] Ang1, Ang2, and Ang3/Ang4 have all been shown to stimulate lymphangiogenic sprouting, with Ang1 having the highest activity.[12]

S.G. Rockson
Division of Cardiovascular Medicine, Stanford University School of Medicine,
Falk Cardiovascular Research Center, Stanford, CA, USA

B.-B. Lee et al. (eds.), *Lymphedema*,
DOI 10.1007/978-0-85729-567-5_59, © Springer-Verlag London Limited 2011

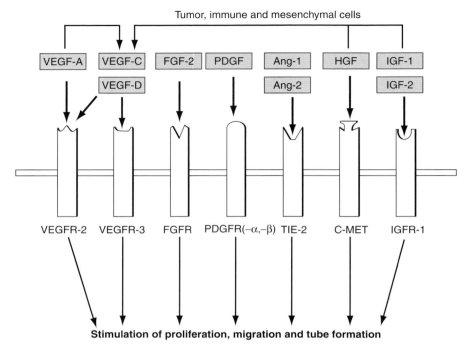

Fig. 59.1 Lymphangiogenic growth factors and their cognate receptors. (Adapted from Van der Auwera et al.[3])

Postnatal Lymphangiogenesis

Beyond the subject of embryonic development, lymphangiogenesis has been best studied in the context of tumor biology. Nevertheless, secondary (i.e., postnatal) lymphangiogenesis also plays a role in the setting of wound healing and of inflammation.[13] Human pathological states of chronic inflammation are associated with an exuberant stimulation of new lymphatic vascular development.[14-16]

By implication, much work in the realm of tumor biology would also seem to support the therapeutic utility of growth factor and endothelial receptor modulation to alter the expression of disease. Recent evidence suggests that active up-regulation of VEGFR-3 and VEGF-C expression and signaling promotes the process of metastatic transformation.[17-20]

Tumor-mediated expression of VEGF-C and VEGF-D correlates with progression to metastasis[21,22] and blocking signaling through VEGFR-3 suppresses cancerous spread.[23] A number of clinical studies underscore the prognostic value of VEGF-C, VEGF-D, and VEGFR-3 expression profiles and resultant lymphatic hyperplasia with regard to tumor progression, regional lymph node metastasis, patient survival, and mortality.[2]

Angiogenic revascularization of the lymphatics is an emerging research area that may have translational implications for the future therapeutics of the edematous conditions that can arise from lymphatic maldevelopment or acquired dysfunction.[1] In various animal models of lymphedema, both administration of recombinant VEGF-C[24] and gene therapy, using either naked plasmid, or virus-associated gene transfer, can produce the desired lymphangiogenic response, accompanied by a diminution in edema.[25-27]

Molecular Therapy for Primary Lymphedema

The primary lymphedemas are those in which developmental disorders of the lymphatic vasculature result in a failure of body fluid homeostasis. Most commonly, this condition emerges clinically after the onset of puberty, a syndrome that has been called hereditary lymphedema praecox, or Meige's syndrome.[28] To date, lymphedema praecox has no identified genetic substrate,[29] but it clinically resembles lymphedema–distichiasis (LD), another pubertal onset syndrome in which the genetic etiology has been delineated.

LD is characterized by the presence of distichiasis at birth and the onset of bilateral lower limb lymphedema at or following puberty.[30] LD has an autosomal dominant mode of inheritance, caused by mutations of the FOXC2 gene.[30,31] FOXC2 knockout mice reproduce the phenotypic and functional alterations of the human disease.[32] In LD, the lymphatic vessels are normal or hyperplastic, suggesting that FOXC2 might participate in the functional integrity of lymphatic vessels rather than in their primary development. Indeed, FOXC2 is a critical transcription factor in pathways of metabolism, perhaps linking lymphatic dysfunction to insulin resistance.[2] A gene-based therapy for this syndrome has not yet been proposed, but it is notable that, in the mutant mice, there is abnormal pericyte recruitment to the lymphatic capillary vasculature and both lymphatics and veins demonstrate defective valve development and maintenance.[33,34] These observations pose distinct challenges for future molecular intervention.

Identification of the role of the SOX18 mutation in recessive and dominant forms of hypotrichosis–lymphedema–telangiectasia syndrome has been achieved recently.[35] This rare disease is characterized by a constellation of childhood hypotrichosis, lymphedema, and telangiectasia or vascular nevi on the palmar surfaces. Again, a molecular intervention is not yet available, but, interestingly, SOX18 is responsible for signaling in lymphatic vascular development (Chap. 4).[36]

Podoplanin/T1α knockout mice also display profound congenital lymphedema.[37] In these animals, though the lymphatic vessels are hyperplastic, there is near absence of lymphatic capillary and plexus formation. The analogous human clinical presentation of this gene knockout has not yet been identified.

Perhaps the most promising scenario for gene therapy surrounds the recent molecular explication for the congenital lymphedema presentation known as Milroy's disease. In many affected family cohorts, congenital hereditary lymphedema has now been associated with mutations in the gene encoding the VEGFR-3 gene.[38,39] In a murine model of Milroy's disease, characterized by a heterozygous inactivating mutation of the tyrosine kinase domain in VEGFR-3, the affected animal subjects exhibit poorly functional lymphatics.[40] These so-called *Chy* mice have a hypoplastic lymphatic vasculature and develop chylous ascites soon after birth, thus mimicking the human disease and its analogous mis-sense mutation. Here, there is clear potential for curative gene therapy[41,42]: induction of functional lymphatic vessel development has been demonstrated in the *Chy* mouse when overexpression of VEGFR-3 ligands is accomplished through adenoviral delivery of recombinant human VEGF-C.

In the future, it is conceivable that, for the inborn, developmental disorders of lymphatic insufficiency, established molecular features, such as the absence or dysfunction of VEGFR-3, FOXC2, SOX18, podoplanin/T1α, and other, as yet undescribed molecular expression targets, can be employed either as biomarkers of disease or as specific targets for therapeutic intervention.[2,43]

Molecular Therapy for Primary Lymphedema

Current treatment strategies for lymphedema do not address the underlying molecular pathophysiology and, therefore, modestly delay the onset of the end-stage sequelae of the disease, including architectural remodeling of tissues, disfigurement, and loss of function.[2]

Just as growth factor therapy has demonstrated potential applicability for the reversal of lymphedema in the *Chy* mouse model of Milroy's disease, an experimentally supported role for therapeutic lymphangiogenesis has been variously described for acquired lymphedema.[24,25,27,44,45]

In the initial descriptions of therapeutic lymphangiogenesis applied to an experimental, rabbit ear model of acquired lymphedema, either direct administration of recombinant VEGFC[24] or plasmid-mediated gene therapy of VEGF-C[25] reverses the established dysfunction of acquired lymphedema. Subsequent applications of growth factor therapy to the dysfunction that accompanies surgical disruption of lymphatic vasculature in the murine tail have been similarly effective.[44,46] The most recently described such model seeks to closely simulate the human setting of breast cancer-associated acquired lymphedema.[27] Here, after surgical extirpation of lymph nodes and lymphatic collecting vessels, the administration of AdVEGF-C or AdVEGF-D reduced edema, with histological documentation of the remodeling of the vasculature to replicate the attributes of newly formed collecting vessels.

Conclusion

Fundamental discoveries in lymphatic development have permitted the design of relevant animal models to simulate the vexatious problem of human lymphedema. Application of genetic and molecular advances to the therapy of both the primary and secondary forms of lymphedema appears to be well underway. Future refinements in both scientific comprehension and biomedical technology will hopefully translate these initial experimental observations into a distinct clinical reality.

Acknowledgment The author gratefully acknowledges the artistic contributions of Shauna Rockson to the development of this chapter.

References

1. An A, Rockson SG. The potential for molecular treatment strategies in lymphatic disease. *Lymphat Res Biol*. 2004;2(4):173-181.
2. Nakamura K, Rockson SG. Molecular targets for therapeutic lymphangiogenesis in lymphatic dysfunction and disease. *Lymphat Res Biol*. 2008;6(3-4):181-189.
3. Van der Auwera I, Cao Y, Tille JC, et al. First international consensus on the methodology of lymphangiogenesis quantification in solid human tumours. *Br J Cancer*. 2006;95(12):1611-1625.
4. Lohela M, Bry M, Tammela T, Alitalo K. VEGFs and receptors involved in angiogenesis versus lymphangiogenesis. *Curr Opin Cell Biol*. 2009;21(2):154-165.
5. Lohela M, Saaristo A, Veikkola T, Alitalo K. Lymphangiogenic growth factors, receptors and therapies. *Thromb Haemost*. 2003;90(2):167-184.
6. Joukov V, Pajusola K, Kaipainen A, et al. A novel vascular endothelial growth factor, VEGF-C, is a ligand for the Flt4 (VEGFR-3) and KDR (VEGFR-2) receptor tyrosine kinases. *EMBO J*. 1996;15(7):1751.
7. Karkkainen MJ, Haiko P, Sainio K, et al. Vascular endothelial growth factor C is required for sprouting of the first lymphatic vessels from embryonic veins. *Nat Immunol*. 2004;5(1):74-80.
8. Wirzenius M, Tammela T, Uutela M, et al. Distinct vascular endothelial growth factor signals for lymphatic vessel enlargement and sprouting. *J Exp Med*. 2007;204(6):1431-1440.
9. Cueni LN, Detmar M. New insights into the molecular control of the lymphatic vascular system and its role in disease. *J Invest Dermatol*. 2006;126(10):2167-2177.
10. Tammela T, Saaristo A, Lohela M, et al. Angiopoietin-1 promotes lymphatic sprouting and hyperplasia. *Blood*. 2005;105(12):4642-4648.
11. Morisada T, Oike Y, Yamada Y, et al. Angiopoietin-1 promotes LYVE-1-positive lymphatic vessel formation. *Blood*. 2005;105(12):4649-4656.
12. Kim KE, Cho CH, Kim HZ, Baluk P, McDonald DM, Koh GY. In vivo actions of angiopoietins on quiescent and remodeling blood and lymphatic vessels in mouse airways and skin. *Arterioscler Thromb Vasc Biol*. 2007;27(3):564-570.
13. Oliver G. Lymphatic vasculature development. *Nat Rev Immunol*. 2004;4(1):35-45.
14. Kunstfeld R, Hirakawa S, Hong YK, et al. Induction of cutaneous delayed-type hypersensitivity reactions in VEGF-A transgenic mice results in chronic skin inflammation associated with persistent lymphatic hyperplasia. *Blood*. 2004;104(4):1048-1057.
15. Baluk P, Tammela T, Ator E, et al. Pathogenesis of persistent lymphatic vessel hyperplasia in chronic airway inflammation. *J Clin Invest*. 2005;115(2):247-257.
16. Cueni LN, Detmar M. The lymphatic system in health and disease. *Lymphat Res Biol*. 2008;6(3-4):109-122.
17. Skobe M, Hawighorst T, Jackson DG, et al. Induction of tumor lymphangiogenesis by VEGF-C promotes breast cancer metastasis. *Nat Med*. 2001;7(2):192-198.
18. Mandriota SJ, Jussila L, Jeltsch M, et al. Vascular endothelial growth factor-C-mediated lymphangiogenesis promotes tumour metastasis. *EMBO J*. 2001;20(4):672-682.
19. Stacker SA, Caesar C, Baldwin ME, et al. VEGF-D promotes the metastatic spread of tumor cells via the lymphatics. *Nat Med*. 2001;7(2):186-191.

20. Goldman J, Conley KA, Raehl A, et al. Regulation of lymphatic capillary regeneration by interstitial flow in skin. *Am J Physiol Heart Circ Physiol.* 2007;292(5):H2176-H2183.
21. Stacker SA, Achen MG, Jussila L, Baldwin ME, Alitalo K. Lymphangiogenesis and cancer metastasis. *Nat Rev Cancer.* 2002;2(8):573-583.
22. Kopfstein L, Veikkola T, Djonov VG, et al. Distinct roles of vascular endothelial growth factor-D in lymphangiogenesis and metastasis. *Am J Pathol.* 2007;170(4):1348-1361.
23. He Y, Kozaki K, Karpanen T, et al. Suppression of tumor lymphangiogenesis and lymph node metastasis by blocking vascular endothelial growth factor receptor 3 signaling. *J Natl Cancer Inst.* 2002;94(11):819-825.
24. Szuba A, Skobe M, Karkkainen M, et al. Therapeutic lymphangiogenesis with human recombinant VEGF-C. *FASEB J.* 2002;16:U114-U130.
25. Yoon YS, Murayama T, Gravereaux E, et al. VEGF-C gene therapy augments postnatal lymphangiogenesis and ameliorates secondary lymphedema. *J Clin Invest.* 2003;111(5):717-725.
26. Saaristo A, Tammela T, Timonen J, et al. Vascular endothelial growth factor-C gene therapy restores lymphatic flow across incision wounds. *FASEB J.* 2004;18(14):1707-1709.
27. Tammela T, Saaristo A, Holopainen T, et al. Therapeutic differentiation and maturation of lymphatic vessels after lymph node dissection and transplantation. *Nat Med.* 2007;13(12):1458-1466.
28. Meige H. Dystophie oedematoeuse hereditaire. *Presse Méd.* 1898;6:341-343.
29. Rezaie T, Ghoroghchian R, Bell R, et al. Primary non-syndromic lymphoedema (Meige disease) is not caused by mutations in FOXC2. *Eur J Hum Genet.* 2008;16(3):300-304.
30. Fang J, Dagenais SL, Erickson RP, et al. Mutations in FOXC2 (MFH-1), a forkhead family transcription factor, are responsible for the hereditary lymphedema-distichiasis syndrome. *Am J Hum Genet.* 2000;67(6):1382-1388.
31. Brice G, Mansour S, Bell R, et al. Analysis of the phenotypic abnormalities in lymphoedema-distichiasis syndrome in 74 patients with FOXC2 mutations or linkage to 16q24. *J Med Genet.* 2002;39(7):478-483.
32. Kriederman BM, Myloyde TL, Witte MH, et al. FOXC2 haploinsufficient mice are a model for human autosomal dominant lymphedema-distichiasis syndrome. *Hum Mol Genet.* 2003;12(10):1179-1185.
33. Petrova TV, Karpanen T, Norrmen C, et al. Defective valves and abnormal mural cell recruitment underlie lymphatic vascular failure in lymphedema distichiasis. *Nat Med.* 2004;10(9):974-981.
34. Mellor RH, Brice G, Stanton AW, et al. Mutations in FOXC2 are strongly associated with primary valve failure in veins of the lower limb. *Circulation.* 2007;115(14):1912-1920.
35. Irrthum A, Devriendt K, Chitayat D, et al. Mutations in the transcription factor gene SOX18 underlie recessive and dominant forms of hypotrichosis-lymphedema-telangiectasia. *Am J Hum Genet.* 2003;72(6):1470-1478.
36. Francois M, Caprini A, Hosking B, et al. Sox18 induces development of the lymphatic vasculature in mice. *Nature.* 2008;456(7222):643-647.
37. Schacht V, Ramirez MI, Hong YK, et al. T1alpha/podoplanin deficiency disrupts normal lymphatic vasculature formation and causes lymphedema. *EMBO J.* 2003;22(14):3546-3556.
38. Ferrell RE, Levinson KL, Esman JH, et al. Hereditary lymphedema: evidence for linkage and genetic heterogeneity. *Hum Mol Genet.* 1998;7(13):2073-2078.
39. Karkkainen MJ, Ferrell RE, Lawrence EC, et al. Missense mutations interfere with VEGFR-3 signalling in primary lymphoedema. *Nat Genet.* 2000;25(2):153-159.
40. Karkkainen MJ, Saaristo A, Jussila L, et al. A model for gene therapy of human hereditary lymphedema. *Proc Natl Acad Sci USA.* 2001;98(22):12677-12682.
41. Rockson S. Preclinical models of lymphatic disease: the potential for growth factor and gene therapy. *Ann NY Acad Sci.* 2002;979:64-75.
42. Shin WS, Rockson SG. Animal models for the molecular and mechanistic study of lymphatic biology and disease. *Ann NY Acad Sci.* 2008;1131:50-74.

43. Nakamura K, Rockson SG. Biomarkers of lymphatic function and disease: state of the art and future directions. *Mol Diagn Ther.* 2007;11(4):227-238.
44. Cheung L, Han J, Beilhack A, et al. An experimental model for the study of lymphedema and its response to therapeutic lymphangiogenesis. *BioDrugs.* 2006;20(6):363-370.
45. Saito Y, Nakagami H, Morishita R, et al. Transfection of human hepatocyte growth factor gene ameliorates secondary lymphedema via promotion of lymphangiogenesis. *Circulation.* 2006;114(11):1177-1184.
46. Jin DP, An A, Liu J, Nakamura K, Rockson SG. Therapeutic responses to exogenous VEGF-C administration in experimental lymphedema: immunohistochemical and molecular characterization. *Lymphat Res Biol.* 2009;7(1):47-57.

Part XV
Oncology and Lymphedema

Chapter 60
Breast Cancer

Sharon L. Kilbreath

In western society, the most common cause of lymphedema is treatment for breast cancer.[1] The incidence of lymphedema depends upon the diagnostic criteria used, but occurs in at least 20% of women treated for breast cancer.[1,2] For the majority of women who develop lymphedema, the complication will present within 3 years of surgery.[2]

Importance of Understanding Risk Factors

The majority of women treated for breast cancer perceive that they are vulnerable to development of lymphedema, even with recent surgical advances and the discontinued routine use of radiotherapy to the axilla.[3,4] Because of this belief, they intend to avoid any strenuous activity with their affected arm. It is these same women, however, that report more arm and chest symptoms than women who did not avoid strenuous arm activity.[4] Identification of risk factors will enable the majority of women to resume their life without fear of developing lymphedema.

Risk Factors

The risk for lymphedema is related, in part, to the surgical and medical management of cancer. Historically, axillary radiation[5-7] was strongly associated with development of lymphedema and so is no longer used routinely. Radiotherapy to the chest

S.L. Kilbreath
Breast Cancer Research Group of the Faculty of Health Sciences,
University of Sydney, Lidcombe, NSW, Australia

B.-B. Lee et al. (eds.), *Lymphedema*,
DOI 10.1007/978-0-85729-567-5_60, © Springer-Verlag London Limited 2011

wall and supraclavicular regions does not seem to be a risk factor for lymphedema.[8] The other major risk factor is axillary surgery[7,9-11]; sentinel node biopsy has reduced the number of women undergoing axillary surgery. However, sentinel node biopsy has not eliminated entirely the occurrence of lymphedema. It is clear that factors other than the type of surgery contribute to the risk of lymphedema.

There is little consensus on what the other risk factors for lymphedema are, in part because the findings are not consistent and in part because of the variety of different factors evaluated. Hayes et al.[12] determined from their prospective study of women treated for unilateral breast cancer that older age, more extensive surgery (i.e., mastectomy), and a sedentary lifestyle significantly increased the odds of developing lymphedema; being overweight or obese was not a risk factor. Clark et al.,[13] in their prospective study of women treated for breast cancer and only including those with level II axillary dissection, identified having a mastectomy, a skin puncture, and body mass index (BMI) ≥ 26 as risk factors for lymphedema; older age was not a risk factor. Other retrospective, case-controlled studies have identified additional factors, such as high BMI, high level of hand use, and previous infection of the affected upper limb as predictors of lymphedema,[14] although these factors have also not been consistently found. For example, Geller et al.[9] did not find obesity (BMI > 30) to be a risk factor. From these examples, it is clear that there is no clear guidance as to what is and is not a risk factor.

Two other factors thought to be associated with the development or exacerbation of lymphedema, physical activity and airplane travel, have recently been challenged. Physical exercise involving the "at risk" limb, e.g., resistance training, has been discouraged by health practitioners for women with lymphedema secondary to breast cancer because it was believed that exercise would either cause lymphedema, or, if already present, exacerbate it.[4,14] Several small studies[15-18] as well as a well-designed randomized controlled trial[19] demonstrated that exercise did not exacerbate lymphedema. Airplane travel may also have been overemphasized as causative of lymphedema, at least for women who participate regularly in upper limb physical activity. Women who had been treated for breast cancer and who were travelling from Canada to Australia as well as within Australia to participate in a dragon boat competition were measured prior to the flight and soon after arrival; a subset of international travelers were also measured 6 weeks after return to Canada.[20] For 95% of women, air travel did not adversely affect their arm. This is contrary to what was found in a single case study of a breast cancer survivor with lymphedema who did not participate in any regular exercise. Although the inter-arm impedance ratio fluctuated over this time, it generally increased and worsened after flying.[21]

The inability to reach consensus on risk factors is that these factors may individually explain relatively little of the overall risk; the major factor may be physiological. Stanton and colleagues[7] used lymphoscintigraphy to explore the lymphatic system in women following treatment for breast cancer. At 7 months after surgery, the indicators of function of the lymphatic system in both the ipsilateral and contralateral subdermis were significantly higher in those women who went on to develop frank lymphedema compared with those women who did not. This was a small study of 36 women, but it does suggest that some women may be predisposed physiologically to developing lymphedema, such that environmental or other stresses may impose a critical load on an already stressed lymphatic system.

Progression of Lymphedema

Lymphedema can occur in the extremity, as well as in the trunk region (i.e., breast and anterior and posterior chest) ipsilateral to the side of surgery. The incidence/prevalence in the trunk region has not been reported, perhaps because there is no easy method of quantifying it other than through observation.[22]

For some women treated for breast cancer, lymphedema may be transient. The percentage of women in whom it is transient varies, ranging from 30% to 60% of women identified as having lymphedema.[12,23] The difference reflects different methods of measurements used and the period of time over which women were followed.[12,23] For example, Hayes et al.[12] used bioimpedance spectroscopy and followed women for 6–18 months; in contrast, Norman and colleagues[23] used self-report and followed women for up to 5 years.

For women in whom the lymphedema is nontransient, little is known about the long-term progression. In two studies in which severity of disease was also noted, women with chronic lymphedema typically presented within the first couple of years after surgery with mild symptoms. In more than half of these women, the lymphedema did not progress beyond the mild stage over the ensuing few years in which they were followed.[23,24]

Women with mild lymphedema (e.g., no obvious swelling; <2-cm interlimb difference) experience symptoms and increased levels of distress compared with women without lymphedema.[1,23,25,26] Symptoms experienced prior to any visible changes include sensations of heaviness, swelling, tightness, and discomfort/pain.[23] These symptoms reflect changes that have commenced, commonly in localized regions.[27,28] These early localized changes can be detected with bioimpedance spectroscopy (BIS), but not by measurement of arm volume.[29]

For up to one half of women with non-transient lymphedema, progression occurs beyond the mild stage. The lymphedematous limb changes in volume as well as in composition. Subcutaneous and subfascial adipose deposition commences early[30] and continues to progress so that, by the advanced non-pitting stage, 73% of the excess volume in the lymphedematous limb is adipose tissue.[31,32] Other changes to the affected limb include cutaneous thickening and hypercellularity,[33] and progressive fibrosis.

Conclusion

For most women treated for breast cancer in whom lymphedema develops the condition is mild, at least in the early years. The challenge for clinicians is to prevent it from becoming established and progressing to a more advanced stage.

References

1. Hayes S, Janda M, Cornish B, Battistutta D, Newman B. Lymphedema secondary to breast cancer: how choice of measure influences diagnosis, prevalence, and identifiable risk factors. *Lymphology*. 2008;41:18-28.
2. Rockson SG, Rockson SG. Diagnosis and management of lymphatic vascular disease. *J Am Coll Cardiol*. 2008;52:799-806.
3. Lee TS, Kilbreath SL, Sullivan G, Refshauge KM, Beith JM. Patient perceptions of arm care and exercise advice after breast cancer surgery. *Oncol Nurs Forum*. 2010;37:85-91.
4. Lee TS, Kilbreath SL, Sullivan G, Refshauge KM, Beith JM, et al. Factors that affect intention to avoid strenuous arm activity after breast cancer surgery. *Oncol Nurs Forum*. 2009;36: 454-462.
5. Nagel PH, Bruggink ED, Wobbes T, Strobbe LJ. Arm morbidity after complete axillary lymph node dissection for breast cancer. *Acta Chir Belg*. 2003;103:212-216.
6. van der Veen PH, De VN, Lievens P, Duquet W, Lamote J, et al. Lymphedema development following breast cancer surgery with full axillary resection. *Lymphology*. 2004;37:206-208.
7. Coen JJ, Taghian AG, Kachnic LA, Assaad SI, Powell SN. Risk of lymphedema after regional nodal irradiation with breast conservation therapy. *Int J Radiat Oncol Biol Phys*. 2003;55: 1209-1215.
8. Lee TS, Kilbreath SL, Refshauge KM, Herbert RD, Beith JM. Prognosis of the upper limb following surgery and radiation for breast cancer. *Breast Cancer Res Treat*. 2008;110:19-37.
9. Geller BM, Vacek PM, O'Brien P, Secker-Walker RH. Factors associated with arm swelling after breast cancer surgery. *J Womens Health*. 2003;12:921-930.
10. Veronesi U, Paganelli G, Viale G, Galimberti V, Luini A, et al. Sentinel lymph node biopsy and axillary dissection in breast cancer: results in a large series. *J Natl Cancer Inst*. 1999;91: 368-373.
11. Armer J, Fu MR, Wainstock JM, Zagar E, Jacobs LK. Lymphedema following breast cancer treatment, including sentinel lymph node biopsy. *Lymphology*. 2004;37:73-91.
12. Hayes SC, Janda M, Cornish B, Battistutta D, Newman B. Lymphedema after breast cancer: incidence, risk factors, and effect on upper body function. *J Clin Oncol*. 2008;26:3536-3542.
13. Clark B, Sitzia J, Harlow W, Clark B, Sitzia J, et al. Incidence and risk of arm oedema following treatment for breast cancer: a three-year follow-up study. *QJM*. 2005;98:343-348.
14. Gillham L. Lymphoedema and physiotherapists: control not cure. *Physiotherapy*. 1994;80: 835-843.
15. Harris SR, Niesen-Vertommen SL. Challenging the myth of exercise-induced lymphedema following breast cancer: a series of case reports. *J Surg Oncol*. 2000;74:95-98.
16. McKenzie DC, Kalda AL. Effect of upper extremity exercise on secondary lymphedema in breast cancer patients: a pilot study. *J Clin Oncol*. 2003;21:463-466.
17. Ahmed RL, Thomas W, Yee D, Schmitz KH. Randomized controlled trial of weight training and lymphedema in breast cancer survivors. *J Clin Oncol*. 2006;24:2765-2772.
18. Turner J, Hayes S, Reul-Hirche H. Improving the physical status and quality of life of women treated for breast cancer: a pilot study of a structured exercise intervention. *J Surg Oncol*. 2004;86:141-146.
19. Schmitz KH, Ahmed RL, Troxel A, Cheville A, Smith R, et al. Weight lifting in women with breast-cancer-related lymphedema. *N Engl J Med*. 2009;361:664-673.
20. Kilbreath SL, Ward LC, Lane K, McNeely M, Dylke ES, et al. Effect of air travel on lymphedema risk in women with history of breast cancer. *Breast Cancer Res Treat*. 2010;120(3): 649-654.
21. Ward LC, Battersby KJ, Kilbreath SL. Airplane travel and lymphedema: a case study. *Lymphology*. 2009;42:139-145.
22. Roberts CC, Levick JR, Stanton AW, Mortimer PS. Assessment of truncal edema following breast cancer treatment using modified Harpenden skinfold calipers. *Lymphology*. 1995;28: 78-88.

23. Norman SA, Localio AR, Potashnik SL, Simoes Torpey HA, Kallan MJ, et al. Lymphedema in breast cancer survivors: incidence, degree, time course, treatment, and symptoms. *J Clin Oncol.* 2009;27:390-397.
24. Bar Ad V, Cheville A, Solin L, Dutta P, Both S, et al. Time course of mild arm lymphedema after breast conservation treatment for early-stage breast cancer. *Int J Radiat Oncol Biol Phys.* 2010;76:85-90.
25. Oliveira MMF, Gurgel MSC, Miranda MS, Okubo MA, Feijo LFA, et al. Efficacy of shoulder exercises on locoregional complications in women undergoing radiotherapy for breast cancer: clinical trial. *Rev Bras De Fisioterapia.* 2009;13:136-144.
26. Cormier J, Xing Y, Zaniletti I, Askew R, Stewart B, et al. Minimal limb volume change has a significant impact on breast cancer survivors. *Lymphology.* 2009;42:161-175.
27. Stanton AW, Mellor RH, Cook GJ, Svensson WE, Peters AM, et al. Impairment of lymph drainage in subfascial compartment of forearm in breast cancer-related lymphedema. *Lymphat Res Biol.* 2003;1:121-132.
28. Ward LC, Czerniec S, Kilbreath SL. Quantitative bioimpedance spectroscopy for the assessment of lymphoedema. *Breast Cancer Res Treat.* 2009;117:541-547.
29. Czerniec S, Kilbreath S, Ward L, Refshauge K, Beith J, et al., editors. Segmental measurement of breast cancer related arm lymphoedema using perometer and bioimpedance spectroscopy. *Sydney Cancer Conference,* Sydney, Australia, 2008.
30. Czerniec S, Ward L, Meerkin J, Refshauge K, Kilbreath S, editors. A Comparison of DEXA and BIS for the Measurement of Breast Cancer Related Arm Lymphoedema. 22nd International Lymphology Society Congress; Sydney, Australia, 2009, 21–25 September.
31. Brorson H, Ohlin K, Olsson G, Karlsson MK. Breast cancer-related chronic arm lymphedema is associated with excess adipose and muscle tissue. *Lymphat Res Biol.* 2009;7:3-10.
32. Brorson H, Ohlin K, Olsson G, Nilsson M. Adipose tissue dominates chronic arm lymphedema following breast cancer: an analysis using volume rendered CT images. *Lymphat Res Biol.* 2006;4:199-210.
33. Rockson SG. Lymphedema. *Am J Med.* 2001;110:288-295.

Chapter 61
Lower Extremity Cancers

Mi-Joung Lee and Stanley G. Rockson

Secondary lower limb lymphedema (LLL) is commonly associated with surgical excision of inguinofemoral lymph nodes and/or radiation of the respective node-bearing areas. The condition of LLL presents as progressive swelling of the leg(s), most typically within the first 12 months after the treatment for cancer. Once it develops, it is typically unremitting and often progressive.

The occurrence of LLL after treatment of reproductive, gastrointestinal, and urinary malignancies and melanoma is reportedly quite common, although reliable incidence estimates vary substantially. LLL as a consequence of genitourinary cancer is a rather neglected subject, despite the fact that it represents a major form of the morbidity after surgery and radiation treatment of these malignancies.

Although many observations have been published regarding the prevalence of upper limb lymphedema (ULL) after breast cancer treatment, estimates of the prevalence of secondary LLL remain somewhat unreliable.[1] The incidence estimates of secondary LLL after cancer treatment seem to be influenced by the type of cancer (Table 61.1). The incidence varies from 1.3–67%, depending on the type of cancer, stage, treatment, and sensitivity of the measurement tool (Table 61.1). The highest relative incidence has been reported after vulvar cancer treatment and the lowest after ovarian cancer.[2,3] The reported incidence of secondary LLL has declined in publications that have appeared since 2000, presumably as a reflection of the adoption of less invasive surgical and radiotherapeutic treatment regimens.

The reported timing of the onset of LLL after the diagnosis of cancer varies considerably.[1] A recent study by Beesley and colleagues reflects that 75% of affected individuals were diagnosed with lymphedema within the first year, 19% in the following year, and 6% between 2 years and 5 years after diagnosis.[2] The initial symptom is usually painless swelling. The patient may also complain of a feeling of

M.-J. Lee (✉)
Division of Cardiovascular Medicine,
Stanford University School of Medicine,
Falk Cardiovascular Research Center, Stanford, CA, USA

B.-B. Lee et al. (eds.), *Lymphedema*,
DOI 10.1007/978-0-85729-567-5_61, © Springer-Verlag London Limited 2011

Table 61.1 Incidence/prevalence of lower limb lymphedema as a consequence of cancer treatment

Primary cancer	Method of diagnosis	N	Incidence/prevalence	Reference
Ovarian cancer	Medical records and subjective symptoms	135	21.1%	19
	Clinical diagnosis and subjective symptoms	234	Total: 20.5%, symptomatic: 15.8%, diagnosed: 4.7%	2
	Retrospective survey	141	7.1%	20
Cervical cancer	Physical examination	228	Stage I–IIA: 31%	21
	Clinical diagnosis and subjective symptoms	197	Total: 26.4%, symptomatic: 14.2%, diagnosed: 12.2%	2
	Retrospective survey	120	17.5%	20
	Clinically detectable finding by patient or physician	192	23.4%	22
	Medical records and subjective symptoms	252	29.8%	19
Endometrial cancer	Limb volume, MFBIA, and self report	60	40% with volume, 67% with MFBIA, 22% with self report	23
	Limb volume, clinical history and physical examination	286	37.8%	24
	Retrospective chart review excluding chronic lower-limb lymphedema related to other medical conditions	670	Uterine corpus cancer follow-up of 3 years: 2.4%	25
	Retrospective survey	141	17.7%	20
Vulvar cancer	Clinical diagnosis and subjective symptoms	243	Total: 22.2%, symptomatic: 14%, diagnosed: 8.2%	2
	Medical records and subjective symptoms	295	27.8%	19
	Retrospective survey	68	47.1%	20
	When swelling persisted for more than 2 months	61	26%	26
	Clinical diagnosis and subjective symptoms	53	Total: 50.9%, symptomatic: 15.1%, diagnosed: 35.8%	2
	Clinically obvious or when elastic bandages were required beyond 3 months postoperatively	172	28%	27
Prostate cancer	Subjective symptoms	16	13%	28
	Subjective symptoms	289	Stage A2–C: 3.1%	29
	Subjective symptoms	372	1.3%	30

Penile cancer	Subjective symptoms, retrospective analysis	53	Scrotal and leg edema: 23%	31
	Circumference measure	10	23%	32
	Unknown, retrospective analysis	234	Inguinal lymph: 25% Ilio-inguinal lymph: 29%	33
	Leg volume difference	66	Inguinal SNB: 6% Inguinal SNB and groin dissection: 64%	34
	Retrospective audit	40	37.5%	35
	Self report, clinical assessment	28	29%	36
Melanoma with inguinal node involvement	Late radiation morbidity scoring system	33	4 weeks of radiation in the groin area: 66%	37

MFBIA multi-frequency bioelectrical impedance analysis, *SNB* sentinel node biopsy

heaviness in the limb, especially at the end of the day and in hot weather. Symptoms may vary throughout the menstrual cycle.[4]

In the earliest stage of the problem, the swelling presents as pitting edema but, with time, classical nonpitting edema will appear.[5] The distribution of lymphedema is asymmetrical and a positive Stemmer sign (inability to tent the skin at the base of the second toe) is a useful clinical sign.[6] LLL can spread proximally (or distally) in the early stages, but this is uncommon after the first year. Nevertheless, the condition can be progressive if treatment is not administered.[7] With time, the affected swollen limb manifests chronic cutaneous changes, with enhanced skin creases, hyperkeratosis, increased skin turgor and papillomatosis.[5,8] Symptomatology may include mild pain or a sense of heaviness or fullness. In severe cases, the skin can break down; lymphorrhea (lymph exuding through any break in the skin) is associated with an increased risk of soft-tissue infection. Indeed, recurrent infections, cellulitis, and lymphangitis are common. Repeated infection can lead to further deterioration in lymphatic function, ending in a vicious cycle of infection and repetitive worsening of the condition. Associated clinical features of LLL include tightness or inability to wear shoes, itching of the legs or toes, burning sensations in the legs, sleep disturbances, and loss of hair in the affected limb. One published study suggests that patients with LLL are more likely to present with swelling, heaviness, tightness, and skin problems when compared to patients with upper limb lymphedema.[9]

While much work has been done on the impact of lymphedema upon quality of life, most of these studies have focused on breast cancer survivors. However, Yost et al.[10] have shown that lymphedema was the most frequent problem impacting on quality of life in 15 women after vulvar cancer treatment. Similarly, in another published study, 82 women with LLL after gynecological cancer treatment reported that their lymphedema had a significant impact on their quality of life, financial state, physical and social activities, the clothes they could wear, and, overall, on their emotional well-being.[3]

One of the major problems associated with LLL after cancer treatment seems to be diminished awareness by the public and among healthcare professionals. Women with LLL after gynecological cancer treatment experienced barriers to the access to treatment, delays in lymphedema diagnosis, and conflicting information on the management of the lymphedema.[3] A recent UK study also suggested that a greater proportion of patients with LLL than ULL may have progressed to a chronic stage before consulting a health professional; in the population studied, only 24.2% of patients with LLL sought treatment within 3 months of symptom onset compared with 56.1% of patients with ULL reporting such behavior.[11] The diagnosis and treatment of LLL may have a lower profile in public consciousness compared with that of ULL after breast cancer treatment.[9] Many cancer treatment centers now have trained breast cancer nurses who provide advice and services to breast cancer survivors regarding lymphedema prevention and early detection, whereas comparable facilities for LLL patients are generally much less readily available.

In clinical practice, the diagnosis of LLL is based upon measures of limb circumference and/or volume. In unilateral presentations, the contralateral leg may be used to assess whether the affected leg is actually swollen. However, the disease often affects both lower limbs, or, alternatively, premorbid asymmetry in the two lower limbs may hamper the ability to accurately compare the limbs in the assessment of edema presence and magnitude. A cloth tape measure can be used to measure circumferential asymmetries between the two limbs, but this technique is unreliable. Water displacement volumetry, although not commonly used, directly measures limb volume[12] and can be more accurate than calculating the leg volume with a tape measure.[13] In lymphedema, the tissue tonicity (degree of tissue resistance to mechanical compression) is either higher or lower than that of the unaffected leg.[14] Measurement of tissue tonometry is more useful in assessing the response to treatment than in the initial assessment of disease. Bioimpedance spectroscopy has been used successfully for the evaluation of swelling in patients with postmastectomy lymphedema, but has not yet been validated for the assessment of leg edema.[15]

The chief aims in treating patients with LLL are to prevent the progression of disease, to achieve mechanical reduction and maintenance of limb size, to ease the symptoms arising from lymphedema, and to prevent skin infection. Treatment depends on the symptoms and the severity of the condition and can be divided into conservative, pharmacological, and surgical approaches. Conservative treatments include manual lymphatic massage, multilayer bandaging and complex decongestive physiotherapy, compression garments, limb exercises and limb elevation, pneumatic bio-compression, and low-level laser therapy.[16] There is scanty published literature to support the specific efficacy of complex decongestive physical therapy in LLL volume reduction for patients who have undergone groin dissection.[17] There is no conclusive published evidence that pharmacological intervention, with agents such as benzopyrones and selenium compounds, adds benefit in the management of secondary LLL.[18] Surgical intervention is generally recommended for only a small subset of such patients.[18]

Both cancer incidence and survival rates continue to increase; thus, the incidence and the public health burden of secondary LLL can be expected to increase in parallel. There is an obvious imperative to provide appropriate guidelines, not only for patients, but also for healthcare professionals. The lack of methodologically sound research on secondary LLL imposes barriers to the development of evidence-based guidelines regarding incidence, risk factors, diagnosis, and treatment. Undoubtedly, there is still much to be learned and studied. However, there is enough knowledge to raise awareness of a condition whose prevalence and population disease burden are likely to be underestimated. During and following cancer treatment, patients can be educated regarding the potential triggers for the onset of overt lymphedema and, thus, the potential strategies for effective prevention. Patients can be informed to make decisions regarding treatments and elective lifestyle behaviors. For those who experience the onset of overt problems, measures should be undertaken to help them appreciate that treatment for secondary LLL can be expected to ameliorate function and that omission of treatment can promote progression and increase the likelihood of complications.

References

1. Radhakrishnan K, Rockson SG. The clinical spectrum of lymphatic disease. *Ann NY Acad Sci.* 2008;1131:155-184.
2. Beesley V, Janda M, Eakin E, Obermair A, Battistutta D. Lymphedema after gynecological cancer treatment: prevalence, correlates, and supportive care needs. *Cancer.* 2007;109: 2607-2614.
3. Ryan M, Stainton MC, Jaconelli C, Watts S, MacKenzie P, Mansberg T. The experience of lower limb lymphedema for women after treatment for gynecologic cancer. *Oncol Nurs Forum.* 2003;30:417-423. Online.
4. Schirger A. Lymphedema. *Cardiovasc Clin.* 1983;13:293-305.
5. Lewis JM, Wald ER. Lymphedema praecox. *J Pediatr.* 1984;104:641-648.
6. Harwood CA, Bull RH, Evans J, Mortimer PS. Lymphatic and venous function in lipoedema. *Br J Dermatol.* 1996;134:1-6.
7. Wolfe JH, Kinmonth JB. The prognosis of primary lymphedema of the lower limbs. *Arch Surg.* 1981;116:1157-1160.
8. Mortimer PS. Swollen lower limb-2: lymphoedema. *BMJ.* 2000;320:1527-1529.
9. Langbecker D, Hayes SC, Newman B, Janda M. Treatment for upper-limb and lower-limb lymphedema by professionals specializing in lymphedema care. *Eur J Cancer Care (Engl).* 2008;17:557-564.
10. Yost KJ, Yount SE, Eton DT, et al. Validation of the Functional Assessment of Cancer Therapy-Breast Symptom Index (FBSI). *Breast Cancer Res Treat.* 2005;90:295-298.
11. Tiwari A, Myint F, Hamilton G. Management of lower limb lymphoedema in the United Kingdom. *Eur J Vasc Endovasc Surg.* 2006;31:311-315.
12. Burnand K, Clemson G, Morland M, Jarrett PEM, Browese NL. Venous lipodermatosclerosis: treatment by fibrinolytic enhancement and elastic compression. *Br Med J.* 1980;280:7-11.
13. Caseley-Smith J. Measuring and representing peripheral oedema and its alterations. *Lymphology.* 1994;27:56-70.
14. Liu NF, Olszewski W. Use of tonometry to assess lower extremity lymphedema. *Lymphology.* 1992;25:155-158.
15. Ward LC. Regarding Edema and leg volume: methods of assessment. *Angiology.* 2000;50: 615-616.
16. Moseley AL, Carati CJ, Piller NB. A systematic review of common conservative therapies for arm lymphoedema secondary to breast cancer treatment. *Ann Oncol.* 2007;18:639-646.
17. Hinrichs CS, Gibbs JF, Driscoll D, et al. The effectiveness of complete decongestive physiotherapy for the treatment of lymphedema following groin dissection for melanoma. *J Surg Oncol.* 2004;85:187-192.
18. Gary DE. Lymphedema diagnosis and management. *J Am Acad Nurse Pract.* 2007;19:72-78.
19. Tada H, Teramukai S, Fukushima M, Sasaki H. Risk factors for lower limb lymphedema after lymph node dissection in patients with ovarian and uterine carcinoma. *BMC Cancer.* 2009;9: 47-52.
20. Ryan M, Stainton MC, Slaytor EK, Jaconelli C, Watts S, Mackenzie P. Aetiology and prevalence of lower limb lymphoedema following treatment for gynaecological cancer. *Aust N Z J Obstet Gynaecol.* 2003;43:148-151.
21. Hong JH, Tsai CS, Lai CH, et al. Postoperative low-pelvic irradiation for stage I-IIA cervical cancer patients with risk factors other than pelvic lymph node metastasis. *Int J Radiat Oncol Biol Phys.* 2002;53:1284-1290.
22. Fuller J, Guderian D, Kohler C, Schneider A, Wendt TG. Lymph edema of the lower extremities after lymphadectomy and radiotherapy for cervical cancer. *Strahlenther Onkol.* 2008;184:206-211.
23. Halaska MJ, Novackova M, Mala I, et al. A prospective study of postoperative lymphedema after surgery for cervical cancer. *Int J Gynecol Cancer.* 2010;20:900-904.

24. Todo Y, Yamamoto R, Minobe S, et al. Risk factors for postoperative lower-extremity lymphedema in endometrial cancer survivors who had treatment including lymphadenectomy. *Gynecol Oncol.* 2010;119(1):60-64.

25. Abu-Rustum NR, Alektiar K, Iasonos A, et al. The incidence of symptomatic lower-extremity lymphedema following treatment of uterine corpus malignancies: a 12-year experience at Memorial Sloan-Kettering Cancer Center. *Gynecol Oncol.* 2006;103:714-718.

26. Judson P, Jonson AL, Paley PJ, et al. A prospective, randomized study analyzing sartorius transposition following inguinal-femoral lymphadenectomy. *Gynecol Oncol.* 2004;95: 226-230.

27. Gaarenstroom KN, Kenter GG, Trimbos JB, et al. Postoperative complications after vulvectomy and inguinofemoral lymphadenectomy using separate groin incisions. *Int J Gynecol Cancer.* 2003;13:522-527.

28. Amdur RJ, Parsons JT, Fitzgerald LT, Million RR. Adenocarcinoma of the prostate treated with external-beam radiation therapy: 5-year minimum follow-up. *Radiother Oncol.* 1990;18:235-246.

29. Greskovich FJ, Sagars GK, Sherman NE, Johnson DE. Complications following external beam radiation therapy for prostate cancer: an analysis of patients treated with and without staging pelvic lymphadenectomy. *J Urol.* 1991;146:798-802.

30. Kavoussi LR, Sosa E, Chandhoke P, et al. Complications of laparoscopic pelvic lymph node dissection. *J Urol.* 1993;149:322-325.

31. Bevan-Thomas R, Slaton JW, Pettaway CA. Contemporary morbidity from lymphadenectomy for penile squamous cell carcinoma: the M.D. Anderson Cancer Center Experience. *J Urol.* 2002;167:1638-1642.

32. Jacobellis U. Modified radical inguinal lymphadenectomy for carcinoma of the penis: technique and results. *J Urol.* 2003;169:1349-1352.

33. Ravi R. Morbidity following groin dissection for penile carcinoma. *Br J Urol.* 1993;72: 941-945.

34. de Vries M, Vonkeman WG, van Ginkel RJ, Hoekstra HJ. Morbidity after inguinal sentinel lymph node biopsy and completion lymph node dissection in patients with cutaneous melanoma. *Eur J Surg Oncol.* 2006;32:785-789.

35. Ballo MT, Zagars GK, Gershenwald JE, et al. A critical assessment of adjuvant radiotherapy for inguinal lymph node metastases from melanoma. *Ann Surg Oncol.* 2004;11:1079-1084.

36. Serpell JW, Carne PW, Bailey M. Radical lymph node dissection for melanoma. *ANZ J Surg.* 2003;73:294-299.

37. Burmeister BH, Smithers BM, Davis S, et al. Radiation therapy following nodal surgery for melanoma: an analysis of late toxicity. *ANZ J Surg.* 2002;72:344-348.

Chapter 62
Radiation Complications

Kathleen C. Horst

The risk and etiology of lymphedema in oncology patients is multifactorial. After a diagnosis of cancer is established, treatment decisions must achieve a balance between tumor eradication and possible treatment-related complications and morbidity. Although radiation treatments alone can sometimes induce lymphedema, the development of lymphedema in oncology patients is more often the result of a combination of injuries, including surgery and postoperative radiotherapy. When evaluating the incremental impact of radiation on the development of lymphedema for various tumor types, it is therefore important to consider the type of surgical procedure performed as well as the radiotherapy treatment techniques utilized.

Pathophysiology of Radiation-Associated Lymphedema

Clinical studies have demonstrated that radiotherapy is an independent risk factor for the development of lymphedema, with postoperative radiation increasing the risk by as much as 10 times compared with surgery alone.[1] The mechanisms by which radiation contributes to this risk, however, are still being elucidated. In animal models, investigators have shown that radiation is associated with cutaneous lymphatic dysfunction[2] whereas in breast cancer patients the increased risk of lymphedema after radiation therapy appears to be associated with decreased numbers of cutaneous lymphatics.[3] Thus, it seems that the disruption of the lymphatic system and the development of lymphedema after radiotherapy may be related to either the depletion or dysfunction of cutaneous lymphatic channels.[4]

Another mechanism by which radiation is thought to increase the risk of lymphedema, particularly after surgery, is by promoting tissue fibrosis via transforming

K.C. Horst
Department of Radiation Oncology, Stanford University, Stanford, CA, USA

B.-B. Lee et al. (eds.), *Lymphedema*,
DOI 10.1007/978-0-85729-567-5_62, © Springer-Verlag London Limited 2011

growth factor (TGF) beta1-dependent mechanisms.[5,6] TGF beta1 has been shown to be a negative regulator of lymphatic regeneration during wound repair,[7] as well as a direct inhibitor of lymphatic endothelial cell (LEC) proliferation and function.[8]

Using irradiated mouse tail models, investigators have demonstrated a dose-dependent, long-term decrease in lymphatic function associated with LEC apoptosis, a long-term decrease in the number of cutaneous lymphatic vessels, and the development of soft tissue fibrosis.[4] Furthermore, even at low doses, radiation causes a significant and dose-dependent increase in LEC senescence compared with controls. The decrease in LEC proliferation and function can be attenuated with short-term inhibition of TGF beta1. Interestingly, radiation-induced lymphatic dysfunction did not seem to cause clinically apparent lymphedema. Prevention of radiation tissue fibrosis may be an avenue of investigation for protection against lymphedema.

Radiotherapy and Disease-Specific Risk of Lymphedema

Breast Cancer

The risk of lymphedema after the treatment of breast cancer can vary according to the type of breast and lymph node surgery performed, as well as the radiotherapy treatment fields delivered. Patients diagnosed with early-stage invasive breast cancer may be candidates for breast conservation therapy, which includes a lumpectomy followed often by postoperative whole-breast radiotherapy to reduce the risk of an in-breast tumor recurrence. Whole-breast radiotherapy consists of tangential radiotherapy fields that target the breast tissue, including the axillary tail of the breast. In patients who have evidence of nodal involvement after a standard lymph node dissection (which includes levels I and II), particularly in those with four or more nodes involved, an additional treatment field is added to target the level III axillary nodes and the supraclavicular lymph nodes.

In patients who receive whole-breast radiotherapy only, the incidence of lymphedema after lumpectomy plus axillary node dissection ranges from 1.8% to 10–16%.[9-11] This risk increases to 18–23% in those receiving whole-breast radiotherapy plus supraclavicular/axillary apical radiotherapy treatment.[10,11] With the addition of a posterior axillary boost field, an additional field that is designed to increase the dose to the axilla in patients with high-risk features, the risk of lymphedema increases to 31%. Thus, compared with treatment to the breast alone, the addition of a supraclavicular field or a posterior axillary boost field increases the risk of lymphedema approximately two- and three-fold respectively.[11]

In contrast, patients with more advanced disease are often treated with mastectomy and level I/II axillary dissection. Postoperative radiotherapy is incorporated if the tumor is ≥5 cm or if four or more lymph nodes are involved, as these patients have been shown to have a high rate of locoregional recurrence without the use of radiotherapy. Treatment fields in the postmastectomy setting target the mastectomy scar and chest wall, the axillary apex (level III) and supraclavicular nodes, and occasionally the internal mammary lymph nodes.

Data from the National Surgical Adjuvant Breast and Bowel Project study B-04 reported the long-term incidence of lymphedema to be 31% in women treated with radical mastectomy (removal of the breast plus level I/II and III dissection), 14.8% in those treated with total mastectomy (removal of the breast tissue without intended nodal dissection or sampling) plus radiotherapy to the chest wall and nodal regions, and 15.5% in women treated with total mastectomy only.[12] Interestingly, these findings suggest that mastectomy alone may cause significant disruption of the lymphatics, and that the extent of lymph node resection is associated with the risk of lymphedema. Although the addition of radiotherapy does not seem to increase the risk of lymphedema when a lymph node dissection is not performed, the use of postmastectomy radiotherapy after lymph node dissection can increase the risk two- or three-fold (i.e., from approximately 3% to 9% in a more modern prospective trial evaluating mastectomy without and with radiotherapy, respectively).[13] Other radiotherapy treatment–related factors, such as total dose, the addition of a posterior axillary boost, radiotherapy treatment techniques before 1999,[14] large daily doses, and overlapping fields,[15] have been shown to be associated with an increased incidence of lymphedema.

With the introduction of sentinel lymph node biopsy in patients who are clinically node-negative, the removal of one or two lymph nodes rather than a complete axillary dissection for staging has led to a reduction in the risk of lymphedema, with women having 3-year incidence of lymphedema of 14% after a complete axillary lymph node dissection compared with 8% in those who only had a sentinel lymph node biopsy.[16]

Because radiotherapy after axillary dissection is a known risk factor for lymphedema, it is important for the radiation oncologist to use conventional fractionation (1.8–2 Gy) to the nodal regions and to spare skin and uninvolved tissues to allow for collateral lymphatic drainage.[17,18] In addition to improvement in the surgical techniques, radiotherapy techniques have also evolved over time. Three-dimensional treatment planning is now routinely used to minimize normal tissue toxicity.

Malignant Melanoma

The additional risk of lymphedema after radiotherapy for melanoma can vary according to the anatomical site. Though the overall incidence of lymphedema after treatment for melanoma has been reported to be approximately 16%, the incidence is much higher after treatment involving the lower extremity (28%) compared with the upper extremity (5%).[19]

Radiotherapy is often recommended after resection of the primary lesion if there are pathological features to suggest a high rate of local recurrence.[20] In addition, radiotherapy has been demonstrated to improve locoregional control after regional lymphadenectomy when there are ≥ four lymph nodes involved, bulky adenopathy, or extracapsular extension.[21] The risk of lymphedema when radiotherapy is incorporated into the treatment plan depends on the site of treatment, the size of the treatment field, and the number of lymph nodes resected. Because early in vitro data suggested that melanoma was radioresistant [22,23] and that there may be a higher likelihood of clinical benefit with larger fraction sizes,[24,25] the dose per fraction and total dose delivered for malignant melanoma are often higher than those used in breast cancer, which can potentially increase the risk of edema. Similar to breast cancer patients, the risk seems to increase over time, with 3-year, 5-year, and 10-year rates of lymphedema reported to be 17%, 19%, and 23%, respectively, after lymphadenectomy and postoperative radiotherapy.

In a series of patients treated with postoperative radiotherapy using a high dose per fraction after axillary lymph node dissection, the incidence of arm edema was reported to be 21%, with those patients receiving extended field irradiation to include the axilla and supraclavicular fossa having a higher incidence than those receiving axillary radiotherapy alone.[26] Because local control did not seem to differ, it is important to consider the risk of lymphedema versus risk of disease recurrence when considering including uninvolved nodal regions in the treatment field.

The risk of lymphedema after lymphadenectomy is higher with inguinal disease than with axillary or cervical nodal treatment.[27] The rate of lymphedema after surgery alone for inguinal or pelvic nodal metastases from melanoma ranges from 7–28%.[28] The rate increases in patients receiving adjuvant irradiation to the groin. In patients treated with postoperative radiotherapy for inguinal and/or pelvic nodal metastases using a high dose per fraction, the 3-year actuarial rate of lymphedema can be as high as 39–48%.[28,29] Interestingly, many patients experience some lymphedema even prior to initiating radiotherapy, suggesting that locally advanced disease as well as aggressive surgical debulking can contribute to risk. Furthermore, the risk of edema has been associated with body mass index (BMI), with a 24% incidence of lymphedema reported in patients with a BMI<30 kg/m², but a 55% incidence in patients with a BMI≥30 kg/m².[28]

When considering radiotherapy treatment fields for high-risk melanoma, it is important to balance the treatment complications with the risk of disease recurrence. The extent of treatment (involved field versus extended field), the treatment site (inguinal versus axillary), the dose per fraction, and the total dose can contribute to radiation-associated lymphedema risk. When designing fields, the radiation oncologist should minimize the dose to normal uninvolved tissues in order to spare lymphatic vessels.

Gynecological Malignancies

The risk of lymphedema after treatment for gynecological malignancies varies according to the disease site, extent of surgical resection and lymphadenectomy, and the radiotherapy treatment fields. Overall, the risk has been reported to be approximately 20%.[19]

Radiotherapy can be used as definitive treatment with chemotherapy in locally advanced cervical cancer or medically inoperable patients. It is also often used postoperatively after resection and lymphadenectomy for cervical, endometrial, and vulvar cancers. Treatment fields and dose differ depending on the disease site. For resected cervical cancer with high-risk pathological features, radiotherapy fields typically cover the pelvic lymph node regions, including the external and internal iliac nodes and the presacral nodes, and occasionally the para-aortic nodal regions. Pelvic radiotherapy is also often used postoperatively after resection of endometrial cancer with adverse pathological features. Occasionally, radiotherapy is delivered to the vaginal cuff using an intracavitary cylinder placed into the vagina. This type of radiotherapy treatment gives local treatment and therefore does not appear to increase the risk of lower extremity lymphedema. After surgical resection of vulvar cancer, however, radiotherapy is often targeting not only the pelvic nodes, but also the inguinal nodal regions, which can indeed increase the risk of lower extremity edema compared with pelvic radiotherapy alone.

In a series of patients with endometrial cancer treated with lymphadenectomy, the incidence of lower extremity lymphedema was 34.5% in patients who did not receive radiotherapy and 67.9% in those patients treated with adjuvant pelvic radiotherapy.[30] Patients with vulvar cancer often undergo surgical resection of the primary as well as inguinofemoral lymphadenectomy. Bilateral lymphadenectomy may be performed in women with higher stage disease or central lesions, which can increase the risk of bilateral lymphedema. Postoperative pelvic and inguinal radiotherapy is recommended in patients with multiple lymph nodes involved.[31] In patients treated with lymph node dissection and postoperative radiotherapy for vulvar cancer, the incidence of lower extremity lymphedema can be as high as 47%.[32] Similar to breast cancer, the sentinel lymph node biopsy is being incorporated into the staging of vulvar cancer with the goal of reducing the risk of lymphedema.

As with other disease sites, it is important to minimize dose to normal lymphatics when designing radiotherapy treatment fields in order to minimize the risk of lymphedema in these patients. Techniques such as intensity modulated radiotherapy (IMRT) are often used to achieve such goals.[33]

Extremity Sarcoma

The risk of lymphedema after treatment for sarcoma depends on the treatment site (upper versus lower extremity), the timing of radiotherapy in relation to surgery (preoperative versus postoperative treatment), the size of the radiotherapy treatment field, and whether the normal compartments of the extremity can be spared. The overall incidence of lymphedema in sarcoma patients has been reported to be approximately 30%.[19]

Surgical resection is an essential component of the treatment of sarcomas; however, local recurrence after excision alone is high, particularly with large tumors or tumors with high-grade features. Although more radical surgery can reduce the risk of recurrence, radiotherapy can maximize the functional outcome without the morbidity and cosmetic deformity that radical surgery creates. Except in select histologies, most adult soft tissue sarcomas carry a low risk of nodal metastasis and therefore do not require lymph node dissections in patients without clinical or radiographic evidence of nodal involvement.

Postoperative radiotherapy increases the risk of extremity edema.[34] Higher doses of radiation, long radiation treatment fields, and irradiation of more than 75% of the extremity diameter have been associated with higher complication rates, including lymphedema.[35] The timing of radiotherapy is also important. Although there was no difference noted in local control or survival in a randomized trial investigating preoperative versus postoperative radiotherapy in the treatment of sarcomas,[36] the risk of lymphedema was more common in the postoperative arm (23.2% versus 15.5%).[37] This is likely due to the larger field sizes required in the postoperative setting as well as the higher doses used in those patients given a boost to the surgical bed. Higher total doses are associated with higher rates of late toxicity.[38] Although preoperative treatment can result in higher rates of reversible acute wound healing complications, preoperative radiotherapy is often used, given the smaller treatment field sizes and lower rates of irreversible late complications, such as lymphedema.

When designing radiotherapy treatment fields, three-dimensional treatment planning is important to allow smaller and more accurate treatment volumes. The use of magnetic resonance imaging (MRI) in the preoperative approach can help define the target volume with more precision than with other imaging modalities to help minimize unnecessary treatment of normal tissues. It is important to irradiate only a portion of the cross-section of the extremity to spare normal lymphatic channels. IMRT can be used to improve dose conformity within the tumor and reduce the dose to normal structures; however, care must be taken to limit larger areas of tissue receiving lower-dose treatment.[39]

Conclusions

The impact of radiotherapy on the development of lymphedema is most striking when used in combination with surgery. The proposed mechanisms involve radiation-induced dysfunction of cutaneous lymphatic vessels via a decreased number of lymphatic channels as well as increased TGF beta1 activity that promotes tissue fibrosis and inhibits lymphatic endothelial cell proliferation and function. The risk of lymphedema can vary according to the disease site and type of surgery performed, as well as the size of the radiotherapy treatment fields, the dose to normal tissues, the dose per fraction, the total dose, and the technical quality of the radiotherapy treatment plan.

References

1. Petrek JA, Senie RT, Peters M, et al. Lymphedema in a cohort of breast carcinoma survivors 20 years after diagnosis. *Cancer.* 2001;92:1368-1377.
2. Mortimer PS, Simmonds RH, Rezvani M, et al. Time-related changes in lymphatic clearance in pig skin after a single dose of 18 Gy of X rays. *Br J Radiol.* 1991;64:1140-1146.
3. Jackowski S, Janusch M, Fiedler E, et al. Radiogenic lymphangiogenesis in the skin. *Am J Pathol.* 2007;11:338-348.
4. Avraham T, Yan A, Zampell JC, et al. Radiation therapy causes loss of dermal lymphatic vessels and interferes with lymphatic function by TGF-{beta}1-mediated tissue fibrosis. *Am J Physiol Cell Physiol.* 2010;299:589-605.
5. Martin M, Lefaix J, Delanian S. TGF-beta1 and radiation fibrosis: A master switch and a specific therapeutic target? *Int J Radiat Oncol Biol Phys.* 2000;47:277-290.
6. Yarnold J, Brotons MC. Pathogenetic mechanisms in radiation fibrosis. *Radiother Oncol.* 2010;97(1):149-161.
7. Clavin NW, Avraham T, Fernandez J, et al. TGF-beta1 is a negative regulator of lymphatic regeneration during wound repair. *Am J Physiol Heart Circ Physiol.* 2008;295:H2113-H2127.
8. Oka M, Iwata C, Suzuki HI, et al. Inhibition of endogenous TGF-beta signaling enhances lymphangiogenesis. *Blood.* 2008;111:4571-4579.
9. Powell SN, Taghian AG, Kachnic LA, et al. Risk of lymphedema after regional nodal irradiation with breast conservation therapy. *Int J Radiat Oncol Biol Phys.* 2003;55(5):1209-1215.
10. Meric F, Buchholz TA, Mirza NQ, et al. Long-term complications associated with breast-conservation surgery and radiotherapy. *Ann Surg Oncol.* 2002;9(6):543-549.
11. Hayes SB, Freedman GM, Li T, et al. Does axillary boost increase lymphedema compared with supraclavicular radiation alone after breast conservation? *Int J Radiat Oncol Biol Phys.* 2008;72(5):1449-1455.
12. Deutsch M, Land S, Begovic M, et al. The incidence of arm edema in women with breast cancer randomized on the National Surgical Adjuvant Breast and Bowel Project study B-04 to radical mastectomy versus total mastectomy and radiotherapy versus total mastectomy alone. *Int J Radiat Oncol Biol Phys.* 2008;70(4):1020-1024.
13. Ragaz J, Olivotto IA, Spinelli JJ, et al. Locoregional radiation therapy in patients with high risk breast cancer receiving adjuvant chemotherapy: 20-year results of the British Columbia randomized trial. *J Natl Cancer Inst.* 2005;97(2):116-126.
14. Hinrichs CS, Watroba NL, Rezaishiraz H, et al. Lymphedema secondary to postmastectomy radiation: incidence and risk factors. *Ann Surg Oncol.* 2004;11(6):573-580.
15. Johansson S, Svensson H, Denekamp J. Dose response and latency for radiation-induced fibrosis, edema, and neuropathy in breast cancer patients. *Int J Radiat Oncol Biol Phys.* 2002;52(5):1207-1219.
16. Ashikaga T, Krag DN, Land SR, et al. Morbidity results from the NSABP B-32 trial comparing sentinel lymph node dissection versus axillary dissection. *J Surg Oncol.* 2010;102:111-118.
17. Leitch A, Meek A, Smith R, et al. Workgroup I: treatment of the axilla with surgery and radiation-preoperative and postoperative risk assessment. *Cancer.* 1998;S83:2877-2879.
18. Graham P, Jagavkar R, Browne L, et al. Supraclavicular radiotherapy must be limited laterally by the coracoid to avoid significant adjuvant breast nodal radiotherapy lymphoedema risk. *Australas Radiol.* 2006;50(6):578-582.
19. Cormier JN, Askew RL, Mungovan KS, et al. Lymphedema beyond breast cancer. A systematic review and meta-analysis of cancer-related secondary lymphedema. *Cancer.* 2010;116(22):5138-5149.
20. Ballo MT, Ang KK. Radiotherapy for cutaneous malignant melanoma: rationale and indications. *Oncology.* 2004;18(1):99-107.
21. Lee RJ, Gibbs JF, Proulx GM, et al. Nodal basin recurrence following lymph node dissection for melanoma: implications for adjuvant radiotherapy. *Int J Radiat Oncol Biol Phys.* 2000;46(2):467-474.

22. Barranco SC, Romsdahl MM, Humphrey RM. The radiation response of human malignant melanoma cells grown in vitro. *Cancer Res.* 1971;31:830-833.
23. Dewey DL. The radiosensitivity of melanoma cells in culture. *Br J Radiol.* 1971;44:816-817.
24. Overgaard J. The role of radiotherapy in recurrent and metastatic malignant melanoma: a clinical radiobiological study. *Int J Radiat Oncol Biol Phys.* 1986;12(6):867-872.
25. Seegenschmiedt MH, Keilholz L, Altendorf-Hofmann A, et al. Palliative radiotherapy for recurrent and metastatic malignant melanoma: prognostic factors for tumor response and long-term outcome: a 20-year experience. *Int J Radiat Oncol Biol Phys.* 1999;44(3):607-618.
26. Beadle BM, Guadagnolo BA, Ballo MT, et al. Radiation therapy field extent for adjuvant treatment of axillary metastases from malignant melanoma. *Int J Radiat Oncol Biol Phys.* 2009;73(5):1376-1382.
27. Agrawal S, Kane JM, Guadagnolo BA, et al. The benefits of adjuvant radiation therapy after therapeutic lymphadenectomy for clinically advanced, high-risk, lymph node-metastatic melanoma. *Cancer.* 2009;115:5836-5844.
28. Ballo MT, Zagars GK, Gershenwald JE, et al. A critical assessment of adjuvant radiotherapy for inguinal lymph node metastases from melanoma. *Ann Surg Oncol.* 2004;11(12):1079-1084.
29. Burmeister BH, Smithers BM, Davis S, et al. Radiation therapy following nodal surgery for melanoma: an analysis of late toxicity. *ANZ J Surg.* 2002;72:344-348.
30. Todo Y, Yamamoto R, Minobe S, et al. Risk factors for postoperative lower-extremity lymphedema in endometrial cancer survivors who had treatment including lymphadenectomy. *Gynecol Oncol.* 2010;119:60-64.
31. Homesley HD, Bundy BN, Sedlis A, et al. Radiation therapy versus pelvic node resection for carcinoma of the vulva with positive groin nodes. *Obstet Gynecol.* 1986;68:733.
32. Ryan M, Stainton MC, Slaytor EK, et al. Aetiology and prevalence of lower limb lymphoedema following treatment for gynaecological cancer. *Aust N Z J Obstet Gynaecol.* 2003;43(2):148-151.
33. Ahamad A, D'Souza W, Salehpour M, et al. Intensity-modulated radiation therapy after hysterectomy: comparison with conventional treatment and sensitivity of the normal-tissue-sparing effect to margin size. *Int J Radiat Oncol Biol Phys.* 2005;62(4):1117-1124.
34. Yang JC, Chang AE, Baker AR, et al. Randomized prospective study of the benefit of adjuvant radiation therapy in the treatment of soft tissue sarcomas of the extremity. *J Clin Oncol.* 1998;16:197.
35. Stinson SF, Delaney TF, Greenberg J, et al. Acute and long-term effects on limb function of combined modality limb sparing therapy for extremity soft tissue sarcoma. *Int J Radiat Oncol Biol Phys.* 1991;21:1493.
36. O'Sullivan B, Davis AM, Turcotte R, et al. Preoperative versus postoperative radiotherapy in soft-tissue sarcoma of the limbs: a randomized trial. *Lancet.* 2002;359:2235.
37. Davis AM, O'Sullivan B, Turcotte R, et al. Late radiation morbidity following randomization to preoperative versus postoperative radiotherapy in extremity soft tissue sarcoma. *Radiother Oncol.* 2005;75:48.
38. Robinson M, Cassoni A, Harmer C, et al. High dose hyperfractionated radiotherapy in the treatment of extremity soft tissue sarcomas. *Radiother Oncol.* 1991;22:118-126.
39. Alektiar KM, Brennan MF, Healey JH, et al. Impact of intensity-modulated radiation therapy on local control in primary soft-tissue sarcoma of the extremity. *J Clin Oncol.* 2008;26:3440.

Part XVI
Phlebolymphedema

Chapter 63
Pathophysiology of Phlebolymphedema and a Physiologic Approach to 'Chronic Veno-lymphatic Insufficiency'

Claude Franceschi, Erica Menegatti, and Paolo Zamboni

Introduction

Chronic venous insufficiency can be defined as an impairment of the venous system so that it cannot adequately fulfill its main function, which consists of the drainage of venous blood flow from the periphery to the heart; similarly, chronic lymphatic insufficiency is described as a fault of the lymphatic system impairing its ability to perform its major mechanical function, which is to clear the interstitial space of large molecules and excess fluid.[1,2]

Often, the two systems offset each other; otherwise, they can be both involved, represented by the so-called phlebolymphedema, which is characterized by mixed venous and lymphatic insufficiency.[1]

Consequently, these conditions lead to an increase in interstitial fluids due to protein accumulation; these trapped proteins retain water, and edema develops. Because of the gravitational effect, such an edema is greater in the lower part of the body; moreover, depending on the individual tissue reaction, it can lead to different alterations in soft tissue and skin, subcutaneous tissue, muscles and fascia, as well as the periosteum and bone.

These changes are clinically manifested as a number of well known stasis injuries: dermatitis eczema, atrophy, cutaneous papillomatosis, skin hyperpigmentation or depigmentation, chronic skin ulceration, and acute and chronic hypodermitis with hardening of the subcutaneous layer to a lipodermatosclerosis.[1,3,4]

C. Franceschi (✉)
Dispensaire Marie Therese, Hopital Saint Joseph, Paris, France

B.-B. Lee et al. (eds.), *Lymphedema*,
DOI 10.1007/978-0-85729-567-5_63, © Springer-Verlag London Limited 2011

Pathophysiological Background

Chronic Venous Insufficiency

In hemodynamic terms, we can define chronic venous insufficiency (CVI) as the incapacity of the venous system to provide blood flow and pressure suitable for drainage, thermoregulation, and heart filling, whatever the subject's posture or muscular activity.[2] It is the consequence of a permanent or transitory dysfunction of one or more of the components of the venous system. Insufficiency is generally identified by particular clinical symptoms according to the impaired function. Slight and/or early forms of insufficiency are often asymptomatic and can be detected only through instrumental testing.[2]

Chronic venous insufficiency has an incidence in western countries ranging from 20% to 50%; this is because the disease severity is subdivided in several classes according to a new international classification, CEAP (clinical severity, etiology, anatomy, pathophysiology): C0 (Class 0) no visible or palpable signs of venous disease; C1 (Class 1) telangiectases, reticular veins, malleolar flare; C2 (Class 2) varicose veins; C3 (Class 3) edema without skin changes; C4 (Class 4) skin changes ascribed to venous disease (e.g., pigmentation, venous eczema, lipodermatosclerosis); C5 (Class 5) skin changes as defined above with healed ulcers; C6 (Class 6) skin changes as defined above with active ulcers.[5]

Pure Chronic Lymphatic Insufficiency and Phlebolymphedema

Lymphedema is usually the abnormal accumulation of interstitial, protein-rich fluid caused either by congenital malformation (primary lymphedema) or the result of lymphatic obstruction or surgical damage (secondary lymphedema). In lymphedema, the chronic accumulation of fluid in the interstitium leads to damage in the skin and subcutaneous tissue, interference with wound healing, and bacterial overgrowth, because the edema provides a culture medium for bacteria that can result in cellulitis.[1]

Secondary lymphedema has multiple causes, including resections for cancer, other trauma, conventional vein stripping, and/or harvesting procedures such as those for coronary bypass or other vascular surgery.[1]

The coexistence of venous insufficiency overloads the interstitium and has an impact on the lymphatic transport capacity. The condition of a combined status of venous and lymphatic insufficiency is usually termed "phlebolymphedema."[1]

The lymphatic and venous systems are intimately functionally integrated, especially in the presence of venous hypertension, a parameter characteristic of CVI. The increase in lymphatic flow becomes greater than the physiological lymph transport. Such a compensatory function of the lymphatic system in the course of CVI can be measured by the means of lymphoscintigraphy. In the early stage, the lymphatic

Fig. 63.1 Typical clinical presentation of phlebolymphedema: hyperpigmentation and lipodermatosclerosis suggest the coexistence of chronic venous insufficiency (CVI). This is confirmed in (**a**) by a reflux detected in the popliteal vein, whereas B-mode imaging of the soft tissue in (**b**) clearly depicts the dilation of the lymph collectors

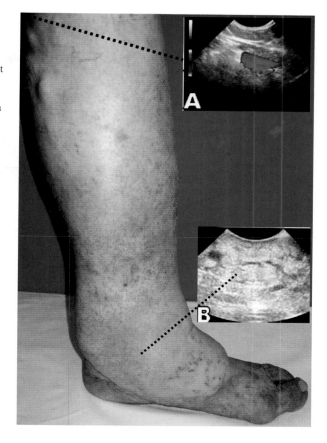

vasculature compensates by increased lymph drainage and the result is low protein edema. Lymphatics may fail for a number of reasons under these circumstances.[1,3]

First, there may be a reduced number of lymph-conducting pathways, either because there is a congenitally determined reduction or because there is an acquired obliteration of lymphatic vessels, concomitant to CVI. Sometimes, this picture can be clinically insignificant, but, when an interstitial overload appears as a consequence of CVI, a reduction in these pathways may occur. The same happens in cases of postoperative lymphedema after venous surgery, a described complication of vein stripping in which the lymphatic vessels are removed through the procedure.[6] From this point of view, the reason for chronic swelling after vein stripping is likely to be a pre-existing subclinical lymphatic insufficiency, suddenly worsened by lymphatic ablation.

Phlebolymphedema also occurs when a severe CVI coexists with subclinical, or clearly clinical, manifestations of lymphedema. The additional effects may create severe pictures of chronic edema (Fig. 63.1). However, the possible resolution of CVI, especially in primary cases, may in turn improve the clinical condition.

528   C. Franceschi et al.

Fig. 63.2 Positive "Stemmer sign" consisting of the inability of the examiner to "tent" the skin at the base of the digits in the involved extremity. This suggests the lymphatic origin of the edema despite the eventual coexistence of CVI assessed by duplex

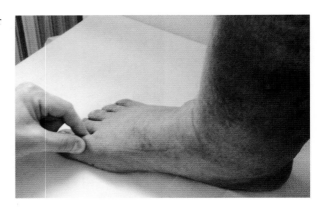

Clinical and Instrumental Assessment

The diagnosis of phlebolymphedema is based on a detailed history and physical examination. Chronic venous insufficiency and lymphedema are not difficult to distinguish from one another. Patients with phlebolymphedema frequently have skin changes characteristic of CVI, such as ankle hyperpigmentation or corona phlebectatica (Fig. 63.1). The distribution of the former in venous disease begins as perimalleolar, retromalleolar, and supramalleolar, but may in time become circumferential. Hyperpigmentation is the result of the extravasation of chronic red blood cells and consequent subcutaneous hemosiderin stores.[2]

These clinical signs confirm the venous dysfunction element related to venous hypertension; moreover, more advanced is the venous disease and other lymphedema hallmarks are associated.[4]

With time, the edema increases and the clinical features of lymphedema begin to appear, including the characteristic skin changes of hyperkeratosis and papillomatosis, particularly in the submalleolar and retromalleolar regions and the lateral border of the foot.

On the contrary, when duplex examination reveals a picture of CVI (Fig. 63.1a), it is practically impossible to see under clinical inspection because of the "peau d'orange" and cutaneous fibrosis, and the clinician is faced with a picture of phlebolymphedema with pre-existing or prevalent lymphatic insufficiency. In our clinical practice we adopt a positive "Stemmer sign" (the inability of the examiner to "tent" the skin at the base of the digits in the extremity involved), as shown in Fig. 63.2, in order to corroborate a clinical diagnosis of pure lymphedema complicated by CVI. Conversely, the presence of hyperpigmentation favors a diagnosis of CVI complicated by lymphatic failure complicated by venous interstitial overload. Both pictures represent phlebolymphedemas, but with different pathophysiological sequences.

Duplex ultrasound should be used to confirm suspected venous insufficiency, identify reflux, and reveal associated proximal or distal chronic venous obstruction, as well.

Furthermore, under the same examination, the B-mode echo high-resolution imaging of soft tissue allows the presence of a lymphatic overload to be assessed that is of different severity, starting from simple suffusion of subcutaneous tissue to abnormal dilatation of the lymphatic ducts (Fig. 63.1b).

In patients affected by phlebolymphedema, confirmed through echo color Doppler examination, the CVI component has to be treated with minimally invasive nonsurgical or surgical procedures in order to avoid the inevitable lymphatic injuries caused by vein stripping. Injuries are also possible through the transmission of energy through the venous wall to the lymphatics encircling the saphenous vein, when endovascular procedures, like laser and radiofrequency are contemplated.

Several studies in the literature report that foam sclerotherapy seems to be more effective than traditional surgery, in the event of signs, even benign ones, of lymphatic insufficiency, with added manual lymphatic drainage and carefully tailored elastic and/or nonelastic compression.[1,6]

Recently, it has been proven by randomized controlled long-term trials that a minimally invasive, surgical technique like hemodynamic correction (CHIVA) is more effective than ablative technique stripping.[7,8] These results reiterate that, in the case of phlebolymphedema, the CVI should be treated using this conservative surgical approach.

CHIVA Definition and Hemodynamic Background

CHIVA is a French acronym for a type of treatment: Conservatrice et Hemodynamique de l'Insuffisance Veineuse en Ambulatoire, which means conservative and hemodynamic treatment of venous insufficiency in ambulatory care. Two main considerations led to the concept of this treatment. The first is clinical. Since varices and most other venous disorders are treated by lying down and, above all, by raising the legs, any treatment that can control hydrostatic pressure, including positioning, would deserve great medical interest. The second consideration is experimental. Venous pressure measurements at the ankle in normal individuals show a maximal pressure while standing still, but it collapses when walking, thanks to the valvulo-muscular pump (VMP), which, by closing alternately the venous valves, fractionates dynamically the hydrostatic blood column (dynamic fractionation of hydrostatic pressure [DFHSP]). Conversely, in most venous patients, the more incompetent the valves are, the less the ankle venous pressure decreases (Fig. 63.3).

Varices and venous insufficiencies are due to an excessive transmural pressure (TMP), i.e., an excessive difference between intra- and extravenous pressure. The intravenous pressure consists of three forces, gravitational for the hydrostatic pressure (HSP) and two motive forces provided respectively by the left heart ventricle (residual pressure [RP]) and the valvulo-muscular pump (VMP). Few varices and venous insufficiencies are due to RP excess: venous blocks, arteriovenous fistulae. Most of them are due to valve incompetence, which impairs the DFHSP and the correct distribution of the VMP pressure.

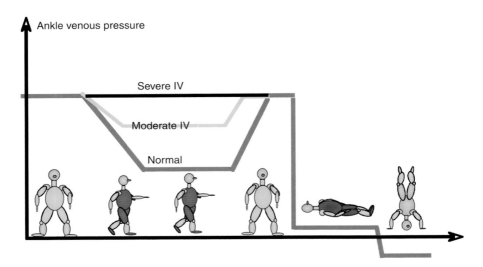

Fig. 63.3 Ankle venous pressure according to posture and movement. No difference between normal and incompetent when standing still, lying down, and lower limb lifting. Conversely, there is a dramatic difference when walking, where the greater the incompetence, the less the pressure reduction

In addition to the disruption of the DFHSP control by the VMP, valve incompetence may provide hemodynamic conditions for a supplementary increase in TMP due to shunts that divert back the TMP flow/pressure.

Such impairment is usually caused by superficial and deep closed shunts (CS) or superficial derived open shunts (DOS) due to venous incompetence that disrupts DFHSP control by the valvulo-muscular pump (VMP). Venous shunts are made of veins overloaded with blood coming from other territories in addition to their physiological draining flow (Fig. 63.4).

A CS is a deep or superficial vein overloaded with deep exogenous blood in a closed circuit by the effect of VMP diastole. A DOS is a superficial vein overloaded with superficial exogenous blood by the effect of the VMP diastole, but without the closed circuit effect. Thus, every shunt consists of a shunting vein that is overloaded with exogenous blood through an escape point EP and drains back through a re-entry point (REP). A shunt classification was made according to the different anatomo-functional features (Fig. 63.5).

Since valve repair or prosthesis has been neither easy nor feasible to date, interruption at or immediately under the escape points should repair the VMP and suppress pathological shunt flow. At the same time, these interruptions fractionate permanently and dynamically the column of pressure. Furthermore, and in order to fragment better the hydrostatic column in long incompetent superficial veins, other interruptions immediately under possible competent perforators connected with those veins are performed. This means that CHIVA restores venous physiology in walking patients by maintaining a low distal venous pressure due to renewed VMP efficiency and its effect on DFHSP and blood drainage. Ultimately, venous disorders and varices are supposed to heal. Edema and trophic disorders caused by

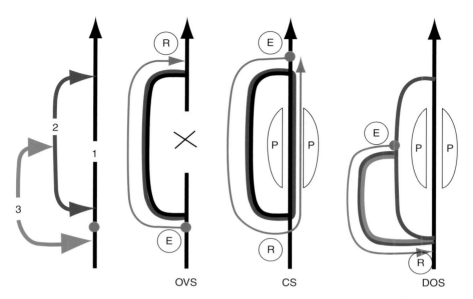

Fig. 63.4 Venous shunt principles. *1, 2, 3* Competent interconnected veins draining their own territory without shunts. *E* escape point, *R* reentry point, *P* valvulo-muscular pump at the diastolic phase, *A* venous shunt is made of a vein overloaded by any flow depending on other territories. *OVS* open vicarious shunt: vein 2 bypasses an obstacle in a collateral vein 1 and so carries out two flows: its physiological draining flow and an overloading flow from the vein 1 territory distal to the obstacle. The escape point E is distal to re-entry R. VOS flow is permanent, but enhanced by P systole. No re-circulation. *CS* closed shunt during P diastolic aspiration, incompetent vein 2 allows a retrograde flow so that vein 2 drains properly its own physiological flow despite its retrograde direction plus vein 1 flow refluxing through E, which is proximal to R. Thus, vein 1 flow recirculates at each P diastole. *DOS* derived open shunt: during P diastolic aspiration, incompetent vein 3 allows a retrograde flow so that vein 3 drains properly its own physiological flow despite its retrograde direction plus vein 2 flow refluxing through E. There is no recirculation because the distal re-entry R is not connected with vein 2, but rather with vein 1

excessive transmural pressure (TMP) should heal because of the restoration of DFHSP and venous drainage repair. Varicose calibres should decrease to normal thanks to TMP decrease, aggressive shunt flow suppression, and efficient VMP blood aspiration. These theoretical hypotheses have been confirmed by numerous publications since their initial presentation at Precy-sous-thil France in October 1988, at which time a text was published entitled *Theorie et pratique de la Cure Conservatrice et Hemodynamique de l'Insuffisance Veineuse en Ambulatoire.*[2]

CHIVA Strategy and Tactics

Strategy is the intellectual concept of the actions that have to be taken in order to reach a goal according to a theoretical model. Tactics are the material means selected to perform the actions according to the strategy. In this field, a successful strategy

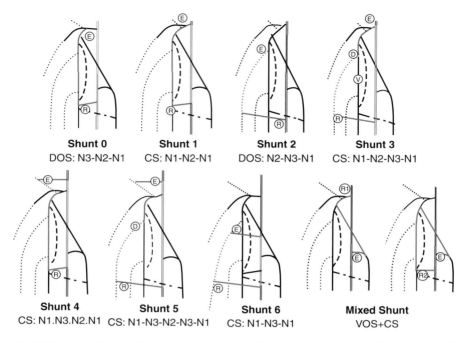

Fig. 63.5 Schematic classification of venous shunts. *N1* deep venous network, *N2* great and small saphenous trunk and the Giacomini vein located in the fascia duplication, *N3* suprafascial tributaries

relies on understanding venous pathophysiology, and the efficiency of the tactics depends on the quality of the material means. Many CHIVA failures are either due to disrespect or misunderstanding of the strategy or to inadequate material means. For this reason, both a clear understanding of the theory and adequate training are necessary to perform CHIVA.

Fundamental Rules of Strategy

The Final Purpose Is to Normalize the TMP

Transmural pressure can be reduced by several means according to the hemodynamic pathophysiological model. TMP will decrease thanks to extravenous pressure enhancement, e.g., compression (banding, elastic stocking) and/or intravenous pressure reduction like lower limb lifting, which reduces the HSP. CHIVA reduces the intravenous pressure at the same time by HSP reduction thanks to DFHSP restoration and VMP pressure/flow diversion.

Preservation of Deep and Superficial Draining Flows Even in Varicose Veins

Any venous flow, even in varicose veins, is composed totally or partially of the physiological draining of blood from tissues. Any blockage of that draining flow involves upstream tissue suffering, including capillaro-venular overload (telangiectasias and micro-varicosities). Collateral veins, overloaded and dilated by the force of draining flow, act as natural venous by-passes that circumvent a blockage and allow for physiological drainage of the upstream tissues. In this way, a vicarious open shunt (VOS) is formed. VOS can be elicited by a functional block, thrombosis, sclerosis, ligation or removal, the latter two being the reason for recurrent varices after disrespect of draining flows. There is no indication for VOS destruction, even if VOS is an unsightly varice. However, it is obvious that removal or occlusion of nondraining or redundant veins is compatible with the CHIVA strategy. At the same time, this venous drainage preservation relieves the lymphatic drainage and the limited and precise venous disconnections prevent the collateral damage of the lymphatic nodes and vessels.

Correction of Deep and Superficial Valve Incompetence Pathogenic Effects

The CHIVA strategy is conservative, not only to preserve the venous capital for further arterial by-pass, but also because vein destruction involves hemodynamic disorders. In fact, venous destruction precludes the drainage that causes tissue suffering and varicose recurrence by a vicarious effect. CHIVA strategy is hemodynamic because it restores proper distal venous pressure. As a matter of fact, CHIVA reduces lateral pressure and consequently transmural pressure (TMP) by restoring DFHSP through disconnection of closed shunts, suppressing pathogenic shunt flows, and preserving beneficial vicarious shunts. CHIVA strategy is focused on the re-entry quality, that is, on its ability to drain the venous network properly in order to avoid the effects of drainage preclusion. For this reason, limited venous interruptions are preferable to extensive ones, even if the immediate aesthetic outcomes are less satisfactory. Actually, aesthetic outcomes improve with time, long-term results are much better, and recurrences are much fewer with limited interventions. Long term RCT clearly show the superiority of CHIVA on ablative techniques, assuming stripping as gold standard, in terms of recurrences.[7,8] Clearly, however, any removal or occlusion of nondraining or redundant veins is not contrary to CHIVA strategy, which consists of the following principles:

(a) Preservation of deep and superficial draining flows, even in varicose veins
(b) Disconnection of deep and superficial CS and superficial DOS in a way that blocks the shunting flow WITHOUT precluding the draining flow

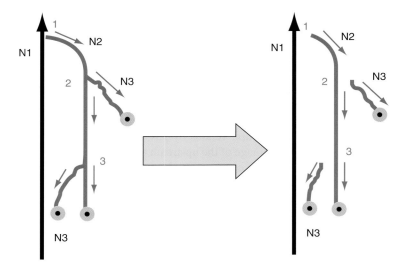

Fig. 63.6 Shunt type 1+2 and associated CHIVA I procedure

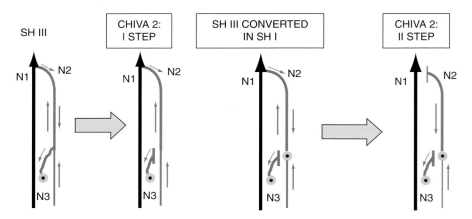

Fig. 63.7 CHIVA II first and second step for shunt type 3

(c) Fractionation of the hydrostatic pressure column WITHOUT precluding the draining flow
(d) Adaptation of the re-entry efficiency to the needs of draining flow
(e) Minimization of venous interruptions. The less the veins are interrupted, even in extended varicose, the better the long-term results. The more the veins are destroyed, even if varicose, the better the short-term results, but the worse the long-term outcome (Figs. 63.6 and 63.7).

Fundamental Rules of Tactics

Which are the best procedures to achieve the strategic decisions? In other words, which are the most accurate, efficient, and lasting material means of performing flow interruptions in the right places according to strategic needs? How not to confuse tactic failure with strategic error? Is a forced or by-passed interruption due to an inappropriate tactic or a mistaken strategy?

Surgical Requirements

Minimally invasive, the CHIVA strategy consists of mini-incisions under local anesthesia regarding superficial veins. Sometimes, only when required, the great or small saphenous arch has to be disconnected.[9] Under local anesthesia, their dissection is eased and limited thanks to the previous duplex marking and the respect of tributaries, surrounding tissues, and lymphatic nodes and vessels.

Therefore, previous precise marking under duplex ultrasound by an operator aware of the surgical necessities is indispensable. Venous short resection (1–4 cm) associated with nonabsorbable ligation and nonabsorbable closure of the perforated fascia seems to be the most precise, efficient, and long-lasting material means to date. Simple nonabsorbable ligations are seldom forced and reopened. Multiple ligations with nonabsorbable thick thread seem to offer better resistance. Absorbable venous ligation after section could favor recanalization because of inflammatory angiogenetic effects.

Nonsurgical Procedures

So far, endovenous procedures (foam, RF, laser) have not demonstrated sufficient capability to fulfill the requirements of the CHIVA strategy, in terms of limitation, precision, and durability of the disconnections.

References

1. Bunke N, Brown K, Bergan J. Phlebolymphedema: usually unrecognized, often poorly treated. *Perspect Vasc Surg Endovasc Ther*. 2009;21(2):65-68; Review.
2. Franceschi C, Zamboni P. *Principles of Venous Haemodynamics*. New York: Nova Publisher; 2009.
3. Mortimer PS. Implications of the lymphatic system in CVI-associated edema. *Angiology*. 2000;51(1):3-7.
4. Rockson SG. Diagnosis and management of lymphatic vascular disease. *J Am Coll Cardiol*. 2008;52:799-806.

5. Eklöf B, Rutherford RB, Bergan JJ, et al. American Venous Forum International Ad Hoc Committee for Revision of the CEAP Classification. Revision of the CEAP classification for chronic venous disorders: consensus statement. *J Vasc Surg*. 2004;40(6):1248-1252.

6. Ouvry PA, Guenneguez H, Ouvry PA. Lymphatic complications from variceal surgery. *Phlebologie*. 1993;46(4):563-568.

7. Carandina S, Mari C, De Palma M, et al. Varicose vein stripping vs haemodynamic correction (CHIVA): a longterm randomised trial. *Eur J Vasc Endovasc Surg*. 2008;35(2):230-237.

8. Parés JO, Juan J, Tellez R, et al. Varicose vein surgery: stripping versus the CHIVA method: a randomized controlled trial. *Ann Surg*. 2010;251(4):624-631.

9. Zamboni P, Gianesini S, Menegatti E, Tacconi G, Palazzo A, Liboni A. Great saphenous varicose vein surgery without saphenofemoral junction disconnection. *Br J Surg*. 2010;97(6): 820-825.

Chapter 64
Diagnosis and Management of Primary Phlebolymphedema

Byung-Boong Lee, James Laredo, and Dirk A. Loose

Definition and Classification

Phlebolymphedema is a unique condition of combined insufficiency of both the venous and lymphatic systems, with various causes.[1-3]

Primary phlebolymphedema, caused by a congenital defect of the venous and lymphatic systems, represents one aspect of the clinical manifestation of Klippel–Trenaunay syndrome (KTS).[4,5] KTS is characterized by having both vascular malformation components, venous malformation (VM) and lymphatic malformation (LM).[6,7]

In contrast, secondary phlebolymphedema is an acquired condition that begins with chronic venous insufficiency (CVI) of various causes. CVI then results in lymphatic dysfunction leading to chronic lymphatic insufficiency (CLI) as a complication.[8-10]

Therefore, the CLI of secondary phlebolymphedema is generally limited as a regional/local condition (e.g., indolent venous stasis ulcer) as a complication of CVI,[11,12] whereas the CLI of primary phlebolymphedema is a diffuse condition of lymphedema caused by a truncular LM[13,14] from the outset together with the CVI caused by the VM[15,16] (Fig. 64.1).

Therefore, proper understanding of the relationship between two different venodynamics and lymphodynamics is required for proper interpretation of this "dual" outflow system failure: CVI+CLI.

Although the venodynamics and lymphodynamics are based on totally different hemodynamic mechanisms, the venous and lymphatic systems are a mutually dependent dual outflow system of the circulation. Therefore, they are one inseparable system and the insufficiency or overload of one or both systems allows the other to play an auxiliary role in compensating fluid return through micro- and macro-anastomotoses.[17,18]

B.-B. Lee (✉)
Department of Surgery, Division of Vascular Surgery,
George Washington University School of Medicine, Washington, DC, USA

B.-B. Lee et al. (eds.), *Lymphedema*,
DOI 10.1007/978-0-85729-567-5_64, © Springer-Verlag London Limited 2011

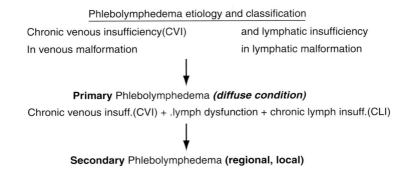

Phlebolymphedema etiology and classification

Chronic venous insufficiency(CVI)   and lymphatic insufficiency

In venous malformation   in lymphatic malformation

Primary Phlebolymphedema *(diffuse condition)*

Chronic venous insuff.(CVI) + .lymph dysfunction + chronic lymph insuff.(CLI)

Secondary Phlebolymphedema **(regional, local)**

Fig. 64.1 Phlebolymphedema etiology and classification

However, both systems are "mutually complementary" *only* when they are functioning normally. When one of the two systems loses its normal function (e.g., chronic venous hypertension, lymphedema), such mutual interdependence generates a new problem in the other.

Failure of one system gives additional burden/load to the other system. Long-term single- system failure results in total failure of this "inseparable" dual system, resulting in the unique clinical condition of phlebolymphedema.

When CVI results in an excessive fluid load at the tissue level, it disrupts the check and balance function of the capillary system, giving an additional load to the lymphatic system. When this overload exceeds the maximum capacity of normal lymphatic compensation, it results in CLI. CLI becomes more prominent, especially in a compromised lymphatic drainage system because of lymphatic dysfunction due to various etiologies (e.g., surgery and radiotherapy associated with cancer treatment).

Secondary phlebolymphedema occurs during the advanced stages of CVI of nonhealing venous stasis ulcer when it reaches its end stage and becomes indolent. This complication has been well known for many decades. Its related problems and issues are well reviewed in Chaps. 63 and 65.

In contrast, "primary" phlebolymphedema is still a relatively unknown condition and is the most common manifestation of the "hemolymphatic" malformation (HLM). The HLM consists of a VM and LM, and represents the clinical condition of the KTS in the majority of cases (Fig. 64.2).

When an arteriovenous malformation (AVM)[19,20] is present in a patient with KTS, this condition is also known as Parkes–Weber Syndrome.[21,22] The presence of an AVM makes the overall condition of primary phlebolymphedema much harder to manage (Fig. 64.3).

Diagnosis and Clinical Evaluation

The clinical manifestation of phlebolymphedema (PLE) is quite variable depending on the etiology (primary and secondary) and the degree and extent of both the CVI and CL. Phlebolymphedema is clinically more distinct in the lower extremities in general.[11,23]

Fig. 64.2 Primary phlebolymphedema as a clinical manifestation of Klippel–Trenaunay syndrome by its vascular malformation component: VM+LM

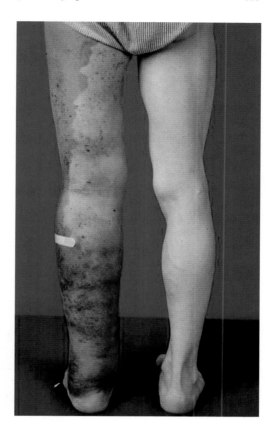

Therefore, simultaneous evaluation of both the venous and lymphatic systems is required. There are various laboratory tests available for venous and lymphatic system assessment. The appropriate combination of tests is dependent on the individual case of PLE and can be selected from among the available tests.[24-30]

The assessment of the extent and severity of the CVI should begin with duplex ultrasound and may include various plethysmographic studies in addition to ascending/descending phlebography to identify the etiology (e.g., marginal vein; Fig. 64.4).[31,32]

The most common VM that causes CVI in patients with primary PLE is the "lateral embryological or marginal vein"[1,33,34] causing venous reflux and venous hypertension. The second most common VM is deep vein dysplasia (e.g., iliac vein agenesis, hypoplastic femoral vein) or defective vein (e.g., web, stenosis, vein valve agenesia, aneurysm, ectasia) with venous outflow obstruction and venous hypertension.

If the extratruncular VM lesion is thought to be involved in the development of CVI and to contribute to PLE, investigation to exclude other VM components of the KTS should be considered. Detailed information on truncular and extratruncular VMs in primary PLE is available elsewhere.[10,15,31]

Fig. 64.3 Primary phlebolymphedema
as a clinical manifestation of Parkes–
Weber syndrome by its vascular
malformation component:
VM + LM + AVM

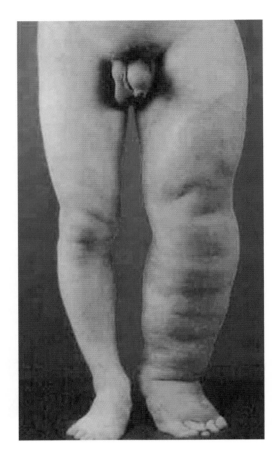

In the evaluation of CLI, the functional status of the lymphatic system should be determined first with radionuclide lymphoscintigraphy as the initial baseline investigation to delineate excessive fluid accumulation in the tissues of the limb or affected lymphatic territories. Additional tests are also required when the extratruncular LM is involved in KTS.

CLI because of primary PLE is mostly due to "primary lymphedema by truncular LM lesions (e.g., lymphatic dysplasia, aplasia, hypoplasia, or hyperplasia). Extratruncular LM lesions (e.g., lymphangioma), on the other hand, are seldom involved in CLI. However, when present, the extratruncular LM may be evaluated with MRI and/or whole body blood pool scintigraphy.[11,23] Other optional tests may be included depending upon the overall CVM components (e.g., AVM; Table 64.1).

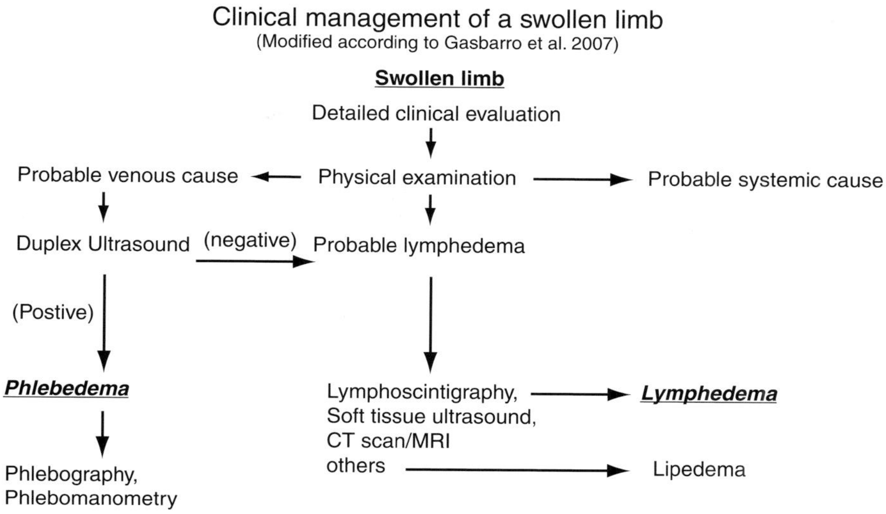

Clinical management of a swollen limb
(Modified according to Gasbarro et al. 2007)

Swollen limb

Detailed clinical evaluation

Probable venous cause ◄—— Physical examination ——► Probable systemic cause

Duplex Ultrasound (negative) Probable lymphedema

(Postive)

Phlebedema

Lymphoscintigraphy, ——► ***Lymphedema***
Soft tissue ultrasound,
CT scan/MRI

Phlebography,   others ——————————► Lipedema
Phlebomanometry

Fig. 64.4 Clinical management of a swollen limb

Table 64.1 Laboratory evaluation for the phlebolymphedema

Venous system
- Venous duplex ultrasound – test of choice
- Air plethysmography: functional assessment
- CT with/without contrast
- MRI study; standard and MR venography (MRV)
- Radioisotope venography
- Ascending and descending venography
- Percutaneous direct puncture phlebography
- Volumetry
- Whole-body blood pool scintigraphy (WBBPS)[a]
- Transarterial lung perfusion scintigraphy (TLPS)[a]

Lymphatic system
- Lymphoscintigraphy – test of choice
- CT – exclude underlying malignancy
- Standard MRI – potentially most useful
- Lymphangiography (oil contrast): optional for the candidate for venolymphatic reconstructive surgery
- Volumetry
- MR lymphangiography: optional
- Ultrasound lymphangiography: optional
- Miscellaneous: dermascan, tonometry, fluorescence microlymphography, ultrasound measurement of subcutaneous edema: optional

[a]For the congenital vascular malformation assessment

Clinical Management

General principle of primary PLE management should remain within the guidelines for the KTS and its vascular malformation component management. It has been well outlined in Chap. 52.

However, this combined venous–lymphatic disorder by two independent VM and LM conditions results in an extremely delicate mutual interdependency; their management mandates proper interpretation of this complicated interrelationship between them.

The management of the CVI should have priority over that of the CLI unless there is a serious complication of the LM component (e.g., leakage with or without sepsis). This is because the degree and extent of negative impact on CLI by the CVI is much more severe than the effect of the CVI on the CLI in our experience. Effective control of the CVI often results in a much improved CLI condition.

Baseline therapy for the CLI component of primary PLE is compression therapy, because the absolute majority of the CLI is limited to lymphedema. Reinforced gradient compression therapy based on complex decongestive therapy (CDT) is required to control the CVI and CLI together.

However, lymphedema caused by CLI in primary PLE is more difficult to control than CLI because of independent primary lymphedema with no CVI component. The CLI and CVI are often resistant to conventional treatment based on CDT, and the disease has a distinct tendency to progress. Therefore, aggressive care with a strict prevention regimen (e.g., infection) is warranted, even for maintenance compared with the solitary condition of primary lymphedema.

When this truncular LM causing primary lymphedema is combined with the extratruncular LM (lymphangioma), additional treatment with sclerotherapy of the coexisting extratruncular LM is rarely required. When such a lesion is present, it has direct communication with the lymph transporting system, which produces a significant burden to the truncular LM and is the underlying cause of the CLI.

Management of the CVI in primary PLE is dependent on its etiology. When the reflux of the marginal vein (MV) is the source of the CVI, the MV should be treated either with open surgical resection or endovascular obliteration. Treatment of the MV requires a normal deep venous system that can tolerate the sudden influx of diverted blood volume from obliteration of the MV system. [31-35]

The CVI of primary PLE is occasionally due to deep vein dysplasia, which would require more conservative management, unless there is clear evidence for significant hemodynamic gain by bypass surgery of the hypoplastic, aplastic iliac and femoral veins to relieve venous hypertension in patients with chronic venous ulcers with indolent ulcers.[8]

However, the benefit of surgery over the basic conservative therapy of CVI in patients with primary PLE (e.g., MV resection) should be carefully weighed against the potential deleterious effects on the coexisting LM with a marginally compensated CLI, which would make the clinical condition worse.

Therefore, primary PLE generated by hemolymphatic malformation (HLM) as the vascular malformation component of KTS should be handled by a multidisciplinary team to manage the extremely delicate interdependency between the VM and LM safely.

Clinical Experience

Group A (n = 9)

Chronic venous insufficiency by the marginal/lateral embryonic vein (MV); 6 have only MV, while 3 have another truncular VM, hypoplasia of the deep vein system plus MV.

Chronic lymphatic insufficiency by lymphatic malformation (LM): 6 with primary lymphedema by truncular LM lesion alone, and 3 with both truncular and extratruncular LM.

All are fall under clinical Stage II of chronic lymphedema. Five have healed (2) or active (3) ulcers.

Group B (n = 4)

Chronic venous insufficiency by deep vein hypoplasia/aplasia alone; CLI is solely due to primary lymphedema (truncular LM). No ulcers. Three belong to clinical Stage II and 1 to Stage I of chronic lymphedema.

Groups A and B underwent diagnostic and therapeutic assessment of the VM and LM with the standard protocol of MRI/MRV, duplex ultrasound, and/or CT angiography in addition to ascending phlebography and air plethysmography of the venous system.

Radionuclide lymphoscintigraphy with and without percutaneous lymphangiography was performed for the lymphatic system.

Groups A and B received identical treatment of the CVI with the compression therapy in addition to leg ulcer care with daily wound dressing. All groups received reinforced compression therapy for the lymphedema based on CDT and followed a standard protocol for chronic lymphedema.

But 6 patients of Group A received additional treatment with surgical excision of the MV. Two patients of Group A with extratruncular LM received OK 432 sclerotherapy for multiple macrocystic lymphangioma lesions in addition to the CDT for CLI.

Treatment outcome assessment was made based on the objective evaluation and findings of the ulcer as well as measurement of limb swelling using a sliding scale. Its score was combined with those of subjective improvement of the symptoms.

Average follow-up assessment at 6-month intervals was a minimum of 4 years (range 4.1–6.2 years)

Results

Group A Patients

The best outcome of the care was obtained in 5 out of 6 patients with MV resection, who had only MV as the cause of CVI and primary lymphedema for CLI with an average scale of 8/10 with two healed ulcers.

The worst outcome with no improvement was observed in one patient who underwent MV resection and sclerotherapy for the combined extratruncular lymphangioma (LM) lesion with no ulcer healing and further increase in symptoms, showing the scale of 2/10.

Group A patients in general had satisfactory improvement of the CVI by aggressive control with MV resection, especially when primary lymphedema was the sole cause of CLI.

Combined lesions of another VM, such as deep system dysplasia, does not seem to affect the outcome of the care of the CVI when MV is taken care of properly.

Group B Patients

All four showed subjective (e.g., aches/pains) as well as objective (e.g., swelling, recurrence of ulcers) improvement within 6 months of proper treatment of CVI as well as CLI and remained throughout the follow-up period on the scale of 8/10.

In Group B CVI due to deep vein dysplasia alone seemed to be easy to control as well as CLI with conventional compression therapy alone, with good long-term results.

Conclusion

- Phlebolymphedema can be managed more effectively when open and/or endovascular therapy is added to the basic compression therapy to control the CVI and CLI together.
- Primary PLE with CVI by the reflux of MV can be treated successfully with MV resection, while CVI by deep vein dysplasia can be treated with conventional compression therapy alone in the majority of cases.

References

1. Bunke N, Brown K, Bergan J. Phlebolymphemeda: usually unrecognized, often poorly treated. *Perspect Vasc Surg Endovasc Ther.* 2009;21(2):65-68.

2. Weissleder H, Waldermann F, Kopf W. Familial venous dysplasia and lymphedema. *Z Lymphol.* 1996;20(1):36-39.
3. Gasbarro V, Michelini S, Antignmani PL, Tsolaki E, Ricci M, Allegra C. The CEAP-L classification for lymphedemas of the limbs: the Italian experience. *Int Angiol.* 2009;28(4):315-324.
4. Klippel M, Trenaunay J. Du noevus variqueux et osteohypertrophique. *Arch Gén Méd.* 1900;3:641-672.
5. Gloviczki P, Driscoll DJ. Klippel–Trenaunay syndrome: current management. *Phlebology.* 2007;22:291-298.
6. Lee BB, Bergan J, Gloviczki P, et al. Diagnosis and treatment of venous malformations: consensus document of the International Union of Phlebology (IUP)-2009. *Int Angiol.* 2009;28(6):434-451.
7. Lee BB, Villavicencio L. General considerations: congenital vascular malformations. In: Cronenwett JL, Johnston KW, eds. *Rutherford's Vascular Surgery.* 7th ed. Philadelphia: Saunders Elsevier; 2010:1046-1064; Section 9. Arteriovenous Anomalies.
8. Raju S, Owen S Jr, Neglen P. Reversal of abnormal lymphoscintigraphy after placement of venous stents for correction of associated venous obstruction. *J Vasc Surg.* 2001;34(5):779-784.
9. Szuba A, Razavi M, Rockson SG. Diagnosis and treatment of concomitant venous obstruction in patients with secondary lymphedema. *J Vasc Interv Radiol.* 2002;13(8):799-803.
10. Loose DA. Contemporary treatment of congenital vascular malformations. In: Dieter RS, Dieter RA Jr, Dieter RA III, eds. *Peripheral Arterial Disease.* New York: McGrawHill Medical; 2009:1025-1040.
11. Silva JH, Janeiro-Perez MC, Barros N, Vieira-Castiglioni ML, Novo NF, Miranda F. Venous-lymphatic disease: lymphoscintigraphic abnormalities in venous ulcers. *J Vasc Bras.* 2009;8(1):33-42.
12. Bull RH, Gane JN, Evans JE, Joseph AE, Mortimer PS. Abnormal lymph drainage in patients with chronic venous leg ulcers. *J Am Acad Dermatol.* 1993;28(4):585-590.
13. Lee BB, Villavicencio JL. Primary lymphedema and lymphatic malformation: Are they the two sides of the same coin? *Eur J Vasc Endovasc Surg.* 2010;39:646-653.
14. Lee BB, Andrade M, Bergan J, et al. Diagnosis and treatment of primary lymphedema: consensus document of the International Union of Phlebology (IUP)-2009. *Int Angiol.* 2010;29(5):454-470.
15. Lee BB. Current concept of venous malformation (VM). *Phlebolymphology.* 2003;43:197-203.
16. Mortimer PS. Evaluation of lymphatic function: abnormal lymph drainage in venous disease. *Int Angiol.* 1995;14(3 Suppl 1):32-35.
17. Tiedjen KU. Detection of lymph vessel changes in venous diseases of the leg using imaging procedures. *Z Lymphol.* 1989;13(2):83-87.
18. Lee BB, Laredo J, Neville R. Arterio-venous malformation: How much do we know? *Phlebology.* 2009;24:193-200.
19. Lee BB. Mastery of vascular and endovascular surgery. In: Zelenock GB, Huber TS, Messina LM, Lumsden AB, Moneta GL, et al., eds. *Arteriovenous Malformation.* Philadelphia: Lippincott; 2006:597-607. Chap. 76.
20. Lee BB, Laredo J, Lee TS, Huh S, Neville R. Terminology and classification of congenital vascular malformations. *Phlebology.* 2007;22(6):249-252.
21. Ziyeh S, Spreer J, Rossler J, Strecker R, Hochmuth A, et al. Parkes Weber or Klippel-Trenaunay syndrome? Non-invasive diagnosis with MR projection angiography. *Eur Radiol.* 2004;14(11):2025-2029; Epub 2004 Mar 6.
22. Piller N. Phlebolymphoedema/chronic venous lymphatic insufficiency: an introduction to strategies for detection, differentiation and treatment. *Phlebology.* 2009;24(2):51-55.
23. Lee BB, Choe YH, Ahn JM, et al. The new role of magnetic resonance imaging in the contemporary diagnosis of venous malformation: Can it replace angiography? *J Am Coll Surg.* 2004;198(4):549-558.

24. Lee BB, Mattassi R, Kim BT, Kim DI, Ahn JM, Choi JY. Contemporary diagnosis and management of venous and AV shunting malformation by whole body blood pool scintigraphy (WBBPS). *Int Angiol.* 2004;23(4):355-367.
25. Lee BB, Mattassi R, Choe YH, et al. Critical role of duplex ultrasonography for the advanced management of a venous malformation. *Phlebology.* 2005;20:28-37.
26. Lee BB, Laredo J, Lee SJ, Huh SH, Joe JH, Neville R. Congenital vascular malformations: general diagnostic principles. *Phlebology.* 2007;22(6):253-257.
27. Lee BB, Mattassi R, Kim BT, Park JM. Advanced management of arteriovenous shunting malformation with transarterial lung perfusion scintigraphy for follow-up assessment. *Int Angiol.* 2005;24(2):173-184.
28. Bräutigam P, Földi E, Schaiper I, Krause T, Vanscheidt W, Moser E. Analysis of lymphatic drainage in various forms of leg edema using two compartment lymphoscintigraphy. *Lymphology.* 1998;31(2):43-55.
29. Franzeck UK, Haselbach P, Speiser D, Bollinger A. Microangiopathy of cutaneous blood and lymphatic capillaries in chronic venous insufficiency. *Yale J Biol Med.* 1993;66(1):37-46.
30. Mattassi R, Vaghi M. Vascular bone syndrome-angio-osteodystrophy: current concept. *Phlebology.* 2007;22:287-290.
31. Weber J, Daffinger N. Congenital vascular malformations: the persistence of marginal and embryonal veins. *Vasa.* 2006;35:67-77.
32. Loose DA. Surgical management of venous malformations. *Phlebology.* 2007;22(6):276-282.
33. Kim YW, Lee BB, Cho JH, Do YS, Kim DI, Kim ES. Haemodynamic and clinical assessment of lateral marginal vein excision in patients with a predominantly venous malformation of the lower extremity. *Eur J Vasc Endovasc Surg.* 2007;33(1):122-127.
34. Lee BB, Laredo J, Kim YW, Neville R. Congenital vascular malformations: general treatment principles. *Phlebology.* 2007;22(6):258-263.
35. Loose DA. Surgical treatment of predominantly venous defects. *Semin Vasc Surg.* 1993;6(4): 252-259.

Chapter 65
Diagnosis and Management of Secondary Phlebolymphedema

Attilio Cavezzi

Premise

Phlebolymphedema (PLE) is characterized by an accumulation of fluid in the interstitial tissues that is caused by a combination of venous (primarily) and of subsequent lymphatic disorders. The chronic venous-lymphatic insufficiency is the common ground for the clinical manifestation of PLE, which is a result of an imbalanced tissue–capillary homeostasis.

At a microcirculatory level the physiological homeostasis was studied and detailed a long time ago by Starling, Landis, and Pappenheimer.[1] In the last few years a significant revision of this proposed balance has been provided by a few authors and especially Levick and Michel,[2] although in vivo and in vitro experimental studies have "overshadowed" the traditional view of the filtration–reabsorption balance, at least in most tissues, while major emphasis has been finally placed on lymphatic function for fluid balance.

Whichever vein impaired drainage (because of obstruction and/or reflux and/or functional impairment without any organic vein lesion) may lead to an increase in the lymph load, which overcomes the lymphatic transport capacity, but also in the advanced stages venous stasis may lead to organic changes in the previously healthy (though overloaded) lymphatic vessels and nodes.[3]

It has been somehow demonstrated that there is often a mutual involvement of both venous and lymphatic systems in the aetiopathogenesis of many primary or secondary vascular edemas and the term PLE has become more familiar.[1,4-11] Typically, postthrombotic syndrome (PTS), which occurs in 20–50% of the patients after deep vein thrombosis (DVT), has been studied in detail by Partsch[12] and subsequently by other authors[3,8,13] by means of lymphoscintigraphy (LSG); a constant progressive degeneration of the lymphatic collectors/nodes has been highlighted,

A. Cavezzi
Vascular Unit, Poliambulatorio Hippocrates and Clinica Stella Maris,
San Benedetto del Tronto (AP), Italy

B.-B. Lee et al. (eds.), *Lymphedema*,
DOI 10.1007/978-0-85729-567-5_65, © Springer-Verlag London Limited 2011

especially in the later stages and mainly in the subfascial layers, all of which results in a secondary PLE of the lower limb (analog changes occur in the upper limb).

Similarly, in the later stages of varicosis of the lower limbs, clinical and ultrasound investigations may elicit the presence of some distal PLE, which may be attributed to decompensation of the lymphatic system,[3,8,13] to outbalanced microcirculatory flow and tissular mechanisms. More generally, in many cases of secondary chronic venous insufficiency in the lower limbs, the lymphatic system is involved in any tissue changes, starting from edema to venous ulcer. The lymphatic component makes the PLE richer in protein content than cardiac–renal, liver edema or pure venous edema,[7] which may result in a cascade of detrimental events toward tissue trophism deterioration.

Secondary PLE is related to a few pathological clinical conditions where an accumulation of negative effects on the interstice and thus on the lymphatic flow is highlighted: PTS, posttraumatic edema (with or without DVT), cancer/surgery/radiotherapy-related fibrosis, and/or compression on the venous and lymphatic axes (mainly in the abdominal and pelvic regions); other compressions caused by cysts or arterial/venous aneurysms (mainly at the popliteal level); the underestimated[14] abdominopelvic vein compression/obstruction (such as May–Thurner syndrome); all those musculoskeletal–neurological–joint–ligament diseases that lead to a plantar–calf pump dysfunction; and morbid obesity, which may correlate with several vein and lymphatic dysfunctions. Finally, the so-called revascularization edema of the lower limb, which is a result of the venolymphatic contingent thrombosis/disruption,[15] but also of the overloaded and dysregulated microcirculation, is to be considered a secondary PLE.

In the case of a primary lymphedema (LYM), the venous participation has been elucidated in a few clinical conditions, such as the breast cancer–related LYM of the upper extremity, where several authors[16-18] have highlighted hemodynamics impairment in the subclavian–axillary venous axis, through color duplex ultrasound or venography in up to 31% of the breast-cancer patients who underwent an operation. The presence of venous insufficiency with limb LYM, if not addressed, may result in poorer outcomes of the typical complex decongestive treatment.[19]

Diagnosis and Treatment of Secondary Phlebolymphedema

A few basic common steps are undertaken when facing a swollen limb, more specifically when a secondary PLE is suspected. Anamnesis or history-taking is of paramount importance, because of the extreme relevance of an antecedent event, which may have caused the venolymphatic impairment. Hence, any data on known DVT or suspicious "phlebitis" episodes, or on any acute/subacute swelling of the limb should be properly addressed. Many other specific disorders or conditions should be known in detail, including: active/antecedent cancer, surgical operations (with relative intra-/postoperative details); traumas; concomitant relevant cardiac–renal–liver diseases; and intake of edema-favoring drugs such as calcium blockers,

Fig. 65.1 Clinical appearance of an advanced post-thrombotic syndrome, with phlebolymphedema and skin dystrophic changes

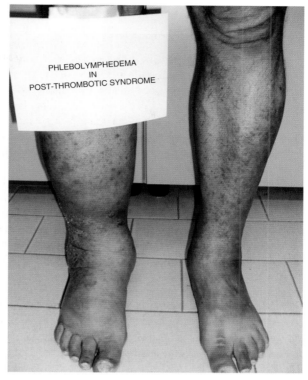

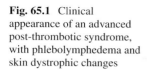
PHLEBOLYMPHEDEMA
IN
POST-THROMBOTIC SYNDROME

alpha-lytics, nitro-derivates. Concerning the edema itself, the patients should report the time of onset and edema reversibility after a night's rest because of the remarkable prognostic value of these data.

The physical examination of a phlebolymphedematous limb (Fig. 65.1) may include inspection of any vein disease signs, such as varices, skin discoloration, and dystrophic changes, unilateral (more specific) or bilateral edema; and localization of the edematous areas (an edema that is visible only at the root of the limb must address the diagnostic pathways toward research of any proximally located vein/lymphatic obstruction, which sometimes turns out to be an unknown cancer). Other useful signs to be collected are degree of edema pitting, skin temperature, palpable dilated lymph node collections (more commonly at the groin/axilla/popliteal areas), evoked pain, Stemmer sign, main arterial pulse palpation, and last but not least, the signs of dysfunction of the plantar–calf muscle–vascular pump.

From the instrumental diagnostic point of view, color duplex ultrasound (CDU) represents the gold standard and may address the vast majority of the necessary issues and provide the information needed for a tailored and proper treatment of PLE.

CDU may highlight with great accuracy several findings in cases of PTS, where a combination of refluxing and obstructed/occluded veins is usually imaged (Fig. 65.2), together with ectatic collateral vein pathways[19]; similarly,

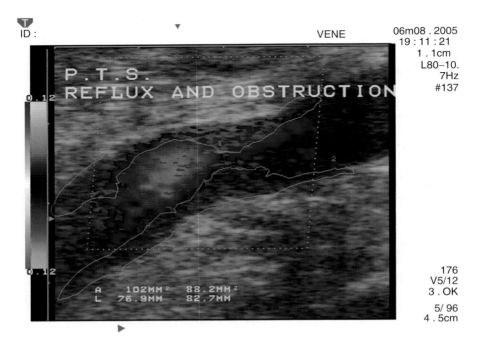

Fig. 65.2 Colour duplex ultrasound image in a case of post-thrombotic syndrome with residual obstruction and reflux in the popliteal vein

CDU may reliably provide information about the morpho-hemodynamic changes that characterize varicose vein disease[20,21] and about the associated lymph stasis (Fig. 65.3).

When an antecedent trauma, surgery, or radiotherapy may have caused PLE, CDU may address any venous flow alterations with good reliability in the veins of the lower and upper limbs, whereas a lower accuracy in the abdominal–pelvic area has been acknowledged. Pathological lymphatic findings (lymph collections, lymphocele, lymphatic collector dilation, hyperechogenic tissues) in the conditions mentioned above are also elicited through ultrasound investigation (refer to subsection chap. 20).

Any cavailiac vein abnormality is more properly investigated through intravascular ultrasound (IVUS), or through venography,[14,22] because of the complexity of the abdominal region and the decreased diagnostic power of CDU. In recent years, Raju and Neglen[14] have focused on the obstruction-related diseases of the pelvic–abdominal veins, thus highlighting a much higher degree of underestimated cava–iliac pathological features in cases of DVT and of primary/secondary PLE.

Plethismographic methods are currently used to assess venous function and, more specifically, the plantar–calf muscular–vascular pump dysfunction.[22]

The diagnostic approach to PLE may include in most cases the use of LSG to detail the functional pathological conditions of the lymph vessels/nodes; this diagnostic method has undergone several reappraisals in the last 20 years to refine modalities, standardization, and possibly to strengthen its accuracy, reproducibility, and finally to get more qualitative and quantitative data. The swollen limb, both in

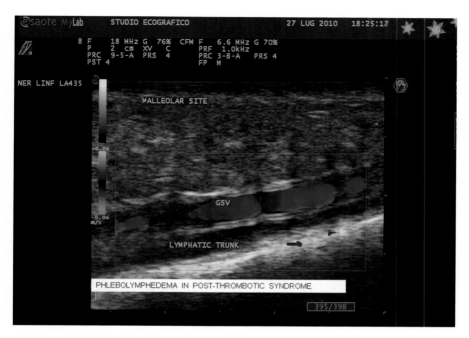

Fig. 65.3 Ultrasound image of phlebolymphedema at the ankle site in a case of post-thrombotic syndrome: lymphatic "lakes" and dilated great saphenous vein

cases of vascular edema and in cases of edema of non-vascular origin, is currently investigated by means of CDU with the usual implementation of LSG in case of any lymphatic flow impairment; although a major lack of morphological information exists for this method, therapies for PLE (especially manual lymphatic drainage and compression) may be targeted according to the LSG findings.

Several other methods have been proposed to complement the diagnostic approach to PLE (see Table 65.1), but most are of purely scientific, experimental value, being of little use in common practice. Computed tomography (CT) and magnetic resonance (MR) technologies have been employed in LYM[23,24] and proposed as essential investigations when any neoplasm/neoformation is involved in PLE, but also in any case of suspected abdominal–pelvic abnormality in venous/lymphatic outflow, to overcome the objective limitations of CDU and to complement LSG data. MR/CT images in PLE are characterized in most cases by the "honeycomb" appearance of the lymphedema component,[23] and these two methods objectively help in the differential diagnosis of pure venous edema, lipedema, and others.

With reference to IVUS and venography, again the abdominal–pelvic vein diseases may benefit from these technologies to achieve a more reliable diagnosis, but their costs and invasiveness enforce the selective use of these investigations. When an endovenous treatment is required in PTS, in any abdominal–pelvic vein segments, these two investigations become fundamental to depicting the pre-, intra-, and postoperative morpho-functional states.[14,22,25]

Table 65.1 List of the possible diagnostic investigations in phlebolymphedema (PLE)

Colour-duplex ultrasound
Lymphoscintigraphy
Computed tomography
Magnetic resonance
Venography
IVUS
Air/strain gauge/reflection light plethysmography
Fluorescence microlymphography
Laser-Doppler flowmetry
Tonometry
Intra-lymphatic pressure measurement
Patent blue (dye)
(Direct lymphography)
Water volumetry
Tape measurement
Multi-frequency bioimpedance
Laser volumetry
Optoelectronic volumetry

Fluorescence microlymphography has been used in a few centers to study lymphatic microcirculation before and after LYM treatment[26] and a possible diagnostic role in edematous conditions has been postulated,[27] but its complexity and costs limit this method to mainly scientific applications.

Tonometry[24,28] data seem to correlate with the degree of fibrosis of the skin/subcutaneous tissues, hence with the higher or lower lymphatic component of PLE.

The proper measurement of fluid accumulation in a phlebolymphedematous limb is crucial to have an accurate idea of the severity of the disease and especially to monitor treatment over time. Among the possible tools that have been validated to measure edema in the lower and upper limbs, the following each has specific possibilities and limitations[29]: water volumetry, tape measurement, multi-frequency bioimpedance analysis (BIA), laser volumetry, and optoelectronic volumetry. The relatively new technology of BIA has gained a scientific validation in segmental unilateral edema assessment, and especially in early (preclinical) detection of fluid retention, although some limitations are objectively linked to bilateral edema and to the presence of fibrosis in the edematous tissues.

Differential diagnosis of primary or secondary PLE may include DVT (in the case of acute onset), acute dermatolymphangioadenitis, lipedema (abnormal fat deposition and fluid retention in both limbs), mixedema (bilateral distal lower limb edema characterized by "viscous" interstitial tissue with fluid retention, due to thyroid disease), any edema of the lower limbs generated by severe cardiac/renal/liver disease or by hypo-dysprotidemia, or finally by edema-favoring drugs.

Classification and/or staging of PLE has never been finalized, although mediation among CEAP (clinical severity, etiology, anatomy, pathophysiology),[30] lymphological CEAP,[31] and "old" proposals,[1] remains in the auspices of the scientific community.

Therapy of PLE may be basically addressed at the possible (venous) causal disease/s and at the fluid stagnation, within the context of a holistic, integrated therapeutic protocol.

The basic treatment strategy of secondary PLE includes a few common therapies that are currently employed under the form of an integrated holistic decongestive therapy for LYM patients,[1,32,33] according to consensus documents[22,24] and current best clinical practice.[34] The therapies that are more commonly employed are: (a) compression (bandages and/or garments), which represents the cornerstone treatment of any vascular edema[35] and which must include medium/low elasticity material as well as inelastic material in the worse cases,[36] (b) drugs (anticoagulants, phlebo-lymphotropic drugs such as coumarin, diosmin, rutins, antibiotics, and NSAIDs or corticoids when needed), (c) manual lymphatic drainage (MLD), (d) electro-medical devices such as sequential intermittent pneumatic compression, electro-(ultra)sound wave devices,[37] calf-pump stimulators, laser-based treatments, (e) topical treatments, (f) rehabilitation exercises and veno-lymphatic hygiene rules (limb elevation!), (g) possible psychological support, (h) skin care to reduce and to prevent infections and to improve skin trophism.

Most of the treatments listed above are detailed in the literature and in this book elsewhere, with respect to their use in LYM patients; some peculiarities may pertain to "venous" drugs, which are used especially in PTS and more generally in chronic venous insufficiency.[22,38] Life-lasting anticoagulation with dicumarols is provided to patients with relevant residual vein occlusions and/or with recurrent venous thromboembolism and especially in patients with significant thrombophilia or active cancer. Fractionated or unfractionated heparins are currently used in clinically "decompensated" limbs with PLE and ulcer, to enhance microcirculation collateral flow and to provide some angiogenesis in the dystrophic skin areas.

Alternative, less frequently applied and less validated treatments in PLE may include: mesotherapy, ablative or reconstructive surgery for lymphatics and/or for fat deposition, vibrational therapy, heat wave therapy, etc.

In cases of PLE related to PTS, a few reconstructive surgical treatments have been proposed in the last few years,[39] achieving interesting outcomes in properly selected patients, although better results are obtained in primary deep vein diseases, and most data need to be validated through larger scale protocols; similarly, endovenous (percutaneous transluminal angioplasty (PTA) ± stent) treatments have gained great popularity,[14,25,39] with cumulative hemodynamics and clinically promising data at mid-term for patients with iliac–caval obstruction/occlusion; some lymphoscintigraphic improvement has been documented after correction of the venous lesions as well.[40] Secondary varicose veins (VV) in PTS may be treated with (ultrasound-guided) foam sclerotherapy (FS),[41,42] which has a very low impact on the fragile limb tissues, and endovenous treatments have been proposed in selective cases. Minimally invasive surgery still holds a place and the proper indications for these treatments are still debated, although patency of the deep veins is recognized as the basic prerequisite. In the presence of an active leg venous ulcer, therapy of PLE must comprehend the typical loco-regional treatments devoted to debridement, granulation enhancement, and second-intention healing of the ulcerated area.

In the last 100 years several treatment modalities have been proposed for primary VV, although the suboptimal knowledge of the morphology and hemodynamic mechanisms that subside in varicose degeneration make any treatment still palliative and the recurrence rate still unacceptably high in the long term. A tailored, minimally invasive surgical approach has been advocated in the last 20 years, on the basis of a detailed pre-operative CDU and local anesthesia usage.[43] In the meantime three main endovenous treatments have been validated, questioning the role of surgery as the gold standard for these patients with PLE and primary VV: laser, radiofrequency, and FS. Notwithstanding a lack of agreement on the indications for these therapies, when facing larger varices, minimally invasive surgery may be beneficial in the mid- to long term; on the other hand, endovenous treatments (FS in primis) may result in a higher recanalization rate when dealing with large caliber (e.g., over 12–15 mm) veins. The extremely cheap and minimally invasive combination of phlebectomy and long catheter FS,[42] combined with tumescence infiltration, seems to produce interesting short- to mid-term outcomes, even in those cases of larger veins associated with PLE. The presence of the LYM component of PLE raises the issue of possible lymphatic complications after treatment of VV;[44,45] hence, minimal invasiveness and specific technical precautions have to be taken into consideration in the case of surgery[46] and in the case of endovenous treatments. CHIVA treatment may be well indicated in similar cases as well.

Conclusions

The diagnostic–therapeutic approach to PLE is usually of a multi-faceted nature, in order to assess the related vascular diseases and the fluid accumulation with the possible tissue dystrophic changes; CDU represents the basic diagnostic method for highlighting most venous and lymphatic abnormalities, especially if combined with LSG; the physical rehabilitation approach is the cornerstone of treatment for the edema component, but several vein-directed therapies are necessary as well, in order to achieve a better and longer lasting outcome. Patient compliance is in fact the key factor in achieving more durable results, and as a matter of fact the LYM component makes any treatment complex and often, but not always, palliative, in nature.

Acknowledgments   Thanks to Dr.C.Elio for her contribution and to Prof. B.B.Lee for his patience.

References

1. Cavezzi A, Michelini S. *Phlebolymphoedema, from Diagnosis to Therapy*. Bologna: Ed. P.R.;1998, ISBN 88-900300-1-1.
2. Levick JR, Michel CC. Microvascular fluid exchange and the revised Starling principle. *Cardiovasc Res*. 2010;87(2):198-210.

3. Mortimer PS. Evaluation of lymphatic function: abnormal lymph drainage in venous disease. *Int Angiol*. 1995;14(3):32-35.
4. Casley-Smith J, Casley-Smith JR. Lymphaticovenous insufficiency and its conservative treatment. *Phlebolymphology*. 1995;6:9-13.
5. Michelini S, Failla A, Sterbini GP, Micci A, Santoro A, Valle G. Limb phlebolymphoedema: diagnostic noninvasive approach and therapeutic implications. *Eur J Lymphol Relat Probl*. 1995;5(20):103-108.
6. Villavicencio JL, Hargens AR, Pikoulicz E. Latest advances in edema. *Phlebolymphology*. 1996;12:9-15.
7. Casley-Smith J, Casley-Smith JR. Pathology of oedema – causes of oedemas: modern treatment for lymphoedema. 5th ed. Adelaide: Lymphoedema Association of Australia; 1997.
8. Bräutigam P, Földi E, Schaiper I, Krause T, Vanscheidt W, Moser E. Analysis of lymphatic drainage in various forms of leg edema using two compartment lymphoscintigraphy. *Lymphology*. 1998;31(2):43-55.
9. Piller N. Phlebolymphoedema/chronic venous lymphatic insufficiency: an introduction to strategies for detection, differentiation and treatment. *Phlebology*. 2009;24(2):51-55.
10. Bunke N, Brown K, Bergan J. Phlebolymphemeda: usually unrecognized, often poorly treated. *Perspect Vasc Surg Endovasc Ther*. 2009;21(2):65-68.
11. Rockson SG. The lymphaticovenous spectrum of edema. *Lymphat Res Biol*. 2009;7(2):67.
12. Partsch H, Mostbeck A. Involvement of the lymphatic system in post-thrombotic syndrome. *Wien Med Wochenschr*. 1994;144(10-11):210-213.
13. Mortimer PS. Implications of the lymphatic system in CVI-associated edema. *Angiology*. 2000;51(1):3-7.
14. Neglen P, Thrasher TL, Raju S. Venous outflow obstruction: an underestimated contributor to chronic venous disease. *J Vasc Surg*. 2003;38(5):879-885.
15. Tiwari A, Cheng KS, Button M, Myint F, Hamilton G. Differential diagnosis, investigation, and current treatment of lower limb lymphedema. *Arch Surg*. 2003;138(2):152-161.
16. Mukhamedzhanov IKh, Drozdovskiĭ BIa, Dergachev AI. Lymphophlebographic studies in arm edema. *Med Radiol (Mosk)*. 1984;29(2):20-24.
17. Pain SJ, Vowler S, Purushotham AD. Axillary vein abnormalities contribute to development of lymphoedema after surgery for breast cancer. *Br J Surg*. 2005;92(3):311-315.
18. Svensson WE, Mortimer PS, Tohno E, Cosgrove DO. Colour Doppler demonstrates venous flow abnormalities in breast cancer patients with chronic arm swelling. *Eur J Cancer*. 1994;30A(5):657-660.
19. Gironet N, Baulieu F, Giraudeau B, et al. Lymphedema of the limb: predictors of efficacy of combined physical therapy. *Ann Dermatol Vénéréol*. 2004;131(8–9):775-779.
20. Coleridge-Smith P, Labropoulos N, Partsch H, Myers K, Nicolaides A, Cavezzi A. Duplex ultrasound investigation of the veins in chronic venous disease of the lower limbs-UIP consensus document. Part I: basic principles. *Eur J Vasc Endovasc Surg*. 2006;31(1):83-92.
21. Cavezzi A, Labropoulos N, Partsch H, et al. Duplex ultrasound investigation of the veins in chronic venous disease of the lower limbs – UIP consensesus document. Part II: anatomy. *Eur J Vasc Endovasc Surg*. 2006;31(1):288-299.
22. Nicolaides AN, Allegra C, Bergan J, et al. Management of chronic venous disorders of the lower limbs: guidelines according to scientific evidence. *Int Angiol*. 2008;27(1):1-59.
23. Hadjis NS, Carr DH, Banks L, Pflug JJ. The role of CT in the diagnosis of primary lymphedema of the lower limb. *AJR Am J Roentgenol*. 1985;144:361-364.
24. International Society of Lymphology. The diagnosis and treatment of peripheral lymphedema. 2009 Consensus Document of the International Society of Lymphology (ISL). *Lymphology*. 2009;42:51-60.
25. Meissner MH, Eklof B, Smith PC, et al. Secondary chronic venous disorders. *J Vasc Surg*. 2007;46(suppl S):68S-83S.
26. Franzeck UK, Haselbach P, Speiser D, Bollinger A. Microangiopathy of cutaneous blood and lymphatic capillaries in chronic venous insufficiency (CVI). *Yale J Biol Med*. 1993;66(1):37-46.

27. Bollinger A, Amann-Vesti BR. Fluorescence microlymphography: diagnostic potential in lymphedema and basis for the measurement of lymphatic pressure and flow velocity. *Lymphology*. 2007;40(2):52-62.
28. Liu NF, Olszewski W. Use of tonometry to assess lower extremity lymphedema. *Lymphology*. 1992;25:155-158.
29. Cavezzi A, Schingale F, Elio C. Limb volume measurement: from the past methods to optoelectronic technologies, bioimpedance analysis and laser-based devices. *Int Angiol*. 2010; 29(5):392-394.
30. Eklof B, Rutherford RB, Bergan JJ, et al. Revision of the CEAP classification for chronic venous disorders: consensus statement. *J Vasc Surg*. 2004;40(6):1248-1252.
31. Gasbarro V, Michelini S, Antignani PL, Tsolaki E, Ricci M, Allegra C. The CEAP-L classification for lymphedemas of the limbs: the Italian experience. *Int Angiol*. 2009;28(4):315-324.
32. Foldi E, Foldi M, Weissleder H. Conservative treatment of lymphoedema of the limbs. *Angiology*. 1985;36:171-180.
33. Leduc O, Leduc A, Bourgeois P, Belgrado J-P. The physical treatment of upper limb edema. *Cancer*. 1998;83:2835-2839.
34. Lymphoedema Framework. *Best Practice for the Management of Lymphoedema. International Consensus*. London: MEP Ltd; 2006.
35. Partsch H, Flour M, Smith PC. International Compression Club. Indications for compression therapy in venous and lymphatic disease consensus based on experimental data and scientific evidence. Under the auspices of the IUP. *Int Angiol*. 2008;27(3):193-219.
36. de Godoy JM, De Godoy Mde F. Godoy & Godoy technique in the treatment of lymphedema for under-privileged populations. *Int J Med Sci*. 2010;7(2):68-71.
37. Ricci M, Paladini S. Demonstration of Flowave's effectiveness through lymphoscintigraphy. *Eur J Lymphol Relat Probl*. 2006;16(49):14-18.
38. Kearon C, Kahn SR, Agnelli G, Goldhaber SZ, Raskob G, Comerota AJ. Antithrombotic therapy for venous thromboembolic disease: ACCP evidence-based clinical practice guidelines (8th ed). *Chest*. 2008;133(6 suppl):454S-545S.
39. Lurie F, Kistner R, Perrin M, Raju S, Neglen P, Maleti O. Invasive treatment of deep venous disease: a UIP consensus. *Int Angiol*. 2010;29(3):199-204.
40. Raju S, Owen S Jr, Neglen P. Reversal of abnormal lymphoscintigraphy after placement of venous stents for correction of associated venous obstruction. *J Vasc Surg*. 2001;34(5): 779-784.
41. Tessari L, Cavezzi A, Frullini A. Preliminary experience with a new slerosing foam in the treatment of varicose veins. *Dermatol Surg*. 2001;27(1):58-60.
42. Cavezzi A, Tessari L. Foam sclerotherapy techniques: different gases and methods of preparation, catheter versus direct injection. *Phlebology*. 2009;24(6):247-251.
43. Cavezzi A, Carigi V, Collura M. Colour flow duplex scanning as a preoperative guide for mapping and for local anaesthesia in varicose vein surgery. *Phlebology*. 2000;15:24-29.
44. Timi JR, Zanoni MF, Stacheski Riesemberg M, Yamada AS. Lymphatic damage after operations for varicose veins: a lymphoscintigraèhic study. *Eur J Lymphol Relat Probl*. 1999;26: 43-44.
45. Suzuki M, Unno N, Yamamoto N, et al. Impaired lymphatic function recovered after great saphenous vein stripping in patients with varicose vein: venodynamic and lymphodynamic results. *J Vasc Surg*. 2009;50(5):1085-1091.
46. Cavezzi A, Jakubiak I, Puviani V, Castellani Tarabini C. Varicose vein surgery and lymphoedema. *Lymphology*. 2002/3;35(suppl. 2):380-387.

Chapter 66
Management of Phlebolymphedema Ulcers

Takki A. Momin and Richard F. Neville

Introduction

Lymphedema is a progressive condition of excessive protein edema, which in time leads to chronic inflammation and irreversible fibrosis. Ulcers associated with phlebolymphedema are a consequence of long-standing lymphedema combined with underlying venous insufficiency. The true incidence of this condition remains unknown, because it is seldom correctly recognized. Identification of the etiology of ulcerogenesis is a key step in successful treatment of all ulcers of the lower extremity. This step is especially important for ulcers caused by phlebolymphedema to guide appropriate therapy.

Pathophysiology

The intimate relationship between the lymphatic and venous systems consequently may lead to lymphatic dysfunction in the presence of underlying venous insufficiency. Hence, an in-depth understanding of the lymphatic system is necessary to properly diagnose and treat phlebolymphedema. The lymphatic vasculature consists of a network of vessels that is essential both to fluid hemostasis and mediation of the regional immune response.[1] The lymphatic system is a unique component of the circulatory system in that it begins peripherally and lacks a central pump mechanism.[1] The lymphatic system functions as a transport system for interstitial fluid, intercellular fluid, and extracellular elements such as transport proteins, macromolecules, cytokines, immunoglobulins, and blood elements.[1] This lymphatic fluid

T.A. Momin (✉)
Vascular Surgery Fellow, Georgetown University/Washington Hospital Center,
Washington, DC, USA

B.-B. Lee et al. (eds.), *Lymphedema*,
DOI 10.1007/978-0-85729-567-5_66, © Springer-Verlag London Limited 2011

passes through abundant and strategically positioned lymph nodes throughout the body before emptying into the thoracic duct, which delivers the material to the circulatory system.

Phlebolymphedema is a condition of mixed venous and lymphatic insufficiency that is poorly recognized and thus often difficult to treat. The underlying pathophysiology is thought to be a type of secondary lymphedema resulting from venous insufficiency and consequent venous hypertension. In the presence of severe venous hypertension, excessive interstitial fluid sequestration leads to a lymphatic load that exceeds the capacity for transport. Initially, the lymphatic system compensates with increased transport; a period characterized by low protein fluid as seen with edema associated with pure venous insufficiency edema.[1] However, chronic lymphedema leads to protein extravasation and high protein fluid characteristic of pure lymphedema. The resultant excessive interstitial and lymphatic fluid stimulates fibroblasts, keratinocytes, and adipocytes resulting in deposition of collagen and glycosaminoglycans within the skin and subcutaneous tissue.[1] This creates an environment of poor skin nutrition and reduced oxygen tension. Moreover, in the presence of venous insufficiency, exorbitant hydrostatic pressure results in capillary rupture with erythrocyte sequestration and destruction. Heme, a by-product of this process, is also deposited within the skin, leading to hyperpigmentation. The process can eventually result in nutrient and oxygen deprivation in the skin envelope with subsequent breakdown and ulcer formation.

Diagnosis

A detailed history and physical examination enables proper identification of phlebolymphedema. Edema secondary to lymphatic dysfunction is differentiated from that related to venous insufficiency by involvement of the dorsum of the foot and the toes. Corona phlebectatica or ankle hyperpigmentation in the presence of lymphedema is a hallmark of phlebolymphedema.[1] Duplex ultrasound is utilized to confirm venous insufficiency. An extensive examination of the deep, superficial, and perforator veins of the extremity is conducted. Vein patency and valvular competence are noted at each level.[2] Indirect radionuclide lymphoscintigraphy (IRL) may be utilized to confirm lymphatic insufficiency.[3] The association between chronic venous ulcers of the lower extremities and qualitative findings on lymphoscintigraphy has been identified in a recent study.[4] In a comparison of lymphoscintigraphy among three groups with varying degrees of venous pathology, 72.5% of patients classified as CEAP classes 5 and 6 had abnormal findings on lymphoscintigraphy versus 31% classified CEAP classes 2, 3, and 4.[4] Seven percent of patients classified as CEAP classes 0 and 1 were found to have abnormalities on lymphoscintigraphy.[4] Significant findings in this study included the presence of dermal reflux, inguinal adenomegaly, and radiopharmaceutical retention (Figs. 66.1 and 66.2). However, IRL is time-consuming, expensive, and often fraught with poor resolution images. It is seldom used as a routine diagnostic tool.

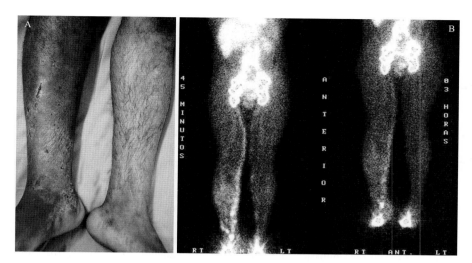

Fig. 66.1 (**a**) A 42-year-old male patient with a right lower limb ulcer lasting for 18 months with two recurrences. (**b**) Lymphoscintigraphy with dermal reflux and radiopharmaceutical retention in the right lower limb. Left lower limb with normal aspect (Courtesy of Jose Humberto Silva, Maria del Carmen Janeiro Perez, Newton de Barros Jr., Mario Luiz Vieira Castiglioni, Neil Ferreira Novo, and Fausto Miranda Jr. Sao Paulo and Santo Amaro, Brazil)

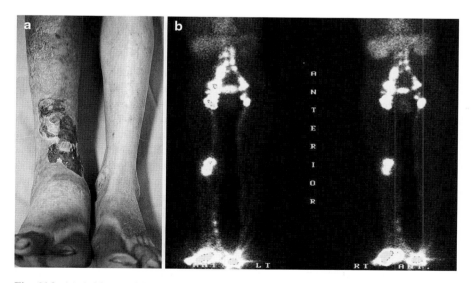

Fig. 66.2 (**a**) A 66-year-old male patient with right lower limb ulcer lasting for 120 months and three recurrences. (**b**) Lymphoscintigraphy showing popliteal lymph node, inguinal adenomegaly, and contrast material retention at the ulcer site on the right. Left lower limb with normal aspect (Courtesy of Jose Humberto Silva, Maria del Carmen Janeiro Perez, Newton de Barros Jr., Mario Luiz Vieira Castiglioni, Neil Ferreira Novo, and Fausto Miranda Jr. Sao Paulo and Santo Amaro, Brazil)

A recent study compared IRL with magnetic resonance lymphangiography (MRL).[5] MRL was found to be more sensitive and accurate than lymphoscintigraphy in the detection of anatomical and functional abnormalities in the lymphatic system in patients with extremity lymphedema.[6] Mixed forms of lymphedema are best diagnosed with axial T2-weighted fat-suppressed (SPIR) sequences in conjunction with coronal T1 spin echo (SE) magnetic resonance imaging (MRI) sequences.[5] No improvement in diagnostic accuracy is noted with the addition of gadolinium contrast material to MRI for this purpose. The coronal T1 SE sequence is most sensitive for demonstrating the honeycomb pattern that characterizes the subcutaneous tissue in lymphedema.[5] T2 SPIR sequences enable elucidation of the honeycomb pattern as fluid or fibrosis in origin.[5]

Indocyanine green (ICG) fluorescence lymphography has been recently developed as a novel imaging modality to visualize lymphatic flow.[7] In this imaging technique, a near-infrared camera system is used to direct morphological changes in lymphatic vessels in patients with secondary lymphedema.[7] Lymphatic function is further assessed by calculating the transit time (TT) of dye as it moves from the dorsum of the foot to the knee or groin in healthy volunteers versus patients with suspected lymphatic dysfunctions.

Management

The mainstay of therapy for phlebolymphedema ulcer is accurate assessment and treatment of the underlying venous insufficiency. Compression therapy and wound management are critical to effect healing of the ulcer. Compressive therapy addresses both the lymphatic and venous components of the underlying pathophysiology. Traditional techniques are centered on compression bandaging at weekly intervals until complete resolution of the ulcer. Patients are then fitted for compression stockings to aid in symptom relief and ulcer recurrence prevention. Venous occlusive disease amenable to angioplasty and stent deployment should be considered for intervention if possible. Venous reflux in patients with phlebolymphedema ulcer is best managed with sclerotherapy, radiofrequency ablation, or laser treatment. It is vital to avoid vein stripping as a management technique in patients with phlebolymphedema for fear of further damage to the lymphatic vessels.

References

1. Bunke N, Brown K, Bergen J. Phlebolymphedema: usually unrecognized, often poorly treated. *Perspect Vasc Endovasc Ther.* 2009;21(2):65-68.
2. Robert K. Diagnosis of chronic venous insufficiency. *J Vasc Surg.* 1986;3(1):185-188.
3. Rockson SG. Diagnosis and management of lymphatic vascular disease. *J Am Coll Cardiol.* 2008;52:799-806.

4. Silva HJ, Perez JMC, Barros N, Castiglioni MLV, Novo NF, Miranda F. Venous-Lymphatic disease: lymphoscintigraphic abnormalities in venous ulcers. *J Vasc Brasil.* 2009;8(1):33-42.
5. Astrom KGO, Abdsaleh S, Brenning GC, Ahlstrom KH, Uppsala MR. Imaging of primary, secondary, and mixed forms of lymphedema. *Acta Radiol.* 2001;42:409-416.
6. Liu N-F et al. Comparison of radionuclide lymphoscintigraphy and dynamic magnetic resonance lymphangiography for investigating extremity lymphoedema. *Br J Surg.* 2010;97:359-365.
7. Minoru S, Naoki U, Naoto Y, Motohiro N, Daisuke S. Impaired lymphatic function recovered after great saphenous vein stripping in patients with varicose vein: venodynamic and lympho-dynamic results. *J Vasc Surg.* 2009;50(5):1085-1091.

Part XVII
Lymphedema Health Care Delivery

Chapter 67
Lymphedema Management by the Therapists

Saskia R.J. Thiadens

This chapter is aimed at introducing the crucial contribution of nurses and hands-on therapists in recognition of the need, development, standardization, provision of care, and patient advocacy for chronic lymphedema.

Recognition of Lymphedema as a Nursing Problem

In the mid 1980s, nurses were increasingly seeing patients with lymphedema, particularly in the emerging cancer centers. As they searched for more information and education, it was recognized that the lymphedema often had been neglected by the medical field because of a lack of sufficient knowledge. This void left nurses without options with regard to quality care for their patients, which was often carried out independently with no proper support by the medical community.

As a consequence, patients with lymphedema were often misdiagnosed, underdiagnosed, or simply neglected. They often became frightened, with many experiencing serious complications and at times devastating lifestyle and psychological changes, all of which could have been mitigated.

It was this need presented by patients that led to the lymphedema clinic in the United States and such a clinic was often organized by nurses for the care of patients all by themselves.

It became apparent that there was a great need for more clinics along with education, awareness, and most importantly, effective multimodal treatments for patients with lymphedema.

Such a movement was started by a dedicated nursing group led by Saskia Thiadens et al. in early 1988: the National Lymphedema Network (NLN®)[1] soon became a leading non-profit providing much needed information on lymphedema to medical professionals, lymphedema patients, and the general public throughout the country.

S.R.J. Thiadens
National Lymphedema Network, Inc., San Francisco, CA, USA

B.-B. Lee et al. (eds.), *Lymphedema*,
DOI 10.1007/978-0-85729-567-5_67, © Springer-Verlag London Limited 2011

As a patient advocate group, it also offered a training program for patients who want to become advocates for clinical and basic research and a parents' network for families that have children with lymphedema, focusing on treatment options as well as diagnostic approaches and basic and clinical research focused on patients with lymphedema.

In the early 1990s, when complex decongestive therapy (CDT) was introduced to the USA, hundreds of dedicated physical therapists and nurses took on a crucial role in accepting it as standard of care on a day-to-day basis.

Indeed, such extraordinary efforts and devotion by the specialized nurse group gave a new opportunity for the right care for the first time to the patients, who either received no care, had inappropriate treatment, or both, which often made their condition worse.

Later, in 1998, the newly organized Lymphology Association of North America (LANA)[2] started to provide new sets of the standards/guidelines for appropriate treatment and training of professionals to become lymphedema therapists to maintain appropriate knowledge fundamental to the treatment of lymphedema.

The Specialized Role of Nurses in Lymphedema Care

Over the last two decades, nurses (especially those who work in the oncology field) have expressed interest in the swollen limb and are often frustrated not knowing how to educate and treat patients after lymph node removal and radiation. Some nurses have become certified lymphedema therapists and are hoping to bring more nurses to the forefront to be involved with patients who are at risk of developing or who already have lymphedema.

However, sometimes nurses have to resist the notion that only physical and occupational therapists should be treating patients with lymphedema, and that nurses should only educate patients.

Another dilemma for nurses is that at the moment there is no reimbursement for nurses treating patients with lymphedema.

Many nurses are working in breast centers or other cancer-related areas, and meet with patients pre- and postoperatively and are in an excellent position to educate patients in risk reduction practices[1] and provide behavioral training, resources, and obtain baseline measurements of both arms.

Educated nurses are capable of assessing lymphedema-related symptoms, such as heaviness, tightness, firmness, pain, and numbness or decreased mobility, and diagnose latent stage lymphedema.[3] In practice, many women treated for breast cancer do not receive appropriate information about lymphedema and risk reduction,[4] and the educated oncology nurse is in a prime position to provide these guidelines.

Nurses are also frequently in the best position to identify patients' needs and provide emotional support and effective counseling.[5] We are fortunate to also have a growing group of nurse researchers in this country who are greatly contributing to multiple areas of clinical and basic research in the treatment of patients with lymphedema and receiving peer-reviewed funding for their work.[3-10]

Legislation, Reimbursement, and Patient Advocacy by Therapists

Although the reimbursement issue is set aside as a separate chapter in this book, its importance cannot be overemphasized. Hence, we will reiterate its basic issues here in this chapter as a mission for the nurse dedicated to lymphedema management.

Despite the increased awareness and education among patients and professionals, access to care and reimbursement continues to be problematic. Patients often cannot receive treatment and have to fight for reimbursement. Many therapists and organizations led by therapists are at the forefront of introducing and promoting new legislation, such as the Women's Health and Cancer Rights Act of 1998.[11]

There have been successes in securing a lymphedema treatment mandate in the Commonwealth of Virginia in 2003 and in the state of North Carolina in 2009 and Congressman Larry Kissel has sponsored HR 4662, the Lymphedema Diagnosis and Treatment Cost Saving Act of 2010, which was officially introduced in the House on 23 February 2010. One of the significant provisions of HR 4662 is to allow Medicare to reimburse lymphedema-trained registered nurses for lymphedema services, which is not currently provided

Now, lymphedema is identified as a legitimate condition in the United States, and CDT-based treatment is fully recognized as the most current standard treatment by most of the university-based clinics, hospitals, rehabilitation centers, and freestanding facilities.

It also has been recognized as an effective treatment protocol by the Medicare Evidence Development Coverage Advisory Committee (MEDCAC).[12]

Nurses and therapists have encouraged more patient advocates to step up and work for patient rights. Currently, awareness and education among the multidisciplinary teams in these breast centers is expanding throughout the United States and has facilitated the gathering of much needed data on lymphedema in general, outcomes of early diagnosis and breast cancer treatment, and follow-up measurements of affected limbs.

Summary

Today, skilled nursing is invaluable in the care of patients with lymphedema. The largest and oldest patient-centered organization for patients with lymphedema (NLN) was founded by and is still run by a nurse. Most quality of life research in the United States is led by nurses.

Multiple National Institutes of Health (NIH; and other) funded research programs are led by nurses, including genomic and microarray studies, as well as studies exploring the latest assessment and treatment technologies.

In many cancer centers and clinics across the nation, a nurse is frequently the point person to inform, assess, and even treat patients with lymphedema. Although nursing care for lymphedema may have had its origins with a single nurse impelled by patient advocacy, today, nurses are a critical part of all aspects of care for patients with lymphedema.

References

1. National Lymphedema Network. Risk reduction practices. Available at: http:www.lymphnet. org. june 2010.
2. The Lymphology Association of North America. Available at: http://www.clt-lana.org. june 2010.
3. Armer JM, Radina ME, Porock D, Culbertson SD. Predicting breast cancer related lymphedema using self-reported symptoms. *Nurs Res*. 2003;52(6):370-379.
4. Fu MR, Ridner SH, Armer J. Post breast cancer lymphedema: risk reduction and management. *Am J Nurs*. 2009;109(8):34-41.
5. Fu MR, Axelrod D, Haber J. Breast cancer-related lymphedema: information, symptoms, and risk reduction behaviors. *J Nurs Scholarsh*. 2008;40(4):341-348.
6. Ridner SH. The psycho-social impact of lymphedema. *Lymphat Res Biol*. 2009;7(2):109-112.
7. Ridner SH, Dietrich MS, Deng J, Bonner CM, Kidd N. Bioelectrical impedance for detecting upper limb lymphedema in nonlaboratory settings. *Lymphat Res Biol*. 2009;7(1):11-15.
8. Ridner SH, McMahon E, Dietrich MS, Hoy S. Home-based lymphedema treatment in patients with cancer-related lymphedema or noncancer-related lymphedema. *Oncol Nurs Forum*. 2008;35(4):671-680.
9. Fu MR, Chen CM, Haber J, Guth AA, Axelrod D. The effect of providing information about lymphedema on the cognitive and symptom outcomes of breast cancer survivors. *Ann Surg Oncol*. 2010;17(7):1847-1853.
10. Wanchai A, Armer JM, Stewart BR. Complementary and alternative medicine use among women with breast cancer: a systematic review. *Clin J Oncol Nurs*. 2010;14(4):E45-E55.
11. US Department of Health and Human Services. Centers for Medicare and Medicaid Services. The Women's Health & Cancer Rights Act. Available at: http://www.cms.gov/HealthInsReformfor Consume/06_TheWomensHealthandCancerRightsAct.asp. Accessed September 11, 2010. Information available from: http://www.cancer.org/Treatment/FindingandPayingforTreatment/ ManagingInsuranceIssues/womens-health-and-cancer-rights-act.
12. Scoresheet from November 18, 2009 MEDCAC meeting on Lymphedema (document #51a), posted November 30, 2009 and available from CMS MEDCAC meetings webpage http:// www.cms.gov/med/viewmcac.asp?where=index&mid=51.

Chapter 68
Education of the Patient

Emily Iker

Lymphedema is a chronic, debilitating condition resulting from a dysfunctional lymph transporting system of the lymphatic vessels and/or lymph nodes. Regardless of its etiology, it remains a generally incurable condition with steady progress through the rest of life. Therefore, a lifetime commitment to its management warrants a proper understanding of the nature of the condition by the patient, the family, as well as the healthcare personnel involved.

Hence, proper education of the patient is so critical in understanding the magnitude of the problem; detailed information on its definition, classification, and clinical and laboratory diagnosis should be provided, in addition to its management and prognosis.

To encourage full commitment of the patient, such dedication to education is so important and its importance in maintaining compliance cannot be overemphasized.

When primary lymphedema is diagnosed, full information should be given as a general orientation on what this should mean to the patient with regard to its long-term care. Basic information on various types of primary lymphedema should be included, and is classified based on the onset of the clinical manifestation: the congenital type when it occurs at birth, the praecox type when it appears at puberty, and the tarda type when it appears later in life after the age of 35. Full instructions for daily self-care should be given as soon as possible after receiving a series of complex decongestive therapy (CDP) sessions to reach a plateau.

Also, the plain fact that frequently the onset of swelling follows simple events like a mosquito bite, trauma, or a long flight, should be emphasized from a preventive point of view. Further information on proper education should include the fact that the swelling of primary lymphedema usually involves one or both lower extremities, but never symmetrically. Additionally, about 20% of primary lymphedema is of the familial type, which draws attention to the proper investigation when needed.

After all, the most important aspect is to make a correct diagnosis of the lymphedema, since appropriate daily treatment can manage this chronic disorder quite

E. Iker
Lymphedema Center of Santa Monica, California, CA, USA

B.-B. Lee et al. (eds.), *Lymphedema*,
DOI 10.1007/978-0-85729-567-5_68, © Springer-Verlag London Limited 2011

well when the patient is fully educated to be aware of the critical importance of compliance.

Secondary lymphedema is also no exception. It is much more common than the primary form, for various reasons; the postoperative/postradiation lymphedema is the most common cause, especially in developed countries, as well as known complications/side effects experienced by cancer patients.[1]

Therefore, cancer patients should be thoroughly informed about the risk of developing lymphedema before and after surgery through appropriate education.[2,3] Intense orientation should emphasize that prompt communication with a physician or a nurse is the most critical action to the patient whenever new symptoms/signs of swelling, tension, heaviness, and/or pressure should develop, suggesting a new condition of chronic lymphedema.

This is because early intervention with proper treatment will lead to a favorable outcome and abort the rapid progress of the condition, with the patient responding better to the lymphedema treatment.

The patient should be aware that a series of lymphedema treatments by well-trained healthcare professionals is mandatory. After completion, there should be clinical improvement in volume reduction and softening of the tissue consistency. The patient should be fitted with a compression garment to be worn daily as a part of the maintenance care, which should be initiated by the patient oneself through appropriate home care. Therefore, during the intensive course of the treatment, the patient should be instructed in daily self-care in order to maintain well-reduced lymphedema following hospital care. To maintain manual lymphatic drainage (MLD)-based complex decongestive therapy (CDT), including compression therapy of the lymphedema through home-orientated maintenance regimens, proper compliance in the treatment, and daily self-care is the most important factor for the management of all forms of chronic lymphedema regardless of etiology, extent, and severity.

However, as a part of general orientation, the patients should be informed about the crucial role of periodic reassessment on the efficacy of the maintenance care; when there is evidence of resistance to the therapy and the condition deteriorates, thorough re-evaluation should be encouraged including possible precipitating factors (e.g., recurrence of the cancer). It is also fair to the patients to provide all the optional therapies to improve CDT-based conservative therapy (e.g., reconstructive and/or excisional surgery) as supplemental therapy if the condition fails to respond to the CDT.

The following guidelines can be given to the patient as part of the basic education with instructions that they must follow closely.

Skin Care

- Maintain well-moisturized skin
- Avoid dry skin, cracks, open lesions, hangnails, and punctures
- Avoid excessive cuticle cuts, blood pressure cuffs on the arm involved, and venipuncture

- If bilateral arms are involved, draw the blood from the hands.
- Avoid constrictive garments, and or jewelry.
- Wear gloves when gardening or during household cleaning.
- An open cut/wound should be cleaned immediately with alcohol and antibiotic cream should be applied to the area.
- After each shower/bath dry your toes carefully to avoid fungal infection from excessive moisture.
- Apply antifungal spray or lotion on your toenails to prevent fungal infection.
- Wear enclosed shoes to protect your feet when suffering from leg lymphedema.

Exacerbation of Lymphedema Usually Follows

- Excessive heat – avoid hot jacuzzis, hot baths, prolonged sun exposure.
- Inappropriate diet – avoid salty/spicy food and excessive alcohol intake.
- Vigorous activity – avoid heavy lifting, carrying, pulling heavy objects, and prolonged repetitious activity.

Activity

If active before surgery, you should return to 50% of the usual activity and progress very gradually. If you experience any adverse reaction, the activity amount should be reduced further. Swimming is the best exercise. If your lymphedema involves your lower extremities, nonweight-bearing exercises are the best (cycling, stair master, elliptical machines).

Travel Advice

When traveling to distant areas, take antibiotics along just in case there are any signs of infection. Wear the compression sleeve/stocking when flying. Avoid prolonged sitting when flying/driving by stretching exercises and short walks.

In Case of an Infection

Sudden onset of swelling, burning, itching, red and hot lymphedema of an arm or leg may indicate an infection. Contact your physician immediately.

References

1. Lawenda BD, Mondry TE, Johnstone PAS. Lymphedema: A primer on the identification and management of a chronic condition in oncologic treatment. *CA Cancer J Clin*. 2009;59:8-24.
2. Ridner SH. Pretreatment lymphedema education and identified educational resources in breast cancer patients. *Patient Educ Couns*. 2006;61(1):72-79.
3. Rumowitz CD. Lymphedema: patient and provider education: current status future trends. *Cancer*. 1998;83(12 suppl):2874-2876.

Chapter 69
Patient/Family Advocacy

Wendy Chaite

Lymphedema – how does one feel, what does one do when given this diagnosis? I know because our daughter was born in 1993 with a complex lymphatic disease – including lymphedema. We were told at the time that there is insufficient scientific/medical knowledge to make a precise diagnosis, there are grossly inadequate treatment options, and there is no cure. Like many, we felt ignorant, isolated, frightened, powerless, and hopeless. The months and years following were filled with the diligent pursuit of a definite diagnosis and optimal medical care. Like many patients we have traveled the country and even sought expertise abroad – frustrated by the limitation of the basic knowledge of the lymphatic system – let alone diseases thereof. Though we've been able to control our daughter's leg lymphedema with complex decongestive therapy and compression, we have had less success with other swollen areas (face, arm, genitals, and trunk) and her underlying disease (diffuse lymphangiomatosis) continues to progress, causing serious, life threatening medical complications.

Pushing past the disappointment and frustration we faced searching for answers, our family started a new search for empowerment – a journey that we hoped would make us feel less powerless and more able to bring genuine change into our daughter's life and the lives of others. We were able to do this in two important ways: (1) successfully advocating for the best medical care possible for our child (and as she develops and matures, enabling her ultimately to manage her own care); and (2) advocating for the advancement of lymphatic research to find improved treatments and cures for lymphatic diseases, lymphedema and related disorders through the Lymphatic Research Foundation.

Set forth below are some concepts we learned along the way that may prove helpful to others who share a similar journey. While we employed the vast majority

W. Chaite
Lymphatic Research Foundation, 40 Garvies Point Road, Suite D, Glen Cove, NY, 11542, USA

B.-B. Lee et al. (eds.), *Lymphedema*,
DOI 10.1007/978-0-85729-567-5_69, © Springer-Verlag London Limited 2011

of these ideas with great success, some items we did not necessarily incorporate into our lives (e.g., charting symptoms), but in hindsight, we wish we had:

- Take control of your disease; don't allow it to control you. Who you are is far beyond your medical problem and physical issues. Speak to your wellness, not your illness.
- Develop and preserve a strong sense of self. Identify your talents, skills, strengths, passions and pursue them with fervor. If you are bright, creative, compassionate, athletic, kind, a team player, insightful, a good family member, and/or a hard worker, for example, these are the areas of strength that help define you – your lymphedema or lymphatic disease, no matter how severe – should not.
- Engage in and foster interests and activities that provide secondary benefits for your underlying condition and which can serve as lifelong leisure activities (e.g., yoga, swimming, etc.).
- Recognize that each patient and circumstance is unique and that a cookie cutter approach to your care may not serve you well. Quality of life is an important factor to consider. Find out as much as you can about all therapeutic treatments available, assess the quality and objectivity of the information, weigh the risks/benefits of the treatment, proceed cautiously, and most important – use common sense. No doubt you will receive varying opinions from professionals, often at odds with one another. Step back, sort through the facts, trust your intuition, and make the best educated decision you can, given your particular circumstance. Monitor your body's response to any and all therapies, and adjust as needed. If you are disappointed in the effectiveness of your treatment, don't beat yourself up if it turns out you could have made a better choice. It serves no purpose; just move forward continuing to make, to the best of your ability, informed decisions given the information and facts you have at hand.
- For parents of young patients, it is best to incorporate compliance-related tasks into your lives *as early as possible* and with limited negotiation (e.g., dietary restrictions, daily/nightly compression, etc.). We made the mistake of being too flexible and paid the price when our child became a teenager, when it is natural for teens to test boundaries. Had her medical compliance tasks been treated as expected and ordinary since infancy, we could have avoided many headaches, heartaches, and of course, a few gray hairs.
- For medical appointments, come prepared with written questions/issues to discuss (in priority order in case not all are addressed). Consider using bulleted points and sub-points instead of writing out formal questions. This allows for flexibility and promotes productive communication exchange. If you have a particular question or require specific information make sure that is a separate, expressly stated bulleted point so it is not overlooked.
- Some individuals feel intimidated when speaking with health care providers. It is important to develop a basic knowledge and understanding of your condition. This will help build your competence and confidence. Your voice matters and is important for achieving the best care possible. Speak up, yet be sensitive to time constraints by being organized and concise; be assertive (but not aggressive) in your approach. Your healthcare is a partnership; take an active (but not obnoxious) role.

- Ask a relative/friend to accompany you for medical consultations. Two sets of ears hear much more than one, providing an opportunity to review and clarify details of the conversation.
- Keep a medical journal or log for health concerns as they arise. If you are tracking a particular symptom (e.g., infection, pain, increase in symptoms, etc.) this will be helpful in reporting accurate information to your health care provider. Take note of influences that may be a contributing factor (e.g., changes in diet, stress, hormones, medications, etc.). Keeping track can help identify patterns, flare ups, etc., so you and your health care provider can make adjustments, modifications, and address issues prophylactically, as needed. Having such a log can prove invaluable in future years as your medical status changes. For some, this can be a burdensome task so be creative (use a calendar with large boxes to make notations, cellular telephone notepad, etc.). This is something we did from time to time for acute situations, but failed to do long term. Needless to say, we wish we had. It is never too late to start. Even if you don't complete religiously – something is always better than nothing.
- Keep an ongoing file of important medical records. At the time of service (especially with specialists, radiology, lab work, hospitalizations, etc.), request a copy of key reports, imaging films (often available digitally on CD), consultations, etc. Store hard copies in an accordion-like folder by categories, in reverse chronological order. It may require several files, and you may even consider keeping a second set of documents stored off premise in case of loss or damage. Note if you decide to maintain your medical records electronically instead of hard copies, be sure to back up your computer files. (We lost irreplaceable information when our laptop computer was stolen without adequate back-up.) With advancements in technology there are several companies that provide fee-based electronic personal health record storage. Over the years, maintaining a full set of important medical records becomes invaluable, especially if you have numerous specialists and/or complex medical issues. It is very difficult to go back and recreate your medical history since often times you may lose track of the who, what, where, and when. When providing information to other health care providers, share *copies only* – no originals (we had the unfortunate experience of having a specialist lose original imaging films before digital technology became available).
- When you need a letter from a health care provider, for any purpose – draft it. It is unrealistic to expect a busy professional to write an effective letter exactly how you would want it expressed. It must be concise, objective, and professional. Allow sufficient time for processing. Providing the signing health care provider with an electronic version can save time. Keep copies of all correspondence.

While it is my hope that at least one, some or even all of the basic tips I've shared will prove helpful to others, my greatest desire is to provide patients and their families with a sense of hope. Hope is the elevating feeling we experience when we see – in the mind's eye – a path to a better future. While hope acknowledges the significant obstacles and deepest falls along the way, it can flourish only when you believe that what you do can make a difference; that your actions can bring a future different than the present.

That is why, in 1998, with the support of my husband, I left my successful legal career to found the Lymphatic Research Foundation (www.lymphaticresearch.org).

The Lymphatic Research Foundation (LRF) is an internationally recognized 501(c) (3) not-for-profit organization whose mission is to advance research of the lymphatic system and to find improved treatments and cures for lymphatic diseases, lymphedema, and related disorders. The LRF's immediate goal is to increase public awareness as well as public and private funding for lymphatic research. Through collaborations and strategic partnerships, the LRF has played a major role in accelerating lymphatic research and is helping make progress toward the development of improved treatments for lymphatic diseases and lymphedema. Because of the LRF, the importance of the lymphatic system and its role in health and disease is finally being recognized by mainstream science and medicine. Achievement highlights include:

- Securing ongoing United States Congressional and National Institutes of Health (NIH) support for lymphatic research and lymphatic diseases and expanding the role of the Trans-NIH Coordinating Committee for the Lymphatic System. Both have resulted in creating and progressively increasing national programmatic and funding initiatives for lymphatic biology and disease.
- Establishing the premiere, biennial Gordon Research Conference Series entitled, *Molecular Mechanisms in Lymphatic Function and Disease* (preceded by organizing ground-breaking, seminal National Institutes of Health "Think Tank" conferences).
- Launching *Lymphatic Research and Biology*, an international peer-reviewed scientific journal published by a leading biomedical publisher and indexed in MEDLINE (United States National Library of Medicine).
- Funding an international grants and awards program for lymphatic research that is attracting scientists and clinicians from distinguished research centers around the world, expanding the pool of researchers and encouraging research that will lead to therapeutic advances.
- Creating the first-ever Endowed Chair of Lymphatic Research and Medicine (at Stanford University School of Medicine, California, USA).
- Progressing toward the LRF's long range goal of establishing a National Lymphatic Disease and Lymphedema Patient Registry and Tissue Bank (at The Feinstein Institute for Medical Research at North Shore-Long Island Jewish Health System, New York, USA) to stimulate research and support clinical trials.

It is my genuine belief that each and every patient/family has the potential for empowerment – not just for you and your family, but for the betterment of mankind. Start by taking simple steps to avail yourself of optimal health by choosing self-empowering and self-fulfilling activities and behaviors. Become involved with and/or support organizations that are meaningful to you.

For our family, the Lymphatic Research Foundation has provided the ultimate sense of empowerment. By promoting and supporting lymphatic research, we are changing the status quo. Only through continued research can there be new treatment options in clinical care. We are creating a healthier tomorrow for our daughter, and the millions of others challenged by lymphatic disease and lymphedema. The transformation from feeling helpless and hopeless to proactive and hopeful is extraordinarily empowering. You too can become empowered. You too can make a difference.

> One person can have a dream; when joined by others it becomes a vision; when put into action it becomes a movement. Movements change history.

Chapter 70
Reimbursement of CDT-based Care

Cheryl L. Morgan

Though knowledge about lymphedema and treatment options has drastically increased, reimbursement issues continue to hinder patients' access to successful treatment.

Lymphedema, specifically related to breast cancer treatment, has garnered the attention of national associations and agencies, increasing the momentum of efforts to improve insurance coverage. This has led to legislative efforts that may eventually improve compensation.

For primary lymphedema (congenital or hereditary) and other secondary forms, such as postsurgical cases or phlebolymphedemas, it remains difficult for patients to obtain a correct diagnosis.[1] Lower extremity cases are often more costly to treat and are frequently complicated by conditions such as chronic wounds, obesity, and peripheral neuropathy.[2]

Patients continue to report seeking diagnosis and appropriate treatment for years. Many describe being referred to numerous specialists before obtaining answers. Some are even hospitalized for complications from untreated symptoms of lymphedema. Numerous patient support groups, advocacy networks, websites, and organizations have sprung up across the United States.[3] These organized efforts by patients and health care professionals are now focused primarily on reimbursement for therapy and supplies necessary to manage the disease.

Initially, most of the efforts to obtain reimbursement were driven by manufacturers of the products used in the treatment of lymphedema. These efforts continue today, but are now more accessory to measures being taken by groups and individuals committed to securing improved reimbursement for all components of care for lymphedema patients.

In the 1980s, only a handful of lymphedema clinics existed in North America. In the 1990s, patient awareness, interested therapists, and physicians stimulated an

C.L. Morgan
Department of Rehabilitation Medicine,
Therapy Concepts Inc., Leawood, KS, USA

B.-B. Lee et al. (eds.), *Lymphedema*,
DOI 10.1007/978-0-85729-567-5_70, © Springer-Verlag London Limited 2011

increase in treatment centers in the United States. In 1992, Medicare (Kansas) approved reimbursement for CDT treatment for lymphedema. By 1997, the state of Florida had approved the protocol. The Women's Health and Cancer Rights Act of 1998 was passed, which stipulated provision of treatment and supplies for those receiving benefits in connection with a mastectomy and/or subsequent breast reconstruction.[4] In 1999, the new CPT code describing manual therapies, including manual lymph drainage (97140) was approved by the American Medical Association.[5] Other CPT codes reportedly used across the country include those for therapeutic exercise (97110), therapeutic activity (97530), and activities of daily living (97535). An application for a CPT code that describes the provision of skilled services for the compression bandaging component of lymphedema therapy is currently in development.

In February 2010, a bill was introduced in the House of Representatives as H.R. 4662, the *Lymphedema Diagnosis and Treatment Cost Saving Act of 2010.*[6] The Centers for Medicare and Medicaid Services (CMS) requested a Technology Assessment to be performed through the Department of Health and Human Services (HHS) and Agency for Healthcare Research and Quality (AHRQ). This document, entitled *Diagnosis and Treatment of Secondary Lymphedema*, was published on 28 May 2010.

The Technology Assessment concluded that although a great deal of research into the diagnosis and treatment of secondary lymphedema has already been undertaken, there is no evidence to suggest the optimal diagnostic test or treatment. Additionally, there is no evidence to suggest whether certain tests or treatments might benefit some types of patients more than others. The field of research into secondary lymphedema is ripe for advancement and the contents of the report may serve as a springboard to guide future scientific endeavors in this domain.[7]

Setting reimbursement schedules requires consensus about the diagnosis and treatment protocols supported by data, neither of which exists. The need for better reimbursement is not disputed. It is regrettable that the determined actions of many efforts to date will not soon enough improve compensation for treatment or supplies. Until consensus occurs, there is no guide to successful billing or coding for reimbursement available.

Lymphedema treatment is primarily provided by physical therapists and occupational therapists.[8] The codes utilized for reimbursement are those in the Rehabilitation Medicine section of the Current Procedural Terminology (CPT) manual. Despite years of effort by individuals and associations, many qualified nurses, massage therapists, and other allied healthcare professionals are not able to treat and bill insurance for reimbursement. While national policy may allow for licensed massage therapists or nurses to provide treatment, it is regulated by each state.

Currently, for massage therapists, the educational requirements vary from state to state. Some states do not recognize the profession within the regulations of their Board of Healing Arts. There are no standards of education formally recognized and few physicians in the United States have had training in the specialty of lymphology to properly provide oversight or know what results to expect from treatment performed.[9]

A similar scenario occurred in the late 1960s. Nurses took the lead in developing wound care protocols and established a curriculum and credential that recognized them as wound care specialists that reflected the training, experience level, and designation for subsequent reimbursement.[10] There now are more than eight separate organizations for health care professionals interested in the field of wound care in the United States. Wound care supplies are covered by Medicare and most insurance companies. Coding for reimbursement of these services correlating with wound care is differentiated among the professionals delivering the care.

In 2006, there was a watershed change in the ownership of medical practices; for the first time, more were owned by hospitals and other health care providers than by the physicians themselves. That figure, medical professionals predict, could rise to 80% within a few years.[11] Most remaining in private practice are specialists. Phlebologists, oncologists, dermatologists, and physiatrists are among the specialists who have included lymphedema services in their practice. This is a tremendous opportunity for specialists interested in expanding their services and improving patients' quality of life.

There is an established need for continuing medical education courses for physicians to learn more about lymphedema and other functions and disorders of the lymphatic system.[12] Several curriculums are being developed at the time of writing. This will provide better evaluation of treatment protocols and assist in the collection of necessary data toward more reliable and measurable outcomes.

From the staging and treatment of the disease, to supplies, the opportunity is here to establish guidelines for care, professional education requirements, and subsequent insurance reimbursement. It is recommended that until these are in place, physicians and allied health care professionals establish a direct relationship with their insurance carriers or find a knowledgeable consultant who can direct them through the establishment, provision, and billing for the services of a lymphedema program.

References

1. Burt J, White G. *Lymphedema: A Breast Cancer Patient's Guide to Prevention and Healing*. Alameda, CA: Hunter House; 2000.
2. Browse N, Burnand KG, Mortimer P. *Diseases of the Lymphatics*. London: Arnold; 2003.
3. Ehrlich A, Vinjé-Harrewijn A, McMahon E. *Living Well with Lymphedema: Lessons from Lymphnotes.com*. San Francisco: Lymph Notes; 2005.
4. Tredbar LL, Morgan CL, Lee BB, et al. *Lymphedema Diagnosis and Treatment*. London: Springer-Verlag; 2008.
5. *Steadman's CPT Dictionary*Stedman's medical dictionary, illustrated. 27th ed. Philadelphia: Lippincott Williams & Wilkins, 2000.
6. URL for GovTrack.US: Website for tracking the United States Congress http://www.govtrack.us/congress/bill.xpd?bill=h111-4662.
7. URL for AHRQ: Agency for Healthcare Research and Quality. Technology assessment produced for the Centers for Medicare and Medicaid Services (CMS) for Diagnosis and Treatment of Secondary Lymphedema. http://www.ahrq.gov/clinic/techix.htm.
8. Zuther J. *Lymphedema Management: The Comprehensive Guide for Patients and Practitioners*. New York: Thieme Medical and Scientific Publishers; 2005.

9. Consensus Document Meeting, American Society of Lymphology Conference; Kansas City, Missouri. Nov27th, 2008.

10. Baxter H. How a discipline came of age: a history of wound care. *J Wound Care*. 2002;11(10):383-386.

11. Bodenheimer T. Primary care – will it survive? *N Engl J Med*. 2006;355(9):861-864.

12. Stewart PJ. When it isn't lymphedema. *Lymph Link*. 2004;16(3):1.

Part XVIII
Epilogue

Epilogue

Almost 30 years have passed since I made my first casual commitment to lymphatic reconstruction without knowing that I was walking into a minefield. My cavalier approach at the time, along with my limited knowledge as a clinical vascular surgeon, resulted in a disastrous failure among the first patient group. After much soul-searching and a self-imposed moratorium, it took me almost a decade to figure out what went wrong and why it went wrong.

It was painful and embarrassing to air my dirty laundry in front of more experienced colleagues around the world and get their merciless peer reviews. But, I felt extremely lucky to receive so many opinions, well-informed advice, and timely assistance, and was able to reorganize a new group with a new strategy and confront the same challenge a second time, a decade later. It has taken years for me to finally figure out what I know, what I do not know, and what I should know to build momentum and establish a clear trajectory in the complex field of lymphology.

Recently, I became humbled once again in reluctantly deciding to follow the advice of many of my senior colleagues. They urged me to use my hard-earned experience as a lymphatic surgeon to organize a compendium that would provide a bird's-eye view on lymphedema-oriented lymphology to share with colleagues.

Without the constant help of my two co-editors, John Bergan and Stanley Rockson, I would not have been able to finish such a daunting task. I also owe a lot to my respected Austrian colleague and friend Professor Hugo Partsch for his timely encouragement. In addition, I would like to thank my mentor, Professor Leonel Villavicencio, for all of his support throughout the years.

And last of all, I salute each of the contributors of this book. I invited these experts from the four corners of the world to share their valuable experience with us in this compendium. Without their tireless efforts in revising and delivering chapters best suited to our aims, this compendium might have become a dull, forbidding textbook. We three editors are deeply grateful to the authors for their engaging and illuminating work.

B.-B. Lee et al. (eds.), *Lymphedema*,
DOI 10.1007/978-0-85729-567-5, © Springer-Verlag London Limited 2011

I, together with my two co-editors, would like to dedicate this compendium to all our colleagues as a guide for navigating the minefield called lymphology. Hopefully you can safely avoid the same mistakes I once made and gain a more comprehensive understanding of this complicated and ever-evolving field of medicine.

Washington, DC, USA   Byung-Boong Lee

Index

B.-B. Lee et al. (eds.), *Lymphedema*,
DOI 10.1007/978-0-85729-567-5, © Springer-Verlag London Limited 2011